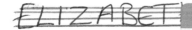

KV-455-708

Contents

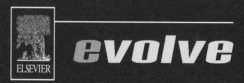

Mosby's

ONCOLOGY
DRUG
REFERENCE

VOLUME EDITORS

Robert J. Ignoffo, PharmD
Professor of Pharmacy
Touro University
Mare Island Vallejo, California
Clinical Professor Emeritus
University of California, San Francisco
Department of Clinical Pharmacy
San Francisco, California

Carol S. Viele, RN, MS
Clinical Nurse Specialist
Hematology-Oncology-Bone Marrow Transplant
Assistant Clinical Professor
Department of Physiological Nursing
University of California, San Francisco
San Francisco, California

Zoe Ngo, PharmD
Investigational Drug Pharmacist
Assistant Clinical Professor
University of California, San Francisco
San Francisco, California

MOSBY
ELSEVIER

11830 Westline Industrial Drive
St. Louis, Missouri 63146

Notice

Knowledge and best practice in this field are constantly changing. As new research and experience broaden our knowledge, changes in practice, treatment and drug therapy may become necessary or appropriate. Readers are advised to check the most current information provided (i) on procedures featured or (ii) by the manufacturer of each product to be administered, to verify the recommended dose or formula, the method and duration of administration, and contraindications. It is the responsibility of the practitioner, relying on their own experience and knowledge of the patient, to make diagnoses, to determine dosages and the best treatment for each individual patient, and to take all appropriate safety precautions. To the fullest extent of the law, neither the Publisher nor the Editors assume any liability for any injury and/or damage to persons or property arising out of or related to any use of the material contained in this book.

The Publisher

Library of Congress Control Number: 2007922302

Executive Publisher: Barbara Nelson Cullen
Senior Editor: Sandra Clark Brown
Senior Developmental Editor: Sophia Oh Gray
Publishing Services Manager: Melissa Lastarria
Senior Project Manager: Joy Moore
Designer: Teresa McBryan

Printed in the United States of America

Last digit is the print number: 9 8 7 6 5 4 3 2 1

**Working together to grow
libraries in developing countries**

www.elsevier.com | www.bookaid.org | www.sabre.org

ELSEVIER   BOOK AID
International   Sabre Foundation

*To those practitioners who help patients and other caregivers
to cope with their disease*

*To our mentors and colleagues who have developed educational
and training programs to enhance our professional skills and knowledge
as well as challenge us to be innovators at the cutting edge
of patient care*

*And finally to our families and significant others
for supporting our efforts to write this book*

—Robert J. Ignoffo, Carol S. Viele, and Zoe Ngo

Preface

This book is designed as both a quick reference on anticancer drugs and a guide to the management of common problems often encountered in cancer patients receiving pharmacotherapy. More than 107 anticancer drugs are highlighted. In each of the drug monographs, we have included information on the pharmacology, clinical use, dosage, and adverse effects of the commercially available agents. We also included a section on drug interactions in each monograph, but Unit 4 goes into greater detail about mechanism and clinical management of specific drug interactions. We did not include investigational agents. In addition, we did not include dosage regimens for specific combinations used in particular cancers because these change too often.

Acknowledgments

We acknowledge Tracy Moran, RN, and Patrick T. Wong, PharmD, for their outstanding work in serving as external reviewers of the contents of our book.
—Robert J. Ignoffo, Carol S. Viele, and Zoe Ngo

Introduction

Mosby's Oncology Drug Reference contains the following:
- **An IV compatibilities chart**
- **Full monographs on more than 107 of the most commonly used drugs in oncology practice**
  The monographs include key information:
  - Generic Name(s) and Brand Name(s)
  - Class of Agent
  - Clinical Pharmacology, including mechanism of action, therapeutic effect, absorption and distribution, half-life, and metabolism and excretion
  - How Supplied/Available Forms
  - Indications and Usage, including dosage adjustments for special patient populations, other existing medical conditions, and use with other drugs
  - Unlabeled Uses
  - Precautions, including pregnancy risk category
  - Contraindications
  - Drug Preparation/Administration/Safe Handling Issues
  - Storage and Stability
  - Interactions, including drug, herbal, and food interactions
  - Lab Effects/Interference
  - Y-Site Compatibles
  - Incompatibles
  - Side effects, including serious reactions and other side effects by frequent, occasional, and rare occurrences
  - Special Considerations, including baseline assessment, interventions and evaluation, and education

  Important information is highlighted within the monographs with a special design: **Note:**
  Critical information is highlighted within the monographs with a special design: ◀ **ALERT** ▶
- **An entire unit focused on Pediatric Oncology**
  This unit outlines incidence, etiology, clinical presentations, prognostic factors, and treatments for acute leukemias, Hodgkin's and non-Hodgkin's lymphoma, and common tumors. In addition, this unit discusses secondary malignancies and late effects (sequelae of the treatment) in pediatric patients.
- **A unit on Supportive Care**
  This unit includes chapters on Hematologic Toxicities, Nausea and Vomiting, Mucositis, Diarrhea and Constipation, Bone Disease, and Cancer Pain.
- **An insert of four full-color illustrations**
  The insert includes images of the chemotherapy exposure during drug preparation, oral mucosa and phases of mucositis, normal bone remodeling, and a cross-sectional diagram of vertebral column structures and corresponding metastases.
- **A unit on Drug Interactions**
  This unit contains drug interactions for over 74 anticancer drugs, with many easy-to-use tables. In addition, the 347 references in this unit provide an in-depth reference for all clinicians.
- **A unit on Preventing Medication Errors**
- **A unit on Occupational Exposure to Hazardous Drugs**

- **An Appendix section**
  The appendix includes useful formulas, chemotherapy regimens and drug information on the Web, and patient assistance programs.
- **A Free Evolve Web site**
  The Web site—http://evolve.elsevier.com/oncologydrug/—features updates on drug information, Web links, commonly used formulas and IV compatibilities, and calculators.
- **A PDA version of the entire book**
  The PDA is offered as a separate purchase and includes all content from the book. The PDA software is available via download or CD purchase.

Mosby's Oncology Drug Reference is a concise source for current oncology drug information. We hope this handbook helps all those in oncology provide care for their patients.

—Robert J. Ignoffo, Carol S. Viele, and Zoe Ngo

Contributors

Maureen A. Cannon, BSN, MS
Oncology Clinical Nurse Specialist
University of California,
  San Francisco
San Francisco, California
  *Unit 3. Chapter 4. Management
    and Treatment of Diarrhea
    and Constipation*

Alexandre Chan, PharmD, BCPS
Oncology Pharmacy Speciality Resident
University of California at Davis
  Medical Center
Sacramento, California
  Unit 1. Cancer Drugs
  *Unit 3. Chapter 1. Management and
    Treatment of Hematologic Toxicities*

Nancy H. Heideman, PharmD, BCPS
Assistant Professor
College of Pharmacy
University of New Mexico
Albuquerque, New Mexico
  Unit 2. Pediatric Oncology

Andrea Iannucci, PharmD, BCOP
Oncology Pharmacy Specialist
Department of Pharmacy
University of California at Davis
  Medical Center
Sacramento, California
Assistant Clinical Professor
Department of Clinical Pharmacy
University of California, San Francisco
San Francisco, California
  Unit 1. Cancer Drugs
  *Unit 3. Chapter 1. Management and
    Treatment of Hematologic Toxicities*

Robert J. Ignoffo, PharmD
Professor of Pharmacy
Touro University
Mare Island Vallejo, California
Clinical Professor Emeritus
University of California, San Francisco
Department of Clinical Pharmacy
San Francisco, California
  Unit 1. Cancer Drugs
  Unit 2. Pediatric Oncology
  Unit 4. Drug Interactions
  *Unit 5. Considerations in Preventing
    Medication Errors*

Masha S. H. Lam, PharmD, BCOP
Clinical Pharmacist, Hematology/
  Oncology
Kaiser Permanente Outpatient
  Oncology Clinic
Walnut Creek, California
  Unit 4. Drug Interactions

Monica Lee, PharmD
Clinical Oncology Pharmacist
University of California,
  San Francisco
San Francisco, California
  *Unit 3. Chapter 3. Management
    and Treatment of Mucositis*

Theresa A. Moran, RN, MS
Medical/Surgical Oncology Clinical
  Nurse Specialist
University of California, San Francisco
  Medical Center
San Francisco, California
  *Unit 3. Chapter 4. Management
    and Treatment of Diarrhea
    and Constipation*

Zoe Ngo, PharmD
Investigational Drug Pharmacist
Assistant Clinical Professor
University of California, San Francisco
San Francisco, California
  Unit 1. Cancer Drugs

Tammy J. Rodvelt, RN, MSN, NP
Urologic Oncology Nurse Practitioner
University of California, San
  Francisco Comprehensive
  Cancer Center
San Francisco, California
  Unit 1. Cancer Drugs
  *Unit 3. Chapter 5. Management
    and Treatment of Bone Disease*

Julie Schwenka, PharmD
Clinical Hematology/Oncology/
  Bone Marrow Transplant
  Pharmacist
University of California, San
  Francisco Medical Center
San Francisco, California
  Unit 1. Cancer Drugs

Dominic A. Solimando, Jr., MA, BCOP, FAPhA, FASHP
President
Oncology Pharmacy Services, Inc.
Arlington, Virginia
*Unit 6. Occupational Exposure
to Hazardous Drugs*

Carol S. Viele RN, MS
Clinical Nurse Specialist
Hematology-Oncology-Bone Marrow
Transplant
Assistant Clinical Professor
Department of Physiological
Nursing
University of California, San
Francisco
San Francisco, California
*Unit 1. Cancer Drugs
Unit 2. Pediatric Oncology*

Patrick T. Wong, PharmD, BCPS
Clinical Pharmacist
Assistant Clinical Professor
University of California, San Francisco
San Francisco, California
*Unit 3. Chapter 6. Management
and Treatment of Cancer Pain*

Helen Wu, PharmD, BCOP
Health Science Associate Clinical
Professor
University of California, San Francisco
San Francisco, California
Unit 1. Cancer Drugs

Courtney W. Yuen, PharmD, BCOP
Assistant Clinical Professor
University of California, San Francisco
San Francisco, California
*Unit 3. Chapter 2. Management
and Treatment of Nausea and Vomiting*

UNIT 1 **Cancer Drugs**

Alexandre Chan, Andrea Iannucci, Robert J. Ignoffo, Zoe Ngo,
Tammy J. Rodvelt, Julie Schwenka, Carol S. Viele, and Helen Wu

ALDESLEUKIN

BRAND NAMES
IL-2, Proleukin

CLASS OF AGENT
Antineoplastic agent, Interleukin

CLINICAL PHARMACOLOGY
Mechanism of Action
The exact mechanism by which aldesleukin
mediates antitumor activity is unknown.
It is a human recombinant interleukin-2 that
is produced by peripheral lymphocytes. It
promotes proliferation, differentiation, and
recruitment of T and B cells, lymphokine-
activated and natural cells, and thymocytes.
It enhances lymphocyte cytotoxicity and
induces lymphokine-activated killer cells
and natural killer cells to engulf abnormal
cells, including tumor cells. In vivo, aldesleukin effects include cellular immunity
with profound lymphocytosis, eosinophilia,
and thrombocytopenia and the production
of cytokines including tumor necrosis
factor, interleukin-1, and γ-interferon.
Aldesleukin targets specific surface receptors that are present on T and malignant
lymphocytes. Therefore, aldesleukin is a
true biologic response modifier which, unlike α-interferon, acts directly, and mediates
its antitumor effects through complex indirect effects on the immune system.
Interleukin-2 has important effects on the
immune system and may be involved in the
regulation of immune tolerance. Interkeukin-
2 has been found to stimulate bone marrow
cell mitosis and to reverse cyclophospha-
mide-, glucocorticoid hormone-, and
cyclosporine-induced immune suppression
in animals. **Therapeutic Effect:** Enhances
cytolytic activity in lymphocytes.
Absorption and Distribution
IM: Absorption is slow and incomplete,
with serum levels that were 2% of those
achieved after IV administration. The area
under the curve after IM dosing was only
30% that achieved after IV dosing. *Subcutaneous:* After subcutaneous administration
of 12 to 18 million International Units/day
of interleukin-2 in 18 patients with HIV infection, maximum absorption was achieved
at an approximate a mean of 4 hrs.

Aldesleukin is primarily distributed into
plasma, lymphocytes, lungs, liver, kidneys,
and spleen. Metabolized to amino acids in
the cells lining the kidneys.
Half-life: 85 mins.
Metabolism and Excretion
Metabolized to amino acids in the cells lining the proximal convoluted tubules of the
kidney. Excreted primarily by the kidney
with a rapid renal clearance of 268 mL/min.

HOW SUPPLIED/AVAILABLE FORMS
Powder for Injection: 22 million units
(1.3 mg).

INDICATIONS AND DOSAGES
Metastatic Melanoma
The Food and Drug Administration–
approved dose of aldesleukin for metastatic
melanoma is 600,000 International Units/
kg/dose administered IV over 15 min every
8 hrs for a maximum of 14 doses. After
9 days of rest, the schedule is repeated for
another 14 doses for a maximum of
28 doses per course, as tolerated. Therapeutic response may be evaluated approximately 4 wks after a course of treatment.
A rest period of at least 7 wks from the
date of hospital discharge should separate
each additional course of therapy.
Renal Cell Carcinoma
Dosing is same as above for melanoma.
Low-dose aldesleukin for renal cell carcinoma is divided into 2-mo courses consisting of 72,000 International Units/kg/dose
administered IV over 15 min every 8 hrs
for a maximum of 15 doses, as tolerated.
Therapy is administered during the remainder of each 2-mo course. After 7 to 10 days
of rest, the schedule is repeated for another
15 doses as tolerated.

UNLABELED USES
Treatment of colorectal cancer, Kaposi's
sarcoma, non-Hodgkin's lymphoma.

PRECAUTIONS
Pregnancy Risk Category: C

CONTRAINDICATIONS
A known history of hypersensitivity to
interleukin-2 or any component of the
aldesleukin formulation; an abnormal

1

Dose Modification

Body System	Hold Dose For	Subsequent Doses May Be Given If
Cardiovascular	Atrial fibrillation, supraventricular tachycardia, or bradycardia that requires treatment or is recurrent or persistent	Patient is asymptomatic with full recovery to normal sinus rhythm.
	Systolic BP <90 mm Hg with increasing requirements for pressors	Systolic BP is 90 mm Hg and stable or improving requirements for pressors.
	Any ECG change consistent with MI, ischemia, or myocarditis with or without chest pain or suspicion of cardiac ischemia.	Patient is asymptomatic, MI and myocarditis have been ruled out, clinical suspicion of angina is low, and there is no evidence of ventricular hypokinesia.
CNS	Mental status changes, including moderate confusion or agitation	Mental status changes completely resolved.
Dermatologic	Bullous dermatitis or marked worsening of preexisting skin condition, avoid topical steroid therapy	Resolution of all signs of bullous dermatitis occurs.
GI	Signs of hepatic failure including encephalopathy, increasing ascites, liver pain, and hypoglycemia	All signs of hepatic failure have resolved.*
	Stool guaiac repeatedly >3-4+	Stool guaiac is negative.
GU	Serum creatinine >4.5 mg/dL or a serum creatinine of 4 mg/dL in the presence of severe volume overload, acidosis, or hyperkalemia	Serum creatinine is <4 mg/dL and fluid and electrolyte status is stable.
	Persistent oliguria, urine output of <10 mL/hr for 16-24 hr with rising serum creatinine	Urine output is >10 mL/hr with a decrease of serum creatinine of >1.5 mg/dL or normalization of serum creatinine.
Respiratory	O_2 saturation <90%	O_2 saturation >90%.
Miscellaneous	Sepsis syndrome, patient is clinically unstable	Sepsis syndrome has resolved, patient is clinically stable, and infection is under treatment.

B/P, blood pressure; ECG, electrocardiogram; MI, myocardial infarction.
*Discontinue all further treatment for that course. Initiate a new course of treatment, if warranted, no sooner than 7 wks after cessation of adverse event and hospital discharge.

thallium stress test or abnormal pulmonary function tests; organ allografts

Retreatment with aldesleukin is contraindicated in patients who have experienced the following drug-related toxicities while receiving an earlier course of therapy:

- Sustained ventricular tachycardia (= 5 beats)
- Cardiac arrhythmias not controlled or unresponsive to management
- Chest pain with ECG changes, consistent with angina or MI
- Cardiac tamponade
- Intubation for greater than 72 hrs
- Renal failure requiring dialysis for greater than 72 hrs
- Coma or toxic psychosis lasting greater than 48 hrs
- Repetitive or difficult-to-control seizures
- Bowel ischemia/perforation
- GI bleeding requiring surgery

DRUG PREPARATION/ADMINISTRATION/ SAFE HANDLING ISSUES

◄ ALERT ►

- Each vial contains 22 million International Units (1.3 mg) of aldesleukin and should be reconstituted aseptically with 1.2 mL of sterile water for injection. When reconstituted as directed, each mL contains 18 million International Units (1.1 mg) of aldesleukin. The resulting solution should be a clear, colorless to slightly yellow liquid. The vial is for single-use only and any unused portion should be discarded.

- During reconstitution, the sterile water for injection should be directed at the side of the vial, and the contents should be gently swirled to avoid excess foaming. DO NOT SHAKE.

- The dose of reconstituted aldesleukin should be diluted aseptically in 50 mL

of D5W and infused over a 15-min period.
- If the total dose of aldesleukin is 1.5 mg or less (e.g., a patient with a body weight of less than 40 kg), the dose of aldesleukin should be diluted in a smaller volume of D5W. Keep concentrations between 30 and 70 mcg/mL. Dilution and delivery of aldesleukin outside of this concentration range should be avoided.
- Glass bottles and plastic (polyvinyl chloride) bags have been used in clinical trials with comparable results. It is recommended that plastic bags be used as the dilution container because experimental studies suggest that use of plastic containers results in more consistent drug delivery.
- In-line filters should NOT be used when administering aldesleukin.
- The solution should be brought to room temperature before infusion in the patient.
- Reconstitution or dilution with bacteriostatic water for injection or 0.9% NaCl injection should be avoided because of increased aggregation.

STORAGE AND STABILITY
Unreconstituted vials of aldesleukin should be stored in a refrigerator at 2-8° C (26-46° F). After reconstitution, aldesleukin is stable for up to 48 hrs at temperatures of 2-25° C (36-77° F). Because there are no preservatives, both the reconstituted and diluted solutions should be stored in the refrigerator. Aldesleukin should not be frozen.

INTERACTIONS
Drug
Antihypertensives: May increase hypotensive effect.
Cardiotoxic, hepatotoxic, myelotoxic, or nephrotoxic medications: May increase the risk of toxicity.
Glucocorticoids: May decrease the effects of aldesleukin and should not be administered concurrently.
Interferon-α: Increased risk of myocardial injury, increased risk of exacerbation or initial presentation of autoimmune or inflammatory disorders.
Live virus vaccines: Should be avoided. May potentiate viral replication, increase side effects, and decrease the patient's antibody response to the vaccine.

Herbal
None known.

LAB EFFECTS/INTERFERENCE
May increase BUN and serum alkaline phosphatase, bilirubin, creatinine, aspartate aminotransferase (serum glutamic oxaloacetic transaminase), alanine aminotransferase (serum glutamic pyruvic transaminase) levels. May decrease serum calcium, magnesium, phosphorus, K, Na levels.

Y-SITE COMPATIBLES
Calcium gluconate, magnesium

INCOMPATIBLES
Dopamine, fluorouracil, ganciclovir (Cytovene), heparin, lorazepam, pentamidine (Pentam), K chloride, prochlorperazine (Compazine), promethazine (Phenergan), rituximab, trastuzumab

SIDE EFFECTS
Serious Reactions
- Anemia, thrombocytopenia, and leukopenia occur commonly. Aldesleukin impairs neutrophil function, and patients are at increased risk of disseminated infections including sepsis and endocarditis
- GI bleeding and pulmonary edema occur occasionally.
- Capillary leak syndrome results in hypotension (systolic pressure less than 90 mm Hg or a 20 mm Hg drop from baseline systolic pressure), extravasation of plasma proteins and fluid into extravascular space, and loss of vascular tone. It may result in cardiac arrhythmias, angina, MI, and respiratory insufficiency.
- Other rare reactions include fatal malignant hyperthermia, cardiac arrest, cerebrovascular accident, pulmonary emboli, bowel perforation, gangrene, and severe depression leading to suicide.
- Even severe side effects are generally self-limiting and reversible within 2-3 days after discontinuing therapy.

Other Side Effects
Frequent (10%-50%): Edema, erythema, rash, stomatitis, anorexia, weight gain, infection (urinary tract infection, injection site, catheter tip), dizziness, fever, chills, nausea, vomiting, hypotension, diarrhea, oliguria or anuria, mental status changes, irritability, confusion, depression, sinus tachycardia, pain (abdominal, chest, back), fatigue, dyspnea, pruritus

Occasional (1%-10%): Dry skin, sensory disorders (vision, speech, taste), dermatitis, headache, arthralgia, myalgia, weight loss, hematuria, conjunctivitis, proteinuria
Rare (Less Than 1%): Coma, psychosis

SPECIAL CONSIDERATIONS
Baseline Assessment
- Obtain CBC with differential, platelet count, electrolyte, BUN, and creatinine levels, and liver function tests.
- Evaluate for any history of GI bleeding or ulcer history.
- Monitor baseline weight.
- Assess patient for any history of diarrhea.

Intervention and Evaluation
- Monitor vital signs on a regular basis if using this agent for inpatient therapy; if for outpatient therapy, monitor vital signs prior to each dose. Hypotension can be significant with this agent in high-dose therapy.
- Weigh daily if for inpatient; if for outpatient weigh with each visit.
- Monitor for any evidence of infection erythema or edema.
- Evaluate patient for signs and symptoms of mental status changes or confusion with high-dose therapy or therapy.
- Assess patient for any new or increasing pain in areas of back, chest, or abdomen.
- Evaluate patient for central venous access device if using high-dose therapy.
- Monitor for skin changes and initiate skin care regimen per institutional guidelines. An example would be the use of frequent moisturizers to prevent skin breakdown.
- Assess patient's respiratory status for any evidence of rales, rhonchi, or diminished breath sounds in bases.

Education
- Instruct patient on when to contact his or her health care provider: fever greater than 38° C (greater than 101° F), chills, shortness of breath, nausea lasting greater than 24 hours, diarrhea lasting greater than 24 hours, or inability to take in at least 1500 mL of fluid in 24 hours.
- Advise patient on a skin care regimen to be done at least twice daily or more often to prevent skin breakdown. Make sure patient is educated on types of moisturizers to utilize; many commercial products contain alcohol, which can be drying.

- Educate patient about the possibility of fluid shifts and how to monitor for weight gain and edema in the lower extremities.
- Instruct patient to contact his or her provider for any evidence of increased pain in the chest, back, or abdomen.
- Advise patient and caregiver to report mental status changes such as confusion, disorientation, or increased somnolence.
- Instruct patient on central venous access care and monitoring and to report any signs of erythema, pain, or drainage.
- Provide patient with information on local resources and support groups available for his or her specific diagnosis.

ALEMTUZUMAB
BRAND NAMES
Campath-1H

CLASS OF AGENT
Monoclonal antibody

CLINICAL PHARMACOLOGY
Mechanism of Action
A recombinant DNA-derived humanized monoclonal antibody directed against CD52 cell surface glycoproteins. CD52 is found on the surface of all B and T lymphocytes, most monocytes, macrophages, natural killer cells, granulocytes, and normal bone marrow stem cells. It is commonly present on malignant lymphocytes evident in chronic lymphocytic leukemia (CLL). Alemtuzumab binds to the CD52 present on the surface of leukemic lymphocytes and induces cell lysis.
Therapeutic Effect: Produces cytotoxicity, reducing tumor size.

Absorption and Distribution
IV administration: Information on the pharmacokinetics (PK) of alemtuzumab is limited. The PK after IV administration is not well characterized. Because this is a large protein that binds to CD52 receptors, the biodistribution and clearance of alemtuzumab is highly dependent on the patient's tumor burden of lymphocytic leukemia cells. In patients without cancer, it is likely that the distribution of the drug will be to lymphoid tissue, bone marrow, and granulocytes throughout the body. A concentration of 1 mcg/mL is considered lympholytic. The mean cumulative dose to reach 1 mcg/mL was 90 mg (range 13-316 mg). An increasing trough concentration was associated with

increasing complete response. Mean troughs of 8-10 mcg/mL were seen in patients achieving minimal residual disease. The apparent steady-state volume of distribution is 0.185 L/kg and the volume of distribution for the terminal phase is 0.252 L/kg.

Subcutaneous administration: The PK after subcutaneous administration is similar to that for IV administration. The rate of absorption, however, is much slower after subcutaneous administration and takes about 6 weeks longer; therefore a higher cumulative dose is needed to achieve the therapeutic threshold concentration of 1 mcg/mL than that with IV administration.

Half-life: Alemtuzumab displays non linear clearance due to reduced CD52 receptor mediated clearance after repeated administrations of the drug. Older studies report a long half-life, ranging between 15 and 20 days after discontinuation of alemtuzumab. Peak and trough levels rise during first few weeks of therapy and approach steady state by about week 6. More recent studies report a shorter half-life ranging between 2 and 8 days, mean of 6.1 days in responding patients. In nonresponders, the half-life is rapid and most of the drug is eliminated in a few days.

Metabolism and Excretion

Clearance of alemtuzumab correlates with residual disease. Those with undetectable CLL had linear clearance and a longer half-life than those with minimal disease. In patients with a large tumor burden, most of the antibody is rapidly cleared from the blood. As the tumor burden shrinks, the drug accumulates and achieves higher trough concentrations.

HOW SUPPLIED/AVAILABLE FORMS
Solution for Injection: 30 mg/1 mL.

INDICATIONS AND DOSAGES
Chronic Lymphocytic Leukemia
IV: The optimal dose and schedule of alemtuzumab have not been fully determined. The following regimens have been used:
1. Initially, 3 mg/day as a 2-hr infusion. When the 3-mg daily dose is tolerated (with only low-grade or no infusion-related toxicities), increase daily dose to 10 mg. When the 10 mg/day dose is tolerated, the maintenance dose may be initiated.
2. Maintenance of 30 mg/day 3 times/wk on alternate days (such as Monday,

Wednesday, and Friday or Tuesday, Thursday, and Saturday) for up to 12 wks. The increase to 30 mg/day is usually achieved in 3-7 days.

Dose Modification for Hematologic Toxicity
Dosage Adjustment in Hepatic Dysfunction
No guidelines are known.
Dosage Adjustment in Renal Dysfunction
No guidelines are known.

UNLABELED USES
Rheumatoid arthritis, prevention of graft-versus-host disease from allogeneic stem cell transplant.

PRECAUTIONS
Pregnancy Risk Category: C

CONTRAINDICATIONS
Active systemic infections, history of hypersensitivity or anaphylactic reaction to the drug, underlying immunodeficiency (e.g., seropositive for HIV).

DRUG PREPARATION/ADMINISTRATION/ SAFE HANDLING ISSUES
◀ ALERT ▶
IV
- Refrigerate vials before dilution. Do not freeze.
- Use the solution within 8 hrs after dilution. The diluted solution may be stored at room temperature or refrigerated.
- Discard the solution if it becomes discolored or contains particulate matter.
- Invert the bag to mix the contents; do not shake it.
- Protect from light.
- Give the 100-mL solution as a 2-hr IV infusion. Do not give alemtuzumab by IV push or bolus.
- Premedication with oral antihistamine and acetaminophen is recommended to prevent infusion-related reactions.
- Antimicrobial prophylaxis is recommended to prevent opportunistic infections (i.e., *Pneumocystis carinii* and herpes virus). In studies, sulfamethoxazole/ trimethoprim double-strength tablet twice daily 3 times/wk plus famciclovir 250 mg twice daily or equivalent were given at initiation of alemtuzumab and for a minimum of 2 mos after therapy or until CD4 = 200 cells/microliter.

Hematologic Toxicity	Dose Modification and Reinitiation of Therapy
For first occurrence of ANC <250/microliters and/or platelet count ≤25,000/microliters	Withhold alemtuzumab therapy. When the ANC is ≥500/microliters and the platelet count is ≥50,000/microliters, resume alemtuzumab therapy at the same dose. If the delay between dosing is ≥7 days, initiate therapy at alemtuzumab 3 mg and escalate to 10 mg and then 30 mg as tolerated.
For second occurrence of ANC <250/microliters and/or platelet count ≤25,000/microliters	Withhold alemtuzumab therapy. When the ANC is ≥ 500/microliters and the platelet count is ≥50,000/microliters, resume alemtuzumab therapy at 10 mg. If the delay between dosing is ≥7 days, initiate alemtuzumab therapy at 3 mg and escalate to 10 mg only.
For third occurrence of ANC <250/microliters and/or platelet count ≤25,000/microliters	Discontinue alemtuzumab therapy permanently.
For a decrease of ANC and/or platelet count to ≤50% of the baseline value in patients initiating therapy with a baseline ANC ≤500/microliters and/or baseline platelet count ≤25,000/microliters	Withhold alemtuzumab therapy. When the ANC and/or platelet count returns to baseline value(s), resume alemtuzumab therapy. If the delay between dosing is ≥7 days, initiate therapy at alemtuzumab 3 mg and escalate to 10 mg and then to 30 mg as tolerated.

STORAGE AND STABILITY
• Refrigerate undiluted solutions; do not freeze.
• Protect from direct sunlight.
• Use the solution within 8 hrs after dilution. The diluted solution may be stored at room temperature or refrigerated.
• Discard the solution if it becomes discolored or contains particulate matter.

INTERACTIONS
Drug
Live-virus vaccines: May potentiate viral replication, increase side effects, and decrease the patient's antibody response to the vaccine.
Herbal
None known.

LAB EFFECTS/INTERFERENCE
May decrease Hgb level, platelet levels, WBC count.

Y-SITE COMPATIBLES
No studies have been reported.

INCOMPATIBLES
Do not mix alemtuzumab with any other medications.

SIDE EFFECTS
Serious Reactions
• Serious infusion-related effects including syncope, pulmonary infiltrates, adult respiratory distress syndrome, respiratory arrest, cardiac arrhythmias, MI, and cardiac arrest have been reported. In some instances, cardiac adverse events have resulted in death. Premedication should be given with an oral antihistamine and acetaminophen before alemtuzumab.
• Neutropenia occurs in 85% of patients, anemia occurs in 80% of patients, and thrombocytopenia occurs in 72% of patients.
• Prolonged, sometimes fatal, pancytopenia may occur.
• Opportunistic infections, sometimes fatal, may be seen.
• A rash occurs in 40% of patients.
• Respiratory toxicity, manifested as dyspnea, cough, bronchitis, pneumonitis, and pneumonia, occurs in 26% of patients.
Other Side Effects
Frequent (10%-50%):
Grade 3 or 4 neutropenia, rigors, tremors, fever, nausea, grade 3 or 4 thrombocytopenia, vomiting, rash, fatigue, hypotension, urticaria, pruritus, skeletal pain, headache, diarrhea, anorexia.
Occasional (1%-10%):
Myalgia, dizziness, abdominal pain, throat irritation, vomiting, neutropenia, rhinitis, bronchospasm, urticaria.
Rare (Less Than 1%):
Idiopathic thrombocytopenic purpura.

SPECIAL CONSIDERATIONS
Baseline Assessment
- Expect to pretreat patient with 650 mg of acetaminophen and 50 mg of diphenhydramine before each infusion to prevent infusion-related side effects.
- Expect to obtain a CBC frequently during and after therapy to assess for anemia, neutropenia, and thrombocytopenia.
- Expect to evaluate patient for any history of hypotension and current antihypertensive therapy if patient is currently on medications.

Intervention and Evaluation
- Monitor patient for infusion-related reactions, including chills, fever, hypotension, and rigors, which usually occur 30 minutes to 2 hours after the first infusion is started. These reactions may resolve by slowing the drip rate. If severe infusion-related events occur, treatment with hydrocortisone 200 mg is used to decrease these effects.
- Monitor for signs and symptoms of hematologic toxicity, including excessive fatigue or weakness, ecchymosis, fever, signs of local infection, sore throat, or unusual bleeding from any site.

Education
- Instruct patient to avoid crowds and those with known infection.
- Educate on importance of continuing antibiotic prophylaxis after alemtuzumab is discontinued for minimum 2 months and per laboratory evidence of recovery of immune function.
- Urge patient to avoid live-virus vaccinations and contact with anyone who has recently received a live-virus vaccine.

ALTRETAMINE

BRAND NAMES
Hexalen

CLASS OF AGENT
Antineoplastic agent

CLINICAL PHARMACOLOGY
Mechanism of Action
A synthetic cytotoxic antineoplastic *S*-triazine derivative with an unknown exact mechanism of action. Altretamine and its metabolites resemble alkylating agents; however, in vitro tests show no alkylating activity. Another possible mechanism may be binding to DNA; however, the relevance of this to cytotoxic activity is unknown. **Therapeutic Effect:** Inhibits DNA and RNA synthesis.

Absorption and Distribution
Altretamine is rapidly and well absorbed. Peak plasma levels are reached in 0.5-3 hr(s). Altretamine and its metabolites are protein bound: free fractions: 6% (parent), 25% (pentamethylmelamine), and 50% (tetramethylmelamine). They are distributed in high concentrations in excretory organs (liver and kidneys) and in the small intestine.
Half-life: 4.7-13 hrs.

Metabolism and Excretion
Extensively metabolized in the liver via demethylation into active metabolites. Excreted primarily in urine (61%-92%).

HOW SUPPLIED/AVAILABLE FORMS
Capsules: 50 mg clear, hard gelatin capsules.

INDICATIONS AND DOSAGES
Second-Line Therapy as Palliative Care in Ovarian Cancer
260 mg/m^2/day orally in 4 divided doses (after meals and at bedtime) for 14 or 21 consecutive days per 28-day cycle.
Hold for 14 days or longer and reinitiate at 200 mg/m^2/day if GI intolerance does not respond to symptomatic interventions, if WBC count is less than 2000/mm^3, if granulocyte count is less than 1000/mm^3, if platelet count is less than 75,000/mm^3, or if progressive neurotoxicity is seen.
Dosage Adjustment in Hepatic/Renal Dysfunction
No recommendations are available.

UNLABELED USES
Breast, cervical, colon, endometrial, head and neck, metastatic, pancreatic, prostatic, and small cell lung cancer; multiple myeloma

PRECAUTIONS
Concurrent administration with monoamine oxidase inhibitors or pyridoxine should be done with caution. Neurologic examinations and CBC with differential should be performed monthly.
Pregnancy Risk Category: D
Be aware that altretamine should not be used during pregnancy, and it is unknown whether the drug is distributed in breast

milk. Breast-feeding is not recommended in this patient population.

CONTRAINDICATIONS
Preexisting severe bone marrow depression; severe neurologic toxicity; hypersensitivity to altretamine or any components of its formulation.

DRUG PREPARATION/ADMINISTRATION/ SAFE HANDLING ISSUES
- Give 4 times daily after meals and at bedtime.

STORAGE AND STABILITY
Store at room temperature: 15-30° C.

INTERACTIONS
Drug
Cimetidine: May increase half-life and toxicity of altretamine.
Live-virus vaccines: May potentiate viral replication, increase vaccine side effects, and decrease the patient's antibody response to the vaccine.
MAOIs: isocarboxazid (Marplan), tranylcypromine (Parnate), phenelzine (Nardil), selegiline (Eldepryl): May increase the risk of severe orthostatic hypotension.
Pyridoxine (vitamin B_6): May reduce the response duration to altretamine.
Herbal
None.

LAB EFFECTS/INTERFERENCE
May reduce WBC and platelet counts. May increase alkaline phosphatase, BUN, creatinine concentrations.

SIDE EFFECTS
Serious Reactions
- Mild to moderate myelosuppression may occur. Get baseline CBC and differential and monitor monthly. Altretamine is contraindicated in patients with preexisting severe bone marrow depression.
- Neurotoxicity has been reported. Neurologic examination should be performed before initiation of each course of therapy. Neurotoxicity has reported to be reversible after drug discontinuation.
- Concomitant administration of MAOI antidepressant drugs with altretamine may result in severe orthostatic hypotension.

Other Side Effects
Frequent (10%-50%):
Anemia, diarrhea, nausea, peripheral neuropathy, vomiting
Occasional (1%-10%):
Elevated BUN, elevated serum creatinine, leukopenia, thrombocytopenia
Rare (Less Than 1%):
Alopecia, anorexia, fatigue, hepatic toxicity, myelosuppression, pruritus, rash, seizures, thrombocytopenia

SPECIAL CONSIDERATIONS
Baseline Assessment
- Obtain CBC with differential, platelet count, electrolyte, BUN and creatinine levels, and liver function tests.
- Evaluate the need for dose reduction if patient's renal function is altered. In elderly patients, age-related decreases in renal function may require decreased dosage and more careful monitoring of blood counts.
- Assess patient for any signs or symptoms of neuropathy.
- Evaluate emetic history with prior chemotherapy agents.
- Assess patient for any history of bowel alterations, i.e., constipation or diarrhea.
- Be aware that the safety and efficacy of altretamine have not been established in children.
Intervention and Evaluation
- Obtain peripheral CBC with differential, electrolyte, BUN, and creatinine levels, and liver function tests at least monthly, before initiation of each course of therapy, and as clinically indicated.
- Assess patient's need for antiemetic therapy before dosing if he or she has a significant history of emesis with prior therapies.
- Monitor for any evidence of anemia, increasing fatigue, shortness of breath, or dyspnea.
- Evaluate patient at each visit for evidence of peripheral neuropathy, numbness, tingling, paresthesia, or dysesthesia.
- Assess for evidence of nausea, vomiting, or diarrhea with this agent.
- Educate patient on when and how to take this agent.
Education
- Instruct patient to take altretamine after meals and at bedtime.
- Educate patient on when to contact his or her primary care provider: fever greater than 38° C (greater than 101° F), nausea

or diarrhea lasting greater than 24 hours, or inability to take in at least 1500 mL fluid daily.
- Educate patient to take antiemetics as needed if he or she has a significant history of emesis with prior therapies.
- Advise patient regarding the possibility of peripheral neuropathy and discuss symptoms to monitor, numbness, and tingling in the hands or feet.
- Instruct patient to report signs and symptoms of anemia, increasing fatigue, shortness of breath, and dyspnea upon exertion.
- Stress to patient that he or she should not receive live-virus vaccinations without the physician's approval because altretamine lowers the body's resistance. Also advise patient to avoid contact with anyone who recently received a live-virus vaccine.
- Provide patient with information on local resources and support groups available for his or her specific diagnosis.

AMIFOSTINE

BRAND NAMES
Ethyol

CLASS OF AGENT
Cytoprotectant, radioprotectant

CLINICAL PHARMACOLOGY
Mechanism of Action
An antineoplastic adjunct and cytoprotective agent that is converted to an active metabolite by alkaline phosphatase in tissues. The active metabolite WR-1065 is taken up readily into normal tissues but less so into malignant cells because of the higher amount of alkaline phosphatase present in normal tissues. WR-1065 acts a scavenger of oxygen-free radicals generated by ionizing radiation or alkylating agent cytotoxic drugs. **Therapeutic Effect:** Reduces the toxic effect of ionizing radiation and cytotoxic drugs on normal renal parenchyma, nerve tissue, mucosa, and bone marrow.
Absorption and Distribution
Amifostine is administered IV and subcutaneously. After subcutaneous administration, the area under the curve of the parent compound ranges from 40% to 50% and the active metabolite (WR-1065) is 68% that of the IV route. The volume

of distribution is equivalent to plasma water. It is rapidly cleared from plasma through conversion in normal tissue to the active free thiol metabolite. Tissue uptake is highest in bone marrow, skin, GI mucosa, and salivary glands. The active metabolite (WR-1065) is very polar and does cross the blood-brain barrier. Although amifostine is not bound serum albumin, WR-1065 is highly protein bound, which allows for delivery of WR-1065 to cell membranes and uptake into the cell.
Half-life: After IV administration: 15 mins. After subcutaneous administration: 49 mins. Less than 10% remains in plasma 6 mins after drug administration.
Metabolism and Excretion
Rapidly converted by alkaline phosphatase, present in many endothelial and capillary cell membranes, to an active metabolite, WR-1065.

HOW SUPPLIED/AVAILABLE FORMS
Powder for Injection: 500 mg in a 10-mL single-use vial.

INDICATIONS AND DOSAGES
To Reduce Cumulative Renal Toxicity from Repeated Administration of Cisplatin in Patients with Advanced Ovarian Cancer
910 mg/m^2 IV once a day as a 15-min infusion, beginning 30 min before chemotherapy. A 15-min or shorter infusion is better tolerated than extended infusions. If the full dose cannot be administered, the dose for subsequent cycles should be 740 mg/m^2.
Treatment of Postoperative Radiation-Induced Xerostomia in Patients with Head and Neck Cancer
200 mg/m^2 IV once a day as a 3-min infusion, starting 15-30 mins before radiation therapy.
Dosage Adjustment in Hepatic Dysfunction
Amifostine has not been studied in this setting.
Dosage Adjustment in Renal Dysfunction
Amifostine has not been studied in this setting.

UNLABELED USES
Subcutaneous: 500 mg/day 20 mins before radiation therapy.
To protect lung fibroblasts from damaging effects of chemotherapeutic agent paclitaxel; Amifostine has been reported to prevent myelosuppression after the use

of cyclophosphamide but has not been adequately tested for this indication.

PRECAUTIONS
Pregnancy Risk Category: C

CONTRAINDICATIONS
Sensitivity to aminothiol compounds or mannitol

DRUG PREPARATION/ADMINISTRATION/ SAFE HANDLING ISSUES
◀ **ALERT** ▶ To prevent severe hypotension during the IV infusion of amifostine, patients should be well hydrated before the infusion of amifostine and placed in a supine position. Antihypertensive therapy or drugs that could potentiate amifostine hypotension should be interrupted at least 24 hrs before administration of amifostine at doses recommended for cytoprotection in patients receiving cisplatin.
Hypotension may occur during or shortly after completion of amifostine infusion, despite adequate hydration and positioning of the patient. B/P should be frequently and carefully monitored during and after IV infusion of the drug in patients whose anti-hypertensive therapy has been temporarily withheld. In addition, B/P should be monitored frequently (e.g., every 5 mins) during amifostine infusion in all patients receiving the drug, and the infusion should be interrupted if a clinically important decline in B/P occurs (e.g., a 20-mm Hg decline for those with pretreatment systolic pressure of less than 100 mm Hg, or a 25-, 30-, 40-, or 50-mm Hg decline for those with a pretreatment systolic pressure of 1001-19, 1201-39, 1401-79, or greater than or equal to 180 mm Hg, respectively). During infusions of less than 5 mins duration, B/P should be monitored at least before and immediately after completion of the infusion and thereafter if needed. If hypotension requiring interruption of the amifostine infusion occurs, the patient should be placed in the Trendelenburg position and an IV infusion of 0.9% NaCl initiated in a separate line. If the patient's B/P returns to normal within 5 mins and the patient is asymptomatic, the amifostine infusion may be resumed.
• Amifostine may be administered by IV infusion or subcutaneous injection. The injection vial is reconstituted by adding 9.7 mL of 0.9% NaCl injection to contain 50 mg/mL. The reconstituted solution

may be further diluted in a compatible IV infusion solution (e.g., 0.9% NaCl injection) in a polyvinyl chloride (PVC) container to a final concentration ranging from 5 to 40 mg of amifostine per mL, which is stable for 5 hrs when stored at room temperature (25° C). When refrigerated at 2-8° C, it is stable for 24 hrs.
• Subcutaneous administration. The drug should be diluted in 2.5 mL of 0.9% NaCl.

STORAGE AND STABILITY
• Amifostine for injection is supplied as a sterile lyophilized powder in 10-mL single-use vials. The lyophilized dosage form should be stored at controlled room temperature (20-25° C; 68-77° F).
• Amifostine is chemically stable when concentrations of 5-40 mg/mL are stored in PVC administration bags for up to 5 hrs at room temperature (25° C, 77° F) or up to 24 hrs if refrigerated at 2-8° C (36-46° F).

INTERACTIONS
Drug
Antihypertensive medications or drugs that may potentiate hypotension: May increase the risk of hypotension.
Herbal
None known.

LAB EFFECTS/INTERFERENCE
May reduce serum calcium levels, especially in patients with nephrotic syndrome.

Y-SITE COMPATIBLES
Cyclophosphamide, cytarabine, dacarbazine, dactinomycin, daunorubicin HCl, dexamethasone Na phosphate, diphenhydramine HCl, dobutamine HCl, docetaxel, dopamine HCl, doxorubicin HCl, doxycycline hyclate, droperidol, enalaprilat, etoposide, famotidine, floxuridine, fluconazole, fludarabine phosphate, fluorouracil, furosemide, gemcitabine HCl, gentamicin sulfate, granisetron HCl, haloperidol lactate, heparin Na, hydrocortisone Na phosphate, hydrocortisone Na succinate, hydromorphone HCl, idarubicin HCl ifosfamide, imipenem-cilastatin Na, leucovorin calcium, lorazepam, magnesium sulfate, mannitol, mechlorethamine HCl, meperidine HCl, mesna, methotrexate Na, methylprednisolone Na succinate, metoclopramide HCl, metronidazole, minocycline HCl, mitomycin, mitoxantrone HCl, morphine sulfate, nalbuphine HCl, netilmi-

cin sulfate, ondansetron HCl, pemetrexed, piperacillin Na, plicamycin, K chloride, promethazine HCl, ranitidine HCl, rituximab, Na bicarbonate, streptozocin, teniposide, thiotepa, ticarcillin disodium, ticarcillin disodium-clavulanate K, tobramycin sulfate, trastuzumab, trimethoprim-sulfamethoxazole, trimetrexate glucuronate vancomycin HCl, vinblastine sulfate, vincristine sulfate, zidovudine

INCOMPATIBLES
Do not mix amifostine in any solution other than 0.9% NaCl.
Acyclovir, amphotericin B colloidal (Amphotec), cefoperazone, cisplatin, ganciclovir Na, hydroxyzine HCl, minocycline, prochlorperazine edisylate

SIDE EFFECTS
Serious Reactions
- A pronounced drop in B/P may require temporary cessation of amifostine and fluid resuscitation.
- Monitor for severe cutaneous hypersensitivity reactions that may include erythema multiforme, Stevens-Johnson syndrome, toxic epidermal necrolysis, toxoderma, and exfoliative dermatitis.

Other Side Effects
Frequent (10%-50%): Flushing or feeling of warmth or chills or feeling of coldness; dizziness, hiccups, sneezing, somnolence, transient reduction in B/P (usually starts 14 mins into infusion, lasts about 6 mins, and returns to normal in 5-15 mins); severe nausea, vomiting.
Occasional (1%-10%): Allergic reactions, fatigue
Rare (Less Than 1%): Clinically relevant hypocalcemia, mild rash

SPECIAL CONSIDERATIONS
Baseline Assessment
- Check vital signs at baseline to evaluate for hypotension.
- Evaluate patient's current medication regimen, checking for diuretic and antihypertensive medications.
- Assess for a potential allergy to thiol derivatives.
- Assess hydration status of patient.

Intervention and Evaluation
- Give premedications for emesis at least 60-90 minutes before amifostine dosing to prevent significant emesis.

- Be aware that premedication with a serotonin antagonist is required for the 740 mg/m^2 dose or for patients receiving combined modality therapy; other antiemetics may be given for the patient's initial doses of radiation therapy, although a serotonin antagonist is usually required.
- Assess hydration status as patient will develop hypotension if not adequately hydrated.
- Place patient in a supine or reclining position to receive this medication to prevent increased hypotension.
- Have patient void preadministration to prevent a syncopal episode upon standing.
- Monitor vital signs preadministration and after hydration
- Deliver agent over less than 1 minute IV at the 500 mg dose or less than 3 minutes at the 740 mg/m^2 dose.

Education
- Educate patient to hold antihypertensive medication until 2 hours after amifostine dosing.
- Instruct patient to drink at least 2 L of fluid per day with only 16 oz in caffeinated beverages as caffeine can induce dehydration.
- Instruct patient to empty the bladder before receiving the agent.
- Have patient maintain a fluid diary to assess hydration status.
- Instruct patient to report any emetic episodes after dosing.
- Instruct patient to take antiemetics 60-90 minutes before amifostine administration.
- Instruct patient on when to contact his or her health care provider: intractable nausea, inability to take at least 1500 mL of fluid per day, fevers after dosing of greater than 38° C (greater than 101° F), or new or worsening cutaneous toxicities.

AMINOGLUTETHIMIDE

BRAND NAMES
Cytadren

CLASS OF AGENT
Adrenal suppressant

CLINICAL PHARMACOLOGY
Mechanism of Action
Aminoglutethimide partially inhibits the conversion of cholesterol to pregnenolone in the adrenal glands and blocks the conversion of androstenedione to estrone and estradiol

in peripheral tissues, preventing the production of cortisol, aldosterone, and estrogens. It also inhibits aromatase enzyme, leading to reduced estrogen levels. Because a reflex rise in adrenocorticotropic hormone (ACTH) will overcome the blockade partially or completely, hydrocortisone supplementation should be given concurrently to keep ACTH levels suppressed and ensure the therapeutic effect of aminoglutethimide (prevent the reflex rise of ACTH, which nullifies the effect of aminoglutethimide). The primary use of aminoglutethimide therapy is for treatment of Cushing's syndrome due to adrenal hyperplasia, ectopic ACTH production, or adrenal carcinoma. **Therapeutic Effect:** In the cancer setting, aminoglutethimide reduces estradiol levels.

Absorption and Distribution

Aminoglutethimide is rapidly and completely absorbed from the GI tract. Protein binding: low (20%-25%).
Half-life: 12.5 ± 1.6 hrs after a single dose. After daily dosing, the half-life is shorter at 7-9 hrs due to hepatic microsomal induction.

Metabolism and Excretion

Metabolized in the liver by acetylation to *N*-acetylaminoglutethimide. Between 34% and 50% of aminoglutethimide is excreted unchanged in the urine. Between 4% and 25% of the *N*-acetyl metabolite is excreted in urine. It is hemodialyzed effectively.

HOW SUPPLIED/AVAILABLE FORMS

Tablets: 250 mg.

INDICATIONS AND DOSAGES

Cushing's syndrome

Initially, 250 mg orally q6h. May increase by 250 mg daily every 1-2 wks. Maximum: 2 g/day.

Dosage Adjustment in Hepatic Dysfunction

Dose adjustments are not required.

Dosage Adjustment in Renal Dysfunction

Dose reduction may be indicated.

PRECAUTIONS

Use cautiously in patients with hematologic abnormalities, hypotension, hypothyroidism, or stress.
Pregnancy Risk Category: D

CONTRAINDICATIONS

Hypersensitivity to glutethimide or aminoglutethimide

DRUG PREPARATION/ADMINISTRATION/SAFE HANDLING ISSUES

Storage and Stability

Keep this medication in a tightly-closed, light-resistant container and do not store above 30° C (86° F).

INTERACTIONS

Drug

Dexamethasone, digitoxin, medroxyprogesterone, tamoxifen, theophylline, warfarin: May decrease effectiveness of these drugs by enhancing metabolism.

Herbal

None known.

LAB EFFECTS/INTERFERENCE

None known.

SIDE EFFECTS

Serious Reactions

Adrenal insufficiency, agranulocytosis, neutropenia, and pancytopenia may occur.

Other Side Effects

Frequent (10%-50%): Drowsiness, rash, loss of appetite, nausea.
Occasional (1%-10%): Depression, dizziness, headache, fever, myalgia, hypotension, tachycardia, pruritus.
Rare (Less Than 1%): Neck tenderness, swelling, increased hair growth in females

SPECIAL CONSIDERATIONS

Baseline Assessment

* Obtain patient's baseline values for CBC with differential, liver function tests, and electrolyte, BUN, creatinine, and cortisol levels.
* Assess patient for any history of depression.
* Evaluate patient's nutritional status.
* Check baseline vital signs to determine evidence of tachycardia.
* Assess patient for history of alcohol use.
* Monitor patient for current medication history as this agent can alter the efficacy of certain agents.

Intervention and Evaluation

* Monitor CBC with differential, liver function tests, and electrolyte, BUN, creatinine, and cortisol levels periodically.
* Evaluate patient for significant weight loss or nausea.
* Monitor for evidence of neutropenia and leukopenia.

- Evaluate for evidence of increasing tiredness and drowsiness; counsel patients not to drive if this symptom occurs.
- Evaluate patient for any symptoms of skin reaction.
- Evaluate vital signs for evidence of orthostatic hypotension or tachycardia.
- Be aware that steroid replacement therapy may be necessary. Hydrocortisone is recommended for glucocorticoid replacement; fludrocortisone is commonly used as a mineralocorticoid replacement.

Education

- Instruct patient on when to contact his or her primary care provider: fever greater than 38° C (greater than 101° F), infection, cough, nausea lasting greater than 24 hours, significant loss of appetite with weight loss of greater than 2 pounds per week, or inability to take at least 1500 mL of fluid in 24 hours.
- Educate patient that feelings of significant fatigue, dizziness upon standing, rapid heart rate, or palpitations need to be treated immediately and to call his or her provider.
- Advise patient to avoid driving if symptoms of drowsiness are associated with taking this agent.
- Educate patient to report any symptoms of skin reactions.
- Instruct patient to avoid alcohol.
- Provide patient with information on local resources and support groups available for his or her specific diagnosis.
- Administer radiation therapy 30-45 minutes after subcutaneous dosing.
- Administer chemotherapy or radiation therapy 30 minutes after dosing.

ANASTROZOLE

BRAND NAMES
Arimidex

CLASS OF AGENT
Aromatase inhibitor

CLINICAL PHARMACOLOGY
Mechanism of Action
In postmenopausal women, an estrogen precursor is produced by the adrenal gland in the form of androstenedione. Androstenedione is further converted in peripheral tissues to estrone and then to estradiol. Anastrozole decreases estrogen levels by inhibiting aromatase, the enzyme that catalyzes the final step in estrogen production. Anastrozole is a nonsteroidal, pure antiestrogen and does not have any estrogenic properties like those of tamoxifen. **Therapeutic Effect:** Deprives estrogen and inhibits the growth of hormone-dependent cancers that are stimulated by estrogens. A 1-mg dose decreases estrogen levels to lower limits of detection. Estrogen is reduced by 70% in 24 hrs and 80% after 14 days. Duration of estrogen suppression is 6 days after drug discontinuation.

Absorption and Distribution
Anastrozole is well absorbed into the systemic circulation (83%-85%). Food reportedly affects the extent of absorption of oral anastrozole. However, patient data assessing the magnitude or significance of this interaction were not provided by the manufacturer. Steady-state plasma levels reached in about 7 days. Protein binding: 40%. *Half-life:* 50 hrs.

Metabolism and Excretion
Extensively metabolized in the liver. Eliminated by the biliary system (85%) and, to a lesser extent, the kidneys (10% unchanged drug).

HOW SUPPLIED/AVAILABLE FORMS
Tablets: 1 mg.

INDICATIONS AND DOSAGES
Adjuvant treatment in postmenopausal women with hormone-receptor positive early breast cancer
1 mg PO once a day
First-line treatment in advanced or metastatic hormone receptor–positive or hormone receptor–unknown postmenopausal women
1 mg PO once a day
Second-line treatment in postmenopausal women with disease progression after tamoxifen therapy
1 mg PO once a day
Dosage Adjustment in Hepatic Dysfunction
Anastrozole has been studied in patients with stable hepatic cirrhosis. No dosage adjustments were necessary because patients had normal plasma anastrozole concentrations.
Dosage Adjustment in Renal Dysfunction
No dose adjustment necessary.

UNLABELED USES
No information.

PRECAUTIONS
Anastrozole has been known to decrease bone mineral density and elevate total cholesterol levels.
Pregnancy Risk Category: D

CONTRAINDICATIONS
Known hypersensitivity to anastrozole or any of its excipients; known or suspected pregnancy

DRUG PREPARATION/ADMINISTRATION/ SAFE HANDLING ISSUES
• Take without regard to food.

STORAGE AND STABILITY
Store at room temperature.

INTERACTIONS
Drug
Anastrozole is known to be a weak cytochrome P450 1A2, 2C8/9, and 3A4 inhibitor. The manufacturer states it is unlikely to affect the metabolism of other P450-mediated drugs.
Herbal
Estrogen-containing herbal supplements may decrease the effect of anastrozole.

LAB EFFECTS/INTERFERENCE
May elevate serum γ-glutamyl transferase level in patients with liver metastasis. May increase serum LDLs, serum alkaline phosphate, AST (SGOT), ALT (SGPT), and total cholesterol levels.

SIDE EFFECTS
Serious Reactions
Cardiovascular events including MI, ischemic cerebrovascular events, ischemic cardiovascular disease, and thrombophlebitis occur rarely.
Other Side Effects
Frequent (10%-50%):
Arthritis, asthenia, back pain, cough, depression, headache, hot flashes, nausea, vomiting, vasodilatation
Occasional (1%-10%):
Abdominal pain, angina, anorexia, bone pain, chest pain, constipation, pharyngitis, diarrhea, diaphoresis dizziness, dry mouth, fractures, hypertension, insomnia, peripheral edema, pelvic pain, depression, osteoporosis, paresthesia, rash, vaginal hemorrhage, weight gain.
Rare (Less Than 1%):
Anaphylaxis, CVA, erythema multiforme, MI, Stevens-Johnson syndrome, thromboembolic events.

SPECIAL CONSIDERATIONS
Baseline Assessment
• Assess patient's CBC with differential, platelet count, activated partial thromboplastin time, prothrombin time, and fibrinogen before commencing therapy with this agent.
• Evaluate patient's history of deep vein thrombosis (DVT) or thromboembolic phenomenon.
• Bone densitometry should be performed to assess for osteoporosis before initiating therapy.
• Evaluate patient for any prior history of hypertension.
• Obtain a lipid panel and baseline bone mineral density before therapy.
Intervention and Evaluation
• Monitor vital signs with each follow-up visit, evaluating for any increase in B/P.
• Assess for side effects of the agent: hot flashes, night sweats, nausea, headaches, irritability, and symptoms of depression.
• Monitor for any signs or symptoms of vaginal bleeding or discharge.
• Obtain bone density follow-up as per institutional protocol.
• Obtain pelvic examinations per protocol to assess for endometrial cancer.
• Evaluate for a possible need for bisphosphonate therapy if patient is at risk for fracture due to significant osteoporosis.
Education
• Instruct patient that if he or she misses a dose, then take the pill as soon as remembered. If patient remembers close to the time for the next dose, then just take the next dose and do not double the dose.
• Instruct patient to report any signs or symptoms of DVT, lower extremity swelling, pain, and tenderness.
• Advise patient to report symptoms such as fatigue, menopausal symptoms, unusual vaginal discharge, or bleeding.
• Instruct patient on when to contact the health care provider with symptoms such as shortness of breath, dyspnea, increasing cough, fatigue, or severe headache.
• Educate patient to avoid all OTC medications or herbal or vitamin supplements without first clearing them with his or her health care provider.
• Instruct patient on the need for bone density scans and the risk of osteoporosis from this agent and with aging.
• Instruct patient to consider therapeutic lifestyle changes and consult with a physician for pharmacologic treatment if the lipid profile worsens.

- Provide patient with information on local resources and support groups available for his or her specific diagnosis.

ARSENIC TRIOXIDE, AS₂O₃
BRAND NAMES
Trisenox

CLASS OF AGENT
Antineoplastic agent

CLINICAL PHARMACOLOGY
Mechanism of Action
An antineoplastic agent that produces morphologic changes and DNA fragmentation, damage, or degradation of the polymorphonuclear leukocyte (PML)/retinoic acid receptor (RAR)-α fusion protein after post-translational modifications, and production of reactive oxygen species by NADPH oxidase in promyelocytic leukemic cells. **Therapeutic Effect:** Produces cell death.
Absorption and Distribution
Arsenic accumulates in the liver, kidney, heart, lung, hair, and nails.
Half-life: $t_{1/2}\ \alpha$ = 1 hr; $t_{1/2}\ \beta$ = 7-13 hrs
Metabolism and Excretion
The metabolism of arsenic trioxide is not related to the cytochrome P450 system. Arsenic pentavalent is reduced to trivalent arsenic and methylation of trivalent arsenic to monomethylarsonic acid. Monomethylarsonic acid is further methylated to dimethylarsinic acid in the liver. Excretion is through urine.

HOW SUPPLIED/AVAILABLE FORMS
Injection:
1 mg/mL preservative-free ampules.

INDICATIONS AND DOSAGES
Acute Promyelocytic Leukemia (APL)
Induction and consolidation therapy for APL in patients whose disease is refractory to or relapsed from retinoid and anthracycline chemotherapy. APL is a subset of acute myeloid leukemia and is characterized by the presence of the t(15;17) translocation or PML/RAR-α gene expression.
Induction: 0.15 mg/kg/day IV until the absence of leukemia cells in bone marrow occurs. Do not exceed 60 induction doses.
Consolidation treatment: Beginning 3-6 wks after completion of induction

therapy, 0.15 mg/kg/day IV for 25 doses over a period of up to 5 wks.
Dosage Adjustment in Hepatic Dysfunction
No recommendations are available.
Dosage Adjustment in Renal Dysfunction
Use with caution in patients with renal impairment.

UNLABELED USES
Chronic myeloid leukemia, acute myelocytic leukemia, multiple myeloma

PRECAUTIONS
Pregnancy Risk Category: D
Arsenic may cause fetal harm when administered during pregnancy. Excretion into human milk is unknown thus breast feeding is not recommended.

CONTRAINDICATIONS
Known hypersensitivity to arsenic trioxide

DRUG PREPARATION/ADMINISTRATION/SAFE HANDLING ISSUES
◀ ALERT ▶ Because arsenic trioxide may be carcinogenic, mutagenic, or teratogenic, wear nitrile or latex, but not vinyl, gloves when handling the drug. If the drug comes in contact with skin, wash the skin thoroughly with soap and water. Do not use waterless hand soap or any antibacterial soap as either can increase the reaction from the agent. If the drug comes in contact with mucous membranes, flush the area with water.
- Dilute with 100-250 mL of D5W or 0.9% NaCl.
- Infuse over 1-2 hrs or up to 4 hrs if patient has acute vasomotor reactions.
- Because of the long duration of therapy, a central venous catheter line may be preferred.

STORAGE AND STABILITY
- Diluted solution is stable up to 24 hrs at room temperature and 48 hrs when refrigerated.
- Store unopened ampules at room temperature, 15°-30° C (59-86° F).

INTERACTIONS
Drug
Amphotericin B, diuretics: May produce electrolyte imbalances.
Antiarrhythmics, thioridazine cisapride, quinolone antibiotics, other drugs that may affect QT interval: May prolong QT interval.
Herbal
None known.

LAB EFFECTS/INTERFERENCE
May decrease Hgb B levels, serum calcium and magnesium levels, platelet and WBC counts. May increase AST (SGOT), and (ALT) SGPT.

Y-SITE COMPATIBLES
No information available.

INCOMPATIBLES
Do not mix arsenic trioxide with any other medications.

SIDE EFFECTS
Serious Reactions
- Torsades de pointes, complete atrioventricular block, and prolonged QT intervals have been reported. Risk factors include extent of QT prolongation, concomitant drugs that cause QT prolongation, hypokalemia or hypomagnesemia, and current and past medical history of cardiac disease. Hospitalize patient if QTc is greater than 500 msec, syncope, or irregular heartbeats develop.
- The APL differentiation syndrome is characterized by fever, dyspnea, weight gain, pulmonary infiltrates, and pleural or pericardial effusions, with or without leukocytosis, and can be fatal. Dexamethasone 10 mg IV twice daily should be administered at the first signs/symptoms for at least 3 days or longer until patient is asymptomatic. Discontinuation of arsenic trioxide may not be necessary during APL differentiation syndrome treatment.
- Overdose: Signs are convulsions, muscle weakness, and confusion. Discontinue therapy and start chelation therapy. Administer dimercaprol 3 mg/kg IM every 4 hrs until the immediate life-threatening toxicity has resolved. May follow-up with penicillamine 250 mg PO up to the maximum frequency of 4 times daily (= 1 g/day).

Other Side Effects
Frequent (10%-50%):
- Cardiac: chest pain, edema, flushing, hypertension, hypotension, palpitations, prolonged QT interval, tachycardia.
- CNS: anxiety, dizziness, fatigue, headache.
- Skin: dermatitis, ecchymosis, hyperpigmentation, pruritus, rash.
- Hematologic: anemia, febrile neutropenia, leukocytosis, neutropenia, thrombocytopenia.
- GI: abdominal pain, anorexia, constipation, diarrhea, dyspepsia, sore throat, nausea, vomiting (high emetic potential).
- Metabolism: anorexia, electrolyte imbalance.
- Respiratory: cough, crackles, diminished breath sounds, dyspnea, epistaxis, hypoxia, pleural effusion, wheezing.
- General: arthralgia, asthenia, blurred vision, eye irritation, insomnia, rigors, fever, herpes simplex, hyperleukosis, infections, injection site pain/erythema, myalgia, nonspecific pain, paresthesia, peripheral neuropathy, sinusitis, tremor, weakness, weight gain/loss.

Occasional (1%-10%):
Coma, convulsion, dry mouth, hemoptysis, hypersensitivity, mucositis, somnolence.

Rare (Less Than 1%):
Confusion, petechiae, oral candidiasis, incontinence.

SPECIAL CONSIDERATIONS
Baseline Assessment
- Monitor CBC with differential, platelet count, electrolyte, BUN, creatinine, and magnesium levels, and liver function tests.
- Obtain a baseline EKG to assess for any cardiac abnormalities, arrhythmias, heart block, or prolongation of the QT interval.
- Correct QTc greater than 500 m/sec, and assessed patient with serial ECGs before arsenic is started.
- Monitor for any history of renal disease, seizures, or pleural or pericardial effusions.
- Assess for any current therapies that may cause QT prolongation or electrolyte abnormalities.

Intervention and Evaluation
- Evaluate CBC with differential, electrolyte, BUN, creatinine, and magnesium levels, and liver function tests before initial dosing and as per institutional protocol. Usual guidelines include daily CBC with differential, electrolyte, BUN, creatinine, and magnesium levels, and at least biweekly liver function tests.
- Be sure K level is greater than 4 mEq/L, and magnesium level is greater than 1.8 mg/dL.
- Obtain ECGs on a scheduled basis to evaluate for the QT interval, before the first dose, and at least weekly.
- Correct QTc greater than 500 m/sec, and reassess the risk/benefits of therapy.
- Discontinue arsenic in symptomatic patients with prolonged QT until QTc interval decreases to less than 460 m/sec, electrolyte abnormalities are corrected,

heart rate normalizes, and syncope ceases.
- Assess for cardiac changes, arrhythmias, tachycardia, palpitations, or chest pain.
- Monitor for arsenic toxicity: prolonged QT interval, unexplained fever, weight gain, or pleural or pericardial effusions. Assess via pulsus paradoxus for pericardial tamponade.
- Although not required, assess patient for central venous access because of the prolonged duration of this therapy.
- Monitor for any signs and symptoms of skin changes, erythema, skin rashes, and dermatitis.
- Administer premedications as ordered and antiemetics as needed.
- Monitor patient for febrile reactions, weight gain, diarrhea, and dyspnea.
- Monitor patient for any signs and symptoms of peripheral neuropathy.

Education
- Educate patient to report any signs and symptoms of shortness of breath, unexplained fever, palpitations, or dyspnea upon exertion.
- Instruct patient to report any nausea, fatigue, abdominal pain, paresthesias, increasing anxiety, or insomnia.
- Advise patient to report any new symptoms of headache, dizziness, or blurred vision.
- Instruct patient to contact the health care provider in case of fever greater than 38° C (greater than 101° F), shaking chills, or rigors.
- Educate patient on the possibility of developing arthralgias, profound myalgias, and fatigue from this agent.
- Instruct patient to refrain from taking any OTC product or herbal or vitamin supplements without first checking with his or her health care provider.

ASPARAGINASE

BRAND NAMES
Elspar

CLASS OF AGENT
Antineoplastic agent, enzyme

CLINICAL PHARMACOLOGY
Mechanism of Action
Asparaginase inhibits protein synthesis by hydrolyzing asparagine to aspartic acid and ammonia. Leukemia cells, especially lymphoblasts, require exogenous asparagines

because they lack asparagine synthetase; normal cells can synthesize asparagine. Asparaginase is cycle-specific for the G_1 phase.
Therapeutic Effect: Blocks asparagine-dependent protein synthesis, resulting in inhibition of tumor cell proliferation.
Absorption and Distribution
IM administration produces peak blood levels 50% lower than those from IV administration. Volume of distribution = 4-5 L/kg; 70-80% of plasma volume; the drug does not penetrate CSF. Protein binding: 30%.
Half-life: IM 39-49 hrs and IV 8-30 hrs.
Metabolism and Excretion
Metabolized by the reticuloendothelial system through slow sequestration. The drug is systemically degraded. Excretion: trace amounts are detectable in urine. Clearance is not affected by age or renal or hepatic function.

HOW SUPPLIED/AVAILABLE FORMS
Powder for Injection: 10,000 International Units in 10 mL.

INDICATIONS AND DOSAGES
Refer to individual disease protocols. Doses and schedules vary according to each protocol. Modifications are based on patient's response to therapy and tolerability.
Acute Lymphocytic Leukemias
IV: infusion as single agent for induction: 200 units/kg/day for 28 days or 500-10,000 units/m$_2$/day for 7 days every 3 wks or 10,000-40,000 units every 2-3 wks
IM: as single agent: 6000-12,000 units/m^2; reconstitution to 10,000 units/mL may be necessary
A test dose is often recommended before the first dose of asparaginase or before restarting therapy after a hiatus of several days. Most commonly, 0.1-0.2 mL of a 20-250 units/mL (2-50 units) is injected intradermally, and the patient is observed for 15-30 mins. False-negative rates of up to 80% to test doses of 2-50 units are reported. Desensitization may be performed in patients found to be hypersensitive by the intradermal test dose or those who have received previous courses of therapy with the drug. Some institutions recommended the following precautions for asparaginase administration: Have parenteral epinephrine, diphenhydramine, and hydrocortisone available at the bedside. Have a freely running IV line in place. Have a physician readily accessible. Monitor patient closely for 30-60 mins.

Dosage Adjustment in Hepatic Dysfunction
No dosage adjustment guideline is available. However, discontinuing asparaginase treatment or lowering doses is warranted in the scenario of rising liver enzyme concentrations or any hepatic dysfunction.

Dosage Adjustment in Renal Dysfunction
No information available.

UNLABELED USES
Treatment of acute myelocytic leukemia, acute myelomonocytic leukemia, chronic lymphocytic leukemia, Hodgkin's disease, lymphosarcoma, melanosarcoma, and reticulum cell sarcoma

PRECAUTIONS
Pregnancy Risk Category: C
Based on limited reports in humans, the use of asparaginase does not seem to pose a major risk to the fetus when used in the second and third trimesters, or when exposure occurs before conception in either females or males. Because of the teratogenicity observed in animals and the lack of human data regarding first trimester exposure, asparaginase should be used cautiously, if at all, during this period.

CONTRAINDICATIONS
History of hypersensitivity to asparaginase and pancreatitis. Patients with a hypersensitivity reaction to *Escherichia coli* asparaginase may be rechallenged with *Erwinia* asparaginase. Use caution because cross-sensitivity exists.

DRUG PREPARATION/ADMINISTRATION/ SAFE HANDLING ISSUES
◀ ALERT ▶ Asparaginase may be irritating to eyes, skin, and the upper respiratory tract. It has also been shown to be embryotoxic and teratogenic by the IV route in animal studies. Because of the drug's toxic properties, appropriate precautions including the use of appropriate safety equipment are recommended for the preparation of asparaginase for administration. Inhalation of dust or vapors and contact with skin or mucous membranes, especially those of the eyes, must be avoided. The National Institutes of Health presently recommends that the preparation of injectable antineoplastic drugs should be performed in a class II laminar flow biologic safety cabinet. Personnel preparing drugs of this class should wear chemical-resistant, impervious gloves, safety goggles, outer garments, and shoe covers. Additional body garments should be used on the basis of the task being performed (e.g., sleevelets, apron, gauntlets, or disposable suits) to avoid exposed skin surfaces and inhalation of vapor and dust. Appropriate techniques should be used to remove potentially contaminated clothing.

STORAGE AND STABILITY
- Intact vials of powder should be refrigerated (less than 8° C, 46° F).
- Vials are allowed to be at room temperature for up to 48 hrs with retained stability if returned to refrigeration.
- Shake well but not too vigorously; use of a 5-micron in-line filter is recommended to remove fiber-like particles in the solution (not a 0.2-micron filter, which has been associated with some loss of potency).
- Solutions for IV infusion are stable for 8 hrs at room temperature or under refrigeration.

INTERACTIONS
Drug
Live-virus vaccines: May potentiate viral replication, increase vaccine side effects, and decrease the patient's antibody response to the vaccine.
Methotrexate: May decrease the effects of methotrexate.
Steroids, vincristine: May increase the risk of neuropathy and disturbances of erythropoiesis; may enhance the hyperglycemic effect of asparaginase.
Cyclophosphamide: May decrease metabolism of cyclophosphamide.
Mercaptopurine: May increase hepatotoxicity of mercaptopurine.
Herbal
No information available.

LAB EFFECTS/INTERFERENCE
May increase BUN, blood ammonia, and blood glucose levels; serum alkaline phosphatase, bilirubin, uric acid, AST (SGOT), and ALT (SGPT) levels; prothrombin time; aPTT; thrombin time. May decrease blood-clotting factors (including antithrombin, plasma fibrinogen, and plasminogen) as well as serum albumin, calcium, and cholesterol levels. May interfere with the interpretation of thyroid function tests by reducing concentrations of thyroxine-binding globulin.

Y-SITE COMPATIBLES
Methotrexate, Na bicarbonate

INCOMPATIBLES
None known. Consult pharmacy.

SIDE EFFECTS
Serious Reactions
- Hepatotoxicity usually occurs within 2 wks of initial treatment.
- The risk of an allergic reaction, including anaphylaxis, increases after repeated therapy.
- Myelosuppression may be severe.

Other Side Effects
Frequent (10%-50%):
Allergic reaction (rash, urticaria, arthralgia, facial edema, hypotension, and respiratory distress), pancreatitis (severe abdominal pain, nausea, and vomiting), fevers, chills, hematologic toxicity (hypofibrinogenemia and depression of clotting factors V and VIII, variable decreased in factors VII and IX, severe protein C deficiency, and decrease in antithrombin III may be dose-limiting or fatal), prenatal azotemia.

Occasional (1%-10%):
CNS effects (confusion, drowsiness, depression, anxiety, and fatigue), stomatitis, hypoalbuminemia or uric acid nephropathy (manifested as pedal or lower extremity edema), hyperglycemia

Rare (Less Than 1%):
Hyperthermia (including fever or chills), thrombosis, seizures, myelosuppression, renal failure, leukopenia, anemia, thrombocytopenia

SPECIAL CONSIDERATIONS
Baseline Assessment
- Assess patients for CBC with differential, electrolyte, BUN, serum creatinine, lipase, amylase, and albumin levels, liver function tests, and coagulation tests including prothrombin time, PTT, and fibrinogen.
- Evaluate patient for multiple allergies.

Intervention and Evaluation
- Administer premedication as ordered per protocol.
- Assess patient's CBC with differential, platelet count, electrolyte, BUN, creatinine, lipase, and amylase levels, and liver function tests before dosing.
- Monitor vital signs before and during IV dosing to evaluate for hypotension.
- Have an anaphylaxis kit at bedside before dosing as patients have an increased risk of anaphylaxis. The anaphylaxis kit should contain the following:
    Hydrocortisone 50 mg
    Diphenhydramine 50 mg
    Epinephrine 1:1000 1 mL; use 0.3 mL for each dose IV, which may be repeated as necessary
    Syringes and needles
    Alcohol wipes
    2-by-2 gauze pads to break ampule.
- Set up oxygen and make sure an Ambu bag is available in the room.
- Evaluate for any skin reaction before dosing.
- Assess for any signs and symptoms of pancreatitis, nausea, abdominal pain, or cramping.
- Monitor patient for signs and symptoms of somnolence syndrome, confusion, depression, drowsiness, and profound fatigue.
- Provide emotional support to patient and family.

Education
- Instruct patient to report any signs or symptoms of a hypersensitivity reaction, shortness of breath, difficulty breathing, rash or pruritus.
- Instruct patient to contact his or her health care provider with any signs or symptoms of pancreatitis, nausea, or vomiting lasting greater than 24 hours, abdominal pain, nausea, or pain after eating, or any evidence of the somnolence syndrome.
- Educate patient and caregiver on signs and symptoms of the somnolence syndrome, confusion, drowsiness, depression, and profound fatigue with patient sleeping all the time and never feeling rested or able to stay awake.
- Provide patient with information on local resources nd support groups available for his or her specific diagnosis.

AZACITIDINE
BRAND NAMES
Vidaza

CLASS OF AGENT
Antineoplastic agent; pyrimidine nucleoside analog of cytidine

CLINICAL PHARMACOLOGY
Mechanism of Action
An antineoplastic agent that exerts a cytotoxic effect on rapidly dividing cells by causing demethylation or hypomethylation of DNA in abnormal hematopoietic cells in the bone marrow. **Therapeutic Effect:** Restores normal function to tumor-suppressor

genes regulating cellular differentiation and proliferation.

Absorption and Distribution

Azacitidine is rapidly absorbed after subcutaneous administration. Subcutaneous injection bioavailability is 89% relative to IV administration. Volume of distribution: 76 ± 26 L. *Half-life:* 4 hrs. **Peak:** 30 mins.

Metabolism and Excretion

Metabolized by the liver. Azacitidine and its metabolites are eliminated mostly in urine.

HOW SUPPLIED/AVAILABLE FORMS

Powder for Injection: 100-mg vial.

INDICATIONS AND DOSAGES

Myelodysplastic Syndromes with Subtypes Including Refractory Anemia and Chronic Myelomonocytic Leukemia

Adults: 75 mg/m^2/day subcutaneously for 7 days every 4 wks. Dosage may be increased to 100 mg/m^2 if the initial dose is insufficient and toxicity is manageable. Each cycle should be repeated every 4 wks for a minimum of 4 cycles.

Alternate regimens: 105 mg/m^2/day subcutaneously for 5 consecutive days or 75 mg/m^2/day subcutaneously on days 1 through 5, off on days 6 and 7, and resume on days 8 and 9. These regimens are used for outpatient clinics that are not open 7 days per wk.

Dosage Adjustment in Hepatic Dysfunction

Not recommended for use in patients with metastatic hepatic disease or albumin less than 3 g/dL.

Dosage Adjustment in Renal Dysfunction*

The next cycle should be held for unexplained elevations in serum creatinine (SCr) or BUN. Once SCr or BUN returns to baseline, the next cycle should be resumed at 50% of normal dose. If serum bicarbonate less than 20 mEq/L, the dose should be reduced 50% with the next cycle. **Note: if your facility does not run serum bicarbonate, this value is equal to the total carbon dioxide level, i.e., 1 mmol/L of carbon dioxide = 1 mEq/L of serum bicarbonate.*

Dosage Adjustment Based on Hematology Laboratory Values

- For patients with baseline WBC greater than 3×10^9/L, ANC greater than 1.5×10/L, and platelet count greater than 75×10^9>/L, adjust the dose as follows, based on nadir counts for any given cycle:

NADIR COUNTS

ANC ($\times 10^9$/L)	Platelets ($\times 10^9$/L)	% Dose in the Next Course
<0.5	<25	50
0.5-1.5	25-50	67
>1.5	>50	100

- For patients whose baseline counts are WBC greater than 3×10^9/L, ANC less than 1.5×10^9/L, or platelet count less than 75×10^9/L, dose adjustments should be based on nadir counts and bone marrow biopsy cellularity at the time of the nadir as noted below, unless there is clear improvement in differentiation at the time of the next cycle, in which case the dose of the current treatment should be continued.

UNLABELED USES

Resistant acute myeloid leukemia, β-thalassemia, sickle cell disease, malignant mesothelioma

PRECAUTIONS

Use azacitidine cautiously in patients with hepatic or renal impairment, serum albumin less than 3 g/dL, serum bicarbonate less than 20 mEq/L, or elevations in BUN/SCr. Closely monitor patients with renal impairment and preexisting liver disease.

Pregnancy Risk Category: D

Azacitidine may be embryotoxic, causing developmental abnormalities in the fetus. Women of childbearing age should avoid becoming pregnant while taking azacitidine. Patients should avoid breast-feeding while taking azacitidine.

CONTRAINDICATIONS

Advanced malignant hepatic tumors, hypersensitivity to mannitol or azacitidine

DRUG PREPARATION/ADMINISTRATION/ SAFE HANDLING ISSUES

- Use aseptic technique and chemotherapy precautions when preparing the drug.
- Reconstitute azacitidine with 4 mL of sterile water for injection. The reconstituted suspension will appear cloudy. Final concentration is 25 mg/mL.
- Use the suspension within 1 hr after reconstitution.
- Divide doses greater than 4 mL equally into two syringes.

- Resuspend the contents by inverting the syringe 2 or 3 times and rolling it between the palms for 30 secs immediately before administration.
- Do not draw up azacitidine and give the injection with the same needle. Replace the used needle with a new needle. This is to prevent clogging.
- Rotate injection sites among the abdomen, upper arms, and thighs for each injection.
- Administer each new injection at least 1 inch from a previous injection site.
- Do not apply heat or ice packs to the injection sites for 1 hr before and 1 hr after injection due to possible altered drug absorption.

STORAGE AND STABILITY
- Store vials at room temperature.
- The reconstituted suspension may be stored for up to 1 hr at room temperature or up to 8 hrs if refrigerated.
- Allow the drug suspension to return to room temperature and use it within 30 mins after removal from refrigeration.

INTERACTIONS
Drug
Bone marrow suppressants: May increase myelosuppression.
Live-virus vaccines: May result in an increased risk of infection by the live vaccine.
Herbal
None known.

LAB EFFECTS/INTERFERENCE
May decrease Hgb level, Hct, WBC, RBC, platelet counts. May increase serum creatinine.

SIDE EFFECTS
Serious Reactions
Hematologic toxicity, manifested most commonly as anemia, leukopenia, neutropenia, and thrombocytopenia, is a common adverse effect.
Other Side Effects
Frequent (10%-50%):
Nausea, anemia, thrombocytopenia, vomiting, pyrexia, leukopenia, diarrhea, fatigue, injection site pain/reactions/erythema, constipation, neutropenia, ecchymosis, cough, dyspnea, weakness, rigors, arthralgia, headache, anorexia, back pain, confusion, dizziness,

peripheral edema, febrile neutropenia, myalgia, abdominal pain, nasopharyngitis, skin lesion, rash, anxiety, hypokalemia, upper respiratory tract infection, pruritus, depression, insomnia, malaise, pneumonia, and increased sweating
Occasional (1%-10%):
Gingival bleeding, lymphadenopathy, herpes simplex, hematoma, night sweats, tachycardia, cellulites, dysuria, lethargy, dyspepsia, hemorrhoids, hypotension, abdominal distension, muscle cramps, postnasal drip, syncope, nasal congestion, dry skin, dysphagia, injection site pigmentation changes, mouth hemorrhage, and tongue ulceration
Rare (Less Than 1%):
Bone marrow suppression, atrial fibrillation, cardiac failure, diverticulitis, cholecystitis, hypersensitivity, bacterial infections, dehydration, muscle weakness, seizures, confusion, renal failure, orthostatic hypotension

SPECIAL CONSIDERATIONS
Baseline Assessment
- Obtain CBC with differential, platelet count, electrolytes including serum bicarbonate (or CO_2), BUN, and creatinine levels, and liver function tests.
- Assess for any prior emetic episodes from other chemotherapy received.
- Age-related renal impairment may increase the risk of renal toxicity in elderly patients.
- Be aware that the safety and efficacy of azacitidine have not been established in children.
Intervention and Evaluation
- Premedicate for nausea and vomiting.
- Monitor complete blood count with differential and platelet count before each dose.
- Assess patient for signs and symptoms of fever greater than 38° C (greater than 101° F) weight loss, fatigue, arthralgias, myalgias, and any evidence of thrombocytopenia—epistaxis, petechiae, easy bruising, or bleeding.
- Initiate neutropenic precautions per institutional protocol as necessary.
- Observe patient's response to the treatment. Notify the health care provider if the patient develops significant diarrhea, nausea, or vomiting.
- Avoid measures that may induce bleeding, such as taking a rectal temperature or using rectal probes, enemas, or suppositories and any IM injections.

- Provide patient and family with education and emotional support.

Education

- Educate patient regarding the possibility of neutropenia and interventions to follow: strict handwashing, avoiding crowds, and monitoring all visitors for signs and symptoms of infection.
- Avoid all IM injections, suppositories, enemas, and rectal temperatures, and to stop flossing teeth when platelets drop below 50,000.
- Instruct patient when to contact his or her health care provider: fever greater than 38° C (greater than 101° F), nausea or diarrhea unrelieved in 24 hours, or inability to take in at least 1500 mL of fluid per day.
- Instruct patient in signs and symptoms of dehydration: feeling dizzy or lightheaded especially when changing positions, increased nausea when changing positions, feeling faint, skin cool, and clammy feeling.
- Advise patient not to receive immunizations without the physician's approval because azacitidine lowers the body's resistance to infection.
- Advise patient to avoid pregnancy and use barrier contraception while receiving azacitidine.
- Instruct patient on community resources and support groups available.

BEVACIZUMAB

BRAND NAMES
Avastin

CLASS OF AGENT
Monoclonal antibody (recombinant, human/murine), vascular endothelial growth factor (VEGF) inhibitor

CLINICAL PHARMACOLOGY
Mechanism of Action
An antineoplastic agent that binds to and inhibits VEGF, a protein that plays a major role in the formation of new blood vessels associated with tumor growth and metastases. Bevacizumab binds and neutralizes all human VEGF forms via recognition of binding sites for the two human VEGF receptor types (flt-1 and flk-1). In animal models, the antibody has been shown to stabilize established tumors or suppress tumor growth by inhibiting angiogenesis induced by VEGF.

Therapeutic Effect: Inhibits metastatic disease progression.

Absorption and Distribution
This drug should only be given via IV. Clearance varies by body weight, gender, and tumor burden and ranges. Volume of distribution is similar to plasma volume and averaged 2.66 and 3.25 L in females and males, respectively. It is unknown whether bevacizumab is excreted into breast milk, but the manufacturer recommends that breast-feeding be ceased during therapy.
Half-life: After usual dose of bevacizumab, the elimination half-life is about 20 days (range, 11-50 days).

Metabolism and Excretion
The clearance of bevacizumab appears to be higher in men than women (0.262 L/day vs. 0.207 L/day). Also, patients with a higher tumor burden had a higher clearance than those with less disease (0.249 L/day vs. 0.199 L/day). Metabolism is unknown but presumably involves binding of the drug to VEGF receptors.

HOW SUPPLIED/AVAILABLE FORMS
Injection: 100- and 400-mg preservative-free, single-use vials.

INDICATIONS AND DOSAGES
First- or Second-Line Treatment of Metastatic Carcinoma of the Colon or Rectum in Combination with 5-Fluorouracil
5 mg/kg IV once every 14 days.
Dosage Adjustment in Hepatic Dysfunction
No studies have been performed to determine whether doses need to be adjusted in patients with hepatic dysfunction.
Dosage Adjustment in Renal Dysfunction
No studies have been performed to determine whether doses need to be adjusted in patients with renal dysfunction.

UNLABELED USES
Adjunctive therapy in breast cancer, renal cell carcinoma, non-small cell lung cancer, and prostate cancer at doses ranging from 3 to 15 mg/kg once every 14-21 days. Intravitreal injections for age-related macular degeneration

PRECAUTIONS
Bevacizumab should be discontinued in the event of GI perforation, wound dehiscence requiring medical intervention, severe bleeding, nephrotic syndrome, hypertensive crisis, or severe arterial thromboembolism

Bevacizumab should be used cautiously in patients with CHF, epistaxis, hypertension, proteinuria, and renal insufficiency and those with squamous cell carcinoma of the bronchus.

Pregnancy Risk Category: C
Bevacizumab is teratogenic and has the potential to impair fertility. Its use by pregnant women may decrease maternal and fetal body weight and increase the risk of fetal skeletal abnormalities. Breast-feeding women should not take bevacizumab.

CONTRAINDICATIONS
No specific contraindications have been provided by the manufacturer of Avastin.

DRUG PREPARATION/ADMINISTRATION/ SAFE HANDLING ISSUES
◄ ALERT ►
* Do not give by IV push or IV bolus.
* Refrigerate vials.
* Withdraw the amount needed for a dose of 5 mg/kg, and dilute it in 100 mL of 0.9% NaCl. Discard any unused portion.
* Diluted solution may be refrigerated for up to 8 hrs.
* Infuse the initial dose over 90 mins after chemotherapy.
* If patient tolerates the first infusion well, the second infusion may be administered over 60 mins.
* If patient tolerates the 60-min infusion well, all subsequent infusions may be administered over 30 mins.

STORAGE AND STABILITY
* Store vials protected from light, under refrigeration at 2-8° C (36-46° F). Do not freeze or shake. This product contains no preservative.
* Diluted solutions in 100 mL of 0.9% NaCl injection may be stored for up to 8 hrs under refrigeration (2-8° C [36-46° F]). Dextrose inactivates bevacizumab.

INTERACTIONS
Drug
None known.
Herbal
None known.

LAB EFFECTS/INTERFERENCE
May decrease serum K, Na, Hgb levels; Hct; WBC and platelet counts.

Y-SITE COMPATIBLES
No information available

INCOMPATIBLES
Do not mix bevacizumab with dextrose solutions.

SIDE EFFECTS
Serious Reactions
* *Cardiac:* Congestive heart failure and arterial thromboembolic events such as myocardial and stroke may occur.
* *Pulmonary:* Life-threatening or fatal pulmonary hemorrhage occurred in 31% of patients with non–small cell lung cancer (4% nonsquamous cell histology) receiving bevacizumab in combination with chemotherapy compared with 0% in the chemotherapy-alone group.
* *GI perforations/wound-healing complications:* GI perforation and wound dehiscence in some instances have been fatal. GI perforation may be associated with intra-abdominal abscess. In patients receiving bolus irinotecan/5-fluorouracil/ leucovorin (IFL) with bevacizumab, the incidence was 2%. The typical presentation includes symptoms of constipation and vomiting. Bevacizumab therapy should be discontinued permanently in patients with GI perforation or wound dehiscence requiring medical intervention.
* *Hemorrhage:* Serious, and in some cases fatal, hemoptysis has been reported in patients with non-small cell lung cancer. The incidence of serious or fatal hemoptysis was 31% in patients with squamous histology and 4% in patients with adeno-carcinoma receiving bevacizumab compared with no cases in patients treated with chemotherapy alone. Patients with recent hemoptysis should not receive bevacizumab. Use caution in patients with CNS metastases. Serious but uncommon CNS events include subarachnoid hemorrhage and hemorrhagic stroke.
* *Urologic or renal:* Urinary tract infections, manifested as urinary frequency or urgency and proteinuria, occur frequently. Nephrotic syndrome with varying degrees of proteinuria has been reported on rare occasions
* Hypersensitivity during infusion including anaphylactoid-like reactions can occur.
* *Reversible Posterior Leukoencephalopathy Syndrome (RPLS):* RPLS is a neurological disorder that manifests as

headache, seizure, lethargy, confusion, blindness, and other visual and neurological symptoms. It has been reported in less than 0.1% and must be diagnosed with MRI. Discontinue bevacizumab and treat hypertension if present. Symptoms usually resolve or improve within days. Safety of bevacizumab rechallenge in patients with previous incidence of RPLS is unknown.

Other Side Effects
Frequent (10%-50%):
Asthenia, vomiting, anorexia, hypertension, epistaxis, stomatitis, constipation, headache, dyspnea, altered taste, dry skin, exfoliative dermatitis, dizziness, flatulence, excessive lacrimation, skin discoloration, weight loss, myalgia, proteinuria
Occasional (1%-10%):
Nail disorder, skin ulcer, alopecia, confusion, abnormal gait, dry mouth, venous thrombosis
Rare (Less Than 1%):
Hypersensitivity reactions, e.g. nasal septum perforation

SPECIAL CONSIDERATIONS
Baseline Assessment
- Evaluate patient's current medications, assessing for antihypertensive medications.
- Evaluate patient's baseline vital signs; CBC with differential, electrolyte, BUN, and creatinine levels before and regularly during bevacizumab treatment. Monitor closely for any sign or symptoms of hyponatremia.
- Assess patient for any prior history of renal alterations, and monitor the patient's urine for proteinuria. Patients with a urine dipstick reading of 2+ or more should have a 24-hour urine collection for protein levels.
- Evaluate date of patient's last major surgical procedure, and assess the incision line for wound healing. Do not administer this agent if the major surgery has been within 28 days.
- Assess patient for any history of deep vein thrombosis (DVT) or other thromboembolic complications.

Intervention and Evaluation
- Assess patient's vital signs before each dose, obtain a dipstick reading of patient's urine for protein, and evaluate B/P for any signs of hypertension.
- Evaluate any incision lines from prior major surgery sites for changes, erythema, drainage, or evidence of dehiscence.
- Premedicate patient if ordered.
- Assess patient for any new symptoms of cardiac changes such as rapid heart rate or rhythm, evidence of DVT such as swelling of legs, erythema, or calf pain.
- Monitor patient's nutritional status; obtain a nutrition consultation as necessary.
- Monitor for any signs of epistaxis, hemolysis, or bleeding episodes.
- Evaluate patient for presence of nausea, diarrhea, constipation, or pain.
- Assess patient for any evidence of rashes.
- Monitor patient for signs and symptoms of fever, fatigue, asthenia, weakness, or any other constitutional symptoms.

Education
- Educate patient on usual side effects of this drug.
- Instruct patient when to contact his or her health care provider: fever greater than 38° C (greater than 101° F), chills, changes in incision area, diarrhea lasting greater than 24 hours, nausea lasting greater than 24 hours, epistaxis lasting greater than 10 minutes or any evidence of bleeding from other sites, headache, urinary difficulty, evidence of weakness, chest pain or shortness of breath, or lower extremity edema, erythema, or pain.
- Encourage patient to use appropriate contraception as this agent poses a risk to fetal development.
- Provide patient with information on local resources and support groups available for his or her specific diagnosis.
- Be aware that the safety and efficacy of bevacizumab have not been established in children.
- Be aware that patients older than 65 years have a higher incidence of serious adverse reactions.

BEXAROTENE
BRAND NAMES
Targretin

CLASS OF AGENT
Antineoplastic retinoid

CLINICAL PHARMACOLOGY
Mechanism of Action
This retinoid antineoplastic agent binds to and activates retinoid X receptor subtypes, which regulate the genes that control cellular differentiation and proliferation. It binds minimally to retinoic acid receptors

(RAR). Activation of the RXR pathway leads to the induction of programmed cell death (apoptosis) and other cellular activities (e.g., enhanced insulin effects). Its exact mechanism of action in cutaneous T-cell lymphoma is unknown. **Therapeutic Effect:** Inhibits growth of tumor cell lines of hematopoietic and squamous cell origin and induces tumor regression.

Absorption and Distribution

Bexarotene is moderately absorbed from the GI tract. Food significantly enhances the absorption of bexarotene, especially fat. Administration of bexarotene 300 mg/m^2 after a fat-containing meal resulted in a 35% increase in the area under the curve and a 48% increase in peak plasma concentrations, compared with these values after administration of bexarotene with a glucose solution. The manufacturer recommends administration of bexarotene with a meal.

Gel applied topically is sporadically absorbed systemically, and low to moderate doses have low potential for significant plasma concentrations of bexarotene. Protein binding: greater than 99% in patients with normal renal function. Protein is significantly altered in patients with renal failure. Bexarotene is metabolized in the liver.

Half-life: 7 hrs.

Metabolism and Excretion

Metabolized primarily by hepatic cytochrome P450 (CYP) 3A4 enzymes, which produce oxidative metabolites (6- and 7-hydroxybexarotene and 6- and 7-oxobexarotene) that are eventually glucuronidated and eliminated through the hepatobiliary system. Hepatic dysfunction may lead to accumulation of the drug. Renal excretion is less than 1%.

HOW SUPPLIED/AVAILABLE FORMS

Capsules (Soft Gelatin): 75 mg.
Gel: 1% 60-g tubes.

INDICATIONS AND DOSAGES

Cutaneous T-Cell Lymphoma Refractory to at Least One Prior Systemic Therapy

Oral: 300 mg/m^2/day orally as a single dose with a meal. If no response after 8 wks and initial dose is well tolerated, may be increased to 400 mg/m^2/day. If not tolerated, may decrease to 200 mg/m^2/day, then to 100 mg/m^2/day or temporarily held.
Topical: Initially, apply topically once every other day. May increase at weekly intervals up to qid.

Dosage Adjustment in Hepatic Dysfunction

The dose of bexarotene may require adjustment in patients with hepatic dysfunction.

Dosage Adjustment in Renal Dysfunction

Although protein binding is altered in severe renal dysfunction; no dose adjustment is recommended by the manufacturer.

UNLABELED USES

Head, neck, lung, and renal cell carcinomas, Kaposi's sarcoma

PRECAUTIONS

- Concurrent intake of vitamin A (greater than 15,000 International Units/day)
- Concurrent use of gel with products containing DEET (*N,N*-diethyl-*m*-toluamide), a common ingredient of insect repellents
- Concurrent use of insulin or insulin potentiators
- Hepatic dysfunction
- Photosensitivity to retinoids
- Lipid abnormalities
- Pancreatitis
- Women of childbearing age: a hormonal contraceptive with an additional barrier method of birth control or two forms of birth control (1 nonhormonal) should be used for 1 mo before treatment, during treatment, and for 1 mo after discontinuation of therapy.

CONTRAINDICATIONS

Hypersensitivity to retinoids or any components of the bexarotene formulation
Pregnancy Risk Category: X

DRUG PREPARATION/ADMINISTRATION/ SAFE HANDLING ISSUES

- Take oral capsule with a meal around the same time each day.
- Gel: Be careful to not apply to normal skin areas. Allow gel to dry before covering with clothes. Occlusive dressings are not required. Wash hands after topical applications.

STORAGE AND STABILITY

Oral Capsules

- Store capsules between 2 and 25° C (36 and 77° F). Exposure to humidity should be avoided after the bottle has been opened. Protect from light.

Topical Gel

- Store gel at 25° C (77° F). Temperature excursions are permitted to 15-30° C (59-86° F). Avoid exposure to humidity after the tube has been opened. Protect from light.

INTERACTIONS
It is unknown whether the interactions below are of clinical significance when the gel preparation is used.
Drug
Antidiabetics: May enhance the effects of these drugs.
Erythromycin, gemfibrozil, itraconazole, ketoconazole: May increase bexarotene blood concentrations by inhibiting its hepatic metabolism.
Phenytoin, fosphenytoin, phenobarbital, Rifampin: May decrease bexarotene blood concentrations.
Methotrexate: May increase the risk of hepatic toxicity from bexarotene.
Tamoxifen: May decrease the effect of tamoxifen.
Vitamin A: Because of similar characteristics, high doses of vitamin A should be avoided to minimize the risk of retinoid toxicity.
Herbal
St John's Wort: Induces CYP 3A4 enzymes and can potentially inhibit bexarotene effects.
Food
Grapefruit inhibits CYP 3A4 enzymes and can potentially enhance the effects of bexarotene.

LAB EFFECTS/INTERFERENCE
• May increase serum cholesterol, triglyceride, total and LDL cholesterol levels. May decrease serum HDL cholesterol levels.
• May increase CA-125 assay value in patients with ovarian cancer.
• May produce abnormal liver function test results.

SIDE EFFECTS
Serious Reactions
• May cause hyperlipidemia in approximately 80% of patients. Pancreatitis due to hypertriglyceridemia has been reported. Monitor triglyceride, total cholesterol, HDL levels.
• Hypothyroidism occurs in about one third of patients.
Other Side Effects
Frequent (10%-50%):
Headache, hyperlipidemia, hypothyroidism, asthenia, rash, nausea, peripheral edema, dry skin, abdominal pain
Occasional (1%-10%):
Chills, exfoliative dermatitis, diarrhea

Rare (Less Than 1%):
No information

SPECIAL CONSIDERATIONS
Baseline Assessment
• Obtain baseline CBC with differential, platelet count, electrolyte, BUN, and creatinine levels, liver function tests, and serum cholesterol and triglyceride levels.
• Evaluate for any evidence of hypothyroidism before initiating therapy with this agent.
• Assess for any history of skin rashes from any other agents received.
• Be aware that bexarotene is a form of retinoid and may cause fetal harm. Perform pregnancy test before initiating therapy.
Intervention and Evaluation
• Monitor lipid levels on a quarterly basis to assess need for therapeutic intervention with medications, diet or exercise, and other lifestyle changes.
• Assess for any evidence of headaches, weakness, weight gain, or peripheral edema.
• Evaluate patient for any evidence of skin changes, significant abdominal pain, or increased nausea with this agent as pancreatitis can be a rare but serious side effect.
• Perform a pulmonary assessment to evaluate for any signs or symptoms of pneumonia.
• Monitor for pregnancy.
Education
• Instruct patient to monitor for any signs or symptoms of significant abdominal pain or nausea after eating and to report to his or her health care provider if these do not resolve in a few hours as they may be evidence of pancreatitis, a rare but serious side effect of this agent.
• Educate patient on the need for laboratory follow-up of liver function tests and cholesterol and triglyceride levels.
• Advise patient to report any signs or symptoms of significant weight gain, fatigue, or weakness as these can be an indication of hypothyroidism.
• Educate patient to monitor for any skin changes or new rashes with this agent and edema.
• Instruct patient to avoid pregnancy and to use appropriate contraception during receipt of this agent. The manufacturer recommends two forms of contraception. Educate males who have partners of childbearing age to use contraception also.

- Instruct patient to avoid receipt of live-virus vaccinations while receiving this chemotherapy.
- Provide patient with information on local resources and support groups available for his or her specific diagnosis.

BICALUTAMIDE
BRAND NAMES
Casodex

CLASS OF AGENT
Antineoplastic agent, antiandrogen

CLINICAL PHARMACOLOGY
Mechanism of Action
A nonsteroidal antiandrogen that competitively inhibits androgen action by binding to androgen receptors in target tissue. **Therapeutic Effect:** Decreases growth of androgen-sensitive prostate carcinoma.
Absorption and distribution
Well absorbed from the GI tract. Bioavailability is unknown. Protein binding: 96%. *Half-life:* 5.9 days, 10.4 days (severe liver dysfunction)
Metabolism and Excretion
Metabolized extensively in the liver to an inactive metabolite. Excreted in urine and feces. Not removed by hemodialysis.

HOW SUPPLIED/AVAILABLE FORMS
Tablets: 50 mg.

INDICATIONS AND DOSAGES
Metastatic Prostate Carcinoma
50 mg PO daily, given concurrently with a luteinizing hormone-releasing hormone (LHRH) analog or after surgical castration.
Dosage Adjustment in Hepatic Dysfunction
Use with caution in patients with moderate to severe hepatic dysfunction. Discontinue drug if jaundice or (ALT) SGPT 2 times the UNL occurs.
Dosage Adjustment in Renal Dysfunction
No adjustments necessary.

UNLABELED USES
150 mg PO daily as monotherapy

CONTRAINDICATIONS
Hypersensitivity to bicalutamide or any of its excipients
Pregnancy Risk Category: X
Bicalutamide is not indicated for females. Drug excretion in breast milk is unknown. Thus, breast feed should not be performed during treatment.

DRUG PREPARATION/ADMINISTRATION/SAFE HANDLING ISSUES
- Take without regard to food and at same time daily.
- Use in combination with an LHRH/gonadotropin-releasing hormone analog agonist.

STORAGE AND STABILITY
Store in room temperature.

INTERACTIONS
Drug
Warfarin: May increase effects of warfarin. Monitor prothrombin time or international normalized ratio.
Herbal
None known.

LAB EFFECTS/INTERFERENCE
May increase BUN level and serum alkaline phosphatase, bilirubin, AST (SGOT), ALT (SGPT) levels. May decrease Hgb level and WBC count.

SIDE EFFECTS
Serious Reactions
- Hepatitis or marked increases of liver enzymes caused 1% of patients to discontinue the drug in clinical trials. Use with caution in patients with moderate to severe hepatic dysfunction. Hepatotoxicity generally occurs in the first 3-4 mos of treatment. Immediately discontinue the drug with follow-up on liver function if the ALT (SGPT) is 2 times the UNL and signs or symptoms of liver dysfunction occur.
- Rare cases of interstitial pneumonitis and pulmonary fibrosis have been reported.
Other Side Effects
Frequent (10%-50%):
Asthenia, constipation, diarrhea, hot flashes, nausea, gynecomastia, pain (back, breast, muscle, pelvic)
Occasional (1%-10%):
Abdominal pain, dizziness, dyspnea, elevated liver enzymes, impotence, insomnia, libido decrease, nocturia, peripheral edema, rash, sweating, vomiting, weight loss/gain
Rare (Less Than 1%):
Alopecia, asthma, dry skin, interstitial pneumonitis, leg cramps, neuropathy, pruritus, pulmonary fibrosis, somnolence

CANCER DRUGS

SPECIAL CONSIDERATIONS
Baseline Assessment
- Obtain CBC with differential, platelet count, electrolyte, BUN, creatinine, and alkaline phosphatase levels, and liver function tests.
- Assess patient for any prior history of liver disease.
- Evaluate patient for any history of pulmonary disease.
- Assess patient's pain score at the initial visit.
- Evaluate patient's baseline weight.
- Assess patient for any history of deep vein thrombosis or warfarin use.

Intervention and Evaluation
- Monitor patient's laboratory data at each visit; assess for anemia, hepatic dysfunction, or evidence of neutropenia.
- Assess patient's pulmonary status and pain score at each visit.
- Monitor for evidence of increasing fatigue, nausea, constipation, or diarrhea at each visit.
- Evaluate patient for symptoms of hot flashes, night sweats, irritability, or insomnia.
- Monitor for evidence of changes in sexual function, gynecomastia, decreased libido, or impotence.
- Weigh patient at each visit and assess for evidence of peripheral edema.

Education
- Instruct patient on when to contact health care provider: fever greater than 38° C (greater than 101° F), chills, shortness of breath, dyspnea upon exertion, significant weight gain, peripheral edema, nausea, vomiting, or diarrhea lasting greater than 24 hrs.
- Instruct patient on signs and symptoms of anemia and neutropenia, increased fatigue, and shortness of breath.
- Advise patient to use good handwashing techniques and to avoid individuals with cold or flu.
- Educate patient on sexual changes that may occur: gynecomastia, decreased libido, and impotence.
- Instruct patient on usual side effects of hot flashes, night sweats, irritability, and insomnia that may occur with this agent.
- Educate patient to not take any over-the-counter medications or herbal or vitamin supplements without first checking with his or her health care provider.
- Provide patient with information on local resources and support groups available for his or her specific diagnosis.

BLEOMYCIN SULFATE

BRAND NAMES
Blenoxane

CLASS OF AGENT
Antineoplastic agent, antibiotic

CLINICAL PHARMACOLOGY
Mechanism of Action
A glycopeptide antibiotic whose mechanism of action is unknown. The drug is most effective in the G_2 phase of cell division. **Therapeutic Effect:** Appears to inhibit DNA synthesis and, to a lesser extent, RNA and protein synthesis.

Absorption and Distribution
IM and intrapleural administration is 30-50% of IV administration. Volume of distribution: 22 L/m²; high concentration in skin, kidney, lung, heart tissues; lowest in testes and GI tract.
Half-life: Biphasic. Normal renal function: initial 1.3 hrs, terminal 9 hrs. End-stage renal disease: initial 2 hrs, terminal 30 hrs.

Metabolism and Excretion
Drug is metabolized in the blood, intestine, kidney, liver, and lung. Renal excretion: 50%. Not removed by hemodialysis.

HOW SUPPLIED/AVAILABLE FORMS
Powder for Injection: 15 units, 30 units.

INDICATIONS AND DOSAGES
Cervical Cancer, Choriocarcinoma, Embryonal Cell Carcinoma, Head and Neck Cancer, Hodgkin's Lymphoma, Lymphoma, Malignant Pleural Effusion, Nasopharyngeal Carcinoma, Squamous Cell Carcinoma, Teratocarcinoma, Testicular Cancer
Maximum lifetime dose: 400 units (or 400 mg) due to risk of pulmonary toxicity. Patients with renal or pulmonary dysfunction should be given less and with caution. Consider intraperitoneal and intrapleural dose as half. Refer to disease individual protocols.
IM, IV, Subcutaneous: 10-20 units/m² 1-2 times/wk
Continuous IV: 15 units/m² over 24 hrs daily for 4 days
Pleural effusion: 50-60 units mixed in 50-100 mL of D5W, 0.9% NaCl, or sterile water for injection given as a single infusion. Periodically reposition the patient before removal. Usual position changes are done every 15 mins. Positions include right side, left side supine, prone, and modified Trendelenburg if patient is able to tolerate it to allow for distribution in the apical

areas. Try to keep the patient in the same position for 15 mins if possible. May repeat in intervals of several days if fluid continues to accumulate. May add lidocaine 100-200 mg to reduce discomfort.
Lymphoma patient test dose: Administer before the first two doses of bleomycin to reduce risk or quickly detect anaphylactoid reaction. Bleomycin less than 2 units IM, IV, or subcutaneous. Monitor vital signs every 15 mins. If no reaction occurs in 1 hr, then the regular dosing schedule may be followed.

Dosage Adjustment in Renal Dysfunction
Ccr 10-50 mL/min: give 75% of normal dose.
Ccr less than 10 mL/min: give 50% of normal dose.

UNLABELED USES
Treatment of mycosis fungoides, osteosarcoma, ovarian tumors, renal carcinoma, soft tissue sarcoma

PRECAUTIONS
Patients at high risk for pulmonary fibrosis include those with decreased pulmonary function, elderly patients, patients receiving greater than 400 units total lifetime dose of bleomycin or single doses greater than 30 units, smokers, and patients with prior radiation therapy or receiving concurrent oxygen (refer to manufacturer package insert for oxygen administration recommendations). Anaphylactoid reactions occur in 1% of patients with lymphoma; administer a test dose for the first and second doses. Nursing staff should be at the patient's bedside for at least 30 mins after the test dose administered. Recommendations for test doses are not universally accepted.

CONTRAINDICATIONS
Hypersensitivity to bleomycin or any component of the formulation; severe pulmonary disease; pregnancy.

Pregnancy Risk Category: X
Drug excretion of bleomycin in breast milk is unknown. Thus, breast feeding should not be performed during treatment.

DRUG PREPARATION/ADMINISTRATION/ SAFE HANDLING ISSUES
◀ ALERT ▶ Because bleomycin may be carcinogenic, mutagenic, or teratogenic, wear nitrile or latex, but not vinyl, gloves when handling the drug. If the drug comes in contact with skin, wash the skin thoroughly with regular soap and water, do not use waterless soap as alcohol can increase the skin reaction in the area. If the drug comes in contact with mucous membranes, flush the area with water. If any amount of the drug splashes in the eyes, wash with copious amounts of water or saline until no more irritation is felt.

• Bleomycin is not a vesicant or irritant.
• IM or subcutaneous injection: Reconstitute a 15-units vial with 1-5 mL of sterile water, 0.9% NaCl, bacteriostatic water for injection, or bacteriostatic 0.9% NaCl. A 30-unit vial should be reconstituted with 2-10 mL. The final concentration will be 3-15 units/mL. Do not use D5W.
• IV: Reconstitute 15- and 30-units vials, respectively, with 5 or 10 mL to make a final concentration of 3 units/mL. Dose has been diluted in 5-1000 mL of 0.9% NaCl or D5W. Administer over at least 10 mins.

STORAGE AND STABILITY
• Bleomycin powder stable at refrigeration (2-8° C, 36-46° F) for 24 mos and should not be used after expiration date.
• After reconstitution in sodium chloride 0.9%, bleomycin is stable for 24 hrs.
• Although reconstituted solution (sodium chloride, 5% dextrose) was stable for 2 wks at room temperature and at 4 weeks refrigerated, contamination is possible. Unused solution should be discarded after 24 hrs.

INTERACTIONS
Drug
Cisplatin: May decrease bleomycin clearance and increase the risk of bleomycin toxicity (from cisplatin-induced renal impairment).
Digoxin: May decrease serum digoxin levels; monitor cardiac parameters and increase dose as necessary.
Phenytoin: May decrease serum phenytoin levels; monitor phenytoin serum levels and adjust dose accordingly.
Live-virus vaccines: May potentiate viral replication, increase vaccine side effects, and decrease the patient's antibody response to the vaccine.
Oxygen: May increase risk of pulmonary toxicity.
Other antineoplastics: May increase the risk of bleomycin toxicity.
Herbal
None known.

LAB EFFECTS/INTERFERENCE
None known.

Y-SITE COMPATIBLES
Cisplatin (Platinol), cefepime (Maxipime), cyclophosphamide (Cytoxan), dacarbazine (DTIC), dexamethasone (Decadron), diphenhydramine (Benadryl), etoposide, fludarabine (Fludara), gemcitabine (Gemzar), ondansetron (Zofran), paclitaxel (Taxol), piperacillin and tazobactam (Zosyn), vinblastine (Velban), vinorelbine (Navelbine)

INCOMPATIBLES
Amphotericin liposomal (AmBisome), aminophylline, ascorbic acid injection, cefazolin, diazepam, hydrocortisone Na succinate, methotrexate, mitomycin, nafcillin, penicillin G Na, terbutaline

SIDE EFFECTS
Serious Reactions
- Pulmonary toxicities may occur in up to 10% of patients with approximately 2% of pneumonitis progressing to pulmonary fibrosis and death. This condition appears to be dose- or age-related, occurring more often in patients receiving a total dose greater than 400 units and those older than 70 years.
- Nephrotoxicity and hepatotoxicity occur infrequently.

Other Side Effects
Frequent (10%-50%):
Anorexia, weight loss, erythematous skin swelling, urticaria, rash, striae, vesiculation, hyperpigmentation (particularly at areas of pressure, skin folds, cuticles, IM injection sites, and scars), stomatitis (usually evident 1-3 wks after initial therapy), nausea, vomiting, alopecia, pain at injection site, and, with parenteral form, fever or chills (typically occurring a few hours after a large single dose and lasting 4-12 hr)
Occasional (1%-10%):
Anaphylactic reaction, onycholysis
Rare (Less Than 1%):
Coronary artery disease, MI, arterial thrombosis, cerebrovascular accidents, pulmonary fibrosis, Raynaud's phenomenon

SPECIAL CONSIDERATIONS
Baseline Assessment
- Obtain pulmonary function studies before initial dosing, paying particular attention to the diffusing capacity of carbon monoxide. Carbon monoxide diffusing capacity should be greater than 60%.
- Be aware that patients may have chest radiographs performed every 1-2 weeks during bleomycin therapy. Chest radiographs do not show the progression of

pulmonary fibrosis, so many institutions do not do them.
- Premedicate patient as ordered at least 30 minutes before administering drug.
- Set up an Ambu bag and anaphylaxis kit at bedside. The anaphylaxis kit should contain the following:
  - Diphenhydramine 50 mg
  - Epinephrine 1:1000
  - Hydrocortisone 50 mg
  - Syringes and alcohol swabs
  - Needles for epinephrine ampule
  - 2-by-2 gauze pads to break ampule
- Record all vital signs before dose administration: temperature, B/P, respirations, and oxygen saturation.
- Administer acetaminophen as ordered; many institutions use 650 mg every 4 hours for two doses, then every 4 hours as needed or 1000 mg every 6 hours. Acetaminophen is administered for the first 24 hours only.
- Inspect skin for any areas or erythema or rashes.
- Assess pulmonary status for any signs and symptoms of rales and rhonchi. Assess for any dyspnea; if any new pulmonary changes are noted, notify the physician or health care provider before administration of dose.

Intervention and Evaluation
- Monitor the patient's breath sounds for pulmonary toxicity as evidenced by dyspnea, fine crackles, and rhonchi.
- Observe the patient for any difficulty in breathing and dyspnea.
- Monitor the patient's CBC with differential, platelet count, and liver and renal function test results, including BUN, serum bilirubin, serum creatinine, AST (SGOT), and ALT (SGPT) levels.
- Assess the patient's skin daily for signs of cutaneous toxicity. More than 50% of patients will experience skin toxicity 2-4 weeks after the dose.
- Monitor the patient for signs and symptoms of anemia (excessive fatigue and weakness), hematologic toxicity (easy bruising, fever, signs of local infection, sore throat, and unusual bleeding), and stomatitis (burning or erythema of the oral mucosa of the lips, palate, and tongue).
- Instruct the patient on oral hygiene; initiate an oral care regimen to be completed three times per day.
- Make sure all staff know that patient has received bleomycin, and, if required, oxygen therapy should be at the lowest

flow possible due to the possibility of oxygen toxicity with the drug.
- Premedicate patient as ordered, if patient has lymphoma a test dose should be administered before the first dose is given. Emergency kit to be available at bedside
  - Diphenhydramine 50 mg
  - Acetaminophen 650 mg
  - Hydrocortisone 50 mg
  - Epinephrine 1:1000. Draw up and deliver only 0.3 mL at one time IM or IV; repeat as necessary
  - Oxygen
  - AMBU bag
  - Albuterol inhaler

Education
- Inform patient that fever and chills occur less frequently with continued bleomycin therapy.
- Instruct patient to report any signs or symptoms of pulmonary toxicity, shortness of breath, or difficulty breathing.
- Make sure patient has a 24-hour number to contact his or her health care provider about any new signs or symptoms.
- Make sure patient has a thermometer at home and to call if fever greater than 38.5° C (greater than 101.5° F) occurs.
- Instruct patient to pay particular attention to skin and nail bed changes and to call if erythema, pain, or edema occurs.
- Instruct patient to call if any unusual symptoms of bleeding, bruising, or extreme fatigue occur.
- Instruct patient to tell all practitioners and in particular before going to surgery that he or she has had bleomycin as they should deliver the lowest flow possible of oxygen.
- Urge patient not to receive live-virus vaccinations and to avoid contact with anyone who has recently received a live-virus vaccine.

BORTEZOMIB
BRAND NAMES
Velcade

CLASS OF AGENT
Antineoplastic agent, proteasome inhibitor

CLINICAL PHARMACOLOGY
Mechanism of Action
A proteasome inhibitor and antineoplastic agent that inhibits the degradation of conjugated proteins required for cell-cycle progression and mitosis, disrupting cell proliferation. **Therapeutic Effect:** Produces antitumor and chemosensitizing activity and cell death.

Absorption and Distribution
Onset: Peak response inhibition is 1 hr. Duration: 48-72 hrs.
Distributed to tissues and organs, with highest level in the GI tract and liver. Protein binding: 83%. Does not get into the CNS.
Half-life: 9-15 hrs.

Metabolism and Excretion
Primarily metabolized by cytochrome P450 enzymes 3A4, 2D6, 2C19, 2C9, and 1A2 in the liver. Rapidly cleared from plasma in 15 mins. Drug levels are not useful for monitoring efficacy. Significant biliary excretion, with lesser amount excreted in the urine.

HOW SUPPLIED/AVAILABLE FORMS
Powder for Injection: 3.5-mg single-dose vials.

INDICATIONS AND DOSAGES
Multiple Myeloma
Treatment cycle consists of 1.3 mg/m2 on days 1, 4, 8, and 11 followed by a 10-day rest period on days 12-21. Consecutive doses are separated by at least 72 hrs. Maintenance cycle is given wkly (days 1, 8, 15, and 22) followed by a rest period on days 23-35 (13 days).

Montle Cell Lymphoma
Dosage is the same as that for Multiple Myeloma.

Dosage Adjustment Guidelines
Therapy is withheld at onset of grade 3 nonhematologic or grade 4 hematologic toxicities, excluding neuropathy. When symptoms resolve, therapy is restarted at a 25% reduced dosage.

Neuropathic Pain, Peripheral Sensory Neuropathy
Adults: For grade 1 with pain or grade 2 (interfering with function but not ADL), 1 mg/m². For grade 2 with pain or grade 3 (interfering with ADL), withhold drug until toxicity is resolved, then reinitiate at 0.7 mg/m². For grade 4 (permanent sensory loss that interferes with function), discontinue bortezomib.

Dosage Adjustment in Hepatic Dysfunction
Clearance may be decreased in patients with hepatic dysfunction. Monitor closely.

Dosage Adjustment in Renal Dysfunction
Not studied in patients with Ccr less than 13 mL/min. Mild to moderate impaired renal function does not seem to affect response rates or toxicities.

UNLABELED USES

Currently being studied in mantle cell lymphoma, leukemias, B-cell lymphomas, Waldenström's macroglobulinemia, solid tumors, as first-line therapy for multiple myeloma, and in combination with other chemotherapy agents

PRECAUTIONS

• Use cautiously in patients with a history of syncope, preexisting heart disease, and electrolyte or acid-base disturbances.
• Use cautiously in patients receiving any medication that increases the risk of dehydration, hypotension, peripheral neuropathy, or myelosuppression.
• Hepatic or renal function impairment.
• History of GI toxicities.
• Allergies, asthma, or hypersensitivity to other drugs can increase risk of hypersensitivity to bortezomib.
• Monitor patients at risk for tumor lysis syndrome closely.
Pregnancy Risk Category: D

CONTRAINDICATIONS

Hypersensitivity to bortezomib, boron, or mannitol

DRUG PREPARATION/ADMINISTRATION/ SAFE HANDLING ISSUES

◀ ALERT ▶ Because bortezomib may be carcinogenic, mutagenic, or teratogenic, wear nitrile or latex, but not vinyl, gloves when handling the drug. If the drug comes in contact with skin, wash the skin thoroughly with soap and water. Do not use waterless hand soap or any antibacterial soap as either can increase the reaction from the agent. If the drug comes in contact with mucous membranes, flush the area with water.
• Reconstitute the vial with 3.5 mL of 0.9% NaCl to a final concentration of 1 mg/mL.
• Give bortezomib as a bolus IV injection over 3-5 secs.
• Be aware that bortezomib is not a vesicant.

STORAGE AND STABILITY

• Store unopened vials at room temperature and protect from light.
• Contains no preservatives so the reconstituted solution must be used within 8 hrs.
• Some studies have shown that if stored in the refrigerator and protected from light, reconstituted bortezomib is clinically stable for 5 days.

INTERACTIONS
Drug

May alter the efficacy of oral hypoglycemic agents, requiring medication adjustment. Monitor patients using concomitant drugs that may cause myelosuppression or peripheral neuropathy. Monitor for efficacy or toxicity when patient is taking other medications metabolized by the cytochrome P450 system.
Herbal
None known.

LAB EFFECTS/INTERFERENCE

May significantly decrease blood Hgb, Hct, and neutrophil, platelet, and WBC counts.

Y-SITE COMPATIBLES
No information

INCOMPATIBLES
No information

SIDE EFFECTS
Serious Reactions

• Thrombocytopenia occurs in 40% of patients. Platelet count peaks at day 11 and returns to baseline by day 21. GI and intracerebral hemorrhages are associated with drug-induced thrombocytopenia.
• Anemia occurs in 32% of patients.
• Neuropathy occurs in 37% of patients. Symptoms usually improve when bortezomib is discontinued, which takes approximately 6 mos.
• Pneumonia occurs occasionally.
Other Side Effects
Frequent (10%-50%):
Abdominal pain, anorexia, anxiety, arthralgia, asthenia, back pain, blurred vision, bone pain, cough, dehydration, diarrhea, dizziness, dyspepsia, edema, fever, headache, hypotension, insomnia, limb pain, muscle cramps, myalgia, nausea, neutropenia, paresthesia, peripheral neuropathy, pneumonia, pruritus, rash, rigors, taste alteration, thrombocytopenia, vomiting
Occasional (Less Than 10%):
From clinical trials and post-trial reports
GI disorders: ascites, paralytic ileus, intestinal obstruction, stomatitis, melena, pancreatitis
Immune system disorders: anaphylactic reactions, hypersensitivity
Infections: aspergillosis, bacteremia, herpes viral infection, septic shock, urinary tract infections, oral candidiasis

Metabolism/nutrition: hypocalcemia, hyperuricemia, hypokalemia, hyperkalemia, hyponatremia, hypernatremia
Nervous system disorders: coma, grand mal convulsion, motor dysfunction, transient ischemic attack, encephalopathy
Renal disorders: bladder spasms, renal failure
Respiratory and chest disorders: acute respiratory distress syndrome, acute diffuse infiltrative pulmonary disease, pneumonia, dyspnea, hypoxia, respiratory distress
Vascular disorders: CVA, deep vein thrombosis, pulmonary embolism, disseminated intravascular coagulation, pulmonary hypertension

Rare (Less Than 1%): Bone marrow suppression
Comparison of Adverse Effects in patients with multiple myeloma versus mantle cell lymphoma:

• Nausea occurs more often in patients with multiple myeloma (57%) compared to patients with mantle cell lymphoma (44%)
• Thrombocytopenia occurs more often in patients with multiple myeloma (38%) compared to patients with mantle cell lymphoma (21%). The incidence of ≥Grade 3 thrombocytopenia higher in patients with multiple myeloma (32%) compared to those with mantle cell lymphoma (11%).
• The incidence of peripheral neuropathy appears to occur more frequently among patients with mantle cell lymphoma (55%) than those with multiple myeloma (37%).
• The incidence of hypotension is about the same in patients with multiple myeloma (12%) and those with mantle cell lymphoma (15%).
• The incidence of neutropenia was higher in patients with multiple myeloma (18%) compared to patients with mantle cell lymphoma (6%). The incidence of ≥Grade 3 neutropenia occurs more frequently in patients with multiple myeloma (14%) than those with mantle cell lymphoma (4%).
• The incidence of fever was higher among patients with multiple myeloma (37%) compared to patients with mantle cell lymphoma (19%). The incidence of ≥Grade 3 fever was 3% in patients with multiple myeloma and 1% in patients with mantle cell lymphoma.

SPECIAL CONSIDERATIONS
Baseline Assessment
• Keep in mind that bortezomib is used to treat patients with refractory or relapsed multiple myeloma, who have received at least two prior therapies and who have demonstrated disease progression with the last therapy.
• Assess patient's prior chemotherapeutic regimens for toxicities such as nausea, diarrhea, fatigue, neuropathy, and myelosuppression.
• Monitor patient's CBC with differential, platelet count, and electrolyte, BUN, and creatinine levels.

Intervention and Evaluation
• Administer premedications for nausea as ordered.
• Evaluate CBC with differential and platelet count before each dose of this agent.
• Assess patient's vital signs and B/P for signs and symptoms of dehydration, orthostatic changes, tachycardia, fever, and infection before each dose. Monitor patient for signs and symptoms of orthostatic hypotension.
• Closely monitor I&O and weight changes.
• Monitor patient's temperature and be alert for fever.
• Avoid all IM injections, rectal temperature, and suppositories when the platelet count is less than 50,000/microliter.
• Assess for peripheral neuropathy before each dose: numbness, tingling, feelings of warmth, or any leg weakness, paresthesia, or hyperesthesias.

Education
• Instruct patient on the usual side effects of this agent (fever, chills, fatigue, neuropathy, and dehydration), what symptoms to monitor, and when to contact his or her health care provider. Make sure patient has a 24-hour number for the provider. Do not floss when the platelet level is less than 50,000.
• Instruct patient to contact his or her health care provider as soon as possible for fever greater than 38° C (greater than 101° F), nausea lasting greater than 24 hour, diarrhea lasting greater than 24 hour, or inability to take at least 1500 mL of fluid in a 24-hour period.
• Instruct patient to drink at least 2 L of fluid per day and no more than 16 oz in caffeinated beverages to prevent dehydration.
• Instruct patient to stay as active as possible and report any signs of increasing weakness.
• Provide patient with nutrition consultations as needed for increased weight loss or inability to take food or fluids.

- Caution women of childbearing age to avoid pregnancy while taking bortezomib. Teach the patient about effective forms of contraception, and stress the importance of pregnancy testing.
- Warn patient to avoid tasks, especially driving, that require mental alertness or motor skills until his or her response to the drug is established.

BUSULFAN
BRAND NAMES
Busulfex; Myleran

CLASS OF AGENT
Antineoplastic agent, alkylating agent

CLINICAL PHARMACOLOGY
Mechanism of Action
Reacts with N-7 position of guanosine and interferes with DNA replication and transcription of RNA. Busulfan interferes with the normal function of DNA by alkylation and cross-linking the strands of DNA. It is a cell cycle phase-nonspecific agent. **Therapeutic Effect:** Disrupts DNA nucleic acid function.
Absorption and Distribution
Well absorbed with peak levels within 2-4 hrs. Volume of distribution: approximate 1 L/kg; the drug is well distributed into CSF and saliva with levels similar to those in plasma. Protein binding: 14-32.4%. *Half-life:* Varies. In a series of doses, elimination after the first dose is about 3.4 hrs; elimination after the last dose is about 2.3 hrs. Clearance is higher in children.
Metabolism and Excretion
Busulfan is metabolized extensively via the liver (may increase with multiple doses). Busulfan is excreted in urine, 10%-50% as metabolites within 24 hrs (less than 2% as unchanged drug).

HOW SUPPLIED/AVAILABLE FORMS
Injection, Solution (Busulfex): 6 mg/mL (10 mL).
Tablet (Myleran): 2 mg.

INDICATIONS AND DOSAGES
Bone Marrow Transplant (BMT)-Ablative Conditioning Regimen
Busulfan dose should be based on adjusted ideal body weight (AIBW) because actual body weight (AW), ideal body weight (IBW), or other factors can produce significant differences in busulfan clearance

among lean, normal, and obese patients; refer to individual protocols. Doses for bone marrow–ablative conditioning regimens are as follows:
Oral: 1 mg/kg/dose (IBW) every 6 hrs for 16 doses.
IV: 0.8 mg/kg (IBW or AW, whichever is lower) every 6 hrs for 4 days (a total of 16 doses).

IV dosing in morbidly obese patients: Dosing should be based on AIBW, which should be calculated as
$$AIBW = IBW + 0.25 \times (AW - IBW).$$

Dosage Adjustment in Hepatic Dysfunction
Although there is no dosage adjustment guideline available for patients with liver dysfunction, busulfan should be used cautiously in these patients.
Dosage Adjustment in Renal Dysfunction
No information available.

UNLABELED USES
Polycythemia vera: PO: 2-6 mg/day
Thrombocytosis: PO: 4-6 mg/day

PRECAUTIONS
Pregnancy Risk Category: D
Busulfan may cause severe fetal defects. Conception within 1 mo of busulfan administration is contraindicated. Breastfeeding is also contraindicated.
Use caution in patients predisposed to seizures. Discontinue if lung toxicity develops. Busulfan has been causally related to the development of secondary malignancies (tumors and acute leukemias). Busulfan has been associated with ovarian failure (including failure to achieve puberty) in females. High busulfan area under the concentration versus time curve values (greater than 1500 µmol/min) are associated with increased risk of hepatic veno-occlusive disease during conditioning for allogeneic BMT.

CONTRAINDICATIONS
Hypersensitivity to busulfan or any component of the formulation; failure to respond to previous courses; pregnancy. Fetal risk is possible with busulfan. Pregnancy within a month of initiating busulfan is contraindicated.

DRUG PREPARATION/ADMINISTRATION/SAFE HANDLING ISSUES
◀ ALERT ▶ Because busulfan may be carcinogenic, mutagenic, or teratogenic, wear

nitrile or latex, but not vinyl, gloves when handling the drug. If the drug comes in contact with skin, wash the skin thoroughly with soap and water. Do not use waterless hand soap or any antibacterial soap as either can increase the reaction from the agent. If the drug comes in contact with mucous membranes, flush the area with water.

- Filter IV busulfan using the 5-micron syringe filter provided, using one filter per ampul. If using the enclosed syringe, filter in the forward flow direction, allow for 0.16 mL of residual busulfan to remain in the filter.
- Dilute busulfan injection in 0.9% NaCl injection or D5W.
- The dilution volume should be 10 times the volume of the busulfan injection, ensuring that the final concentration of busulfan is 0.5 mg/mL.
- IV busulfan should be administered via a central venous catheter as a 2-hr infusion.
- Do not use polycarbonate syringes.
- To facilitate ingestion of high oral doses, insert multiple tablets into clear gel capsules. Have patient take on an empty stomach with an 8-oz glass of water.

STORAGE AND STABILITY
Store unopened ampuls (injection) under refrigeration (2-8° C, 36-46° F). The final solution is stable for up to 8 hrs at room temperature (25° C, 77° F), but the infusion must also be completed within that 8-hr time frame. Dilution of busulfan injection in 0.9% NaCl is stable for up to 12 hrs with refrigeration (2-8° C, 36-46° F), but the infusion must also be completed within that 12-hr time frame.

INTERACTIONS
Drug
CYP 3A4 inducers (aminoglutethimide, carbamazepine, nafcillin, nevirapine, phenobarbital, phenytoin, and rifamycin): May decrease the levels/effects of busulfan.
CYP 3A4 inhibitors (azole antifungals, ciprofloxacin, clarithromycin, diclofenac, doxycycline, erythromycin, imatinib, isoniazid, nefazodone, nicardipine, propofol, protease inhibitors, quinidine, and verapamil): May increase the levels/effects of busulfan.
Acetaminophen: May increase toxicity of busulfan. Acetaminophen use within 72 hrs

of administration may deplete the plasma and tissues of glutathione required for busulfan clearance.
Live-virus vaccines: May potentiate viral replication, increase vaccine side effects, and decrease the patient's antibody response to the vaccine.
Herbal
St John's Wort: May decrease busulfan levels.
Food
Grapefruit inhibits CYP 3A4 enzymes and can potentially enhance busulfan effects.

LAB EFFECTS/INTEREFENCE
May increase alkaline phosphatase, bilirubin, creatinine, and ALT (SGPT) levels.

Y-SITE COMPATIBLES
Docetaxel, granisetron, paclitaxel, palonosetron, rituximab, trastuzumab

INCOMPATIBLES
Thiotepa, voriconazole

SIDE EFFECTS
Serious Reactions
- The major adverse effect of busulfan is myelosuppression resulting in hematologic toxicity, as evidenced by anemia, severe leukopenia, and severe thrombocytopenia.
- Very high busulfan dosages may produce blurred vision, muscle twitching, and tonic-clonic seizures. Prophylactic antiepileptic agents have been used in some protocols.
- Long-term therapy (more than 4 years) may produce a pulmonary syndrome ("busulfan lung"), characterized by persistent cough, congestion, crackles, and dyspnea. This may occur years after therapy has been discontinued.
Other Side Effects
Frequent (10%-50%):
Hematologic: Severe pancytopenia, leukopenia, thrombocytopenia, anemia, and bone marrow suppression are common, and patients should be monitored closely while receiving therapy. In large doses, busulfan is myeloablative and is used in BMT for this reason.
Occasional (1%-10%):
Dermatologic: Hyperpigmentation skin (busulfan tan), urticaria, erythema, alopecia
Endocrine and metabolic: Amenorrhea

GI: Nausea, vomiting, diarrhea; little effect on GI mucosal lining

Rare (Less Than 1%):

Cardiovascular: Endocardial fibrosis

Endocrine and metabolic: Adrenal suppression, gynecomastia, hyperuricemia

GU: Isolated cases of hemorrhagic cystitis reported

Hepatic: Hepatic dysfunction

Ocular: Blurred vision, cataracts

Respiratory: After long-term or high-dose therapy, a syndrome known as "busulfan lung" may occur. This syndrome is manifested by diffuse interstitial pulmonary fibrosis and persistent cough, fever, rales, and dyspnea, which may be relieved by corticosteroids.

SPECIAL CONSIDERATIONS
Baseline Assessment
- Monitor for CBC with differential, platelet count, electrolyte, BUN, and creatinine levels, and liver function tests.
- Monitor patient for any history of seizures, pulmonary symptoms, or kidney stones.
- Evaluate baseline vital signs and oxygen saturation.
- Evaluate patient's current medication list for any new over-the-counter medications or herbal or nutritional supplements.

Intervention and Evaluation
- At high doses evaluate patient's vital signs with oxygen saturation before each dose.
- Monitor CBC with differential, electrolyte, BUN, and creatinine levels, and liver function tests before each high dose or at each visit for patients receiving this agent on a daily basis.
- Administer antiemetics as ordered for high-dose regimens.
- Administer antiseizure medications as ordered before high-dose regimens and deliver busulfan IV over 2 hours.
- If patient is receiving daily oral doses, instruct to take with an 8-oz glass of water and on an empty stomach.
- Monitor patients receiving daily dosing regimens for emesis, and use antiemetics as needed.
- Monitor patient receiving this agent on a daily basis for any pulmonary changes as fibrosis can occur in this patient population.

- Assess patient for mucositis, and visually inspect oral cavity with high-dose regimen.
- Initiate a mouth care regimen for those receiving the high-dose regimen. An example of an oral care regimen is 1 tsp of salt and 1 tsp of baking soda dissolved in 1 glass of tap water to swish and spit after each meal and before bedtime. Instruct patient to use a soft toothbrush if platelet count is less than 50,000 mm^3.
- Evaluate patient's skin for rashes, erythema, or areas of irritation every shift if receiving high-dose regimens. Have patient shower twice daily while receiving high-dose regimens for BMT as a way to lessen skin toxicity as drug can be excreted as patient experiences diaphoresis.
- Offer emotional support to patient and family.

Education
- For patients receiving this agent on a daily basis, educate patient on to take medication on an empty stomach with a 8-oz glass of water.
- Instruct patient on potential side effects of nausea, vomiting, and pulmonary changes, and to notify his or her health care provider if any respiratory changes, shortness of breath, dyspnea, or cough develops.
- Instruct patient to take no over-the-counter medications or herbal or vitamin supplements without checking with his or her health care provider.
- Educate patient on fertility issues and the use of contraception while receiving this agent.
- For patients receiving high-dose regimens, educate patient on number of doses of busulfan to be given. Antiseizure medications may be used as a precaution even in patients without a history of a seizure disorder.
- Instruct patient that premedications for nausea will be given.
- Educate patient on the oral care regimen per institutional protocol.
- Instruct patient on the skin care protocol of showers twice daily until 48 hours after the last dose of agent or the skin care protocol per institutional guidelines.
- Provide patient with information on local resources and support groups available for his or her specific diagnosis.

CAPECITABINE

BRAND NAMES
Xeloda

CLASS OF AGENT
Antineoplastic

CLINICAL PHARMACOLOGY
Mechanism of Action
Activated via a three-step sequential process using the enzymes carboxylesterase and cytidine deaminase and ultimately thymidine phosphorylase, which generate fluorouracil (FU) intracellularly. FU is then activated to fluorodeoxyuridine monophosphate (FdUMP) and fluorouridine triphosphate (FUTP). FdUMP inhibits thymidylate synthesis and subsequently DNA synthesis. FUTP gets incorporated into RNA as a false nucleotide, inhibiting RNA synthesis and function. It is hypothesized that DNA inhibition is responsible for antitumor activity and RNA inhibition is associated with toxicity.

Absorption and Distribution
About 80% of the parent compound, capecitabine, is absorbed intact through the gastric mucosa, resulting in peak FU concentrations in about 1.5 hrs. Food reduces both the rate and extent of absorption. About 35% of capecitabine is bound to serum albumin. Capecitabine distributes to the liver, where carboxyesterase metabolizes it to 5'-deoxyfluorocytidine (inactive), which is then converted by hepatic tumoral cytidine deaminase to 5'-deoxyfluorouridine (inactive) and finally by thymidine phosphorylase (TP) to 5-FU (active). Because concentrations of TP are higher in tumor cells than in normal tissue, higher concentrations of FU are produced intracellularly.
Half-life: Ranges from 38 to 45 mins. Its major metabolite, 5-fluorouracil, has a half-life of about 45 mins.

Metabolism and Excretion
About 60% of capecitabine and its metabolites is bound to plasma proteins. FU is subsequently catabolized by dihydropyrimidine dehydrogenase (DPD) to the less toxic 5-fluorodihydrofluorouracil and 5-fluoroureidopropionic acid (FUPA). β-Ureidopropionase converts FUPA to α-fluoro-β-alanine (FBAL) (inactive). About 95% of capecitabine and its metabolites are excreted in the urine, 50% as FBAL.

HOW SUPPLIED/AVAILABLE FORMS
Tablets: 150 and 500 mg.

INDICATIONS AND DOSAGES
Breast Cancer
In combination with docetaxel, capecitabine is indicated for the treatment of patients with metastatic breast cancer after failure of prior anthracycline-containing chemotherapy.
Capecitabine monotherapy is also indicated for the treatment of patients with metastatic breast cancer resistant to both paclitaxel and an anthracycline-containing chemotherapy regimen or resistant to paclitaxel and for whom further anthracycline therapy is not indicated, e.g., patients who have received cumulative doses of 400 mg/m^2 of doxorubicin or doxorubicin equivalents.

Colorectal Cancer
First-line treatment of patients with metastatic colorectal carcinoma when treatment with fluoropyrimidine therapy alone is preferred.
Capecitabine adjuvant therapy is also indicated for the treatment of patients with Duke's C colon cancer after complete resection when fluoropyrimidine therapy alone is preferred.

Usual Dosage (All Indications)
- The recommended starting dose of capecitabine is 1250 mg/m^2 administered orally in morning and evening; equivalent to 2500 mg/m^2 total daily dose.
- Administered in a 21-day cycle consisting of 14 days of therapy followed by a 7-day rest period.
- Dosage is based on a patient's BSA (see table below).

Dosage Based on Body Surface Area (BSA) 1250 mg/m^2

BSA	Total Daily Dose	150-mg Tablets	500-mg Tablets
<1.25	3000	0	3
1.26-1.37	3300	1	3
1.38-1.51	3600	2	3
1.52-1.65	4000	0	4
1.66-1.77	4300	1	4
1.78-1.91	4600	2	4
1.92-2.05	5000	0	5
2.06-2.17	5300	1	5
>2.18	5600	2	5

From Product Information, Xeloda. Roche Pharmaceuticals, 2005.

Dosage Based on BSA 1000 mg/m²

BSA	Total Dose	150-mg Tablets	500-mg Tablets
<1.25	2000	0	2
1.26-1.37	2600	2	2
1.38-1.51	3000	0	3
1.52-1.65	3150	0 in AM & 1 in PM	3
1.66-1.77	3300	1	3
1.78-1.91	3600	2	3
1.92-2.05	3900	3	3
2.06-2.17	4150	0 in AM & 1 in PM	4
<2.18	4300	1	4

From Product Information, Xeloda. Roche Pharmaceuticals, 2005.

Dosage Adjustment for Grade 2 or 3 Toxicities

- Dosage modifications are not recommended for grade 1 events.
- Therapy with capecitabine should be interrupted upon the occurrence of a grade 2 or 3 adverse event. Once the adverse event has resolved or decreased in intensity to grade 1, then capecitabine therapy may be restarted at the full dose or as adjusted according to the previous table, except for grade 3 hand-and-foot syndrome in which case the dose should be reduced to 75% of the original. If a grade 4 adverse event occurs, therapy should be discontinued or interrupted until the event is resolved or decreased to grade 1, and therapy should be restarted at 50% of the original dose. Doses of capecitabine omitted for toxicity are not replaced or restored; instead the patient should resume the planned treatment cycles.

Dosage Adjustment in Hepatic Dysfunction
No dose adjustment is necessary.

Dosage Adjustment in Renal Dysfunction
Dose reductions to 75% of original dose (e.g., 1250 mg/m² twice daily is reduced to 950 mg/m² twice daily is required for patients with moderate renal impairment (Ccr = 30-50 mL/min). Contraindicated in patients with severe renal impairment (Ccr less than 30 mL/min).

UNLABELED USES
Gastric cancer, esophageal cancer, pancreatic cancer

PRECAUTIONS
Use capecitabine cautiously in patients with hepatic impairment, those receiving warfarin therapy, those having grade 3 or 4 hand-and-foot syndrome, patients with evidence of coronary artery disease, those suspected of dihydropyrimidine dehydrogenase (DPD) deficiency, and those who have myelosuppression with docetaxel. For patients with ANCs less than 1500/mm³ or platelet counts less than 100,000/mm³, withhold treatment until neutrophil counts recover to greater than 1500/mm³ and platelet counts to greater than 100,000/mm³.

Pregnancy Risk Category: D

CONTRAINDICATIONS
Documented DPD deficiency and severe renal insufficiency (Ccr less than 30 mL/min)

Dosage Adjustment for Toxicity Recommended Dose Modifications

Toxicity NCIC Grades*	During a Course of Therapy	Dose Adjustment for Next Treatment (% of Starting Dose)
Grade 1	Maintain dose level	Maintain dose level
Grade 2		
1st appearance	Interrupt until resolved to grade 0-1	100
2nd appearance	Interrupt until resolved to grade 0-1	75
3rd appearance	Interrupt until resolved to grade 0-1	50
4th appearance	Discontinue treatment permanently	
Grade 3		
1st appearance	Interrupt until resolved to grade 0-1	75
2nd appearance	Interrupt until resolved to grade 0-1	50
3rd appearance	Discontinue treatment permanently	
Grade 4		
1st appearance	Discontinue permanently or if the physician deems it to be in the patient's best interest to continue, interrupt until resolved to grade 0-1	50

*National Cancer Institute of Canada (NCIC) Common Toxicity Criteria were used except for the hand-and-foot syndrome.

DRUG PREPARATION/ADMINISTRATION/ SAFE HANDLING ISSUES
- Take 30 mins after a meal.
- Tablets should be swallowed with water only.

STORAGE AND STABILITY
Tablets should be stored at room temperature 20-25° C (68-77° F).

INTERACTIONS
Drug
Warfarin: Clearance is usually decreased by 37%. The international normalized ratio (INR) was increased 2.8-fold in four patients studied. Because of the schedule of capecitabine administration, frequent monitoring of INR should be performed within cycles. Altered coagulation parameters may be seen for mos after discontinuation of capecitabine.

Capecitabine or its metabolites: May inhibit metabolism of drugs by the CYP 2C9 pathway.

Aluminum-magnesium antacids: Increase capecitabine area under the curve and maximum concentrations by 16% and 35%, respectively. However, antacids do not affect capecitabine metabolism in vivo. The clinical significance of this interaction is not known.

Leucovorin: May increase toxicity of capecitabine, leading to severe myelosuppression, mucositis, diarrhea, and other adverse events.

SIDE EFFECTS
Serious Reactions
- *Diarrhea:* Capecitabine can cause diarrhea, sometimes severe. NCIC grade 2 diarrhea is defined as an increase of 4-6 stools/day or nocturnal stools, grade 3 diarrhea as an increase of 7-9 stools/day or incontinence and malabsorption, and grade 4 diarrhea as an increase of greater than or equal to 10 stools/day, grossly bloody diarrhea, or the need for parenteral support. Patients with severe diarrhea should be given fluid and electrolyte replacement if they become dehydrated. In the overall clinical trial safety database of capecitabine monotherapy (n = 875), the median time to first occurrence of grade 2 to 4 diarrhea was 34 days (range from 1 to 369 days). The median duration of grade 3 to 4 diarrhea was 5 days. If grade 2, 3, or 4 diarrhea occurs, administration of capecitabine should be immediately interrupted until the diarrhea

resolves or decreases in intensity to grade 1. After a reoccurrence of grade 2 diarrhea or occurrence of any grade 3 or 4 diarrhea, subsequent doses of capecitabine should be decreased. Standard antidiarrheal treatments (e.g., loperamide) are recommended.
- *Cardiac toxicity:* Capecitabine has been associated with MI, angina, and dysrhythmias.
- Necrotizing enterocolitis (typhlitis) has been reported.

Other Side Effects
Frequent (10%-50%):
Abdominal pain, alopecia, anemia, anorexia, constipation, dermatitis, diarrhea, fatigue, fever, hand-and-foot syndrome, hyperbilirubinemia, lymphopenia, myelosuppression (neutropenia, thrombocytopenia), nausea, paresthesia, stomatitis, vomiting

Occasional (1%-10%):
Dehydration, dizziness, dyspepsia, edema, headache, insomnia, myalgia, nail disorders, limb pain

Rare (Less Than 1%):
Necrotizing enterocolitis, pancreatitis

SPECIAL CONSIDERATIONS
Baseline Assessment
- Record baseline laboratory data, obtain CBC with differential, check ANC, monitor liver function and renal function tests, and assess for dose reduction if creatinine is rising.
- Inspect oral cavity and assess skin thoroughly, paying particular attention to hands, feet, and areas of diaphoresis.
- Evaluate compliance with the oral agent, have patient bring medication to each visit, check the medication diary, and assess for appropriate timing of dosing
- Evaluate all current medications; for patients taking warfarin, check prothrombin time and INR more frequently due to altered metabolism by capecitabine.
- Check for any other OTC medications or herbals or vitamins supplements patient may be taking.

Intervention and Evaluation
- Monitor for signs and symptoms of neutropenia, anemia, or thrombocytopenia.
- If patient is taking warfarin, evaluate any bleeding tendency.
- Evaluate skin of patient, in particular, hands, feet, areas of diaphoresis, axilla, groin, and back of knees.

- Monitor for signs and symptoms of abdominal pain, constipation, and diarrhea
- Evaluate oral hygiene and instruct patient on oral care: use of salt and baking soda mouth washes three times per day and at bedtime or institutional protocol.
- Monitor for continued compliance with oral medication.
- Evaluate any signs and symptoms of nausea, vomiting, or diarrhea.
- Evaluate for any new medications patient may be taking; instruct patient NOT to take any new medications or supplements unless instructed by his or her health care provider.

Education
- Instruct patient to take dose 30 minutes after meals.
- Instruct patient to take medication only take with water, not with other fluids.
- Instruct patient on signs and symptoms of infection: fever and chills.
- Instruct patient on signs and symptoms of bleeding, especially if patient is taking warfarin.
- Make sure patient has thermometer at home and knows how to use it.
- Instruct patient on oral care regimen, per institutional protocol. Remind patient that most commercial mouthwashes have alcohol and may irritate mucosa. Advise patient to try alcohol-free mouthwash.
- Instruct patient on skin assessment, making sure patient is aware of when to call his or her health care provider. Monitor for any signs and symptoms of erythema, pain, or blisters. Patient may use moisturizer on hands and feet at least twice daily. Aquaphor, Eucerin, Absorbase, or an institutional agent is preferred. Other products have significant alcohol content, which can dry skin and enhance breakdown.
- Instruct patient to take NO medications or OTC products unless approved by his or her health care provider.
- Make sure patient has a 24-hour number to reach his or her health care provider.
- Provide patient with information on local resources and support groups available for his or her specific diagnosis.

CARBOPLATIN

BRAND NAMES
Paraplatin

CLASS OF AGENT
Antineoplastic agent, alkylating agent

CLINICAL PHARMACOLOGY
Mechanism of Action
A platinum coordination complex that inhibits DNA synthesis by cross-linking with DNA strands, preventing cell division. It is a cell cycle phase-nonspecific agent. **Therapeutic Effect:** Interferes with DNA function.

Absorption and Distribution
Protein binding: low. Volume of distribution: 16 L.
Half-life: 2.55-0.9 hr with a Ccr greater than 60 mL/min.

Metabolism and Excretion
Hydrolyzed in solution to the active form. Excreted primarily in urine (60%-90%) within 24 hrs. Removed by hemodialysis.

HOW SUPPLIED/AVAILABLE FORMS
Powder for Injection: 50 mg, 150 mg, 450 mg.
Injection Solution 10 mg/mL: 50 mg, 150 mg, 450 mg, 600 mg.

INDICATIONS AND DOSAGES
Ovarian Carcinoma
Target Area Under the Curve (AUC)-Based Carboplatin Dose:
- AUC 4-7 mg/mL/min: based on disease protocol and q2-4wk dosing cycle.
- AUC 2 mg/mL/min: based on disease protocol and qwk dosing cycle.
- Dosages may be delayed, reduced, or discontinued due to myelosuppression or other toxicities.

Use the Calvert formula to determine dose:

$$\text{Dose (in mg)} = \text{AUC} + (\text{GFR} + 25)$$

where GFR is glomerular filtration rate. May use the Cockcroft-Gault formula to determine CrCl that estimates GFR:

$$\text{CrCl (mL/min)} = (140 - \text{age}) \text{ weight (kg)} \times 0.85 \text{ (for females)}/72 \times \text{Scr}$$

The Cockcroft-Gault formula may overpredict CrCl in patients with ascites or muscle-wasting or in obese patients. Adjusted or ideal body weight may be used to adjust for excess fluids or fat. The Calvert formula is derived using ^{51}Cr-EDTA clearance to estimate GFR.

BSA-Based Carboplatin Dose
- Interpatient variability in AUC with BSA dosing.
- Ovarian cancer: 300-360 mg/m^2 IV every 3-4 wks.
- Autologous bone marrow transplantation: 1600 mg/m^2 total dose IV divided over

4 days. (Inclusion criteria mandate CrCl greater than 50 mL/min for patients receiving transplants).
- Intraperitoneal: 200-650 mg/m^2 in 2 L administered into the peritoneum of patients with ovarian cancer.

Hemodialysis Dose
The literature supports the use of the Calvert formula with a GFR of zero. AUC 4-7 mg/mL/min is based on the disease protocol. Dialyze 16-24 hrs after chemotherapy.

Dosage Adjustment in Renal Dysfunction
Carboplatin may accumulate with decreased renal function. The Calvert formula accounts for dosage adjustment to renal impairment based on the patient's decreased GFR. Refer to the package insert for BSA-based dosage adjustment.

Dosage Adjustment in Hepatic Dysfunction
No adjustments required.

Dosage Adjustment in Myelosuppression
Dosage adjustment for single-agent or combination therapy is based on the lowest post-treatment platelet or neutrophil counts.

Platelets	Neutrophils	Adjustment Dose (from Prior Course)
>100,000	>2000	125%
50,000-100,000	500-2000	No adjustment
<50,000	<500	75%

UNLABELED USES
Treatment of bladder cancer, breast cancer, bony and soft-tissue sarcomas, cervical cancer, endometrial cancer, esophageal cancer, germ cell tumors, head and neck cancer, lung cancer, neuroblastoma

PRECAUTIONS
Use carboplatin cautiously in patients with chickenpox, herpes zoster, infection, or renal impairment.

Pregnancy Risk Category: D
Carboplatin use should be avoided during pregnancy, if possible, especially in the first trimester because it may cause fetal harm. Drug excretion into human breast milk is unknown/not recommended.

CONTRAINDICATIONS
Hypersensitivity to carboplatin, cisplatin, mannitol, or any component of the formulation. Carboplatin should not be used in patients with severe bone marrow suppression or significant bleeding.

DRUG PREPARATION/ADMINISTRATION/ SAFE HANDLING ISSUES
◀ **ALERT** ▶ Carboplatin dosage is individualized on the basis of the patient's GFR using the Calvert formulation, clinical response, and tolerance of the drug's adverse effects. In general, allow recovery of platelet count to greater than 100,000/mm^3 and neutrophil count to greater than 2000/mm^3 before giving repeat dosage.

◀ **ALERT** ▶ Because carboplatin may be carcinogenic, mutagenic, or teratogenic, wear nitrile or latex, but not vinyl, gloves when handling the drug. If the drug comes in contact with skin, wash the skin thoroughly with soap and water. Do not use waterless hand soap or any antibacterial soap as either can increase the reaction from the agent. If the drug comes in contact with mucous membranes, flush the area with water.

- Carboplatin is not a known vesicant or irritant.
- Do not use aluminium needles or administration sets that come in contact with drug because this may produce black precipitate and a loss of potency.
- Lyophilized powder: Reconstitute the 50-mg vial with 5 mL, the 150-mg vial with 15 mL, and the 450-mg vial with 45 mL of sterile water for injection, D5W, or 0.9% NaCl to provide a concentration of 10 mg/mL.
- Further dilute the solution with D5W or 0.9% NaCl to provide a concentration as low as 0.1 mg/mL, if needed.
- Infuse the solution over 15-60 mins. Refer to individual protocols; some protocols call for 24 hrs continuous infusion.
- Hydration is not required.
- When given as a sequential infusion, administer a taxane derivative (e.g., paclitaxel or docetaxel) before carboplatin to limit myelosuppression.
- Coadministration of carboplatin and topotecan may result in severe myelosuppression. Coadminister carboplatin on day 1 of the topotecan series.
- Be aware that an anaphylactic reaction may occur minutes after administration. Use epinephrine, diphenhydramine, and corticosteroid, as prescribed, to alleviate symptoms.

STORAGE AND STABILITY
- Store vials at room temperature and protect from light.
- Reconstitute the drug immediately before use.
- After reconstitution, the solution is stable for 8 hrs. Discard any unused portion after 8 hrs because the formulation is preservative-free.

INTERACTIONS
Drug
Aminoglycosides: Concomitant use may increase the risk of nephrotoxicity and/or ototoxicity.
Bone marrow depressants: May increase myelosuppression.
Live-virus vaccines: May potentiate virus replication, increase vaccine side effects, and decrease the patient's antibody response to the vaccine.
Nephrotoxic, ototoxic medications: May increase the risk of nephrotoxicity or ototoxicity, respectively.
Phenytoin: May decrease bioavailability of phenytoin, resulting in decreased effectiveness; monitor phenytoin levels.
Taxanes (docetaxel, paclitaxel): Carboplatin should be administered after taxanes to decrease risk of myelosuppression.
Warfarin: May increase effect of warfarin. Monitor thrombin or the international normalized ratio.
Herbal
None known.

LAB EFFECTS/INTEREFENCE
May decrease serum electrolyte levels, including calcium, magnesium, K, Na. High dosages (more than 4 times the recommended dosage) may elevate BUN and serum alkaline phosphatase, bilirubin, creatinine, and AST (SGOT) levels.

Y-SITE COMPATIBLES
Amifostine, amphotericin B liposomal (AmBisome), etoposide (VePesid), filgrastim (Neupogen), gemcitabine (Gemzar), granisetron (Kytril), ondansetron (Zofran), paclitaxel (Taxol), palonosetron (Aloxi), sargramostim (Leukine), vinorelbine (Navelbine)

INCOMPATIBLES
Amphotericin B lipid cholesteryl (Amphotec), amphotericin B lipid complex (Abelcet), diazepam, fluorouracil, lansoprazole, leucovorin, mesna, phenytoin, Na bicarbonate

SIDE EFFECTS
Serious Reactions
- Myelosuppression may be severe, resulting in anemia, infection (sepsis and pneumonia), and bleeding. Thrombocytopenia is most common.
- Prolonged treatment may result in peripheral neurotoxicity.
- Severe hypersensitivity reactions have occurred in later cycles (e.g., 6th-8th dose cycle.). Use diphenhydramine 50-100 mg IV, hydrocortisone succinate 100 mg IV, epinephrine 1:1000 (1 mg/mL) 0.3 mL IV, albuterol inhaler 2-4 puffs, and oxygen as necessary. Rechallenge of carboplatin is not recommended for severe reactions. However, for patients with limited treatment options, several variations of carboplatin desensitization protocols described in the literature have successfully been used.
Other Side Effects
Frequent (10%-50%):
Anemia, dose-limiting bone marrow suppression (particularly thrombocytopenia), hypersensitivity, increases in creatinine and BUN levels (mostly mild and reversible; less nephrotoxic than cisplatin), nausea and vomiting (moderate to high potential), pain.
Occasional (1%-10%):
Alopecia, asthenia, constipation, diarrhea, electrolyte imbalances, peripheral neuropathy
Rare (Less Than 1%):
Acute renal failure, anaphylaxis, ototoxicity (less than cisplatin), visual disturbances

SPECIAL CONSIDERATIONS
Baseline Assessment
- Be aware that treatment should not be administered until the patient's CBC recovers from previous therapy. Monitor patient's platelets carefully after dosing and do not readminister until platelet recovery occurs (platelets greater than 100,000/mm^3).
- Evaluate for any signs or symptoms of peripheral neuropathy, numbness, tingling, sensitivity to heat, cold, altered vibratory sense, or pain, based on patient's comorbidities, such as diabetes mellitus.
- Ensure patient's renal function has been taken into account.
- Consider baseline auditory function tests before high-dose therapy.
- Have an anaphylaxis kit available at bedside before administration of this

agent. The anaphylaxis kit should include the following:

Diphenhydramine 50 mg
Hydrocortisone 50 mg
Epinephrine 1:1000
Albuterol inhaler
Syringes and needles
Alcohol wipes
Oxygen setup
Ambu bag at bedside

Intervention and Evaluation
- Monitor the patient's blood CBC with differential, platelet count, and electrolyte, BUN, and creatinine levels before each dose.
- Be aware that myelosuppression is increased in those who have received previous carboplatin therapy or have impaired renal function.
- Give transfusions as necessary for patients receiving prolonged therapy.
- Monitor patient for signs and symptoms of hematologic toxicity, such as ecchymosis, petechiae, epistaxis, fever, signs of local infection, sore throat, excessive fatigue or weakness, and unusual bleeding from any site.
- Monitor for signs of hypersensitivity, especially after seven doses of therapy or retreatment after prior carboplatin therapy.
- Administer antiemetics, as ordered, to control nausea and vomiting.

Education
- Instruct patient to immediately notify his or her physician or health care provider if he or she experiences signs of infection or bleeding including fever greater than 38° C (greater than 101° F) and flu-like symptoms, sore throat, epistaxis, petechiae, and easy bruising or bleeding.
- Inform the patient that nausea and vomiting may occur, but generally abates in less than 24 hours. Instruct patient to check with his or her health care provider for antiemetic orders after treatment.
- Caution patient to notify his or her physician or health care provide if nausea and vomiting continue for longer than 24 hours after completion of therapy.
- Educate patient about fatigue and its causes and any interventions to promote well-being. Encourage patient to plan a minimal exercise program while undergoing therapy. Studies have demonstrated patients who continue to do some minimal exercise tolerate chemotherapy better with fewer symptoms of nausea and fatigue.

- Urge patient to avoid receiving live-virus vaccinations without his or her physician's approval and to avoid contact with anyone who recently received a live-virus vaccine because carboplatin lowers the body's resistance.
- Provide patient with information on local resources support groups available for his or her specific diagnosis.
- Encourage patient to report any new symptoms.

CARMUSTINE

BRAND NAMES
BiCNU, Gliadel

CLASS OF AGENT
Nitrosourea; antineoplastic alkylating agent

CLINICAL PHARMACOLOGY
Mechanism of Action
The exact mechanism by which the nitrosoureas are cytotoxic is not fully established; however, it is thought that they liberate alkylating moieties that inhibit DNA and RNA synthesis by cross-linking with DNA and RNA strands, preventing cell division. It is cell cycle phase nonspecific.

A polymer form of carmustine (wafer implants) are designed to deliver the drug directly into the resected surgical brain cavity. Within the brain cavity, the copolymer (polifeprosan) releases the carmustine into the surrounding brain tissue. Most of the copolymer (70%) degrades within 3 wks; however, autopsy data have observed wafer remnants up to 232 days from the surgical implantation of the wafers.

Absorption and Distribution
Because of its high lipid solubility, carmustine readily crosses the blood-brain barrier. About 15%-30% of the drug crosses into the CSF after IV administration. It has a large volume of distribution, 2.6 L/kg. It is most effective in the treatment of brain tumors, melanoma, myeloma, and some solid tumors. Carmustine has also been used in the treatment of Hodgkin's disease and meningeal leukemia because of its diffusion into the CSF.

No absorption studies were done in human subjects receiving carmustine wafer implants. In animal studies, no detectable levels of carmustine was measured in the CSF or plasma after carmustine wafer implant insertion.

Half-life: 1.4 mins in the first phase and 17.8 mins in the second.

Metabolism and Excretion

The metabolism of carmustine is not well described. It is rapidly converted to active metabolites. 60% to 70% of the drug in excreted renally as metabolites. Biliary excretion accounts for only 1% of the drug.

HOW SUPPLIED/AVAILABLE FORMS

Powder for Injection (BiCNu): 100 mg.
Wafer (Gliadel): 7.7 mg.

INDICATIONS AND DOSAGES

Disseminated Hodgkin's Disease, Non-Hodgkin's Lymphoma, Multiple Myeloma, and Primary and Metastatic Brain Tumors in Previously Untreated Patients (Monotherapy)

IV (BiCNu): 150-200 mg/m^2 as a single dose or 75-100 mg/m^2 on 2 successive days.
Pediatrics: 200-250 mg/m^2 every 4-6 wks as a single dose.
Implantation (Gliadel): Up to 8 wafers may be placed in resection cavity.
◀ ALERT ▶ Subsequent dosing should be based on clinical and hematologic response to the previous dose and no sooner than 6 wks apart (platelet count greater than 100,000/mm^3 and leukocytes greater than 4000/mm^3).

Dosage Adjustment in Myelosuppression

Guidelines of subsequent dose based on nadir laboratory results

Dosage Adjustment in Hepatic Dysfunction

No dose modification.

NADIR AFTER PRIOR DOSE		Percentage of Prior Dose to Be Given
Leukocytes/mm^3	Platelets/mm^3	
>4000	>100,000	100
3000-3999	75,000-99,999	100
2000-2999	25,000-74,999	70
<2000	<25,000	50

Dosage Adjustment in Renal Dysfunction

No specific guidelines exist, but carmustine may require dose reduction in patients with renal dysfunction.

UNLABELED USES

Treatment of hepatic or GI carcinoma, malignant melanoma, mycosis fungoides

PRECAUTIONS

Pregnancy Risk Category: D

CONTRAINDICATIONS

None known.

DRUG PREPARATION/ADMINISTRATION/SAFE HANDLING ISSUES

◀ ALERT ▶ IV: When preparing this agent, use nitrile or latex, but not vinyl, gloves only. If a splash occurs with this agent, wash with mild soap and water; do not use antibacterial soap or waterless soap as either can increase the skin reaction. If an eye splash occurs, use copious amounts of water or normal saline to flush the eyes. Accidental contact of reconstituted BiCNU with the skin has caused transient hyper-pigmentation of the affected areas.
IV administration of carmustine should be in a glass container. A vial of carmustine contains no preservative and is not intended as a multiple dose use product. Carmustine reconstituted as directed and further diluted to 0.2 mg/mL in D5W injection.
If carmustine appears as an oil film in the bottom of the vial, it is not suitable for use and should be discarded.

STORAGE AND STABILITY

Vials for Parenteral Administration

• Carmustine should appear as dry flakes or a dry congealed mass in the vial. The product has a low melting point (30.5-32° C, 86.9-89.6° F) and will liquefy and decompose if exposed to such temperatures.

• Carmustine has a low melting point (30.5-32.0° C [86.9-89.6° F]). Exposure of the drug to this temperature or above will cause the drug to liquefy and appear as an oil film on the vials. This is a sign of decomposition, and vials should be discarded. If there is a question of ade-quate refrigeration upon receipt of this product, immediately inspect the larger vial in each individual carton. Hold the vial to a bright light for inspection. Carmustine will appear as a very small amount of dry flakes or dry congealed mass. If this is evident, carmustine is suitable for use and should be refriger-ated immediately.

• Reconstituted vials should be stored at room temperature (25° C [77° F]), protected from light, and utilized within 8 hrs.

• Intact vials are stable for up to 3 years if refrigerated (2-8° C [36-46° F]) and protected from light. Room temperature storage results in a slow decomposition, approximately 3% loss of potency within

36 days. Decomposition occurs usually only if drug is grossly mishandled.

- Wafer implants: Carmustine wafers must be stored at or below –20° C (–4° F). Unopened foil pouches may be kept at room temperature for a maximum of 6 hrs.

INTERACTIONS
Drug
Bone marrow depressants, cimetidine: May enhance the myelosuppressive effect of carmustine.
Hepatotoxic, nephrotoxic medications: May increase the risk of hepatotoxicity or nephrotoxicity.
Live-virus vaccines: May potentiate virus replication, increase vaccine side effects, and decrease the patient's antibody response to the vaccine.
Herbal
None known.

LAB EFFECTS/INTERFERENCE
May increase BUN, serum alkaline phosphatase, bilirubin, AST (SGOT), ALT (SGPT) levels.

Y-SITE COMPATIBLES
Amifostine, Aztreonam, Cisplatin, Dacarbazine, Filgrastim, Fludarabine, Granisetron Hydrochloride, Ondansetron, Palonosetron, Piperacillin Na/Tazobactam, Sargramostim, Vinorelbine

INCOMPATIBLES
Allopurinol (Aloprim), Na bicarbonate solution

SIDE EFFECTS
Serious Reactions after IV Administration
- Hematologic toxicity due to myelosuppression occurs frequently. Thrombocytopenia occurs about 4 wks

---

Handling and disposal: Wafers should only be handled by personnel wearing surgical gloves because exposure to carmustine can cause severe burning and hyperpigmentation of the skin. Use of double gloves is recommended and the outer gloves should be discarded into a biohazard waste container after use. A surgical instrument dedicated to the handling of the wafers should be used for wafer implantation. If repeat neurosugical intervention is indicated, any wafer or wafer remnant should be handled as a potentially cytotoxic agent.

GLIADEL® Wafer should be handled with care. The aluminum foil laminate pouches containing GLIADEL® Wafer should be delivered to the operating room and remain unopened until ready to implant the wafers. **The outside surface of the outer foil pouch is not sterile.**

Instructions for opening pouch containing GLIADEL® wafer

Figure 1: To remove the sterile inner pouch from the outer pouch, locate the folded corner and slowly pull in an outward motion.

Figure 4: To open the inner pouch, gently hold the crimped edge and cut in an arc-like fashion around the wafer.

Figure 2: Do NOT pull in a downward motion rolling knuckles over the pouch. This may exert pressure on the wafer and cause it to break.

Figure 5: To remove to GLIADEL® wafer, gently grasp the wafer with the aid of forceps and place it onto a designated sterile field.

Figure 3: Remove the inner pouch by grabbing hold of the crimped edge and pulling upward.

Once the tumor is resected, tumor pathology is confirmed, and hemostasis is obtained, up to eight GLIADEL® Wafers (polifeprosan 20 with carmustine implant) may be placed to cover as much of the resection cavity as possible. Slight overlapping of the wafers is acceptable. Wafers broken in half may be used, but wafers broken in more than two pieces should be discarded in a biohazard container. Oxidized regenerated cellulose (Surgicel®) may be placed over the wafers to secure them against the cavity surface. After placement of the wafers, the resection cavity should be irrigated and the dura closed in a water tight fashion.

From the package information for Gliadel Water, MGI Pharma, 2005.

after carmustine treatment begins and lasts 1-2 wks.
- Leukopenia is evident 5-6 wks after treatment begins and lasts 1-2 wks. Anemia occurs less frequently and is less severe.
- Mild, reversible hepatotoxicity also occurs frequently.
- Prolonged high-dose carmustine therapy may produce impaired renal function.
- Prolonged high-dose carmustine therapy may produce pulmonary toxicity (pulmonary infiltrate or fibrosis).
- CNS toxicity of implant (seizures, brain edema, brain abscess/meningitis, obstructive hydrocephalus, etc.).
- Adverse reactions from Gliadel wafer are similar to those seen after IV administration.
- Healing at the site implantation is higher than that seen with placebo implantation.

Other Side Effects
Frequent (10%-50%):
Nausea and vomiting within minutes to 2 hrs after administration (may last up to 6 hrs).
Occasional (1%-10%):
Diarrhea, esophagitis, anorexia, dysphagia
Pulmonary toxicity: The onset may be several years after drug administration (even up to 17 years, but most conditions present between 1 and 4 years after therapy). High doses used in bone marrow transplantation (600-1200 mg/m² cumulative dose) are associated with a high incidence (9.5%) of fatal interstitial pneumonitis. Elderly patients (greater than 70 years) and patients between 31 and 50 years are at greater risk than others. Concurrent radiation therapy and preexisting lung disease also increases the risk. A baseline measurement of carbon monoxide diffusing capacity (DLCO) should be performed before the administration of carmustine. It is recommended that a CT scan of the chest be performed every 3 mos to monitor for toxicity. This can be done in conjunction with a CT scan used for assessing tumor response.
Rare (Less Than 1%):
Thrombophlebitis

SPECIAL CONSIDERATIONS
Baseline Assessment
- Monitor CBC with differential, electrolyte, BUN, and creatinine levels, pulmonary function tests, and liver function tests before each dose
- Evaluate patient for possible need of central venous access device as this agent can induce thrombophlebitis.

- Assess patient for any evidence of pulmonary or cardiac symptoms or visual or ocular changes.
Intervention and Evaluation
- Obtain CBC with differential, platelet count, electrolyte, BUN, and creatinine levels, and liver function tests before each dose.
- Perform pulmonary function tests every 3 months to assess DLCO. If DLCO is decreased by 25%, carmustine should be discontinued.
- Evaluate for signs and symptoms of neutropenia, thrombocytopenia, and anemia. Initiate neutropenic precautions as needed.
- Be aware that because carmustine contains 10% ethanol, rapid administration may cause flushing and hypotension. This can be controlled with further dilution in saline or D5W and infusion over 1-2 hours.
- Initiate neutropenic precautions.
- Initiate oral care regimen as necessary.
- Initiate skin care regimen as needed per institutional protocol after high-dose regimen.
- Premedicate with antiemetics as ordered.
- Assess patient for pulmonary symptoms of cough, shortness of breath, dyspnea, rales, or rhonchi.
- Obtain EKGs per institutional protocol when used as a preparative regimen for bone marrow transplantation.
- Assess for any cardiac symptoms, tachycardia, tachyarrhythmias, heart block, chest pain, or myocardial ischemia in receiving the high-dose regimen.
- Monitor for any signs of hepatic toxicity, right upper quadrant pain, nausea, vomiting, jaundice, or pruritus.
- Assess diarrhea and administer antidiarrheals as necessary.
- Obtain a nutrition consultation as needed.
- Monitor for any signs or symptoms of thrombophlebitis.
- Monitor for CNS toxicities and complications of craniotomy with implant.
Education
- Instruct patient on when to contact his or her health care provider fever greater than 38° C (greater than 101° F), chills, cough, shortness of breath, chest pain, nausea lasting greater than 24 hours, diarrhea lasting greater than 24 hours, or any evidence of infection or stomatitis.
- Instruct patient on neutropenic precautions:

Practice good handwashing techniques. Avoid all crowds and persons who are ill. Avoid salad bars in restaurants. Cook all foods well and avoid fresh fruits and vegetables while neutropenic.

- Educate patient not to take any new OTC medications or herbal or vitamin supplements without checking with his or her health care provider.
- Instruct patient on use of nutritional supplements for weight loss.
- Educate patient on an oral care regimen, including warm water rinses at least three times per day and at bedtime. A combination of 1 tsp baking soda and 1 tsp salt may be used to rinse the mouth.
- Instruct patient to avoid commercial mouth rinses and to use a soft bristle toothbrush.
- Educate patient to report any signs or symptoms of skin toxicity.
- Instruct patient to report any signs of visual changes.
- Provide patient with information on local resources and support groups available for his or her specific diagnosis.
- Be aware that carmustine is a teratogen and should be used with caution in women of childbearing age. Contraception is recommended during therapy.

CETUXIMAB

BRAND NAMES
Erbitux

CLASS OF AGENT
Monoclonal antibody, epidermal growth factor receptor (EGFR) inhibitor

CLINICAL PHARMACOLOGY
Mechanism of Action
Monoclonal antibody that binds specifically to the transmembrane epidermal growth factor receptor (EGFR, HER1,

or c-ErbB-1) on both normal and tumor cells that express the receptor. Binding of cetuximab to the EGFR blocks phosphorylation and activation of receptor-associated kinases, resulting in inhibition of cell growth, induction of apoptosis, and decreased matrix metalloproteinase and vascular endothelial growth factor production. EGFR is expressed on epithelial tissues, especially skin and hair follicles. **Therapeutic Effect:** Inhibits the growth and survival of tumor cells that overexpress EGFR.

Absorption and Distribution
Cetuximab is administered only by IV infusion. It reaches steady-state levels by the third wkly infusion. Clearance decreases as dose increases and is stable at doses greater than 200 mg/m^2. Volume of distribution for cetuximab appears to be independent of dose and approximates the vascular space of 2-3 L/m^2.
Half-life: Patients receiving 400 mg/m^2, followed by a 250 mg/m^2 maintenance dose, exhibited a half-life ranging from 3 to 7 days.

Metabolism and Excretion
Elimination of cetuximab is extensive and is via EGFR binding/internalization on hepatocytes and skin. Cetuximab metabolism is saturable.

HOW SUPPLIED/AVAILABLE FORMS
Injection: 2 mg/mL; 50-mL vials.

INDICATIONS AND DOSAGES
EGFR-Expressing Metastatic Colorectal Carcinoma in Combination with Irinotecan or Monotherapy in Patients Who Are Intolerant of Irinotecan-based Chemotherapy, Squamous Cell Cancer of the Head and Neck
In combination with radiation therapy for locally or regionally advanced disease. Or as monotherapy in patients in whom head and neck cancer has

CETUXIMAB DOSE MODIFICATION GUIDELINES

Severe Acneform Rash	Cetuximab	Outcome	Cetuximab Dose Modification
First occurrence	Delay infusion 1-2 wks	Improvement	Continue at 250 mg/m^2
		No improvement	Discontinue cetuximab
Second occurrence	Delay infusion 1-2 wks	Improvement	Reduce dose to 200 mg/m^2
		No improvement	Discontinue cetuximab
Third occurrence	Delay infusion 1-2 wks	Improvement	Reduce dose to 150 mg/m^2
		No improvement	Discontinue cetuximab
Fourth occurrence	Discontinue cetuximab		

From Product Information for Erbitux. Bristol-Myers Squibb, March 2006.

spread (metastasized) despite the use of standard chemotherapy.

Initially, 400 mg/m^2 IV as a loading dose. Maintenance 250 mg/m^2 IV infused over 60 mins wkly. Premedication with an H$_1$ antagonist (e.g., 50 mg of diphenhydramine IV) is recommended. Appropriate medical resources for the treatment of severe infusion reactions should be available during cetuximab infusions.

Dosage Modification for Dermatologic Reactions

Patients with a history of severe acneiform rash should have the dose of cetuximab reduced as shown.

Dosage Adjustment in Hepatic Dysfunction

No change necessary.

Dosage Adjustment in Renal Dysfunction

No change necessary.

UNLABELED USES

Metastatic colorectal carcinoma in EGFR-negative tumors by immunohistochemical analysis

PRECAUTIONS

Use cetuximab cautiously in patients with a hypersensitivity to murine proteins.

Pregnancy Risk Category: C

CONTRAINDICATIONS

None known.

DRUG PREPARATION/ADMINISTRATION/ SAFE HANDLING ISSUES

◀ ALERT ▶ Do not give cetuximab by IV push or bolus.

◀ ALERT ▶ When preparing this agent, use either nitrile or latex, but not vinyl, gloves.

◀ ALERT ▶ Premedicate the patient with 50 mg of diphenhydramine IV. Cetuximab may be used as monotherapy or in combination with irinotecan.

- The solution should appear clear and colorless; it may contain a small amount of visible white particulates.
- Do not shake or dilute the vials.
- Infuse the drug using a low protein-binding 0.22-micron in-line filter.
- Give the first dose as a 120-min IV infusion.
- Administer maintenance infusions over 60 mins. The maximum infusion rate is 5 mL/min.
- Flush the line with 0.9% NaCl.

STORAGE AND STABILITY

- Refrigerate vials at 2-8° C (36-46° F).
- Preparations in infusion containers are stable for up to 8 hrs at room temperature or 12 hrs if refrigerated. Discard any unused portion.
- Do not freeze.

INTERACTIONS

Drug

None known.

Herbal

None known.

LAB EFFECTS/INTERFERENCE

Hypomagnesemia occurred in 50% of patients during clinical studies (10%-15% severe). May decrease WBC count, Hct, Hgb level.

Y-SITE COMPATIBLES

No information

INCOMPATIBLES

No information

SIDE EFFECTS

Serious Reactions

- A severe infusion reaction, characterized by rapid onset of airway obstruction, a precipitous drop in B/P, and severe urticaria, occurs rarely.
- Dermatologic toxicity, pulmonary embolus, leukopenia, and renal failure occur rarely.

Other Side Effects

Frequent (10%-50%):

Acneiform rash, malaise, fever, nausea, diarrhea, constipation, headache, abdominal pain, anorexia, vomiting, hypomagnesemia, nail disorder, back pain, stomatitis, peripheral edema, pruritus, cough, insomnia

Occasional (1%-10%):

(9%-5%) Weight loss, depression, dyspepsia, conjunctivitis, hypersensitivity reactions (anaphylactoid-type), alopecia, hepatotoxicity, leukopenia and anemia

Rare (Less Than 1%):

Interstitial lung disease, renal dysfunction (in conjunction with irinotecan), myalgia, arthralgia

SPECIAL CONSIDERATIONS

Baseline Assessment

- Monitor patient' CBC with differential, platelet count, electrolyte, BUN, creati-

nine, and magnesium levels, and liver function tests.
- Assess patient for signs and symptoms of a skin reaction.
- Examine patient's nails on both hands and feet for any skin disorders.
- Assess the patient's pregnancy status.

Intervention and Evaluation
- Premedicate the patient as ordered to include antiemetics and diphenhydramine.
- Educate patient that if a reaction occurs he or she will need to be observed for at least 1 hour or longer after recovery from the reaction, which may prolong the time at the health care provider's office or clinic.
- Evaluate the CBC with differential, electrolyte, BUN, creatinine, and magnesium levels, and liver function tests before each dosing. It is very important to monitor magnesium levels on a regular basis as significant side effects have been reported with this agent when hypomagnesemia has occurred.
- Monitor patient for signs and symptoms of a hypersensitivity reaction, such as rapid onset of bronchospasm, hoarseness, hypotension, stridor, and urticaria during each treatment. Patients may experience their first severe infusion reaction during subsequent infusions. Patients who experience an infusion reaction must be observed for at least 1 hour after the reaction.
- Be sure an anaphylaxis kit is at bedside along with oxygen and an Ambu bag in the room. The anaphylaxis kit should contain the following:
  Diphenhydramine 50 mg
  Hydrocortisone 50 mg
  Epinephrine 1:1000 (1 mg/mL). Administer 0.3 mL IV and repeat as necessary.
  Syringes and needles
  2-by-2 gauze pads
  Alcohol wipes
- Assess patient's skin for evidence of dermatologic toxicity, such as dry skin, exfoliative dermatitis, or rash, and inflammatory sequelae.
- Monitor patient for signs and symptoms of pulmonary toxicity, rales, rhonchi, wheezing, and shortness of breath.

Education
- Instruct the patient on when to contact his or her health care provider: fever greater than 38° C (greater than 101° F), signs or symptoms of infection, sore

throat, cough, rigor, or chills. Make sure patient has a 24-hour number for the provider.
- Instruct patient to report signs and symptoms of skin toxicity and to initiate a skin care program as needed. Remind patient that this is not acne, so drying agents should not be used. Rather, moisturizers, such as Eucerin, Aquaphor, or Absorbase, should be used on skin rashes. Instruct patient that if rash becomes pustular either topical or oral antibiotics may be needed and to contact his or her health care provider. Instruct the family on the skin care program; a number of patients have stopped therapy because of skin reactions so make sure the family knows that the provider should be contacted for questions or concerns about skin reactions.
- Instruct patient to limit sun exposure and wear sunscreen when outdoors during cetuximab therapy because sunlight can exacerbate skin reactions.
- Educate patient to report any new pulmonary symptoms such as cough, shortness of breath, dyspnea, or wheezing and to contact his or her health care provider for new onset of any of the above symptoms.
- Educate patient about nail changes that can occur, including cracking of nail beds cracking, and to note bleeding or infections.
- Instruct patient to avoid taking any new medications, OTC preparations, or herbal or vitamin supplements without prior discussion with his or her health care provider.
- Instruct patient not to receive live-virus vaccinations and to avoid contact with crowds, persons with a known infection, and anyone who has recently received a live-virus vaccine.
- Instruct patient to avoid becoming pregnant during cetuximab therapy because of the potential of the drug to cause fetal harm.

Nursing Considerations
Skin care for dermatologic reactions:
- Wash thoroughly using a mild soap with the active agent pyrithione zinc.
- Use water-based creams, apply to ears and nose.
- Avoid sun exposure, use SPF 3-sunscreen.
- Use hypoallergenic makeup.

- Use nasal spray followed by petroleum jelly to reduce risk of nosebleeds.
- Use 12% Lac-Hydrin or other exfoliating lotions during the dry phase.
- Stay hydrated.
- Apply a zinc barrier to the rectal area after washing to reduce irritation, use some type of baby wipe to reduce irritation from toilet paper.
- Clean all skin folds carefully and monitor for infection in groin, and rectal areas.
- Use plenty of water-soluble lubricant for intercourse.
- Keep fingernails and toenails trimmed, apply liquid bandage for breaks.
- Avoid artificial nails.

CHLORAMBUCIL

BRAND NAMES
Leukeran

CLASS OF AGENT
Antineoplastic agent, alkylating agent

CLINICAL PHARMACOLOGY
Mechanism of Action
Forms covalent cross-links with DNA, thereby resulting in cytotoxic, mutagenic, and carcinogenic effects. The end result of the alkylation process is misreading of the DNA code and inhibition of DNA, RNA, and protein synthesis in rapidly proliferating tumor cells. Chlorambucil is cell cycle phase nonspecific. **Therapeutic Effect:** Interferes with nucleic acid function.
Absorption and Distribution
Rapidly and almost completely absorbed (70%-80%) from the GI tract. Protein binding: 99%. Taking chlorambucil with food significantly decreases its absorption to about 20%. Chlorambucil is widely distributed throughout the body
Half-life: 1.5 hrs; metabolite 2.5 hrs.
Metabolism and Excretion
Rapidly metabolized in the liver to the active metabolite, phenylacetic acid mustard. The parent compound and the metabolite spontaneously degrade to hydroxyl derivatives. Very little of the parent drug or active metabolite appears in the urine. Not removed by hemodialysis.

HOW SUPPLIED/AVAILABLE FORMS
Tablets: 2 mg.

INDICATIONS AND DOSAGES
Palliative Treatment of Advanced Hodgkin's Disease, Advanced Malignant (Non-Hodgkin's) Lymphoma (Including Giant Follicular Lymphoma and Lymphosarcoma), Chronic Lymphocytic Leukemia
For initial or short-course therapy, 0.1-0.2 mg/kg/day as a single or in divided doses for 3-6 wks (average dose, 4-10 mg/day). Alternatively, 0.4 mg/kg initially as a single daily dose every 2 wks and increased by 0.1 mg/kg every 2 wks until response and myelosuppression occur. Maintenance dose is 0.03-0.1 mg/kg/day (average dose, 2-4 mg/day).
Dosage Adjustment in Hepatic Dysfunction
No adjustments required.
Dosage Adjustment in Renal Dysfunction
No adjustments required.

UNLABELED USES
Treatment of hairy cell leukemia, nephrotic syndrome, ovarian or testicular carcinoma, polycythemia vera

PRECAUTIONS
Pregnancy Risk Category: D

CONTRAINDICATIONS
Previous allergic reaction or disease resistance to drug

DRUG PREPARATION/ADMINISTRATION/ SAFE HANDLING ISSUES
◀ ALERT ▶ The tablets should be handled with protective gloves.

STORAGE AND STABILITY
- Chlorambucil tablets (Leukeran) should be refrigerated at 2-8° C (36-46° F).
- Tablets can be stored at temperatures of up to 30° C (86° F) for up to 1 wk.

INTERACTIONS
Drug
Bone marrow depressants: May increase bone myelosuppression.
Live-virus vaccines: May potentiate viral replication, increase vaccine side effects and decrease the patient's antibody response to the vaccine.
Other immunosuppressants (including steroids): May increase the risk of infection or development of neoplasms.
Herbal
None known.

LAB EFFECTS/INTERFERENCE
May increase serum alkaline phosphatase, serum uric acid, AST (SGOT) levels.

SIDE EFFECTS
Serious Reactions
- Hematologic toxicity due to myelosuppression occurs frequently and may include neutropenia, leukopenia, progressive lymphopenia, anemia, and thrombocytopenia.
- Serious myelosuppression may occur if given within 4 wks of other chemotherapy or radiation.
- After discontinuation of short-course therapy, thrombocytopenia and leukopenia usually last for 1-2 wks but may persist for 3-4 wks.
- The neutrophil count may continue to decrease for up to 10 days after the last dose.
- Hematologic toxicity appears to be less severe with intermittent rather than continuous drug administration.
- Overdosage may produce seizures in children.
- Excessive serum uric acid level and hepatotoxicity occur rarely.
- Cross-hypersensitivity manifests as a rash with other alkylating agents, especially melphalan.
- Pulmonary fibrosis may occur after long-term therapy.

Other Side Effects
Frequent (10%-50%):
Myelosuppression, especially neutropenia that may last greater than 10 days, GI effects such as nausea, vomiting, anorexia, diarrhea, and abdominal distress (generally mild, lasting less than 24 hrs and occurring only if single dose exceeds 20 mg)
Occasional (1%-10%):
Rash or dermatitis, pruritus, cold sores
Rare (Less Than 1%):
Alopecia, urticaria, erythema, hyperuricemia, pulmonary fibrosis

SPECIAL CONSIDERATIONS
Baseline Assessment
- Obtain baseline CBC with differential, platelet count, electrolyte, BUN, and creatinine levels, and liver function tests.
- Assess for any history of seizures.
- Evaluate emetic history.
- Assess patient's ability to comply with oral medication regimen.

Intervention and Evaluation
- Monitor laboratory parameters at each visit: CBC with differential, platelet count, electrolyte, BUN, and creatinine levels, and liver function tests.
- Administer premedications for nausea as ordered.
- Monitor for any signs or symptoms of skin changes, rashes, or pruritus.
- Evaluate patient for compliance with oral medication regimen.
- Assess for alopecia.

Education
- Instruct patient on when to contact his or her health care provider: fever greater than 38° C (greater than 101° F), shaking, chills, nausea lasting greater than 24 hours, diarrhea lasting greater than 24 hours, or inability to take at least 1500 mL of fluid in 24 hours.
- Advise patient and caregiver to report any evidence of seizure-like activity.
- Educate patient that nausea may be an issue and to take antinausea medications as needed.
- Instruct patient that alopecia occurs rarely.
- Educate patient to use sunscreen as this agent may produce some photosensitivity.
- Advise patient to use moisturizers as rashes and pruritus have been noted with this agent.
- Instruct patient to avoid all OTC medications or herbal or vitamin supplements without first checking with his or her health care provider.
- Provide patient with information on local resources and support groups available for his or her specific diagnosis.

CISPLATIN
BRAND NAMES
Platinol-AQ

CLASS OF AGENT
Antineoplastic agent, alkylating agent

CLINICAL PHARMACOLOGY
Mechanism of Action
A platinum coordination complex that inhibits DNA and to a lesser extent, RNA, and protein synthesis by cross-linking with DNA strands to prevent cell division. It is cell cycle phase nonspecific.
Therapeutic Effect: Interferes with DNA function.

Absorption and Distribution
Rapidly and widely distributed into tissues. Protein binding: 90%.
Half-life: Initial excretion 20-40 mins; terminal half-life of total platinum is 5 days or longer.

Metabolism and Excretion
Undergoes rapid nonenzymatic conversion to inactive metabolite; covalently binds to glutathione and thiosulfate. Excreted in urine greater than 90%.

HOW SUPPLIED/AVAILABLE FORMS
Solution for Injection: 1 mg/mL as 50-mL, 100-mL, and 200-mL multidose vials.

INDICATIONS AND DOSAGES
Advanced Bladder Cancer, Metastatic Ovarian Cancer, Testicular Tumors
Daily for 5 days repeated every 3-4 wks: 20-30 mg/m^2/day IV
Every 3-4 wks: 50-100 mg/m^2 IV
Intraperitoneal: 100 mg/m^2 q3wk (Refer to ovarian cancer protocol)
Dosage Adjustment in Renal Dysfunction
Dosage is modified based on Ccr.

Ccr	Administer % of Dose
10-50 mL/min	50-75
>10 mL/min	50 or hold

UNLABELED USES
Breast, cervical, endometrial, gastric, head and neck, lung, and prostate carcinomas; germ cell tumors; neuroblastoma; osteosarcoma

PRECAUTIONS
Use cisplatin cautiously in patients with impaired renal function and those who have previously been treated with other antineoplastic agents or radiation. Age-related renal impairment may require a dosage adjustment in elderly patients. Patients should be adequately hydrated before and 24 hrs after administration. Ccr and serum electrolyte levels should be monitored.
Pregnancy Risk Category: D
Cisplatin may cause fetal harm when administered during pregnancy, especially in the first trimester. Patients taking this drug should not breast-feed.

CONTRAINDICATIONS
Hearing impairment, myelosuppression, severe renal dysfunction, pregnancy, hypersensitivity to cisplatin or any formulation components

DRUG PREPARATION/ADMINISTRATION/SAFE HANDLING ISSUES
◄ ALERT ► Verify any cisplatin dose exceeding 100 mg/m^2 per course. Cisplatin dosage is individualized on the basis of the patient's clinical response and tolerance of the drug's adverse effects. When administering this drug in combination therapy, consult specific protocols for optimum dosage and sequence of drug administration. Be aware that repeat courses should not be given more often than every 3-4 wks. Also, the course should not be repeated unless the patient's auditory acuity is WNL, serum creatinine is less than 1.5 mg/dL, BUN is less than 25 mg/dL, and platelet and WBC counts are within acceptable levels.
◄ ALERT ► Because cisplatin may be carcinogenic, mutagenic, or teratogenic, wear nitrile or latex, but not vinyl, gloves when handling the drug. If the drug comes in contact with skin, wash the skin thoroughly with soap and water; do not use antibacterial or waterless soap as either can enhance the skin reaction. If the drug comes in contact with mucous membranes, flush the area with copious amounts of water or 0.9% NaCl (NS).
• Cisplatin is considered an irritant; it may cause thrombophlebitis and tissue damage if infiltrated. Extravasation of cisplatin with a concentration less than 0.5 mg/mL may result in tissue necrosis, cellulitis, and fibrosis. Na thiosulfate is an antidote; consult institution policy guidelines.
• Cisplatin is stable in dextrose 5% (D5)-1/4NS, D51/2NS, D5NS, 1/4NS, 1/3NS, 1/2NS, and NS; it is not stable in Na bicarbonate 5%. Do not dilute in plain D5W.
• Prehydrate with 1-2 L of normal saline with or without a diuretic. Adequate hydration and urinary output (greater than 100 mL/hr) should be maintained for 24 hrs after administration.
• Infuse the solution over 1-24 hrs. Avoid rapid infusion less than 1 hr because this increases the risk of nephrotoxicity and ototoxicity.
• When given as a sequential infusion, administer a taxane derivative (e.g., paclitaxel or docetaxel) before cisplatin to limit myelosuppression.

- Monitor patient for an anaphylactic reaction during the first few minutes of the IV infusion.

STORAGE AND STABILITY
- Store intact amber vials at room temperature, 15-25° C (59-77° F) and protect from light.
- Do not refrigerate because precipitation may occur; precipitate may be dissolved without loss of potency by warming solution to 37° C or within hrs to days.
- In-use vials are stable up to 28 days if protected from light or up to 7 days if under fluorescent room light.

INTERACTIONS
Drug
Amifostine: Theoretically may reduce cytotoxicity of cisplatin to tumor cells. Studied in advanced ovarian cancer for the cytoprotective effect. Be cautious if using cisplatin as curative intent in other tumor settings.
Aminoglycosides: Aminoglycosides may cause cumulative renal toxicity.
Anticonvulsants: May reduce anticonvulsant (e.g., carbamazepine or phenytoin) levels. Monitor anticonvulsant plasma levels and adjust accordingly.
Antigout medications: May decrease the effects of these drugs.
Bleomycin: May reduce bleomycin clearance.
Bone marrow depressants: May increase myelosuppression.
Live virus vaccines: May potentiate viral replication, increase vaccine side effects, and decrease the patient's antibody response to the vaccine.
Loop diuretics: Concomitant use may cause additive ototoxicity.
Nephrotoxic, ototoxic medications: May increase the risk of nephrotoxicity or ototoxicity.
Rituximab: Concomitant use has resulted in severe renal toxicity.
Taxanes: Administer taxane before cisplatin in combination therapy to reduce myelosuppression.
Herbal
None known.

LAB EFFECTS/INTERFERENCE
May increase BUN and serum creatinine, uric acid, AST (SGOT) levels. May decrease Ccr and serum calcium, magnesium, phosphate, K, Na levels. May cause a positive Coombs' test result.

Y-SITE COMPATIBLES
Allopurinol, aztreonam, bleomycin (Blenoxane), cimetidine (Tagamet), cyclophosphamide (Cytoxan), cytarabine, dactinomycin, daunorubicin, dexamethasone, dexrazoxane, diphenhydramine, docetaxel, doxorubicin (Adriamycin), doxorubicin liposome (Doxil), droperidol, Etoposide (VePesid), famotidine (Pepcid), filgrastim (Neupogen), fludarabine, fluorouracil, furosemide (Lasix), gemcitabine, granisetron (Kytril), heparin, hydromorphone (Dilaudid), idarubicin, ifosfamide, lorazepam (Ativan), magnesium sulfate, mannitol, methotrexate, metoclopramide (Reglan), mitomycin, mitoxantrone, ondansetron (Zofran), paclitaxel, palonosetron (Aloxi), prochlorperazine (Compazine), sargramostim, trastuzumab, vinblastine (Velban), vincristine (Oncovin), vinorelbine (Navelbine)

INCOMPATIBLES
Amifostine (Ethyol), amphotericin B conventional, amphotericin B liposomal (AmBisome), amphotericin B colloidal (Amphotec), cefepime (Maxipime), dantrolene, diazepam, gallium nitrate, insulin (regular), lansoprazole, morphine, pantoprazole, piperacillin and tazobactam (Zosyn), thiotepa

SIDE EFFECTS
Serious Reactions
- An anaphylactic reaction manifested as angioedema, wheezing, tachycardia, and hypotension, may occur in the first few mins of IV administration in patients previously exposed to cisplatin. Use diphenhydramine 50-100 mg IV, hydrocortisone succinate 100 mg IV, epinephrine 1:1000 (1 mg/mL) 0.3 mL IV, albuterol inhaler 2-4 puffs, and oxygen as necessary. Rechallenge of cisplatin is not recommended for severe reactions. However, for patients with limited treatment options, several variations of platinum desensitization protocols described in the literature have successfully been used.
- Nephrotoxicity occurs in 28%-36% of patients treated with a single dose of cisplatin, usually during the second wk of therapy.
- Ototoxicity, including tinnitus and hearing loss, occurs in 31% of patients treated with a single dose of cisplatin. It may be more severe in children and may become more frequent or severe with repeated doses.

Other Side Effects
Frequent (10%-50%):
Electrolyte disturbances; elevation of liver enzymes, nausea, vomiting (greater than 50 mg/m^2: high emetic potential; may be acute and/or delayed); mild alopecia, myelosuppression (affecting 25%-30% of patients with recovery generally occurring in 18-23 days; nephrotoxicity; ototoxicity
Occasional (1%-10%):
Diarrhea; hyperuricemia; pain or redness at injection site; peripheral neuropathy (with prolonged therapy [4-7 mos]), loss of taste or appetite
Rare (Less Than 1%):
Anaphylactic reaction; arrhythmias; blurred vision, hemolytic anemia, stomatitis

SPECIAL CONSIDERATIONS
Baseline Assessment
- Monitor patient's CBC with differential, platelet count, electrolyte, BUN, creatinine, and magnesium levels, and liver function tests before each dose.
- Evaluate patient's Ccr before dosing.
- Monitor vital signs as well as oxygen saturation.
- Check hydration status before and after each dose to monitor urinary output both before and after each dose for 24 hours. If inadequate, i.e., less than 100 mL/hr, then diuresis may be required. Follow institutional protocol. This will decrease the risk of nephrotoxicity with this agent.
- Assess patient for any prior history of ototoxicity before the initial dose and before each subsequent dose.
- Evaluate for any signs or symptoms of peripheral neuropathy before each dose.

Intervention and Evaluation
- Premedicate patient with antiemetics at least 30 minutes before initiating this agent. If using aprepitant with dexamethasone, reduce steroid dose by 50% as steroid metabolism may be inhibited.
- Assess patient for episodes of nausea and maintain antiemetic therapy for 120 hours after receipt of this agent. Emesis has a bimodal peak with cisplatin, and patients will have severe emesis on day 1 if not appropriately premedicated with a serotonin antagonist, and the emesis will repeat at 48-72 hours. Make sure patient has appropriate antiemetics for treatment of both acute and delayed emesis.
- Provide hydration as ordered with at least 500 mL 0.9% NaCl.

- Monitor I&O at least every 4 hours or per institutional protocol. If urine output less than 100 mL every hour, contact the health care provider; diuretics may be required.
- Monitor vital signs every 4 hours during infusion, especially B/P, as hypotension can occur.
- Monitor BUN, creatinine, electrolyte, and magnesium levels daily if patient is receiving more than one dose of cisplatin and weekly as an outpatient. If patient has severe magnesium and K wasting, more frequent monitoring will be required.
- Assess patient's ability to maintain hydration status after completion of this agent; if patient is unable to take in at least 1500 mL of fluid in 24 hours, IV hydration may be required. Follow institutional guidelines.

Education
- Instruct patient to report any signs and symptoms of infection: fever greater than 38° C (greater than 101° F), chills, nausea lasting greater than 24 hours, diarrhea lasting greater than 24 hours, or inability to take in at least 1500 mL of fluid in 24 hours.
- Make sure patient has the 24-hour number to access his or her health care provider.
- Instruct patient on proper use of antiemetic medications.
- Educate patient to report any difficulty with passing urine or feelings of inability to keep self hydrated.
- Instruct patient on signs and symptoms of hypokalemia and hypomagnesemia such as weakness, feeling lightheaded, palpitations, and rapid heart rate.
- Instruct patient to report any signs or symptoms of high-pitched sounds, ringing or roaring in the ears, or significant hearing loss with the inability to hear or understand normal conversational tones.
- Advise patient to report any signs or symptoms of peripheral neuropathy: numbness, tingling in fingers or toes, loss of coordination, difficulty walking up stairs, or raising feet to meet the curb if walking outside the home.
- Urge the patient to avoid live-virus vaccinations while receiving this agent because cisplatin lowers the body's resistance.

OTHER INFORMATION
Do not confuse cisplatin with carboplatin or Platinol with Paraplatin or Patanol.

CLADRIBINE

BRAND NAMES
Leustatin

CLASS OF AGENT
Antineoplastic agent, antimetabolite

CLINICAL PHARMACOLOGY
Mechanism of Action
A synthetic purine nucleoside that disrupts cellular metabolism by incorporating into DNA. Intracellular accumulation of the active triphosphate deoxynucleotide form prevents cells from properly repairing single-strand DNA breaks. Cytotoxic to both actively dividing and quiescent lymphocytes and monocytes.
Therapeutic Effect: Prevents DNA synthesis and repair.
Absorption and Distribution
Extensively distributed into tissues. Crosses the blood-brain barrier. Protein binding: 20%. Volume of distribution = 9 L/kg.
Half-life: 5.4 hours.
Metabolism and Excretion
Metabolized in all cells with deoxycytidine kinase activity to the active triphosphate deoxynucleotide form. Primarily excreted in urine (18% excreted in 5-day continuous IV infusion of 3.5-8.1 mg/m^2/day).

HOW SUPPLIED/AVAILABLE FORMS
Injection: 1 mg/mL preservative-free single-use 10-mL vials.

INDICATIONS AND DOSAGES
Hairy Cell Leukemia
Single course of 0.09 mg/kg/day as continuous infusion for 7 days.
Dosage Adjustment in Hepatic/Renal Dysfunction
No recommendations available. Use with caution.

UNLABELED USES
Chronic lymphocytic leukemia, chronic myelogenous leukemia, cutaneous T-cell lymphoma, multiple sclerosis, non-Hodgkin's lymphoma

PRECAUTIONS
Use cautiously in patients with impaired liver or renal function and bone marrow suppression. Up to 70% of patients developed severe myelosuppression. Fever occurred in 69% of patients in the first month of treatment. Initiate empiric antibiotics as clinically indicated.

Pregnancy Risk Category: D
Cladribine may cause fetal harm in pregnant women. Excretion into human breast milk is unknown/not recommended.

CONTRAINDICATIONS
Hypersensitivity to cladribine or any of its formulation

DRUG PREPARATION/ADMINISTRATION/SAFE HANDLING ISSUES
◀ ALERT ▶ Because cladribine may be carcinogenic, mutagenic, or teratogenic, wear nitrile or latex, but not vinyl, gloves when handling the drug. If the drug comes in contact with skin, wash the skin thoroughly with soap and water. Do not use waterless hand soap or any antibacterial soap as either can increase the reaction from the agent. If the drug comes in contact with mucous membranes, flush the area with water.
- Must dilute before administration.
- Preparation of 24-hr dose: Add calculated dose (0.09 mg/kg) of cladribine to 500 mL of 0.9% NaCl. Infuse continuously over 24 hrs. Repeat daily for total of 7 consecutive days.
- Preparation of a 7-day infusion: Add calculated dose (7 days × 0.09 mg/kg/day) of cladribine to infusion reservoir using a 0.22-micron hydrophilic syringe filter. Add through filter the calculated amount of bacteriostatic 0.9% NaCl to make a total volume of 100 mL. Discard the used filter. Aseptically aspirate air bubbles from the reservoir with a new syringe and filter. Infuse continuously over 7 days. Use caution in patients weighing greater than 85 kg because of decreased effectiveness of the lower concentration of preservatives.

STORAGE AND STABILITY
- Refrigerate single-use unopened vials. Protect from light.
- Diluted solution is stable in polyvinyl chloride containers for 24 hours at room temperature and 7 days in Pharmacia Deltec cassettes.
- Precipitate may occur due to exposure to low temperatures; resolubilize by allowing solution to warm naturally to room temperature and by shaking vigorously. Do not heat or microwave solution.

INTERACTIONS
Drug
Bone marrow depressants: May increase bone marrow depression.
Live-virus vaccines: May potentiate virus replication, increase vaccine side effects, and decrease the patient's antibody response to vaccine.
Nephrotoxic, neurotoxic medications: May increase toxicity.
Herbal
None known.

LAB EFFECTS/INTERFERENCE
None known.

Y-SITE COMPATIBLES
Carboplatin, cisplatin, cyclophosphamide, cytarabine, dexamethasone, diphenhydramine, doxorubicin, granisetron, idarubicin, leucovorin, mannitol, mesna, methylprednisolone, mitoxantrone, ondansetron, paclitaxel, prochlorperazine, promethazine, teniposide, vincristine

INCOMPATIBLES
Do not mix with other IV drugs or additives; do not infuse concurrently via a common IV line. Avoid D5W (increases degradation of medication).

SIDE EFFECTS
Serious Reactions
- Myelosuppression characterized by severe neutropenia (less than 500 cells/mm^3), severe anemia (Hgb less than 8.5 g/dL), and thrombocytopenia occur commonly.
- High-dose treatment may produce acute nephrotoxicity and/or neurotoxicity manifested as irreversible motor weakness of upper or lower extremities. This is reported rarely with standard dose regimens.

Other Side Effects
Frequent (10%-50%):
Anemia, anorexia, fatigue, fever, headache, infection (6% were serious), injection site reactions, nausea (mild), neutropenia, rash, thrombocytopenia, vomiting
Occasional (1%-10%):
Abdominal/trunk pain, arthralgia, chills, constipation, cough, diaphoresis, diarrhea, dizziness, edema, epistaxis, erythema, insomnia, malaise, myalgia, petechiae, pruritus, purpura, shortness of breath, tachycardia
Rare (Less Than 1%):
Tumor lysis syndrome

SPECIAL CONSIDERATIONS
Baseline Assessment
- Monitor baseline CBC with differential, platelet count, electrolyte, BUN, creatinine levels, and liver function tests.
- Assess patient for any evidence of peripheral neuropathy.
- Evaluate patient for any prior history of renal disease.
- Check whether patient is allergic to benzyl alcohol if being treated with a 7-day continuous infusion.
Intervention and Evaluation
- Premedicate patient as ordered.
- Monitor CBC with differential and platelet count before and after therapy.
- Perform periodic liver and kidney function tests.
- Have anaphylaxis kit available at the bedside before administration of this agent. The kit should contain the following:
  Diphenhydramine 50 mg
  Hydrocortisone 50 mg
  Epinephrine 1:1000
  Syringes
  Needles
  2-by-2 gauze pads to break ampule of epinephrine
  Alcohol wipes
  Oxygen setup
  Ambu bag at bedside
- Monitor vital signs during infusion, especially during the first hour. Observe for hypotension or bradycardia (usually both do not occur during same course).
- Immediately discontinue administration if a severe hypersensitivity reaction occurs.
- Monitor temperature and report fever promptly. Fever occurred in up to 69% of patients during the first month of treatment; only one third had documented infection. Initiate empiric antibiotics as clinically indicated.
- Assess for signs of infection.
- Assess skin for evidence of rash or petechiae.
Education
- Instruct patient on when to contact his or her health care provider: fever greater than 38° C (greater than 101° F), chills, rigors, cough, shortness of breath, symptoms of infection, symptoms of bradycardia, or slowing of heart rate.
- Educate patient regarding neutropenic precautions and good handwashing techniques.

- Educate patient to perform oral hygiene at least three times per day.
- Advise patient to cook all foods and avoid raw food and salad bars if eating out.
- Instruct patient to avoid crowds and individuals with symptoms of colds or flu.
- Educate patient on symptoms of neurotoxicity: numbness and tingling in fingers and toes or pain in upper and lower extremities.
- Instruct patient to avoid immunizations without his or her physician's approval (drug lowers body's resistance).
- Tell patient to avoid contact with those who have recently received a live-virus vaccine.
- Instruct women of childbearing age not to become pregnant during treatment.
- Instruct men to use a condom while receiving this agent to prevent pregnancy in a partner.

CYCLOPHOSPHAMIDE

BRAND NAMES
Cytoxan (USA), Neosar, Procytox (Canada)

CLASS OF AGENT
Antineoplastic agent, alkylating agent

CLINICAL PHARMACOLOGY
Mechanism of Action
Active metabolites of cyclophosphamide covalently bind to the N-7 atom of purine bases, forming DNA adducts and cross-links, inducing programmed cell death. Thus, it is an alkylating agent that inhibits DNA and RNA-directed protein synthesis. It is cell cycle phase nonspecific. **Therapeutic Effect:** Cytotoxic antineoplastic; potent immunosuppressant.

Absorption and Distribution
After oral administration, 70%-75% of the drug is well absorbed from the GI tract. About 24% of the parent compound is bound to plasma proteins. V_d after oral administration is approximately 0.48 L/kg. V_d after IV administration ranges from 0.34 to 1.2 L/kg. Cyclophosphamide crosses the blood-brain barrier.
Half-life: After oral administration the elimination half-life of the parent compound ranges between 1.3 and 6.8 hrs. For the IV route, the half-life ranges from 4.1 to 16 hrs. The half-life for the

alkylating species, phosphoramide mustard and acrolein, when given by either route of administration ranges between 7.7 and 9.9 hrs. The 4-hydroxycyclophosphamide metabolite has a half-life ranging from 2.5 to 5.5 hrs.

Metabolism and Excretion
Cyclophosphamide is a prodrug that is converted by hepatic microsomal cytochrome P450 enzymes (CYP 2B6, 2C9, and 3A4) to the active metabolites aldophosphamide, 4-hydroxycyclophosphamide, phosphoramide mustard, and acrolein. Cyclophosphamide is metabolized in the liver to three inactive metabolites including 4-ketocyclophosphamide, carboxyphosphamide, and dechloroethylcyclophosphamide. Although the parent compound is excreted primarily in urine, it is avidly reabsorbed from the renal tubules, resulting in a large fraction of the drug being metabolized by the liver. The parent compound can be removed by hemodialysis.

HOW SUPPLIED/AVAILABLE FORMS
Tablets (Cytoxan): 25 mg, 50 mg.
Powder for Injection (Neosar): 100 mg, 200 mg.
Powder for Injection (Cytoxan, Neosar): 500 mg, 1 g, 2 g.

INDICATIONS AND DOSAGES
Ovarian Adenocarcinoma, Breast Carcinoma, Hodgkin's Disease, Non-Hodgkin's Lymphoma, Multiple Myeloma, Leukemia (Acute Lymphoblastic, Acute Myelogenous, Acute Monocytic, Chronic Granulocytic, Chronic Lymphocytic), Mycosis Fungoides, Disseminated Neuroblastoma, Retinoblastoma
Oral: In the treatment of cancer, oral doses of 400 mg/m^2/day on days 1-5 every 3-4 wks or 60-120 mg/m^2/day have been used. In breast cancer, the usual dose as part of the CMF (cyclophosphamide, methotrexate, and 5-fluorouracil) regimen is 100 mg/m^2/day for 14 days followed by 14 days of rest. In nonmalignant diseases such as cerebral vasculitis or Wegener's granulomatosis, the dose ranges from 1 to 5 mg/kg daily depending on disease severity. The dose is adjusted to disease response and neutropenia.
IV: In high-dose autologous or allogeneic transplants, the usual total dose ranges from 40 to 50 mg/kg in divided doses over 2-5 days. For a variety of solid tumors, the

dose ranges from 600 to 1,500 mg/m^2 repeated every 3 wks. There are several complex regimens for lymphoma and multiple myeloma. The reader is referred to the primary literature for details on dosing.

Dosage Adjustment in Hepatic Dysfunction
Because of the complexity of cyclophosphamide metabolism, toxicity, and pharmacologic effects, recommendations for dosage adjustment in the presence of hepatic failure have not been established. However, patients with hepatic failure develop more toxicity with cyclophosphamide than patients with normal hepatic function and should be monitored closely.

Dosage Adjustment in Renal Dysfunction
Guidelines for dose adjustment in patients with renal dysfunction have not been established. Micromedex recommends no dose adjustment for mild renal dysfunction (Ccr greater than 50 mL/min). However, patients with moderate renal failure (glomerular filtration rate [GFR] 10-50 mL/min) should receive 75% of the normal dose. Patients with severe renal failure (GFR less than 10 mL/min) should receive 50% of the normal dose. Other compendia suggest less conservative dose reductions or none at all.

UNLABELED USES
Treatment of carcinoma of bladder, cervix, endometrium, lung, prostate, or testicular cancer; germ cell ovarian tumors; osteosarcoma; rheumatoid arthritis; systemic lupus erythematosus

PRECAUTIONS
Pregnancy Risk Category: D

CONTRAINDICATIONS
Patients with severe bone marrow suppression or severe allergy to cyclophosphamide should not receive the drug.

DRUG PREPARATION/ADMINISTRATION/ SAFE HANDLING ISSUES
◀ ALERT ▶ Because cyclophosphamide may be carcinogenic, mutagenic, or teratogenic, wear nitrile or latex, but not vinyl, gloves when handling the drug for IV use. If the drug comes in contact with skin, wash the skin thoroughly with soap and water. Do not use waterless hand soap or any antibacterial soap as either can increase the reaction from the agent. If the drug comes in contact with mucous membranes, flush the area with water.

Lyophilized cyclophosphamide should be prepared for parenteral use by adding bacteriostatic water for injection, USP (paraben preserved only) or sterile water for injection, USP to the vial and shaking to dissolve. Use the quantity of diluent shown in the table to reconstitute the product to a final concentration of 20 mg/mL. Cyclophosphamide has been reconstituted using 0.9% NaCl and D5W solutions as well.

Dose Strength	Quantity of Diluent
100 mg	5 mL
200 mg	10 mL
500 mg	25 mL
1000 mg	50 mL
2000 mg	100 mL

STORAGE AND STABILITY
Storage of both the tablets and powder for injection at or less than 25° C (77° F) is recommended; this product will withstand brief exposure to temperatures up to 30° C (86° F) but should be protected from temperatures above 30° C (86° F). Reconstituted solutions are physically stable for up to 24 hrs at room temperature or for 6 days under refrigeration. It is recommended for the drug to be administered within 6 hrs if reconstituted with any solution other than bacteriostatic water for injection.

INTERACTIONS
Drug
Allopurinol: May increase levels of the cytotoxic metabolites of cyclophosphamide; monitor for increased adverse effects including bone marrow suppression.
Anthracyclines: May increase cardiotoxicity.
Bone marrow depressants: May increase myelosuppression.
CYP 2B6 and CYP 3A4 inhibitors: May decrease metabolism of cyclophosphamide or its metabolites.
CYP 2B6 and CYP 3A4 inducers: May increase metabolism of cyclophosphamide or its metabolites.
Immunosuppressants: May increase the risk of infection and development of neoplasms.
Live-virus vaccines: May potentiate virus replication, increase vaccine side effects, and decrease the patient's antibody response to the vaccine.

Neuromuscular blocking agents: May decrease levels of cholinesterase and prolong/potentiate effects of neuromuscular blocking agents such as succinylcholine.

Pentostatin: Fatal cardiac toxicity has been reported in a few patients receiving concurrent high-dose cyclophosphamide (total dose 6.4 g/m^2 over 4 days) and pentostatin (4 mg/m^2 over 4 hr on day 3).

Herbal

St John's Wort: This herbal product is a known inducer of cytochrome P450 metabolism. Drugs that are substrates for CYP2C9, 3A4, or 2D6 will be affected by St John's wort. It may increase the metabolism of cyclophosphamide or its metabolites, thereby decreasing their cytotoxic effects. Avoid use.

Food

Grapefruit inhibits CYP 3A4 enzymes and can potentially enhance cyclophosphamide effects.

LAB EFFECTS/INTERFERENCE

May increase serum uric acid levels.

Y-SITE COMPATIBLES

Allopurinol Na, amifostine, amikacin sulfate, ampicillin Na, amphotericin B liposomal (AmBisome), anidulafungin, azlocillin Na, aztreonam, bleomycin sulfate, cefamandole nafate, cefazolin Na, cefepime hydrochloride, cefoperazone, cefotaxime, cefoxitin, cefuroxime, chloramphenicol Na, chlorpromazine hydrochloride, cimetidine hydrochloride, cisplatin, cladribine, clindamycin phosphate, cytarabine, dactinomycin, daunorubicin hydrochloride, dexamethasone Na phosphate, doxorubicin hydrochloride, doxycycline hyclate, droperidol, epinephrine hydrochloride, epirubicin hydrochloride, erythromycin lactobionate, etoposide, etoposide phosphate, famotidine, filgrastim, fludarabine phosphate, fluorouracil, furosemide, gallium nitrate, ganciclovir Na, gatifloxacin, gemcitabine hydrochloride, gentamicin sulfate, granisetron hydrochloride (Kytril), heparin Na, hydromorphone hydrochloride (Dilaudid), idarubicin hydrochloride, kanamycin hydrochloride, lansoprazole, leucovorin calcium, levofloxacin, linezolid, lorazepam (Ativan), melphalan hydrochloride, methotrexate Na, methylprednisolone Na succinate, metoclopramide hydrochloride, metronidazole, minocycline hydrochloride,

mitomycin, mitoxantrone hydrochloride, morphine sulfate, nafcillin Na, ondansetron hydrochloride (Zofran), oxacillin Na, oxaliplatin, paclitaxel, pantoprazole Na, pemetrexed disodium, penicillin G K, piperacillin Na, piperacillin-tazobactam Na, prochlorperazine edisylate, promethazine hydrochloride, propofol (Diprivan), ranitidine hydrochloride, rituximab, sargramostim, Na acetate, Na bicarbonate, sulfamethoxazole-trimethoprim, teniposide, thiotepa, ticarcillin disodium, ticarcillin Na-clavulanate K, tobramycin sulfate, topotecan hydrochloride, trastuzumab, vancomycin hydrochloride, vinblastine sulfate vincristine sulfate, vinorelbine sulfate

INCOMPATIBLES

Amphotericin B colloidal (Amphotec), lansoprazole

ADVERSE REACTIONS
Serious Reactions

- The major toxic effect of cyclophosphamide is myelosuppression resulting in blood dyscrasias, such as leukopenia, anemia, thrombocytopenia, and hypoprothrombinemia.
- Expect leukopenia to resolve in 17-28 days. Anemia generally occurs after large doses or prolonged therapy. Thrombocytopenia may occur 10-15 days after drug initiation.
- Hemorrhagic cystitis occurs commonly in long-term therapy, especially in pediatric patients.
- Pulmonary fibrosis and cardiotoxicity have been noted with high doses. High cyclophosphamide concentrations may produce damage to cardiac muscle cells. In addition, cyclophosphamide has been reported to potentiate doxorubicin-induced cardiotoxicity.
- Amenorrhea, azoospermia, and hyperkalemia may also occur.

Other Side Effects
Frequent (10%-50%):

Acute and delayed nausea, vomiting (acute emesis begins about 6 hrs after administration), alopecia (33%), cervical dysplasia (16%), marked leukopenia/neutropenia 8-15 days after initial therapy

Occasional (1%-10%):

Diarrhea, darkening of skin and fingernails, stomatitis, headache, diaphoresis, hemorrhagic cystitis

Rare (Less Than 1%):
Pain or redness at injection site

SPECIAL CONSIDERATIONS
Baseline Assessment
- Evaluate CBC with differential, platelet count, electrolyte, BUN, and creatinine levels, and liver function tests.
- Evaluate the patient for any prior history of bladder problems, infections, dysuria, or recurrent urinary tract infections.
- Discuss fertility issues before high doses of this agent are given.

Intervention and Evaluation
- Monitor CBC with differential, platelet count, electrolyte, BUN, and creatinine levels, and liver function tests before each dose.
- Administer premedications for nausea and vomiting as ordered.
- Instruct patient to take all oral doses before 4 PM (1600 hours).
- Assess patient's ability to take in at least 2 L of fluid per day.
- Assess patient's ability to comply with voiding every 2 hours during the day and every 4 hours at night.
- Evaluate for any side effects post-treatment.
- Dipstick all urine for blood or send daily urinalysis for any high-dose therapy.
- Assess patients for signs and symptoms of infection, fever greater than 38° C (greater than 101° F), chills, fatigue, shortness of breath, dyspnea, or evidence of thrombocytopenia, petechiae, purpura, epistaxis, or bleeding from any sites.

Education
- Instruct patient on signs and symptoms of infection and when to contact health care provider: fever greater than 38° C (greater than 101° F), shaking, chills, fatigue, shortness of breath or difficulty breathing, hematuria, passing clots, or an inability to empty the bladder. Make sure patient has 24-hour number to contact his or her health care provider.
- Inform patient of signs and symptoms of thrombocytopenia: bleeding gums, epistaxis, easy bruising, petechiae, and ecchymoses.
- Instruct patient to drink at least 2 L of fluid per day and to limit the caffeinated products to no more than 16 oz per day.
- Instruct patient to void every 2 hours during the day and to get up at least once during the night or void every 4 hours at night.
- Instruct patient to take all oral doses of this agent before 4 PM (1600 hours).
- Provide patient with information on local resources and support groups available for his or her specific diagnosis.

CYTARABINE, CYTOSINE ARABINOSINE HYDROCHLORIDE
BRAND NAMES
Cytosar-U

CLASS OF AGENT
Antineoplastic agent, antimetabolite

CLINICAL PHARMACOLOGY
Gains entry into cells by a carrier process and then must be converted to its active compound, aracytidine triphosphate. Cytarabine is a purine analog and is incorporated into DNA; however, the primary action is inhibition of DNA polymerase, resulting in decreased DNA synthesis and repair. The degree of cytotoxicity correlates linearly with incorporation into DNA; therefore, incorporation into the DNA is responsible for drug activity and toxicity. Cytarabine is specific for the S phase of the cell cycle. **Therapeutic Effect:** Inhibition of DNA synthesis.
Absorption and Distribution
IM and subcutaneous routes result in considerably lower peak plasma levels. V_d: total body water. Cytarabine crosses blood-brain barrier with CSF levels of 40%-50% of plasma level.
Half-life: Initial: 7-20 mins; Terminal: 0.5-2.6 hrs
Metabolism and Excretion
Metabolism is primarily hepatic; aracytidine triphosphate is the active moiety. About 86%-96% of dose is metabolized to inactive uracil arabinoside. The drug is mostly excreted in urine (about 80% as metabolites) within 24-36 hrs.

HOW SUPPLIED/AVAILABLE FORMS
Injection, Powder for Reconstitution:
100 mg, 500 mg, 1 g, 2 g
Injection, Solution: 20 mg/mL (5 mL, 25 mL, 50 mL); 100 mg/mL (20 mL).

INDICATIONS AND DOSAGES
Acute Nonlymphocytic Leukemia, Acute Lymphocytic Leukemia, Chronic Myelocytic Leukemia, Meningeal Leukemia

IV bolus, IV piggyback, and continuous IV doses of cytarabine are very different. Bolus doses are relatively well tolerated because the drug is rapidly metabolized, but are associated with greater neurotoxicity. Continuous infusion uniformly results in myelosuppression. Refer to individual protocols. Dosages for adults are as follows.

Remission Induction

IV: 100-200 mg/m2/day for 5-10 days; a second course, beginning 2-4 wks after the initial therapy, may be required in some patients.

Intrathecal (IT): 5-75 mg/m2 every 2-7 days until CNS findings normalize or age-based dosing, or *less than 1 year:* 20 mg, *1-2 years*: 30 mg, *2-3 years:* 50 mg, *greater than 3 years:* 75 mg.

Remission Maintenance

IV: 7-20 mg/m^2/day for 2-5 days at mo intervals.

IM, Subcutaneous: 1-1.5 mg/kg single dose for maintenance at 1- to 4-wk intervals.

High-Dose Therapies

Doses as high as 1-3 g/m^2 have been used for refractory or secondary leukemias or refractory non-Hodgkin's lymphoma.

Doses of 1-3 g/m^2 every 12 hrs for up to 12 doses have been used in treating leukemias.

Bone marrow transplant conditioning chemotherapy: 1.5 g/m^2 continuous infusion over 48 hrs.

Dosage Adjustment in Hepatic Dysfunction

No specific recommendation guidelines available. Dose may need to be adjusted since cytarabine is partially detoxified in the liver.

Dosage Adjustment in Renal Dysfunction

Although there is no recommended guideline for cytarabine dosage adjustment in patients with renal failure, cytarabine must be used cautiously because renal dysfunction predisposes patients to neurotoxicity.

Hemodialysis: Supplemental dose is not necessary.

Peritoneal dialysis: Supplemental dose is not necessary.

UNLABELED USES

Malignant tumor of meninges, non-Hodgkin's lymphoma, neuroblastoma, retinoblastoma

PRECAUTIONS

IV doses of 1.5 g/m^2 may produce conjunctivitis that can be ameliorated with prophylactic use of corticosteroid (0.1% dexamethasone) eye drops. Dexamethasone 0.1% ophthalmic drops (or a comparable corticosteroid) should be administered at 1-2 drops every 6 hr during and for 2-7 days after cytarabine treatment. The risk of cerebellar toxicity increases with Ccr less than 60 mL/min, age older than 50 years, preexisting CNS lesion, and alkaline phosphatase levels exceeding 3 times the UNL. Use with caution in patients with impaired renal and hepatic function.

Pregnancy Risk Category: D

Cytarabine may cause fetal harm when administered during pregnancy with the greatest risk occurring in the first trimester. Drug excretion into human breast milk is unknown/not recommended.

CONTRAINDICATIONS

Hypersensitivity to cytarabine or any component of the formulation

DRUG PREPARATION/ADMINISTRATION/ SAFE HANDLING ISSUES

◀ **ALERT** ▶ Because cytarabine may be carcinogenic, mutagenic, or teratogenic, wear nitrile or latex, but not vinyl, gloves when handling the drug. If the drug comes in contact with skin, wash the skin thoroughly with soap and water. Do not use waterless hand soap or any antibacterial soap as either can increase the reaction from the agent. If the drug comes in contact with mucous membranes, flush the area with water.

- *IV:* Reconstitute powder with bacteriostatic water for injection.
- *IT:* Reconstitute with preservative-free saline or preservative-free lactated Ringer's solution.
- Solutions containing bacteriostatic agents should not be used for the preparation of either high doses or IT doses of cytarabine; they may be used for IM and subcutaneous doses and for low-dose (100-200 mg/m^2) IV solutions.
- Cytarabine can be administered IM, by IV infusion, IT, or subcutaneously at a concentration not to exceed 100 mg/mL.
- IV administration can be as a bolus, by IV piggyback (high doses of greater than 500 mg/m^2), or continuous IV infusion (doses of 100-200 mg/m^2).

- High-dose regimens are usually administered by IV infusion over 1-3 hrs or as a continuous IV infusion.

STORAGE AND STABILITY

Powder for reconstitution: Store intact vials of powder at room temperature, 15-30° C (59-86° F). Reconstituted solutions are stable for up to 8 days at room temperature. Solution: Before dilution, store at room temperature, 15-30° C (59-86° F); protect from light.

INTERACTIONS
Drug

Alkylating agents and radiation; purine analogs: Increased risk for toxicity.
Digoxin: Decreases digoxin oral tablet absorption.
Gentamicin, flucytosine: Decreased effect of gentamicin, flucytosine.
Methotrexate: When administered before cytarabine, may enhance the efficacy and toxicity of cytarabine. Some combination treatment regimens (e.g., hyper-CVAD [cyclophosphamide, vincristine, Adriamycin, and dexamethasone]) have been designed to take advantage of this interaction.
Herbal
No information.

LAB EFFECTS/INTERFERENCE

No information available.

Y-SITE COMPATIBILITIES

Amifostine, amsacrine, aztreonam, cefepime, chlorpromazine, cimetidine, cladribine, dexamethasone Na phosphate, diphenhydramine, doxorubicin liposome, droperidol, etoposide phosphate, famotidine, filgrastim, fludarabine, furosemide, gatifloxacin, gemcitabine, gentamicin, granisetron, hydrocortisone Na succinate, hydromorphone, idarubicin, linezolid, lorazepam, melphalan, methotrexate, metoclopramide, morphine, ondansetron, paclitaxel, piperacillin/tazobactam, prochlorperazine edisylate, promethazine, propofol, ranitidine, sargramostim, Na bicarbonate, teniposide, thiotepa, vinorelbine

INCOMPATIBLES

Allopurinol, fluorouracil, ganciclovir, heparin, insulin (regular), methylprednisolone Na succinate, nafcillin, oxacillin, penicillin G Na

SIDE EFFECTS
Serious Reactions

Symptoms of overdose include myelosuppression, megaloblastosis, nausea, vomiting, respiratory distress, and pulmonary edema. A syndrome of sudden respiratory distress progressing to pulmonary edema and cardiomegaly has been reported after high doses. Treatment is symptomatic and supportive.

Other Side Effects
Frequent (10%-50%):
CNS: Fever (greater than 80%)
Dermatologic: Alopecia
GI: Nausea, vomiting, diarrhea, mucositis. GI effects may be more pronounced with divided IV bolus doses than with continuous infusion.
Hematologic: Myelosuppression; neutropenia, and thrombocytopenia are severe; anemia may also occur.
Hepatic: Hepatic dysfunction, mild jaundice, transaminase levels increased (acute)
Ocular: Tearing, ocular pain, foreign body sensation, photophobia, and blurred vision may occur with high-dose therapy; ophthalmic corticosteroids usually prevent or relieve the condition.
Occasional (1%-10%):
CNS: Dizziness, headache, somnolence, confusion, malaise. A severe cerebellar toxicity occurs in about 8% of patients receiving a high dose (greater than 36-48 g/m^2/cycle); it is irreversible or fatal in about 1%.
Dermatologic: Skin freckling, itching, cellulitis at injection site. Rash, pain, erythema, and skin sloughing of the palmar and plantar surfaces may occur with high-dose therapy. Prophylactic topical steroids and/or skin moisturizers may be useful.
GU: Urinary retention
Neuromuscular and skeletal: Myalgia, bone pain
Respiratory: Syndrome of sudden respiratory distress, including tachypnea, hypoxemia, interstitial and alveolar infiltrates progressing to pulmonary edema, pneumonia
Rare (Less Than 1%):
Increases in amylase and lipase levels; isolated cases of pancreatitis; dysphagia (reported with intrathecal use); peripheral neuropathy, neuritis; accessory nerve paralysis (reported with intrathecal use); diplopia (reported with intrathecal use); cough, hoarseness (reported with intrathecal use); aphonia (reported with intrathecal use)

SPECIAL CONSIDERATIONS
Baseline Assessment
- Obtain baseline CBC with differential, platelet count, electrolyte, BUN, creatinine levels, and liver function tests.
- Evaluate for any signs and symptoms of prior cerebellar toxicities
- Assess patient's emetic history,

Intervention and Evaluation
- Administer premedications as ordered.
- Monitor for any signs and symptoms of cerebellar changes, altered finger to nose coordination, dysarthria, aphasia, or gait disturbances before each dose of medication greater than 750 mg/m^2.
- Monitor for signs and symptoms of mucositis. Initiate an oral care regimen consisting of salt and baking soda in 1 glass of water to swish and spit after each meal and at bedtime.
- Evaluate for any skin changes, including rashes or raised areas or blistering especially on the hands and feet. Initiate a skin care regimen if noted, including moisturizers to areas of erythema or silver sulfadiazine to areas of blisters if no allergy to sulfa products. Wrap open areas with soft gauze and pad feet if blisters occur so patient can maintain mobility.
- Evaluate patient for any signs or symptoms of mental status changes, confusion, disorientation, or hallucinations.
- Monitor for any respiratory changes during high-dose therapy.

Education
- Instruct patient to take antiemetics as ordered.
- Educate patient and caregiver on when to contact the primary care provider: fever greater than 30° C (greater than 101° F), shaking, chills, nausea lasting greater than 24 hours, diarrhea lasting greater than 24 hours, inability to take in at least 1500 mL of fluid within 24 hours, any mental status changes, or changes in coordination.
- Instruct patient that alopecia will occur with high-dose therapy and that will recover after 3-4 months, but texture and color may be different.
- Instruct patient on signs and symptoms of infection: any localizing signs of erythema or drainage.
- Educate patient regarding skin changes and advocate for the use of moisturizers and sunscreen as these drugs usually cause photosensitivity.
- Educate patient to report any signs or symptoms of respiratory changes, shortness of breath, cough, or dyspnea upon exertion.
- Instruct patient to use appropriate contraception while receiving this agent.
- Urge patients to avoid individuals who have received live-virus vaccines.
- Provide patient with information on local resources and support groups available for his or her specific diagnosis.

CYTARABINE, LIPOSOMAL

BRAND NAMES
DepoCyt

CLASS OF AGENT
Antimetabolite, antineoplastic agent

CLINICAL PHARMACOLOGY
Mechanism of Action
This is a sustained-release formulation of the active ingredient cytarabine. Cytarabine gains entry into cells by a carrier process and then must be converted to its active compound and incorporated into DNA; however, the primary action is inhibition of DNA polymerase resulting in decreased DNA synthesis and repair. The degree of its cytotoxicity correlates linearly with its incorporation into DNA; therefore, incorporation into the DNA is responsible for drug activity and toxicity. It is cell cycle specific for the S phase of cell division. **Therapeutic Effect:** Inhibition of DNA synthesis.

Absorption and Distribution
The drug distributes in CSF after intrathecal injection. Systemic exposure after intrathecal administration is negligible because the transfer rate from CSF to plasma is slow. *Half-life: CSF:* 100-263 hrs.

Metabolism and Excretion:
The drug is metabolized in plasma to ara-U (an inactive metabolite). It is cleared from CSF at a similar rate to the CSF bulk flow rate. The drug is primarily excreted in urine (as metabolite ara-U).

HOW SUPPLIED/AVAILABLE FORMS
Injection, Suspension: 10 mg/mL (5 mL) (preservative free).

INDICATIONS AND DOSAGES
Lymphomatous Meningitis
Induction: 50 mg intrathecally every 14 days for a total of 2 doses (wks 1 and 3).
Consolidation: 50 mg intrathecally every 14 days for 3 doses (wks 5, 7, and 9), followed by an additional dose at wk 13.
Maintenance: 50 mg intrathecally every 28 days for 4 doses (wks 17, 21, 25, and 29). If drug-related neurotoxicity develops, the dose should be reduced to 25 mg. If toxicity persists, treatment with liposomal cytarabine should be discontinued.
NOTE: Dexamethasone 4 mg twice daily (oral or IV) for 5 days should be started, beginning on the day of liposomal cytarabine injection.
Dosage Adjustment in Hepatic/Renal Dysfunction
No information available.

UNLABELED USES
No information available.

PRECAUTIONS
The incidence and severity of chemical arachnoiditis are reduced by coadministration with dexamethasone. The drug may cause neurotoxicity. Blockage to CSF flow may increase the risk of neurotoxicity. Safety and use in pediatric patients have been evaluated in limited studies.

CONTRAINDICATIONS
Hypersensitivity to cytarabine or any component of the formulation; active meningeal infection; pregnancy

DRUG PREPARATION/ADMINISTRATION/ SAFE HANDLING ISSUES
◀ ALERT ▶ For intrathecal use only. Dose should be removed from the vial immediately before administration (must be administered within 4 hrs of removal). An in-line filter should not be used. Vials are intended for a single use and contain no preservative. Administer directly into the CSF via an intraventricular reservoir or by direct injection into the lumbar sac. Injection should be made slowly (over 1-5 mins). Patients should lie flat for 1 hr after lumbar puncture. Patients should be monitored closely for immediate toxic reactions.
◀ ALERT ▶ Because liposomal cytarabine may be carcinogenic, mutagenic, or teratogenic, wear nitrile or latex, but not vinyl, gloves when handling the drug. If the drug comes in contact with skin, wash the skin thoroughly with soap and water. Do not use waterless hand soap or any antibacterial soap as either can increase the reaction from the agent. If the drug comes in contact with mucous membranes, flush the area with water.

STORAGE AND STABILITY
Store under refrigeration (2-8° C, 36-46° F); protect from freezing and avoid aggressive agitation. Unopened vials are stable at room temperature for up to 72 hrs. Suspensions should be used within 4 hrs of withdrawal from the vial. Particles may settle in diluent over time and may be resuspended by gentle agitation or inversion of the vial.

INTERACTIONS
Drug
No formal studies of interactions with other medications have been conducted. The limited systemic exposure minimizes the potential for interaction between liposomal cytarabine and other medications. Concomitant administration with other antineoplastics may increase the risk of neurotoxicity.
Herbal
No information available.

LAB EFFECTS/INTERFERENCE
Because cytarabine liposomes are similar in appearance to WBCs, care must be taken in interpreting CSF examinations in patients receiving liposomal cytarabine.

Y-SITE COMPATIBLES
No information available.

INCOMPATIBLES
No information available.

SIDE EFFECTS
Serious Reactions
Chemical arachnoiditis may be fatal if untreated. Symptoms include nausea, vomiting, headache, fever, neck rigidity, neck pain, meningismus, back pain, and CSF pleocytosis. No overdosage with liposomal cytarabine has been reported.
Other Side Effects
Frequent (10%-50%):
Confusion, fever, headache, nausea, pain, somnolence, vomiting

Occasional (1%-10%):
Abnormal gait, anemia, back pain, constipation, incontinence, neutropenia, peripheral edema, thrombocytopenia, weakness
Rare (Less Than 1%):
Anaphylaxis, neck pain

SPECIAL CONSIDERATIONS
Baseline Assessment
- Obtain baseline CBC with differential.
- Assess patient for prior neurotoxicity.
- Evaluate patient for any history of diabetes as this agent requires steroids to mitigate the arachnoiditis.
Intervention and Evaluation
- Monitor the patient's CBC with differential for signs of bone marrow depression.
- Premedication with steroids is required before administration of this agent and should be continued for 96 hrs after dosing.
- Make sure only intrathecal medication is at the bedside when delivering this agent to avoid errors.
- Monitor patient for signs or symptoms of thrombocytopenia: easy bruising, bleeding, and epistaxis.
- Assess patient for signs and symptoms of neutropenia: fever, fatigue, sore throat, or cough.
- Assess for neurotoxicity: numbness and tingling, paresthesia, dysesthesias, weakness, and fatigue.
- Evaluate blood glucose on a regular basis while patient is receiving steroids with this agent.
- Assess patient for any signs or symptoms of arachnoiditis, nuchal rigidity, headaches, pain, and changes in mental status.
Education
- Instruct patient on neutropenic precautions to prevent transmission of infection: good handwashing techniques, avoidance of raw or uncooked foods, washing all raw foods well, and cooking all vegetables.
- Instruct patient on when to contact his or her health care provider: fever greater than 38° C (greater than 101° F), fatigue, cough, shortness of breath, bleeding, easy bruising, and epistaxis.
- Educate patient on signs and symptoms of arachnoiditis: neck rigidity, headache, stiff neck, fatigue, and change in mental status.

- Advise patient on when to take steroids and how to take them; monitor for any GI changes or reflux.
- Stress to the patient that he or she should not receive live-virus vaccinations and should avoid crowds and contact with anyone who recently received a live-virus vaccine.
- Provide patient with information on local resources and support groups available for his or her specific diagnosis.

DACARBAZINE
BRAND NAMES
DTIC-Dome

CLASS OF AGENT
Antineoplastic agent, alkylating agent

CLINICAL PHARMACOLOGY
Mechanism of Action
Exact antitumor mechanism of action of dacarbazine is unknown. Presumably, it acts at multiple sites: (1) through inhibition of DNA synthesis (by acting as a purine analog), (2) through action as an alkylating agent attacking nucleophilic groups on DNA, and (3) through interaction with sulfhydryl groups. **Therapeutic Effect:** Inhibits DNA, RNA, and protein synthesis.
Absorption and Distribution
Dacarbazine is used intravenously. Its volume of distribution exceeds body water, suggesting that it enters several tissue compartment in the body, and ranges from 0.6 to 1.49 L/kg. About 15% of the drug crosses the blood-brain barrier. Protein binding: 5%.
Half-life: 5 hrs (increased in impaired renal function).
Metabolism and Excretion
Extensively metabolized in the liver to several metabolites including 5-aminoimidazole-4-carboxamide (inactive) and minor metabolites of adenine, hypoxanthine, xanthine, and uric acid. Extensive biliary excretion occurs. After drug administration, between 18 and 63% of the drug is excreted unchanged in the urine within 6 hrs.

HOW SUPPLIED/AVAILABLE FORMS
Powder for Injection: 100-mg vial, 200-mg vial, 500-mg vial.

INDICATIONS AND DOSAGES
Malignant Melanoma
2-4.5 mg/kg/day IV for 10 days, repeated every 4 wks; or 250 mg/m^2/day for 5 days, repeated every 3 wks.
Hodgkin's Disease
150 mg/m^2/day IV for 5 days, repeated q4wk; or 375 mg/m^2 once, repeated every 14 days (as combination therapy).
Dosage Adjustment in Hepatic Dysfunction
It is unknown to what extent the pharmacokinetic parameters of dacarbazine are altered in hepatic insufficiency. Therefore, specific dosing recommendations cannot be made. However, it is suggested that patients with hepatic insufficiency be carefully monitored.
Dosage Adjustment in Renal Dysfunction
Since a substantial amount an administered dose of dacarbazine is excreted in the urine, dosage adjustment in renal insufficiency may be warranted. No specific guidelines are published either in the literature or the product information.

UNLABELED USES
Treatment of islet cell carcinoma, soft-tissue sarcoma.

PRECAUTIONS
Pregnancy Risk Category: C

CONTRAINDICATIONS
Demonstrated hypersensitivity to dacarbazine

DRUG PREPARATION/ADMINISTRATION/ SAFE HANDLING ISSUES
◀ ALERT ▶ When preparing this agent, use of nitrile or latex gloves for drug preparation is recommended. If a splash occurs, use mild soap and water to wash area. Do not use antibacterial or waterless soap, as this will increase the skin reaction. If an eye splash occurs, rinse with copious amounts of water or 0.9% NaCl.

STORAGE AND STABILITY
- The vials of dacarbazine should be stored in the refrigerator, 2-8° C (36-46° F).
- Solution remaining in the vial after reconstitution may be stored at 4° C (39° F) for up to 72 hrs. At normal room temperature and lighting, the reconstituted solution is good for up to 8 hrs.
- Decomposition of reconstituted solution is detected by a change of color from normal pale yellow to pink.

- Solutions of dacarbazine (after reconstitution) that are diluted further with 50-100 mL of D5W or 0.9% NaCl remain stable under refrigeration (4° C, 39° F) and protected from light for up to 24 hrs. Solutions stored at room temperature under normal conditions are good for 8 hrs.

INTERACTIONS
Drug
Aldesleukin: Increased risk for hypersensitivity reactions (erythema, pruritus, hypotension) within hrs of the combination.
Clinical Management: Patients should be monitored for signs and symptoms of hypersensitivity reactions with concomitant use of dacarbazine agents and aldesleukin. Medical intervention for severe hypotension may be required.
Bone marrow depressants: May enhance myelosuppression.
Cytochrome P450 (CYP) 1A2 and CYP 2E1 inhibitors: May increase levels of dacarbazine and increase toxicity.
CYP 1A2 and CYP 2E1 inducers: May decrease levels of dacarbazine and reduce its efficacy
Live virus vaccines: May potentiate virus replication, increase vaccine side effects, and decrease the patient's antibody response to the vaccine.
Herbal
None known.

LAB EFFECTS/INTERFERENCE
May increase BUN, serum alkaline phosphatase, AST (SGOT), and ALT (SGPT) levels.

Y-SITE COMPATIBLES
Amifostine, aztreonam, docetaxel, doxorubicin HCl liposome injection, etoposide phosphate, filgrastim, fludarabine phosphate, granisetron HCl, melphalan HCl, ondansetron HCl, paclitaxel, sargramostim, teniposide, thiotepa, vinorelbine tartrate

INCOMPATIBLES
Allopurinol (Aloprim), amphotericin B liposomal (AmBisome), cefepime (Maxipime), heparin, hydrocortisone, pantoprazole, pemetrexed, piperacillin, tazobactam (Zosyn)

SIDE EFFECTS
Serious Reactions
- Myelosuppression may result in blood dyscrasias, such as leukopenia and

thrombocytopenia, generally 2-4 wks
after the last dacarbazine dose.
- Hepatotoxicity including the liver
  necrosis.

Other Side Effects
Frequent (10%-50%):
(90%) Nausea, vomiting, anorexia (occurs
within 1 hr of initial dose; may last up to
12 hrs)
Occasional (1%-10%):
Facial flushing, paresthesia, alopecia,
flu-like symptoms (fever, myalgia, malaise),
dermatologic reactions, confusion, blurred
vision, headache, lethargy
Rare (Less Than 1%):
Diarrhea, stomatitis, photosensitivity,
hepatic necrosis, CNS events such as severe
dementia or seizures, and cardiovascular
effects including hypotension and EKG
abnormalities

SPECIAL CONSIDERATIONS
Baseline Assessment
- Obtain baseline CBC with differential,
  electrolyte, BUN, creatinine, and magnesium levels, and liver function tests.
- Assess patient for central venous access
  as this agent is an irritant and can induce
  significant pain upon infusion. It is
  classified as an irritant not a vesicant.
Intervention and Evaluation
- Evaluate CBC with differential, platelet
  count, electrolyte, BUN, creatinine, and
  magnesium levels, and liver function tests
  before each dose.
- Premedicate patient with a serotonin
  antagonist as ordered; patients who have
  anticipatory nausea should receive an
  anxiolytic such as lorazepam.
- Monitor baseline vital signs.
- Evaluate for signs and symptoms of
  pancytopenia.
- Assess for signs and symptoms of infection, fever greater than 38° C (greater than
  101° F), chills, rigors, fatigue, evidence of
  thrombocytopenia (increased bruising,
  epistaxis, and ecchymotic areas) and any
  evidence of bleeding.
- Monitor for signs of prolonged neutropenia and thrombocytopenia occurring
  2-4 weeks after the last dose has been
  given
- Monitor for signs and symptoms of allergic reactions; have an emergency kit
  available at bedside along with an oxygen
  setup and Ambu bag. Anaphylaxis kit
  should include the following:

Diphenhydramine 50 mg
Hydrocortisone 50 mg
Epinephrine 1:1000 mg, use 0.3 mg IV
    and repeat as necessary
Syringes and needles
Alcohol wipes

Education
- Educate patient on when to contact
  health care provider: fever greater than
  38° C (greater than 101° F), shaking,
  chills, nausea lasting for greater than
  24 hours, diarrhea lasting for greater
  than 24 hours, or the inability to drink
  at least 1500 mL fluid in 24 hours.
- Instruct patient on continuing antiemetic
  dosing.
- Instruct patient that alopecia is a usual
  side effect of this agent; although the hair
  will usually grow back, color and consistency may be different when it returns.
- Advise patient of other common side
  effects such as facial flushing, skin rashes,
  and flu-like symptoms such as fever,
  myalgias, and arthralgias.
- If this agent has been given via a peripheral vein, give information on possibility
  of irritation occurring at venipuncture site.
  If erythema develops, instruct patient to
  use warm compresses on the area and
  notify health care provider if pain or erythema does not resolve within 24-48 hours.
- Instruct patient to use sunscreen (at least
  SPF greater than 15) as photosensitivity
  can occur with this agent.
- Educate patient on neutropenic precautions
  as necessary:
    Practice good handwashing technique.
    Avoid individuals who are ill.
    Wash and cook all foods well.
    Avoid crowds.
    Avoid fresh fruits and vegetables.
- Educate patient on thrombocytopenic
  precautions:
    Use of a soft bristle toothbrush.
    No flossing if platelet count is less than
        50,000/mm^3.
    No IM injections.
    No rectal suppositories.
    No aerobic exercise.
- Instruct patient to take no over-the-counter
  medications or herbal or vitamin supplements without checking with his or her
  health care provider.
- Educate patient on available local
  resources and advise of support groups
  available for the patient's specific
  malignancy.

DACTINOMYCIN

BRAND NAMES
Cosmegen

CLASS OF AGENT
Antitumor antibiotic

CLINICAL PHARMACOLOGY
Mechanism of Action
Antibiotic obtained from cultures of *Streptomyces parvulus*. It acts by forming complexes with DNA and selectively inhibiting the DNA-directed synthesis of RNA. Dactinomycin is thought to inhibit protein synthesis by inhibiting the synthesis of messenger RNA. Dactinomycin inhibits DNA synthesis but in much higher concentrations than are required to inhibit RNA synthesis. Cell cycle phase-nonspecific agent. **Therapeutic Effect:** Inhibits DNA-dependent RNA synthesis.
Absorption and Distribution
Administered via IV. It is extensively distributed into leukocytes, granulocytes, and several tissue types. Dactinomycin is concentrated in nucleated cells, with poor penetration into RBCs and cerebrospinal fluid; concentrations are higher in bone marrow and tumor cells than in plasma. Dactinomycin does not cross blood-brain barrier. *Half-life:* 36 hrs.
Metabolism and Excretion
Dactinomycin is minimally metabolized. About 30% of the drug has been recovered in the urine and feces 1 wk after administration. Biliary excretion accounts for 50-90% of drug elimination.

HOW SUPPLIED/AVAILABLE FORMS
Powder for Injection: 500 mcg

INDICATIONS AND DOSAGES
Ewing's Sarcoma, Childhood Rhabdomyosarcoma, Wilms' Tumor
15 mcg/kg/day IV for 5 days (in combination with other chemotherapy).
Gestational Trophoblastic Neoplasia
12 mcg/kg/day IV for 5 days as a single agent or 500 mcg on days 1 and 2 in combination with etoposide, methotrexate, folinic acid, vincristine, cyclophosphamide, and cisplatin.
Metastatic Nonseminomatous Testicular Carcinoma
1000 mcg/m^2 IV on day 1 in combination with cyclophosphamide, bleomycin, vinblastine, and cisplatin.

Regional Perfusion in Solid Malignancies
50 mcg/kg of body weight for lower extremities/pelvis; 35 mcg/kg of body weight for upper extremities.
Dosage Adjustment in Hepatic Dysfunction
Dactinomycin has not been studied in the setting of hepatic dysfunction. The drug should be used with caution in patients with elevated liver function tests.
Dosage Adjustment in Renal Dysfunction
Dactinomycin has not been studied in the setting of renal dysfunction. The drug should be used with caution in patients with severe renal failure.

UNLABELED USES
Childhood germ cell tumors, endodermal sinus tumors, melanoma, ovarian carcinoma

PRECAUTIONS
Use cautiously within the first 2 mos of radiation therapy.
Pregnancy Risk Category: D

CONTRAINDICATIONS
Do not give dactinomycin at or around the time of chickenpox or herpes zoster infection or exacerbation.

DRUG PREPARATION/ADMINISTRATION/ SAFE HANDLING ISSUES
◀ ALERT ▶ Know that dosage is individualized based on clinical response and tolerance to adverse effects. When used in combination therapy, consult specific protocols for optimum dosage and sequence of drug administration. The dose intensity per 2-wk cycle should not exceed 15 mcg/kg/day for 5 days or 400-600 mcg/m^2/day for 5 days. Dosage for obese or edematous patients is based on surface area. Repeat dosage at least at 3-wk intervals, provided all signs of toxicity have disappeared.
◀ ALERT ▶ The use of nitrile or powderless latex gloves when handling and preparing drug is recommended. The drug may be carcinogenic, mutagenic, or teratogenic. Handle with extreme care during preparation/ administration. If a splash occurs, wash with mild soap and water; do not use antibacterial or waterless soap as either can enhance skin reaction. If an eye splash occurs, use only water or 0.9% NaCl to copiously flush eyes. Flushing should be done from inner to outer canthus.
• Prepare solution immediately before use.
• Discard unused portion.
• Solution should be clear or gold.

- Reconstitute a 500-mcg vial with 1.1 mL of sterile water for injection without preservative (avoids precipitate) to provide concentration of 500 mcg/mL.
- Infuse over 15 min.
- Extravasation usually but not necessarily produces immediate pain and severe local tissue damage. Aspirate as much infiltrated drug as possible; then apply cold compresses.

STORAGE AND STABILITY

- Store unopened vials of dactinomycin at controlled room temperature, 15-30° C (59-86° F). Protect from light, humidity, and excessive heat.
- Unused portions of reconstituted solutions should be discarded.
- Dextrose 5% in water and 0.9% NaCl (without preservatives) can be used as diluents for the reconstituted drug.
- Dactinomycin (9.8 mcg/mL) is stable for at least 24 hrs at room temperature (less than 10% decrease in potency) in D5W (glass and polyvinyl chloride containers).

INTERACTIONS
Drug
Live-virus vaccines: May potentiate viral replication, increase vaccine side effects, and decrease the patient's antibody response to the vaccine.
Herbal
None known.

LAB EFFECTS/INTERFERENCE
May increase uric acid level. May interfere with antibiotic drug level assays. May worsen liver and renal function tests.

Y-SITE COMPATIBLES
Acyclovir, allopurinol, Amifostine, Amphotericin B colloidal (Amphotec), amphotericin B liposome (AmBisome), cisplatin, cyclophosphamide, cyclosporine, daunorubicin, dexamethasone, dexrazoxane, diphenhydramine, docetaxel, etoposide, gemcitabine, granisetron, heparin, hydrocortisone, idarubicin, ifosfamide, leucovorin, melphalan, mesna, methotrexate, methylprednisolone, mitomycin, mitoxantrone, ondansetron, oxaliplatin, paclitaxel, palonosetron, pemetrexed, rituximab, sargramostim, tacrolimus, teniposide, thiotepa, trastuzumab, vinblastine, vincristine, vinorelbine

INCOMPATIBLES
Dantrolene, diazepam, filgrastim, indomethacin, pantoprazole, phenytoin, riboflavin

SIDE EFFECTS
Serious Reactions

- Hematologic toxicity: Myelosuppression is one of the major and dose-limiting adverse effects of dactinomycin and is manifested primarily by leukopenia and thrombocytopenia. Anemia, pancytopenia, reticulopenia, agranulocytosis, and aplastic anemia may also occur. Myelosuppression, which is often first manifested by a decrease in the platelet count, usually occurs 1-7 days after completion of a course of therapy with dactinomycin. Leukocyte and platelet nadirs generally occur 14-21 days after completion of a course of therapy, and leukocyte and platelet counts usually return to normal levels within 21-25 days. The patient's hematologic status must be carefully monitored. If severe myelosuppression develops in patients receiving dactinomycin, particularly when used in combination with other antineoplastic agents, therapy must be discontinued until these adverse effects have resolved.
- GIand oral mucosal effects: The other major and dose-limiting adverse effects of dactinomycin are GI and oral mucosal toxicities. Severe oropharyngeal mucositis has occurred in patients receiving dactinomycin and radiation therapy directed to the nasopharynx. Nausea and vomiting usually occur within a few hrs after administration of the drug and can last up to 24 hrs. Antiemetics may be effective in preventing or treating nausea and vomiting. Anorexia, abdominal pain, diarrhea, proctitis, and GI ulceration may also occur. Stomatitis, cheilitis, glossitis, dysphagia, and oral ulceration occur often in patients receiving dactinomycin; esophagitis and pharyngitis may also occur. If stomatitis or diarrhea develops in patients receiving dactinomycin, particularly when used in combination with other antineoplastic agents, therapy must be discontinued until these symptoms have subsided.
- Radiation effects: Dactinomycin appears to potentiate the effects of radiation therapy. In patients treated with radiation therapy and dactinomycin, erythema occurs early in normal skin and buccal and pharyngeal mucosa. Erythema at the site of irradiation may be followed rapidly by

hyperpigmentation and/or edema, desquamation, vesiculation, and rarely necrosis. Radiation myelitis has also been associated with the drug. Dactinomycin may reactivate these effects in previously irradiated tissues, especially if the interval between radiation therapy and administration of the drug is brief; however, these effects may recur even if dactinomycin is administered mos after radiation therapy. Reactivation of radiation enteritis by dactinomycin has also been reported. If radiation therapy encompasses regions containing mucous membranes, severe reactions may occur if high doses of both dactinomycin and radiation are used or if the patient is especially sensitive to such combination therapy.

Dactinomycin should be administered with particular caution in the first 2 mos after radiation therapy in patients treated for right-sided Wilms' tumor, because hepatomegaly, elevated serum AST (SGOT) concentrations, and ascites have reportedly occurred in some of these patients. Dactinomycin generally should not be administered concomitantly with radiation therapy in the treatment of Wilms' tumor unless the benefit outweighs the risk.

Increased incidence of GI toxicity and myelosuppression has also been reported with concurrent administration of dactinomycin and radiation therapy.

- Local effects: Pain and erythema may occur at the injection site. Extravasation of dactinomycin can produce severe local tissue damage, necrosis, cellulitis, phlebitis, and inflammation and, in at least one patient, has led to contracture of the arms. Epidermolysis, erythema, and edema, sometimes severe, have been reported with regional limb perfusion. Extravasation is usually accompanied by immediate pain. However, extravasation may occur with or without an accompanying burning or stinging sensation, even if blood returns well on aspiration of the infusion needle. If any signs or symptoms of extravasation occur, the injection or infusion should be terminated immediately and restarted in another vein. If extravasation is suspected, intermittent application of ice to the affected area for 15 min 4 times daily for 3 days may be helpful. The benefit of locally administered drugs has not been clearly established. Because of the progressive nature of extravasation reactions, close observation and plastic surgery consultation are recommended. The occurrence of blistering, ulceration, and/or persistent pain indicate the need for wide excision surgery followed by split-thickness skin grafting.

- Hepatic effects: Hepatotoxicity, including ascites, hepatomegaly, hepatic veno-occlusive disease, hepatitis, and liver function test abnormalities, has been reported in patients receiving dactinomycin.

- Congestive heart failure: Dactinomycin has also been associated with exacerbation of CHF in one patient with doxorubicin-induced cardiomyopathy.

Other Side Effects

Frequent (10%-50%):
Nausea, vomiting, buccal/pharyngeal/skin erythema, rash (particularly when combined with radiation), lethargy, malaise, fatigue, and fever

Occasional (1%-10%):
Anorexia, alopecia, abdominal distress, myalgia

Rare (Less Than 1%):
Hepatitis, hepatic failure, hepatic veno-occlusive disease, and pneumonitis are rare

SPECIAL CONSIDERATIONS

Baseline Assessment

- Obtain baseline laboratory CBC with differential, platelets, electrolytes, BUN, creatinine, and liver function tests.
- Assess GI status and history of significant emesis with prior agents.
- Evaluate oral cavity as this agent can induce significant mucositis.
- Assess for need of venous access device as this agent is a vesicant.

Intervention and Evaluation

- Obtain CBC with differential and platelet counts daily during therapy and for 2 weeks after a course of therapy.
- Monitor renal and hepatic function before each dose.
- Assess pattern of daily bowel activity and stool consistency.
- Monitor for signs or symptoms of pancytopenia, anemia, thrombocytopenia, or neutropenia.
- Evaluate venous access.
- Administer premedications for nausea.

Education
• Instruct patient on when to contact health care provider: fever greater than 38° C (greater than 101° F), chills, epistaxis, easy bruising, bleeding, nausea lasting greater than 24 hours, diarrhea lasting greater than 24 hours, or inability to consume at least 1500 mL of fluid in 24 hours.
• Educate patient to continue taking antiemetics as directed.
• Advise patient to immediately report any signs or symptoms of erythema, pain, or edema at injection site.
• Instruct patient that alopecia occurs with this agent and that the hair may grow back after a few mos off therapy, although color and texture may be different.
• Educate patient on neutropenic precautions as necessary:
    Practice good handwashing technique.
    Avoid individuals who are ill.
    Wash and cook all foods well.
    Avoid crowds.
    Avoid fresh fruits and vegetables.
• Educate patient on available local resources and support groups available related to their particular diagnosis.
• Instruct the patient not to have immunizations without physician's approval (drug lowers body's resistance).
• Instruct patient to take no over-the-counter medications or herbal or vitamin supplements without checking with his or her health care provider.
• Advise the patient to avoid contact with those who have recently received a live-virus vaccine.

DARBEPOETIN ALFA
BRAND NAMES
Aranesp

CLASS OF AGENT
Growth factor, colony-stimulating factor; recombinant human erythropoietin

CLINICAL PHARMACOLOGY
Mechanism of Action
Induces erythropoiesis by stimulating the division and differentiation of committed erythroid progenitor cells; induces the release of reticulocytes from the bone marrow into the bloodstream, where they mature to erythrocytes. **Therapeutic Effect:** Stimulates RBC production and improves anemia.

Absorption and Distribution
Slow absorption after subcutaneous injection. Bioavailability = 37% in chronic renal failure patients. Volume of distribution = 52 mL/kg (IV). *Half-life:* Chronic renal failure patients: subcutaneous: 48.5 hrs. IV: 21 hrs.
Metabolism and Excretion
Minimal renal excretion.

HOW SUPPLIED/AVAILABLE FORMS
Vials and Prefilled Syringes: 25 mcg/mL, 40 mcg/mL, 60 mcg/mL, 100 mcg/mL, 150 mcg/mL, 200 mcg/mL, 300 mcg/mL, 500 mcg/mL.

INDICATIONS AND DOSAGES
Anemia in Chronic Renal Failure
IV bolus, subcutaneous: 0.45 mcg/kg once wkly.
Titration: Increases in dose should not be made more frequently than once a mo. If the Hgb is increasing and approaching 12 g/dL, the dose may be reduced by approximately 25%. If the Hgb continues to increase to greater than 12 g/dL, the drug should be temporarily withheld until the Hgb begins to decrease, at which point therapy should be reinitiated at a dose approximately 25% below the previous dose. If the Hgb increases by more than 1 g/dL in a 2-wk period, the dose should be decreased by approximately 25%. The dose should be adjusted for each patient to achieve and maintain a target Hgb not to exceed 12 g/dL.
Anemia Associated with Chemotherapy
Subcutaneous: 2.25 mcg/kg/dose every week or every 3 weeks in 500 mcg as a subcutaneous injection. Alternatively, it may be given in doses of 100 mcg qwk, 200 mcg q2wk, or 300 mcg q3wk.
Titration: The dose should be adjusted for each patient to achieve and maintain a target Hgb. For wkly administration, if the increase in Hgb is less than 1 g/dL after 6 wks of therapy, the dose should be increased up to 4.5 mcg/kg. If there is no response after 12 wks of therapy, consider patient darbepoetin alfa failure and discontinue therapy. If Hgb increases by greater than 1 g/dL in a 2-wk period or if the Hgb is greater than 11 g/dL, the dose should be reduced by 40% of the previous dose. If the Hgb is greater than 13 g/dL, doses should be temporarily withheld

until the Hgb falls to 12 g/dL. Therapy should be reinitiated at a dose approximately 40% below the previous dose. Dosage requirements for patients with chronic renal failure who do not require dialysis may be less than those in patients requiring dialysis. Monitor patients closely during the time period in which a dialysis regimen is initiated; the dosage requirement may increase. The IV route is recommended for dialysis patients.

Conversion of Epoetin Alfa to Darbepoetin Alfa: Estimated Aranesp starting doses for patients based on previous Epoetin Alfa dose

UNLABELED USES
Prevention of anemia in patients donating blood before elective surgery or autologous transfusion.

PRECAUTIONS
Use darbepoetin alfa cautiously in patients with hemolytic anemia, history of seizures, hypertension, liver disease, sickle cell anemia, hypercoagulable states, porphyria (an impairment of erythrocyte formation in bone marrow), and thrombotic events. Pure red cell aplasia (PRCA) and sudden severe anemia were reported postmarketing. A patient who suddenly develops a loss of response and experiences severe anemia and low reticulocyte count should be evaluated for neutralizing antibodies. Do not switch to other erythropoietic proteins as they may cross-react.

Pregnancy Risk Category: C
Drug excretion into human breast milk is unknown. Caution should be used when administered to a nursing woman.

Adult Previous Weekly Epoetin Alfa Dose (units/week)	DARBEPOETIN DOSE (MCG/WEEK)	
	Adult	Pediatric
<1,500	6.25	See text*
1,500-2,499	6.25	6.25
2,500-4,999	12.5	10
5,000-10,999	25	20
11,000-17,999	40	40
18,000-33,999	60	60
34,000-89,999	100	100
≥90,000	200	200

*For pediatric patients receiving a weekly epoetin alfa dose of less than 1,500 units/week, the available data are insufficient to determine an Aranesp conversion dose. Darbepoetin (Aranesp) Prescribing Information, Amgen Inc., December 2005.

CONTRAINDICATIONS
History of sensitivity to mammalian cell-derived products or human albumin or uncontrolled hypertension

DRUG PREPARATION/ADMINISTRATION/ SAFE HANDLING ISSUES
IV
- Avoid excessive agitation of vial; do not shake because it can cause foaming. Also, vigorous shaking may denature medication, rendering it inactive.
- Reconstitution is not necessary.
- May be given as an IV bolus.

Subcutaneous
- Use one dose per vial; do not reenter vial. Discard unused portion.
- May be mixed in a syringe with bacteriostatic 0.9% NaCl with 0.9% benzyl alcohol or bacteriostatic saline at a 1:1 ratio. Benzyl alcohol acts as a local anesthetic and may reduce injection site discomfort.

STORAGE AND STABILITY
Store at 2-8° C (36-46° F). Do not freeze. Protect from light. Do not shake vials vigorously because doing so may denature medication, rendering it inactive.

INTERACTIONS
Drug
Thalidomide: An increase in the thrombogenic state in patients with myelodysplastic syndromes.
Herbal
No information.

Y-SITE COMPATIBLES
None known.

INCOMPATIBLES
Do not mix with other medications.

SIDE EFFECTS
Serious Reactions
- Vascular access thrombosis, CHF, sepsis, arrhythmias, and anaphylactic reactions occur rarely.
- PRCA and sudden severe anemia were reported postmarketing (see Precautions).

Other Side Effects
Frequent (10%-50%):
Diarrhea, edema, fever, headache, hypertension, hypotension, myalgia, peripheral edema

Occasional (1%-10%):
Asthenia, dizziness, fatigue, injection site reaction, pruritus, pulmonary embolism, rash, seizure, stroke, transient ischemic attack, vomiting
Rare (Less Than 1%):
PRCA or severe anemia

SPECIAL CONSIDERATIONS
Baseline Assessment
• Establish patient's baseline CBC with differential, reticulocytes, electrolytes, BUN, creatinine, and coagulation parameters; especially note the patient's Hgb and Hct levels.
• Assess patient's B/P before administering darbepoetin. Because 80% of patients with chronic renal failure have a history of hypertension, expect that B/P will rise during early therapy.
• Assess patient's serum iron level. Keep in mind that transferrin saturation should be greater than 20%, and the serum ferritin level should be greater than 100 ng/mL before and during therapy.
• Consider that all patients will eventually need supplemental iron therapy.
• Assess baseline weight.
• If patient is a Jehovah's Witness, ensure that he or she is informed that darbepoetin alfa contains albumin.
Intervention and Evaluation
• Monitor patient's Hct level diligently. Reduce the dosage if the Hct level increases more than 4 points in 2 weeks.
• Monitor patient's Hgb level, and adjust dose accordingly but not more frequently than once mo.
• Monitor patient's CBC with differential, Hgb, reticulocyte count, and BUN, phosphorus, K, serum creatinine, and serum ferritin levels.
• Monitor patient's B/P aggressively for an increase because 25% of patients taking darbepoetin alfa require antihypertensive therapy and dietary restrictions.
Education
• Educate patient on when to contact health care provider: fever greater than 38° C (greater than 101° F), chills, cough, shortness of breath, palpitations, or severe headaches or weight gain of greater than 4 pounds per week.
• Stress to patient that frequent blood tests will be needed to determine correct dosage.

• Educate patient for signs and symptoms of deep vein thrombosis and pulmonary embolus.
• Warn patient to report severe headache.
• Warn patient to avoid tasks that require mental alertness or motor skills until his or her response to the drug is established.

DAUNORUBICIN HCL
BRAND NAMES
Cerubidine

CLASS OF AGENT
Anthracycline antitumor antibiotic

CLINICAL PHARMACOLOGY
Mechanism of Action
An anthracycline antibiotic that is cell cycle phase nonspecific. The anthracyclines intercalate between strands of the DNA double helix. This DNA binding blocks DNA, RNA, and protein synthesis. Anthracyclines also produce single- and double-stranded DNA breaks and sister chromatid exchanges. Another mechanism involves oxidation-reduction reactions. Daunorubicin is activated to a free radical intermediate by an enzyme system found throughout the body, producing superoxide radicals, which in turn can create hydrogen peroxide anhydroxyl radicals that are toxic to cells, including the heart. Cardiac tissue lacks the necessary enzymes to break down hydrogen peroxide. Some investigators also feel that DNA breaks and damages that occur in the presence of daunorubicin may result from its ability to become a free radical. **Therapeutic Effect:** Inhibits DNA and DNA-dependent RNA synthesis.
Absorption and Distribution
Administer only by the IV route. Widely distributed but does not cross the blood-brain barrier. The highest levels are seen in the spleen, kidneys, liver, lungs, and heart. Highly protein bound.
Half-life: 18.5 hrs; metabolite: 26.7 hrs.
Metabolism and Excretion
Extensively metabolized in the liver to daunorubicinol (active), 7-deoxy-aglycone daunorubicinol (inactive), and demethyldeoxy-aglycone (inactive). Within several min to 1 hr of daunorubicin administration, the concentration of daunorubicinol exceeds that of the parent. Renal excretion is about 20%. Most of the drug is eliminated by biliary excretion.

HOW SUPPLIED/AVAILABLE FORMS
Injection: 20-mg vial, 50-mg vial (5 mg/mL).
Lyophilized Powder: 20-mg vial, 50-mg vial.

INDICATIONS AND DOSAGES
Induction Therapy for Acute Myelogenous Leukemia (AML) in Patients Younger Than 60 Years of Age
45 mg/m^2/day IV on days 1, 2, and 3 of the first course and on days 1 and 2 of subsequent courses AND cytosine arabinoside 100 mg/m^2/day IV infusion daily for 7 days for the first course and for 5 days for subsequent courses.
Induction Therapy for AML in Patients 60 Years Old
30 mg/m^2/day IV on days 1, 2, and 3 of the first course and on days 1 and 2 of subsequent courses AND cytosine arabinoside 100 mg/m^2/day IV infusion daily for 7 days for the first course and for 5 days for subsequent courses.
Induction Therapy for Adult Acute Lymphocytic Leukemia (ALL)
45 mg/m^2/day IV on days 1, 2, and 3 and vincristine 2 mg IV on days 1, 8, and 15; prednisone 40 mg/m^2/day orally (PO) on days 1 through 22, then tapered between days 22 and 29; L-asparaginase 500 International Units/kg/day for 10 days IV on days 22 through 32.
Induction Therapy for Pediatric ALL
25 mg/m^2 IV on day 1 every wk, vincristine 1.5 mg/m^2 IV on day 1 every wk, and prednisone 40 mg/m^2 PO daily. Generally, a complete remission will be obtained within four such courses of therapy; however, if after four courses the patient is in partial remission, an additional course or, if necessary, two courses may be given in an effort to obtain a complete remission. In children less than 2 years of age or with less than 0.5 m^2 BSA, it has been recommended that the daunorubicin dosage calculation should be based on weight (1 mg/kg) instead of BSA.
Dosage Adjustment in Hepatic Dysfunction
The dose of daunorubicin citrate liposome should be reduced if the serum bilirubin level is elevated as follows:
> For serum bilirubin 1.2-3 mg/dL, give three-fourths the normal dose.
> For serum bilirubin greater than 3 mg/dL, give one-half the normal dose.

Dosage Adjustment in Renal Dysfunction
Based on experience with conventional daunorubicin hydrochloride, it is recommended that the dose of daunorubicin citrate liposome be reduced if the serum creatinine is elevated as follows:
For serum creatinine greater than 3 mg/dL, give one-half the normal dose

UNLABELED USES
Treatment of chronic myelocytic leukemia, Ewing's sarcoma, neuroblastoma, non-Hodgkin's lymphoma, Wilms' tumor

PRECAUTIONS
Use cautiously in patients with biliary, liver, or renal impairment.
Pregnancy Risk Category: D

CONTRAINDICATIONS
Arrhythmias, CHF (CHF), left ventricular ejection fraction less than 40%, preexisting bone marrow suppression

DRUG PREPARATION/ADMINISTRATION/ SAFE HANDLING ISSUES
◀ ALERT ▶ Daunorubicin is a vesicant and must be administered with great caution. In patients without a central line, the preferred method is by IV push. For patients with a central line, it is recommended that daunorubicin (maximum concentration of 5 mg/mL) be infused intravenously in 50 mL of standard IV piggyback fluids (i.e., D5W or 0.9% NaCl) over 15 min.
Be aware that daunorubicin dosage is individualized based on the patient's clinical response and tolerance of the drug's adverse effects. When daunorubicin is used in combination therapy, consult specific protocols for optimum dosage and sequence of drug administration. Do not exceed a total dosage of 500-600 mg/m^2 in adults, 400-450 mg/m^2 in those who have received irradiation of the cardiac region, 300 mg/m^2 in children older than 2 years of age, or 10 mg/kg in children younger than 2 years (increases risk of cardiotoxicity). Expect to reduce dosage in patients with liver or renal impairment. Use body weight to calculate dose in children younger than 2 years of age or with a BSA less than 0.5 m^2.
Because daunorubicin may be carcinogenic, mutagenic, or teratogenic, handle the drug with extreme care during preparation and administration.

• Reconstitute the contents of a daunorubicin 20-mg vial (Cerubidine) with 4 mL of sterile water for injection and agitate gently until the drug is completely dissolved. This provides 20 mg of daunorubicin at a concentration of 5 mg/mL.

STORAGE AND STABILITY
• Refrigerate unopened vials.
• Once reconstituted with 4 mL of sterile water for injection, daunorubicin is stable at room temperature for 24 hrs and for 48 hrs under refrigeration. PROTECT FROM LIGHT.

INTERACTIONS
Drug
Bone marrow depressants: May enhance myelosuppression.
Cyclophosphamide: May increase cardiotoxicity, primarily with high-dose cyclophosphamide.
Live Virus Vaccines: May potentiate viral replication, increase vaccine side effects, and decrease the patient's antibody response to vaccine.
Trastuzumab: May increase cardiotoxicity (like doxorubicin).
Herbal
None known.

LAB EFFECTS/INTERFERENCE
May increase serum alkaline phosphatase, serum bilirubin, serum uric acid, and AST (SGOT) levels.

Y-SITE COMPATIBLES
Amifostine, cyclophosphamide, cytarabine, etoposide, filgrastim, granisetron HCl, hydrocortisone Na succinate, ondansetron HCl, palonosetron, trastuzumab, vinorelbine tartrate

INCOMPATIBLES
Allopurinol, aluminum needles, aminophylline, amphotericin B liposomal (AmBisome), aztreonam, cefepime, dexamethasone Na, fludarabine, heparin Na, lansoprazole, levofloxacin, paclitaxel, pantoprazole, pemetrexed, piperacillin/tazobactam

SIDE EFFECTS
Serious Reactions
• Bone marrow depression manifested as hematologic toxicity (severe leukopenia, anemia, and thrombocytopenia) may occur.

• Decreases in platelet and WBC counts occur in 10-14 days and return to normal levels by the third wk of daunorubicin treatment.
• Cardiotoxicity is noted as either acute with transient abnormal EKG findings or as chronic with cardiomyopathy manifested as CHF. The risk of cardiotoxicity increases when the cumulative dose exceeds 550 mg/m^2 in adults and 300 mg/m^2 in children older than 2 years of age or when the total dosage is greater than 10 mg/kg in children younger than 2 years of age.
Other Side Effects
Frequent (10%-50%):
Mild to moderate nausea, fatigue, fever
Occasional (1%-10%):
Diarrhea, abdominal pain, esophagitis, stomatitis (redness or burning of oral mucous membranes, inflammation of gums or tongue), transverse pigmentation of fingernails and toenails
Rare (Less Than 1%):
Transient fever, chills

SPECIAL CONSIDERATIONS
Baseline Assessment
• Complete blood count with differential platelets, electrolytes, and liver BUN creatine function tests before beginning therapy.
• Give antiemetics, if ordered, to patient to prevent and treat nausea.
• Evaluate patient's veins for risk of extravasation reactions
Intervention and Evaluation
• Monitor patient for signs and symptoms of stomatitis, including burning and erythema of the oral mucosa. Know that stomatitis may lead to ulceration within 2-3 days.
• Monitor for extravasation.
• Monitor cardiac function after obtaining a baseline EKG.
• Assess patient's skin and nail beds for hyperpigmentation.
• Monitor patient's hematologic status, results of liver and renal function studies, and serum uric acid level.
• Assess patient's pattern of daily bowel activity and stool consistency.
• Monitor patient for signs and symptoms of anemia, including excessive fatigue and weakness, and hematologic toxicity, including easy bruising, fever, signs of local infection, sore throat, or unusual bleeding from any site.

Education

* Educate patient on neutropenic precautions as necessary:
  Practice good handwashing technique.
  Avoid individuals who are ill.
  Wash and cook all foods well.
  Avoid crowds.
  Avoid fresh fruits and vegetables.
* Educate patient on thrombocytopenic precautions:
  Use of a soft bristle toothbrush.
  No flossing if platelet count is less than 50,000/mm^3.
  No IM injections.
  No rectal suppositories.
  No aerobic exercise.
* Advise patient that his or her urine may turn a reddish color for 1-2 days after daunorubicin therapy is started.
* Explain to patient that alopecia is reversible, but new hair may have a different color or texture. Tell patient that new hair growth resumes about 5 weeks after the last daunorubicin therapy dose.
* Teach patient to maintain fastidious oral hygiene.
* Stress to patient that he or she should not receive vaccinations and should avoid contact with anyone who recently received a live virus vaccine.
* Warn patient to notify the physician if he or she experiences easy bruising, fever, signs of local infection, sore throat, or unusual bleeding from any site.
* Urge patient to increase his or her fluid intake to help protect against development of hyperuricemia.
* Caution patient to notify his or her physician if nausea and vomiting persist at home.
* Educate patient on local resources available and support groups related to their particular diagnosis.

DAUNORUBICIN LIPOSOMAL

BRAND NAMES
DaunoXome

CLASS OF AGENT
Anthracycline antitumor antibiotic

CLINICAL PHARMACOLOGY
Mechanism of Action
An anthracycline antibiotic that is cell cycle phase nonspecific. The anthracyclines intercalate between strands of the DNA double helix. This DNA binding blocks DNA, RNA, and protein synthesis. Anthracyclines also produce single- and double-stranded DNA breaks and sister chromatid exchanges. Another mechanism involves oxidation-reduction reactions. Daunorubicin is activated to a free radical intermediate by an enzyme system found throughout the body, producing superoxide radicals, which in turn can create hydrogen peroxide anhydroxyl radicals that are toxic to cells, including the heart. Cardiac tissue lacks the necessary enzymes to break down hydrogen peroxide. Some investigators also feel that DNA breaks and damages that occur in the presence of daunorubicin may result from its ability to become a free radical.
Therapeutic Effect: Inhibits DNA and DNA-dependent RNA synthesis.

Absorption and Distribution
Administer only by the IV route. In contrast to daunorubicin HCl, the volume of distribution is 6.4 L. Animal models suggest that it might cross the blood-brain barrier. It is highly protein bound (63%). Liposomal daunorubicin distributes preferentially into tumor tissue.
Half-life: Elimination half-life is 4.4 hrs, and probably reflects distribution half-life.

Metabolism and Excretion
In contrast to therapy with free daunorubicin, a low concentration of the primary metabolite, daunorubicinol, is detected in the plasma after IV administration. Renal excretion is about 20%. Most of the drug is eliminated by biliary excretion.

HOW SUPPLIED/AVAILABLE FORMS
Injection: DaunoXome 2 mg/mL.

INDICATIONS AND DOSAGES
Kaposi's Sarcoma
20-40 mg/m^2 over 1 hr repeated every 2 weeks.
Dosage Adjustment in Hepatic Dysfunction
Reduce dose if the serum bilirubin level is elevated as follows:
  For serum bilirubin 1.2-3 mg/dL, give three-fourths the normal dose.
  For serum bilirubin greater than 3 mg/dL, give one-half the normal dose.
Dosage Adjustment in Renal Dysfunction
On the basis of experience with conventional daunorubicin hydrochloride, it is recommended that the dose of daunorubicin

citrate liposome be reduced if the serum creatinine level is elevated as follows:
> For serum creatinine greater than 3 mg/dL, give one-half the normal dose

UNLABELED USES
Treatment of chronic myelocytic leukemia, Ewing's sarcoma, neuroblastoma, non-Hodgkin's lymphoma, Wilms' tumor

PRECAUTIONS
Use cautiously in patients with biliary, liver, or renal impairment.
Pregnancy Risk Category: D

CONTRAINDICATIONS
Arrhythmias, CHF (CHF), left ventricular ejection fraction less than 40%, preexisting bone marrow suppression

DRUG PREPARATION/ADMINISTRATION/ SAFE HANDLING ISSUES
◀ **ALERT** ▶ Be aware that daunorubicin dosage is individualized on the basis of the patient's clinical response and tolerance of the drug's adverse effects. When daunorubicin is used in combination therapy, consult specific protocols for optimum dosage and sequence of drug administration. Do not exceed total dosage of 500-600 mg/m^2 in adults, 400-450 mg/m^2 in those who have received irradiation of the cardiac region, 300 mg/m^2 in children older than 2 years of age, or 10 mg/kg in children younger than 2 years of age (increases risk of cardiotoxicity).
◀ **ALERT** ▶ Special attention must be given to the potential cardiotoxicity of daunorubicin. Although there is no reliable means of predicting CHF, cardiomyopathy induced by anthracyclines is usually associated with a decrease in the left ventricular ejection fraction (LVEF). Cardiac function should be evaluated in each patient by means of a history and physical examination before each course of DaunoXome and determination of LVEF should be performed at total cumulative dosages of DaunoXome of 320 mg/m^2, and every 160 mg/m^2 thereafter.
◀ **ALERT** ▶ Patients who have received prior therapy with anthracyclines (doxorubicin greater than 300 mg/m^2 or equivalent), have preexisting cardiac disease, or have received previous radiotherapy encompassing the heart may be less "cardiac" tolerant to treatment with DaunoXome. Therefore, monitoring of LVEF at cumulative

DaunoXome doses should occur before therapy and after every 160 mg/m^2 of DaunoXome.
◀ **ALERT** ▶ Expect to reduce dosage in patients with liver or renal impairment. Use body weight to calculate dose in children younger than 2 years of age or with a BSA less than 0.5 m^2.
◀ **ALERT** ▶ Because daunorubicin may be carcinogenic, mutagenic, or teratogenic, handle the drug with extreme care during preparation and administration.
◀ **ALERT** ▶ Triad infusion reactions consisting of back pain, flushing, and chest tightness have been reported in 13.8% of patients (16 of 116) treated with DaunoXome in a randomized clinical trial and in 2.7% of treatment cycles (27 of 994). This triad generally occurs during the first 5 min of the infusion, subsides with interruption of the infusion, and generally does not recur if the infusion is then resumed at a slower rate. This combination of symptoms appears to be related to the lipid component of DaunoXome, as a similar set of signs and symptoms has been observed with other liposomal products not containing daunorubicin.
- In contrast to daunorubicin, DaunoXome has not been reported to cause vesicant reactions if extravasated.
- Daunorubicin citrate liposome should be diluted 1:1 with D5W before administration.
- Each vial of DaunoXome contains daunorubicin citrate equivalent to 50 mg of daunorubicin base, at a concentration of 2 mg/mL. The recommended concentration after dilution is 1 mg/mL.
- The only fluid that may be mixed with DaunoXome is D5W. The drug must not be mixed with saline, bacteriostatic agents such as benzyl alcohol, or any other solution.
- Infuse over 60 min.
- Do not use an inline filter for IV infusion of DaunoXome.

STORAGE AND STABILITY
- Refrigerate unopened vials. Do not freeze, and protect from light.
- Be aware that reconstituted solution is stable for 6 hrs if refrigerated.

INTERACTIONS
Drug
Antigout medications: May decrease the effects of these drugs.

Bone marrow depressants: May enhance myelosuppression.
Live-virus vaccines: May potentiate virus replication, increase vaccine side effects, and decrease the patient's antibody response to the vaccine.
Herbal
None known.

LAB EFFECTS/INTERFERENCE
May increase serum alkaline phosphatase, serum bilirubin, serum uric acid, and AST (SGOT) levels.

Y-SITE COMPATIBLES
Trastuzumab

INCOMPATIBLES
Do not mix with any other solution, especially NaCl or bacteriostatic agents (e.g., benzyl alcohol).

SIDE EFFECTS
Serious Reactions
• Bone marrow depression manifested as hematologic toxicity (severe leukopenia, anemia, and thrombocytopenia) may occur.
• Decreases in platelet and WBC counts occur in 10-14 days and return to normal levels by the third wk of daunorubicin treatment.
• Cardiotoxicity noted as either acute with transient abnormal EKG (ECG) findings or as chronic with cardiomyopathy manifested as CHF can occur. The risk of cardiotoxicity increases when the cumulative dose is greater than 320 mg/m^2 in adults and greater than 300 mg/m^2 in children older than 2 years of age, or when the total dosage is greater than 10 mg/kg in children younger than 2 years of age.
• Monitor LVEF before therapy and at cumulative DaunoXome doses of 320 mg/m^2 and with every 160 mg/m^2 of DaunoXome, thereafter.
Other Side Effects
Frequent (10%-50%):
Mild to moderate nausea, fatigue, fever
Occasional (1%-10%):
Diarrhea, abdominal pain, esophagitis, stomatitis (redness or burning of oral mucous membranes or inflammation of gums or tongue), transverse pigmentation of fingernails and toenails
Rare (Less Than 1%):
Transient fever, chills

SPECIAL CONSIDERATIONS
Baseline Assessment
• Obtain patient's complete blood count with differential platelets before beginning therapy and at frequent intervals during daunorubicin therapy.
• Obtain patient's baseline ECG before beginning daunorubicin therapy.
• Give antiemetics, if ordered, to patient to prevent and treat nausea.
Intervention and Evaluation
• If patient exhibits sign of the triad infusion reaction (back pain, flushing, and chest tightness), stop the infusion and then resume the infusion at a slower rate after the symptoms have abated.
• Observe patient for signs of CHF, including shortness of breath and pulmonary edema. Refer patient to an MD for evaluation.
• Monitor patient for signs and symptoms of stomatitis, including burning and erythema of the oral mucosa. Know that stomatitis may lead to ulceration within 2-3 days.
• Assess patient's skin and nail beds for hyperpigmentation.
• Extravasation kit to bedside if this agent is given peripherally.
• Monitor patient's hematologic status, results of liver and renal function studies, and serum uric acid level.
• Assess patient's pattern of daily bowel activity and stool consistency.
• Monitor patient for signs and symptoms of anemia, including excessive fatigue and weakness, and hematologic toxicity, including easy bruising, fever, signs of local infection, sore throat, or unusual bleeding from any site.
Education
• Instruct patient on when to contact health care provider: fever greater than 38° C (greater than 101° F), chills, shortness of breath, chest pain, nausea lasting greater than 24 hours, diarrhea lasting longer than 24 hours, or the inability to take in at least 1500 mL of fluid in 24 hours.
• Tell patient about the signs of CHF and to seek medical attention if necessary.
• Advise patient that his or her urine may turn a reddish color for 1-2 days after daunorubicin therapy is started.
• Explain to patient that alopecia is reversible, but new hair may have a different color or texture. Tell patient that new hair

growth resumes about 5 weeks after the last daunorubicin therapy dose.
- Educate patient on neutropenic precautions as necessary:
  Practice good handwashing technique.
  Avoid individuals who are ill.
  Wash and cook all foods well.
  Avoid crowds.
  Avoid fresh fruits and vegetables.
- Teach patient to maintain fastidious oral hygiene.
- Stress to patient that he or she should not receive vaccinations and should avoid contact with anyone who recently received a live-virus vaccine.
- Warn patient to notify the physician if he or she experiences easy bruising, fever, signs of local infection, sore throat, or unusual bleeding from any site.
- Urge patient to increase his or her fluid intake to help protect against development of hyperuricemia.
- Caution patient to notify his or her physician if nausea and vomiting persist at home.
- Instruct patient to take no over-the-counter medications or herbal or vitamin supplements without checking with his or her health care provider.
- Educate patient on local resources available and support groups related to their particular diagnosis.

DECITABINE

BRAND NAMES
Dacogen

CLASS OF AGENT
Demethylating pyrimidine antimetabolite

CLINICAL PHARMACOLOGY
Mechanism of Action
A pyrimidine analog of cytarabine and de-oxycytidine that blocks the methylation of newly formed DNA by inhibiting DNA methyltransferase. DNA hypomethylation produces gene activation and differentiation of neoplastic cells, especially leukemia cells. Activation of these genes induces terminal cell differentiation and loss of proliferative capacity. Reduction of DNA methylation appears to activate previously silenced groups of genes that are important in the control of the cell cycle, DNA repair, cell adherence, or detoxification, thus restoring normal cell function. **Therapeutic Effect:** Inhibition of DNA methyltransferase resulting in hypo-methylation may lead to cell apoptosis.
Absorption and Distribution
No information is available on oral absorption. Decitabine distributes into leukemia cells and crosses the blood-brain barrier. *Half-life and protein binding:* After discontinuation of IV administration, the parent compound, decitabine, has α and β plasma half-life of 7 and 35 min, respectively. Plasma protein binding of decitabine is negligible (less than 1%).
Metabolism and Excretion
Eliminated by rapid inactivation by cytidine deaminase, which is present primarily in hepatic tissue but is also in granulocytes, whole red blood, and intestinal epithelial cells. Inactivation also occurs by drug deamination in leukemia cells. The total urinary excretion is less than 1% of the administered dose.

HOW SUPPLIED/AVAILABLE FORMS
Lyophilized Powder for Injection: 50 mg.

INDICATIONS AND DOSAGES
Myelodysplastic Syndrome
15 mg/m^2 administered by continuous IV infusion over 3 hrs repeated every 8 hrs for 3 days. May repeat every 6 wks for at least 4 cycles.
Dosage Adjustment in Hepatic Dysfunction
There are no guidelines to date.
Dosage Adjustment in Renal Dysfunction
There is no alteration in dosage.

UNLABELED USES
Acute myelogenous leukemia, chronic myelogenous leukemia

PRECAUTIONS
Prior hypersensitivity reactions to decitabine. Patients with active infection should not receive decitabine.
Pregnancy Risk Category: D

CONTRAINDICATIONS
Hypersensitivity to prior decitabine

DRUG PREPARATION/ADMINISTRATION/SAFE HANDLING ISSUES
- Reconstitute with 10 mL of sterile water for injection (USP) to produce 5 mg/mL at pH 6.7-7.3.
- Immediately after reconstitution, the solution should be further diluted with

0.9% NaCl injection, 5% dextrose injection, or lactated Ringer's injection to a final drug concentration of 0.1-1 mg/mL.
* The large volume dilution should be administered as continuous infusion over 3 hrs.

STORAGE AND STABILITY
* Store 50-mg vials at 25° C (77° F); excursions are permitted to 15-30° C (59-86° F).
* Decitabine decomposes rapidly upon reconstitution of vials (sterile water); drug concentrations decrease by approximately 10% after 5 hrs at 25° C (77° F) or after 24 hrs at 4°C (39° F).
* The manufacturer of Dacogen recommends that unless it is started within 15 min of reconstitution, the diluted solution must be prepared using cold (2-8° C; 36-46° F) infusion fluids and stored at 2-8° C for up to a maximum of 7 hrs until administration.

INTERACTIONS
Drug
Bone marrow depressants: May increase risk of bone marrow depression.
Live-virus vaccines: May potentiate viral replication, increase vaccine side effects, and decrease the patient's antibody response to the vaccine.
Cytochrome P450: In vitro studies in human hepatic microsomes indicate that decitabine has little effect on relevant enzymes. Thus, it is unlikely that decitabine interacts with other agents that are affected by or affect hepatic microsomal enzymes. Drug displacement is unlikely as the plasma protein binding of decitabine is less than 1%.
Herbal
None known.

LAB EFFECTS/INTERFERENCE
Elevated liver function tests.

Y-SITE COMPATIBLES
No data.

INCOMPATIBLES
Since no data are available on compatibility, it is recommended that decitabine not be infused with any other drugs.

SIDE EFFECTS
Serious Reactions
Severe myelosuppression and febrile neutropenia

Other Side Effects
Frequent (10%-50%):
Nausea, vomiting, diarrhea, anorexia, malaise, abdominal cramping, enteritis, rash, pruritus, localized erythema, myelosuppression manifested mainly as granulocytopenia and thrombocytopenia
Occasional (1%-10%):
Mucositis, alopecia, fatigue
Rare (Less Than 1%):
MI and acute heart failure have been reported but were more likely due to underlying conditions, increased hepatic enzymes, and nephrotoxicity.

SPECIAL CONSIDERATIONS
Baseline Assessment
* Obtain CBC with differential, platelets. electrolytes, BUN, and creatinine, and liver function tests.
* Assess patients for prior MI and heart failure.
* Evaluate patient's history of emesis with prior chemotherapeutic agents.
* Monitor for any prior skin toxicity as this agent can induce rash and erythema.
Intervention and Evaluation
* Assess all laboratory data before each dose, paying particular attention to liver function tests.
* Weigh patient before dosing.
* Monitor vital signs before each dose, assessing for cardiac changes, tachycardia, bradycardia, and palpitations.
* Evaluate patient for any symptoms of chest pain, palpitations, or evidence of cardiac failure, edema, weight gain, shortness of breath, or tachycardia.
* Premedicate patients with antiemetic agents before each dose.
* Monitor for skin changes, evaluating rashes, irritation, pruritus, and desquamation.
* Assess pain before dosing, especially right upper quadrant pain, which may be an indication of altered liver function.
* Monitor patient for number and consistency of stools as diarrhea can result from this agent.
* Initiate neutropenic and thrombocytopenic precautions.
Education
* Instruct patient on when to contact health care provider: fever greater than 38° C (greater than 101° F), chills, shortness of breath, chest pain, nausea lasting greater

than 24 hours, diarrhea lasting greater than 24 hours, or the inability to take in at least 1500 mL of fluid in 24 hours.

- Educate patient on neutropenic precautions:

  Practice good handwashing technique.

  Avoid crowds.

  Avoid all fresh fruits and vegetables.

  Avoid all persons with colds or flu.

- Educate patient on thrombocytopenic precautions:

  Use of a soft bristle toothbrush.

  No flossing if platelet count is less than 50,000/mm^3.

  No IM injections.

  No rectal suppositories.

- Educate patient on the use of antinausea and antidiarrheal agents as needed.

- Advise patient that hair loss may occur.

- Instruct patient on the use of moisturizers Prn for skin rash.

- Instruct patient to take no over-the-counter medications or herbal or vitamin supplements without checking with his or her health care provider.

- Educate patient on local resources available and support groups related to their particular diagnosis.

DENILEUKIN DIFTITOX

BRAND NAMES
Ontak

CLASS OF AGENT
Antineoplastic agent

CLINICAL PHARMACOLOGY
Mechanism of Action

A cytotoxic fusion protein composed of amino acid sequences for diphtheria toxin fragments A and B followed by sequences for interleukin-2 (IL-2) that targets cells expressing IL-2 receptors. After binding to IL-2 receptors, it directs cytocidal action to malignant cutaneous T-cell lymphoma cells. **Therapeutic Effect:** Causes inhibition of protein synthesis and cell death.

Absorption and Distribution

Denileukin diftitox has a two-compartment behavior with a distribution phase (2-5 min) and a terminal phase. Systemic exposure is variable and proportional to dose. A study in rats showed the liver and kidneys to be the primary sites of distribution. Volume of

distribution: ~0.06-0.08 L/kg.

Half-life: 70-80 min.

Metabolism and Excretion

Metabolized by proteolytic degradation. Excretion is less than 25% of total dose and consists of broken by-products.

HOW SUPPLIED/AVAILABLE FORMS
Injection: 150 mcg/mL (2 mL/vial).

INDICATIONS AND DOSAGES
Treatment of Persistent or Recurrent T-Cell Lymphoma Whose Malignant Cells Express the CD25 Component of the IL-2 Receptor

9 or 18 mcg/kg/day IV for 5 consecutive days every 21 days. Infuse over at least 15 min.

Dosage Adjustment in Hepatic/Renal Dysfunction

No information.

UNLABELED USES
HIV infection, chronic lymphocytic leukemia, Hodgkin's lymphoma, non-Hodgkin's lymphoma, psoriasis, rheumatoid arthritis

PRECAUTIONS
Use with extreme caution in patients with cardiovascular disease, hepatic or renal impairment, and preexisting low serum albumin levels. Anaphylaxis reactions and vascular leak syndrome characterized by hypotension, edema, and hypoalbuminemia have been reported. Delay dose if serum albumin levels are less than 3 g/dL.

Pregnancy Risk Category: C

Excretion of drug into breast milk is unknown/not recommended in nursing women.

CONTRAINDICATIONS
Hypersensitivity to diphtheria toxin, IL-2, or denileukin diftitox excipients

DRUG PREPARATION/ADMINISTRATION/ SAFE HANDLING ISSUES
◀ ALERT ▶ When handling this agent, use nitrile or latex gloves only. If a splash occurs, wash with mild soap and water; do not use waterless or antibacterial soap as either can enhance the skin reaction. If an eye splash occurs, use copious amounts of water or 0.9% NaCl to flush the eyes. Flushing should be done from inner to outer canthus.

- Bring drug to room temperature before preparing the dose. The vials may be

thawed in the refrigerator for not more than 24 hrs or at room temperature for 1-2 hrs. Do not heat.
- Gently swirl the vial. Do not shake vigorously. Solution is clear when it is at room temperature.
- Do not refreeze the solution.
- Prepare and hold diluted medication in plastic syringes or soft plastic IV bags. Do not use a glass container.
- The concentration of denileukin diftitox must be at least 15 mcg/mL during all steps in the preparation of the solution for IV infusion. According to the manufacturer, this is accomplished by withdrawing the calculated dose from the vial and injecting it into an empty IV infusion bag. For each 1 mL of denileukin diftitox from the vial, no more than 9 mL of sterile saline without preservative should then be added to the IV bag.
- Infuse over at least 15 min.
- Do not administer as a bolus injection, with other drugs, or through an in-line filter.
- Prepared solutions should be administered within 6 hrs. Discard unused portions.

STORAGE AND STABILITY
Store frozen at or below −10° C (14° F).

INTERACTIONS
Drug
There are no known drug interactions. According to the manufacturer, a dose of denileukin diftitox had no effect on the cytochrome P450 system.
Herbal
None known.

LAB EFFECTS/INTERFERENCE
May decrease serum albumin, calcium, and K levels, WBC count, Hgb, Hct, and platelet count. Increases AST (SGOT) and ALT (SGPT) levels.

Y-SITE COMPATIBLES
Do not mix with other drugs.

INCOMPATIBLES
Do not mix with other drugs.

SIDE EFFECTS
Serious Reactions
- Two distinct syndromes occur very commonly. One syndrome is a hypersensitivity reaction (69%), consisting of at least more than one of the following: hypotension, back pain, dyspnea, vasodilation, vascular leak syndrome (characterized by hypotension, edema, and hypoalbuminemia), rash, chest tightness, tachycardia, dysphagia, and syncope. The other is a flu-like symptom complex (91%), consisting of at least more than one of the following: fever, chills, nausea, vomiting, diarrhea, myalgia, or arthralgia. Management consists of interrupting the infusion, reducing the rate of infusion, and administration of supportive medications such as antihistamine, corticosteroids, and epinephrine. Severe reactions may call for drug discontinuation.
- Vascular leak syndrome characterized by hypotension, edema, and hypoalbuminemia was reported in 27% of patients. The onset of symptoms was delayed and occurred within the first wks. Treatment should be initiated if clinically indicated with some cases being self-limiting. Weight, edema, B/P, and serum albumin levels should be monitored.
- Loss of visual acuity or loss of color vision with or without retinal pigment mottling was reported and in most patients resulted in persistent impairment.
- Development of antibodies to the fusion protein or to the IL-2 portion of the molecule was correlated with a significant increase (2- or 3-fold) in clearance and decreased the mean systemic exposure by 25%. Antibodies did not correlate with risk of hypersensitivity.
Other Side Effects
Frequent (10%-50%):
Anemia, anorexia, chest pain, cough, decreased weight, dehydration, diaphoresis, diarrhea, dizziness, dyspnea, flu-like syndrome, hypersensitivity reaction, hypoalbuminemia (nadirs 1-2 wks after administration), hypotension, infection, injection site reaction, myalgia, nausea and vomiting, pharyngitis, pruritus, rash (both acute and delayed), rhinitis, tachycardia, vasodilation
Occasional (1%-10%):
Arrhythmia, confusion, constipation, dyspepsia, dysphagia, hypertension, leukopenia, thrombocytopenia, thrombotic events
Rare (Less Than 1%):
Acute renal insufficiency, hyperthyroidism, hypothyroidism, microscopic hematuria, oral ulcer, pancreatitis

SPECIAL CONSIDERATIONS
Baseline Assessment
- Assess CBC with differential, electrolyte, BUN, creatinine, and albumin levels, and liver function tests.
- Confirm test result of CD25 expression of the IL-2 receptor on tumor cells.
- Monitor albumin level, which must be greater than 3 mg/dL before administration of this agent.
- Obtain baseline vital signs, oxygen saturation, and weight.
- Black box warning: Patients treated with denileukin diftitox must be managed in a facility equipped and staffed for cardio-pulmonary resuscitation and where the patient can be closely monitored for an appropriate period based on his or her health status.

Intervention and Evaluation
- Evaluate laboratory data prior to each dosing.
- Premedications for hypersensitivity prevention as ordered.
- Have an anaphylaxis kit at bedside before dosing. The anaphylaxis kit should contain the following:
  - Diphenhydramine 50 mg
  - Hydrocortisone 50 mg
  - Epinephrine 1:1000 ampules (1 mg/mL), single use vial 0.3 mL at one time, may repeat doses as necessary
  - Syringes and needles to draw up epinephrine from ampule
  - 2 by 2 gauze pads to break ampules
  - Alcohol wipes
- Set up oxygen and make sure an Ambu bag is available in the room.
- Monitor patient for evidence of side effects of tachycardia, tachypnea, hypertension, febrile reactions, and altered mental status.
- Assess for any visual changes or impairments.
- Assess patient for evidence of third spacing and capillary leak syndrome.
- Monitor patient greater than 65 years more closely for adverse events, i.e., hypotension, confusion, and decreased fluid intake.

Education
- Educate patient to monitor weight for evidence of third spacing or capillary leak syndrome.
- Instruct patient to maintain nutritional status as much as possible.
- Educate patient on neutropenic precautions as necessary:
  - Practice good handwashing technique.
  - Avoid individuals who are ill.
  - Wash and cook all foods well.
  - Avoid crowds.
  - Avoid fresh fruits and vegetables.
- Educate patient on risk for infections, especially avoiding persons with colds, flu, and viral syndromes.
- Educate patient on good handwashing technique to prevent infections.
- Instruct patient on when to contact primary care provider: fever greater than 38° C (greater than 101° F), chills, cough, shortness of breath, edema, nausea lasting greater than 24 hours, diarrhea lasting greater than 24 hours, or the inability to take in at least 1500 mL in 24 hours.
- Advise patient that he or she may experience flu-like symptoms after this agent in the form of arthralgias, myalgias, fever, chills, diarrhea, nausea, and vomiting.
- Warn patient not to have immunizations without physician's approval because denileukin lowers the body's resistance.
- Instruct patient to avoid contact with those who have recently received a live-virus vaccine.
- Instruct patient to take no over-the-counter medications or herbal or vitamin supplements without checking with his or her health care provider.
- Educate patient on availability of local resources and support groups related to their diagnosis.

DOCETAXEL

BRAND NAMES
Taxotere

CLASS OF AGENT
Antineoplastic agent, taxane

CLINICAL PHARMACOLOGY
Mechanism of Action
An antimitotic agent belonging to the taxane family that disrupts the microtubular cell network by promoting assembly and inhibiting depolymerization of microtubules. **Therapeutic Effect:** Inhibits cellular mitosis or cell division, resulting in apoptosis.

Absorption and Distribution
Distributed into peripheral compartments. Mean steady state volume of distribution: 113 L. Protein binding: 94%-97%.

Half-life: Terminal phase 11.1 hrs.
Metabolism and Excretion
Extensively metabolized in the liver.
Excreted primarily in feces (75%), with
lesser amount in urine.

HOW SUPPLIED/AVAILABLE FORMS
Injection: 20-mg vial, 80-mg vial
(10 mg/mL).

INDICATIONS AND DOSAGES
**Breast Cancer, Non-Small Cell Lung
Cancer, Prostate Carcinoma, Advanced
Gastric Adenocarcinoma, Squamous Cell
Carcinoma of the Head and Neck**
Every 3 weeks: 60-100 mg/m^2 IV over 1 hour.
Weekly (unlabeled): 35 mg/m^2 IV over
1 hour.
**Dosage Adjustment in Hepatic
Dysfunction**
Total bilirubin greater than ULN or AST
(SGOT) greater than $1.5 \times$ ULN + alka-
line phosphatase greater than $2.5 \times$ ULN:
manufacturer recommends to hold drug.

UNLABELED USES
Treatment of small cell bladder, head and
neck, and ovarian cancer.

PRECAUTIONS
Severe hypersensitivity reactions have been
reported.
Use docetaxel cautiously in patients with
hepatic impairment, peripheral neuropathy,
myelosuppression, or preexisting pleural
effusion.
Pregnancy Risk Category: D
Avoid use during pregnancy because the
drug may cause fetal harm. It is unknown
whether docetaxel is distributed in breast
milk, and patients receiving docetaxel
should not breast-feed.

CONTRAINDICATIONS
A history of hypersensitivity to docetaxel,
polysorbate 80, or any component of
the formulation or ANC less than
1,500 cells/mm^3

DRUG PREPARATION/ADMINISTRATION/
SAFE HANDLING ISSUES
◀ ALERT ▶ Because docetaxel may be carcinogenic, mutagenic, or teratogenic, wear
nitrile or latex, but not vinyl, gloves when
handling the drug. If the drug comes in
contact with skin, wash the skin thoroughly
with soap and water. Do not use the waterless or antibacterial soap as either can in-

crease the reaction from the agent. If the
drug comes in contact with mucous membranes, flush the area with water.
◀ ALERT ▶ Premedicate the patient with dexamethasone starting 1 day before docetaxel
administration to reduce the risk of peripheral and pulmonary edema. Breast cancer
trial regimen consists of 8 mg orally (PO)
bid for 3 days starting on the day before
docetaxel. Prostate cancer trial regimen
consists of 8 mg PO 12 hrs before, 3 hrs
before, and 1 hrs before docetaxel. These
prostate cancer patients also received prednisone 5 mg PO bid as part of their combination chemotherapy regimen.
• Docetaxel is considered an irritant.
• Transfer the entire amount of diluent into
  the docetaxel vial (1.8 mL for the 20mg
  vial and 7.1 mL for the 80-mg vial). Invert or rotate the vial to promote mixture.
  Do not shake as this will cause foaming.
• The initial diluted solution results in a
  concentration of 10 mg/mL.
• Final dilution should be in 0.9% NaCl
  or D5W with a final concentration of
  0.3-0.74 mg/mL.
• Dispense in either glass or Excel/PAB
  containers. Use nonpolyvinyl chloride
  (non-PVC) tubing (e.g., polyethylene) to
  minimized leaching of **di-2-ethyl hexyl
  phthalate** from PVC infusion bags or
  administration sets.
• With a sequential infusion, administer
  docetaxel before platinum derivatives
  (e.g., cisplatin and carboplatin) to limit
  myelosuppression.
• Monitor patient's vital signs during the
  infusion, especially during the first hr.
• Discontinue docetaxel administration and
  notify the physician if patient experiences
  shortness of breath, tachycardia, tachypnea,
  bradycardia, or a severe hypersensitivity
  reaction.

STORAGE AND STABILITY
• Store intact vials at refrigerated or room
  temperature of 2-25° C (36-77° F).
• The reconstituted solution is stable
  at refrigerated or room temperature
  for up to 8 hrs as it does not contain
  preservatives.
• The fully prepared docetaxel infusion
  solution, in either 0.9% NaCl or 5% D5W
  solution, should be used within 4 hrs.

INTERACTIONS
Drug
Cytochrome (CYP) 3A4 inducers

(carbamazepine, phenytoin, phenobarbital, rifampin): May decrease the levels/effects of docetaxel

CYP 3A4 inhibitors (ciprofloxacin, clarithromycin, cyclosporine, doxycycline, erythromycin, isoniazid, ketoconazole, nifedipine, protease inhibitors, verapamil): May increase the levels/effects of docetaxel

Bone marrow depressants: May increase myelosuppression.

Live-virus vaccines: May potentiate viral replication, increase vaccine side effects, and decrease the patient's antibody response to the vaccine.

Herbal
None known.

Food
Grapefruit inhibits CYP 3A4 enzymes and can potentially enhance docetaxel effects.

LAB EFFECTS/INTERFERENCE
May significantly increase BUN, serum alkaline phosphatase, bilirubin, creatinine, AST (SGOT), and ALT (SGPT) levels. Reduces blood neutrophil, thrombocyte, and WBC counts.

Y-SITE COMPATIBLES
Amifostine, bumetanide (Bumex), busulfan, calcium gluconate, carboplatin, carmustine, cyclophosphamide, cytarabine, dacarbazine, dactinomycin, dexamethasone (Decadron), dexrazoxane, doxorubicin, diphenhydramine (Benadryl), dobutamine (Dobutrex), dopamine (Intropin), epirubicin, etoposide, etoposide phosphate, fludarabine, fluorouracil, furosemide (Lasix), gemcitabine, granisetron (Kytril), heparin, hydromorphone (Dilaudid), ifosfamide, irinotecan, leucovorin, lorazepam (Ativan), magnesium sulfate, mannitol, mesna, methotrexate, mitoxantrone, morphine, ondansetron (Zofran), palonosetron (Aloxi), potassium chloride, rituximab, teniposide, thiotepa, trastuzumab, vincristine, vinorelbine

INCOMPATIBLES
Amphotericin B conventional (Fungizone), amphotericin B liposomal (AmBisome), dantrolene, doxorubicin liposomal (DaunoXome), idarubicin, methylprednisolone (Solu-Medrol), nalbuphine (Nubain), phenytoin

SIDE EFFECTS
Serious Reactions
- In patients with normal liver function tests, neutropenia (neutrophil count less than 2,000 cells/mm^3; nadir 8 days) and leukopenia (WBC count less than 4,000 cells/mm^3) occur in 96% of patients, anemia (Hgb level less than 11 g/dL) occurs in 90% of patients, thrombocytopenia (platelet count less than 100,000 cells/mm^3) occurs in 8% of patients, and infection occurs in 28% of patients.
- A severe hypersensitivity reaction, including dyspnea, severe hypotension, angioedema, and generalized urticaria, occurs rarely. Occurrence usually is within the first 15 min of infusion of the first or second dose and may vary per individual. Premedication may minimize the effect. Use diphenhydramine 50-100 mg IV, hydrocortisone succinate 100 mg IV, epinephrine 1:1000 (1 mg/mL) 0.3 mL IV, albuterol inhaler 2-4 puffs, and oxygen as necessary. Rechallenge of docetaxel is not recommended with severe reactions. However, for patients with limited treatment options, several variations of docetaxel desensitization protocols described in the literature have successfully been used.
- Neurosensory and neuromotor effects, such as distal paresthesias and weakness, occur in 54% and 13% of patients, respectively.
- Peripheral edema or fluid retention are common adverse effects and may exacerbate heart and lung conditions.

Other Side Effects
Frequent (10%-50%):
Alopecia, asthenia, fluid retention, fever, infusion-related reactions, myalgia, nail changes, nausea and diarrhea, stomatitis, vomiting

Occasional (1%-10%):
Anorexia, dizziness, edema, headache, hypotension, infection, peripheral neuropathy, weight gain

Rare (Less Than 1%):
Anaphylaxis, arthralgia, conjunctivitis, dry skin, hematuria, proteinuria, sensory disorders (vision, speech, taste), weight loss

SPECIAL CONSIDERATIONS
Baseline Assessment
- Evaluate patient's CBC with differential and platelets before each dose. The ANC should be greater than 1,500 cells/mm^3 and platelets should be greater than 100,000 cells/mm^3 to deliver a dose of this agent.

- Assess for any drug allergies before dosing.
- Assess for patient's ability to comply with steroid dosing.
- Assess for diabetes in patients receiving this agent.

Intervention and Evaluation
- Give antiemetics, if ordered, to prevent or treat nausea and vomiting.
- Pretreat patient with corticosteroids, as ordered, before initiating docetaxel therapy to reduce the severity of fluid retention and hypersensitivity reactions.
- Assess for hypersensitivity reactions during the first and second dose of this agent.
- Have an anaphylaxis kit at bedside before dosing, along with an oxygen setup and Ambu bag in the room. The anaphylaxis kit should include the following:
    Diphenhydramine 50 mg
    Hydrocortisone 50 mg
    Epinephrine 1:1000 1 ampule 1 mg/mL; use 0.3 mL IV and may repeat as necessary
    Syringe to deliver epinephrine
    2 by 2 gauze to break ampule
    Needle to draw up epinephrine
    Alcohol wipes
- Monitor patient's CBC with differential and, in particular, liver and renal function studies and serum uric acid levels. A neutrophil count of less than 1,500 cells/mm³ requires interruption of docetaxel therapy.
- Evaluate liver function tests before each dose.
- Weigh patient before each dose and assess for any signs of peripheral edema.
- Assess patient for signs and symptoms of peripheral neuropathy.
- Observe patient for cutaneous reactions characterized by a rash with eruptions, mainly on the feet or hands.
- Assess patient for signs of extravascular fluid accumulation, such as dependent edema, dyspnea at rest, crackles, and pronounced abdominal distensions from ascites.
- Offer emotional support to patient, family, and significant others.

Education
- Instruct patient to report any signs or symptoms of infection, fevers greater than 38° C (greater than 101° F), shaking, chills, or mouth sores, and to contact health care provider for any of these symptoms.
- Make sure patient has 24-hour number for the health care provider.

- Educate patient on neutropenic precautions as necessary:
    Practice good handwashing technique.
    Avoid individuals who are ill.
    Wash and cook all foods well.
    Avoid crowds.
    Avoid fresh fruits and vegetables.
- Educate patient on thrombocytopenic precautions:
    Use of a soft bristle toothbrush.
    No flossing if platelet count is less than 50,000/mm³.
    No IM injections.
    No rectal suppositories.
    No aerobic exercise.
- Instruct patient to take no over-the-counter medications or herbal or vitamin supplements without checking with his or her health care provider.
- Educate patient on local resources available and support groups related to their particular diagnosis.
- Instruct patient on an oral care regimen per institutional protocol. An example is 1 tsp each of salt and baking soda dissolved in 1 glass of water to swish and spit at least 4 times/day.
- Educate patient on the possibility of a hypersensitivity reaction, and instruct patient on what signs and symptoms to report.
- Inform patient of the possibility of neuropathy from this agent and to report any numbness or tingling or burning sensations in the hands or feet.
- Urge patient not to receive vaccinations and to avoid contact with anyone who has recently received a live virus vaccine.
- Inform patient that alopecia is a side effect of this agent and hair growth will resume 2-3 months after the last dose of docetaxel, but new hair may have a different color or texture.

DOXORUBICIN

BRAND NAMES
Adriamycin, Caelyx, Rubex

CLASS OF AGENT
Antineoplastic agent, anthracycline

CLINICAL PHARMACOLOGY
Mechanism of Action
Binds tightly to DNA by intercalation where there is a local uncoiling of the double helix as a result of the separation of the stacked bases by the intercalated moiety. After direct binding to DNA (intercalation)

several actions ensue, including blockade of DNA and RNA synthesis, fragmentation of DNA, and inhibition of DNA repair. Doxorubicin significantly alters mitochondrial function by causing mitochondrial swelling, cristolysis, and inhibition of coenzyme Q-dependent mitochondrial electron transfer reactions. Two other mechanisms that may contribute to the mutagenicity and cardiac toxicity of doxorubicin are formation of free radicals and inhibition of topoisomerase II enzymes. Free radical formation occurs after reduction by the microsomal enzyme cytochrome P450 (CYP) reductase. Reduced doxorubicin causes single-strand DNA scission and may contribute to its cardiotoxicity. It appears to produce two waves of DNA single-strand breakage. The initial wave involves protein-linked single-strand breaks that occur within min of drug exposure. Topoisomerase II enzymes normally produce transient, enzyme-linked double-stranded cuts in a DNA molecule to facilitate strand passing, condensation, or even relaxation of DNA supercoils. Antitumor drugs such as doxorubicin inhibit one phase of topoisomerase II activity: ligation of the DNA after double-strand breakage. As a result, the DNA is left broken with topoisomerase II subunits attached covalently to the 5' ends. **Therapeutic Effect:** Prevents cell division.

Absorption and Distribution
Widely distributed with a volume of distribution: 20-30 L/kg. It is highly protein bound in the plasma (74%-76%) and does not cross the blood-brain barrier.
Half-life: 16 hrs; 32 hrs (metabolite).

Metabolism and Excretion
Metabolized rapidly and extensively in the liver to active metabolites, doxorubicinol (active), and doxorubicin aglycones (inactive). Thus, changes in hepatic function may produce different levels of the active metabolite. Eliminated primarily in the bile and feces. It is not removed by hemodialysis.

HOW SUPPLIED/AVAILABLE FORMS
Powder for Injection (Adriamycin RDF): 10 mg, 20 mg, 50 mg, 150 mg.
Lyophilized Powder (Rubex): 50 mg, 100 mg.
Solution for Injection (Adriamycin PFS): 2 mg/mL.
Preservative-Free Solution (PFS) for Injection (Adriamycin PFS): 2 mg/mL.

INDICATIONS AND DOSAGES
Acute Lymphoblastic and Myeloblastic Leukemia; Breast, Bronchogenic, Gastric, Ovarian, Thyroid, and Transitional Cell Bladder Carcinomas; Hodgkin's Disease; Non-Hodgkin's Lymphomas; Neuroblastoma; Hepatocellular Carcinoma; Soft-Tissue and Osteogenic Sarcomas; Wilms' Tumor
60-75 mg/m^2 IV as a single dose every 14 days (dose-dense) or 21 days, 20 mg/m^2 IV once wkly, or 25-30 mg/m^2/day on 2-3 successive days every 4 weeks. Because of the risk of cardiotoxicity, do not exceed a cumulative dose of 550 mg/m^2 (400-450 mg/m^2 for those previously treated with related compounds or irradiation of cardiac region).
Dosage in Hepatic Impairment
Dosage is modified based on serum bilirubin level.

Serum Bilirubin Concentration	% of Normal Dose
1.2-3 mg/dL	50
>3 mg/dL	25

UNLABELED USES
Treatment of cancers of the cervix, head or neck, uterus, liver, ovary, pancreas, prostate, and testes. Other uses include treatment for germ cell tumors and multiple myeloma.

PRECAUTIONS
Use doxorubicin cautiously in patients with impaired hepatic function.
Pregnancy Risk Category: D
Excretion into breast milk is unknown/not recommended in nursing women.

CONTRAINDICATIONS
Cardiomyopathy; preexisting myelosuppression; previous or concomitant treatment with cyclophosphamide, idarubicin, mitoxantrone, or irradiation of the cardiac region; severe CHF

DRUG PREPARATION/ADMINISTRATION/SAFE HANDLING ISSUES
◀ ALERT ▶ Individualized based on the patient's clinical response and tolerance of the drug's adverse effects. When administering this drug, in combination therapy, consult specific protocols for optimum dosage and sequence of drug administration.

◀ **ALERT** ▶ Because doxorubicin may be carcinogenic, mutagenic, or teratogenic, wear nitrile or latex gloves when preparing or administering the drug. If doxorubicin powder or solution comes in contact with your skin, wash the area thoroughly with regular soap and water. Do not use waterless soap as this can enhance the skin reaction. When accessing a vein for infusion, avoid areas overlying joints and tendons, small veins, and swollen or edematous extremities. Use a one-pass technique for this agent.

- Reconstitute each 10-mg vial with 5 mL of preservative-free 0.9% NaCl (20-mg vial with 10 mL, 50-mg vial with 25 mL) to provide a concentration of 2 mg/mL.
- Shake the vial and allow the contents to dissolve.
- Withdraw an appropriate volume of air from the vial during reconstitution to avoid excessive pressure buildup.
- Further dilute the solution with 50 mL dextrose in water (D5W) or 0.9% NaCl, if necessary, and administer it as a continuous infusion through a central venous line.
- For IV push, administer the drug into the tubing of a free-flowing IV infusion of D5W or 0.9% NaCl, preferably through a butterfly needle. To avoid facial flushing and erythematous streaking or flare along the vein, administer over no less than 3-5 min.
- Test for flashback every 30 sec to make sure that the needle remains in the vein during injection.
- Be aware that extravasation usually produces immediate pain, which results in severe local tissue damage. If extravasation occurs, stop drug administration immediately; withdraw as much medication as possible, obtain an extravasation kit, and follow institutional protocol.

STORAGE AND STABILITY

- Store doxorubicin lyophilized powder at room temperature 15-30° C (59-86° F).
- Store doxorubicin HCl solution in refrigerator at 2-8° C (36-46° F).
- Reconstituted solution is stable for up to 7 days at room temperature or 15 days under refrigeration.
- Protect the reconstituted solution from prolonged exposure to sunlight; discard any unused portions.

INTERACTIONS
Drug
Anthracyclines or anthracenediones (daunorubicin, idarubicin, epirubicin, mitoxantrone): May increase the risk of cardiotoxicity.
Bone marrow depressants: May increase myelosuppression.
CYP 344 interacting drugs: Inducers (e.g., phenobarbital) may decrease doxorubicin levels; inhibitors (e.g., azole antifungal agents) may increase doxorubicin levels.
Digoxin: Decreases digoxin levels and may inhibit its cardiac effects. Digoxin levels should be monitored more closely.
Trastuzumab: May increase risk for cardiotoxicity.
Live-virus vaccines: May potentiate viral replication, increase vaccine side effects, and decrease the patient's antibody response to the vaccine.
Herbal
None known.

LAB EFFECTS/INTERFERENCE
May cause EKG (ECG) changes and increase serum uric acid level. Doxorubicin will reduce neutrophil, RBC, and platelet counts.

Y-SITE COMPATIBILITIES
Amifostine, bleomycin, cimetidine, cyclophosphamide, cytarabine, dactinomycin, dexamethasone (Decadron), diphenhydramine (Benadryl), docetaxel, etoposide (VePesid), famotidine, filgrastim, fludarabine, granisetron (Kytril), hydromorphone (Dilaudid), ifosfamide, leucovorin, lorazepam (Ativan), melphalan, mesna, methotrexate, mitomycin, morphine, ondansetron (Zofran), oxaliplatin, paclitaxel (Taxol), sargramostim, teniposide, thiotepa, topotecan, trastuzumab, vinblastine, vincristine, vinorelbine

INCOMPATIBILITIES
Allopurinol (Aloprim), amphotericin B colloidal (Amphotec), cefepime (Maxipime), furosemide (Lasix), ganciclovir (Cytovene), heparin, lansoprazole, levofloxacin, pantoprazole, pemetrexed, piperacillin and tazobactam (Zosyn), propofol (Diprivan), rituximab, voriconazole

SIDE EFFECTS
Serious Reactions
- Myelosuppression may cause hematologic toxicity (manifested principally as

neutropenia and, to lesser extent, anemia and thrombocytopenia), usually within 10-15 days of starting therapy. Blood counts typically return to normal levels by the third wk.

- Cardiotoxicity (either acute, manifested as arrhythmias or CHF, or chronic, manifested as significant CHF or cardiomyopathy) may occur.

Other Side Effects
Frequent (10%-50%):
Complete alopecia (scalp, eyebrows, eyelashes, axillary, and pubic hair), esophagitis (especially if drug is given on several successive days), myelosuppression, nausea, orange-reddish urine, stomatitis, vomiting
Occasional (1%-10%):
Anorexia, cardiomyopathy, diarrhea, hyperpigmentation of skin, nail beds, phalangeal and dermal creases, radiation recall
Rare (Less Than 1%):
Chills, conjunctivitis, excessive lacrimation, fever

SPECIAL CONSIDERATIONS
Baseline Assessment
- Obtain patient's CBC with differential and platelet count, before and periodically during doxorubicin therapy.
- Obtain a baseline EKG or multiple gated acquisition scan before starting doxorubicin therapy. Results must be known before the drug is administered; the usual criterion is an ejection fraction (EF) of 50%.
- Obtain liver function studies and electrolyte levels along with BUN and creatinine levels before administering each dose. If patient is receiving diuretics, make sure K and magnesium are evaluated before giving doxorubicin. Hypokalemia and hypomagnesemia can trigger arrhythmias.
Intervention and Evaluation
- Be aware that there are maximum cumulative doses for this agent that it is important to know the cumulative dose for this patient before administering another dose.
- Know that the maximum lifetime for doxorubicin is 550 mg/m^2 if no chest wall radiation has been given or 450 mg/m^2 if patient has received or will receive chest wall radiation.
- Before administration of doxorubicin know patient's EF; usual protocols call for 50% EF.
- Monitor patient for signs and symptoms of

mucositis and stomatitis, including burning or erythema of oral mucosa and difficulty swallowing. Be aware that mucositis and stomatitis may lead to ulceration of mucous membranes within 2-3 days.
- Instruct patient on oral care, and initiate a mouth care regimen. An example of an oral care regimen is 1 tsp each of salt and baking soda in 1 glass of water to swish and spit after each meal and before bedtime.
- Evaluate patient for evidence of mucositis, which may be viral or fungal in nature.
- Obtain ECG as ordered per institutional protocol, looking for any signs of arrhythmias or heart block.
- Examine patient's nail beds and skin for hyperpigmentation.
- Monitor patient's CBC with differential, along with platelets, liver and renal function test results, and serum uric acid levels.
- Assess patient's pattern of daily bowel activity and stool consistency. Evaluate for any changes in color or consistency.
- Give antiemetics, as ordered to prevent or treat nausea and vomiting.
- Monitor patient for signs and symptoms of hematologic toxicity, including excessive fatigue and weakness, ecchymosis, fever, signs of local infection, sore throat, and unusual bleeding from any site.
Education
- Warn patient to notify health care provider if he or she experiences easy bruising, fever greater than 38° C (greater than 101° F), signs of local infection, sore throat, or unusual bleeding from any site or if nausea and vomiting persist for greater than 24 hours (or greater than 12 hours for those at-risk, e.g., older patients) after dosing that is unrelieved by antiemetics.
- Instruct patient to report any signs or symptoms of cardiac alteration, rapid heart rate, palpitations, or lightheadedness.
- Advise patient to maintain good oral hygiene and educate patient on the institutional oral care regimen.
- Inform patient that total alopecia usually occurs with this agent and that hair growth will resume 2-3 mos after the last dose of doxorubicin, but new hair may have a different color and texture.
- Advise patient that urine will turn a reddish orange color for approximately 24-48 hours after dosing.
- Instruct patient to use sunscreen (SPF greater than 15) when outside as this

agent increases photosensitivity.
- Caution patient not to receive vaccinations and to avoid contact with anyone who has recently received a live-virus vaccine.
- Instruct patient to take no over-the-counter medications or herbal or vitamin supplements without checking with his or her health care provider.
- Instruct patient on local resources available and support groups related to their diagnosis.

DOXORUBICIN HCL LIPOSOME

BRAND NAMES
Doxil

CLASS OF AGENT
Antineoplastic agent, anthracycline

CLINICAL PHARMACOLOGY
Mechanism of Action
An anthracycline antibiotic that inhibits DNA and DNA-dependent RNA synthesis by binding with DNA strands. Liposomal encapsulation increases uptake by tumors, prolongs drug action, and may decrease toxicity. After distribution of liposomes to the tissue compartment, free doxorubicin is released, although the precise mechanism for this effect is unclear. The mechanism of tumor uptake of doxorubicin hydrochloride liposome appears related to the increased permeability of tumor vasculature (which occurs during angiogenesis), enabling localization into the tumor interstitial space; an enhanced vascular permeability coefficient to allow efficient transit across capillaries (paracellular pathway) may also be operative.
Therapeutic Effect: Prevents cell division.
Absorption and Distribution
Confined primarily to the intravascular space, having a volume of distribution of only 2.8 L/m^2. This contrasts with free doxorubicin, which has a larger volume of distribution than doxorubicin hydrochloride liposome and is extensively distributed to body tissues.
Protein binding is unknown. It does not cross the blood-brain barrier and is metabolized rapidly in the liver to the active metabolite.
Half-life: The elimination (second phase) half-life ranges from 45 to 55 hours, without apparent dose dependency over the range of 10-50 mg/m^2. This is longer than the elimination half-life of conventional liposomal doxorubicin formulations (about 15 hours) or equivalent doses of free doxorubicin (10-20 hours)

Metabolism and Excretion
Appears to undergo metabolism by the same pathways as free doxorubicin. However, in contrast to free doxorubicin, the rate of metabolite excretion is more rapid than the rate of metabolite formation, preventing significant plasma accumulation. Plasma concentrations of doxorubicin metabolites are either very low or undetectable after IV doxorubicin hydrochloride liposome. Approximately 2% of a dose of doxorubicin hydrochloride liposome has been recovered in the urine as doxorubicin, doxorubicinol, or other metabolites during the first 24 hours after injection. Excretion increased to approximately 5% after 72 hours. These values are less than after injection of free doxorubicin (11% urinary recovery after 24 hours). Eliminated primarily intact by biliary system and not removed by hemodialysis.

HOW SUPPLIED/AVAILABLE FORMS
Injection Solution: Lipid Complex (Doxil): 2 mg/mL.

INDICATIONS AND DOSAGES
AIDS-Related Kaposi Sarcoma (KS)
Indicated for the treatment of AIDS-related KS in patients with disease that has progressed with prior combination chemotherapy or in patients who are intolerant to such therapy. No controlled trials have been performed to demonstrate either increased survival or an improvement in symptoms of the disease.
Ovarian Cancer
Liposomal doxorubicin is indicated for the treatment of patients with ovarian cancer whose disease has progressed or recurred after platinum-based chemotherapy.

UNLABELED USES
Treatment of breast, cervical, head or neck, uterus, liver, pancreatic, and prostate cancer, and multiple myeloma.
Dosage
Adults: KS 20 mg/m^2 every 3 weeks.
Adults: Ovarian cancer 40-50 mg/m^2. Efficacy in ovarian cancer appears to be equal for 40 and 50 mg/m^2 dosing; however, patients better tolerate a dose of 40 mg/m^2.

Dosage Adjustment in Hepatic Impairment
Dosage is modified based on serum bilirubin level.

Serum Bilirubin Concentration	% of Normal Dose
1.2-3 mg/dL	50
>3 mg/dL	25

Dosage Adjustment in Hand-Foot Syndrome, Hematologic Toxicity, or Stomatitis
Grade 2 or higher toxicities of hand-foot syndrome(HFS), hematologic toxicity, or stomatitis can be managed by dose delay or dose adjustments. The following tables from the Product Information sheet may be used:

PRECAUTIONS
Use cautiously in patients with impaired hepatic function.
Pregnancy Risk Category: D

CONTRAINDICATIONS
Cardiomyopathy; preexisting myelosuppression; previous or concomitant treatment with cyclophosphamide, idarubicin, mitoxantrone, or irradiation of the cardiac region; severe CHF

DRUG PREPARATION/ADMINISTRATION/ SAFE HANDLING ISSUES
◀ ALERT ▶ Dosage is individualized on the basis of the patient's clinical response and tolerance of the drug's adverse effects. When administering this drug, in combination therapy, consult specific protocols for optimum dosage and sequence of drug administration.
◀ ALERT ▶ Because doxorubicin lipid complex may be carcinogenic, mutagenic, or teratogenic, wear nitrile or latex gloves when preparing or administering the drug. If doxorubicin powder or solution comes in contact with the skin, wash the area thoroughly with mild soap and water. Do not use waterless or antibacterial soap as either can increase the skin reaction. If the agent splashes in the eyes, use copious amounts of water or 0.9% NaCl to rinse eyes. When accessing a vein for infusion, avoid areas overlying joints and tendons, small veins, and swollen or edematous extremities.
◀ ALERT ▶ Doxorubicin lipid complex use should be avoided during pregnancy, especially in the first trimester. Avoid breast-feeding as the drug gets into breast milk.
• Dilute each dose in 250 mL of D5W. Do not use any diluent except D5W.

LIPOSOMAL DOXORUBICIN DOSE MODIFICATION FOR HFS

Toxicity grade	Symptoms	Dose adjustment
1	Mild erythema, swelling, or desquamation not interfering with daily activities	Redose unless patient has experienced previous grade 3 or 4 HFS. If so, delay up to 2 wks and decrease dose by 25%. Return to original dosing interval.
2	Erythema, desquamation, or swelling interfering with, but not precluding, normal physical activities; small blisters or ulcerations <2 cm in diameter	Delay dosing up to 2 wks or until resolved to grade 0 to 1. If after 2 wks there is no resolution, liposomal doxorubicin should be discontinued. If resolved to grade 0 to 1 within 2 wks, and there was no prior grade 3 to 4 HFS, continue treatment at previous dose and return to original dosing interval. If patient experienced previous grade 3 or 4 toxicity, continue treatment with a 25% dose reduction and return to original dosing interval.
3	Blistering, ulceration, or swelling interfering with walking or normal daily activities; cannot wear regular clothing	Delay dosing up to 2 wks or until resolved to grade 0 to 1. Decrease dose by 25% and return to original dosing interval. If after 2 wks there is no resolution, liposomal doxorubicin should be discontinued.
4	Diffuse or local process causing infectious complications or a bedridden state or hospitalization	Delay dosing up to 2 wks or until resolved to grade 0 to 1. Decrease dose by 25% and return to original dosing interval. If after 2 wks there is no resolution, liposomal doxorubicin should be discontinued.

LIPOSOMAL DOXORUBICIN DOSE MODIFICATION FOR HEMATOLOGIC TOXICITY

Grade	ANC (cells/mm³)*	Platelet Count (cells/mm³)	Modification
1	1,500-1,900	75,000-150,000	Resume treatment with no dose reduction.
2	1,000-<1,500	50,000-<75,000	Wait until ANC ≥1,500 cells/mm³ and platelet count ≥75,000 cells/mm³; redose with no dose reduction.
3	500-999	25,000-<50,000	Wait until ANC ≥1,500 cells/mm³ and platelet count ≥75,000 cells/mm³; redose with no dose reduction.
4	<500	<25,000	Wait until ANC ≥1,500 cells/mm³ and platelet count ≥75,000 cells/mm³; redose at 25% dose reduction or continue full dose with cytokine support.

*ANC = absolute neutrophil count.

- Infuse liposomal doxorubicin over more than 30 min.
- Do not use in-line filters.

STORAGE AND STABILITY
- Store at room temperature.
- The reconstituted solution is stable for up to 24 hrs at room temperature or up to 48 hrs if refrigerated.
- Protect the reconstituted solution from prolonged exposure to sunlight; discard any unused portions.
- Refrigerate unopened vials.
- Use the solution within 24 hrs of dilution.

INTERACTIONS
Drug
Antigout medications: May decrease the effects of these drugs.
Bone marrow depressants: May increase myelosuppression.
Daunorubicin: May increase the risk of cardiotoxicity.
Live-virus vaccines: May potentiate virus replication, increase vaccine side effects, and decrease the patient's antibody response to the vaccine.
Herbal
None known.

LAB EFFECTS/INTERFERENCE
May cause EKG (ECG) changes and increase serum uric acid level. Liposomal doxorubicin may reduce neutrophil, RBC, and platelet counts.

INCOMPATIBILITIES
Do not mix with any other medications.

SIDE EFFECTS
Serious Reactions
- Myelosuppression may cause hematologic toxicity (manifested principally as neutropenia and, to lesser extent, anemia and thrombocytopenia), usually within 10-15 days of starting therapy. Blood counts typically return to normal levels by the third wk.
- Cardiotoxicity (either acute, manifested as transient ECG abnormalities or a CHF-type picture, or chronic, manifested as significant CHF or cardiomyopathy) may occur.
- Severe HFS manifested by extreme hand or foot blistering, local infections, and local pain may occur.

Other Side Effects
Frequent (10%-50%):
Leukopenia, neutropenia, anemia, thrombocytopenia, mild alopecia (scalp, axillary, and pubic hair), emesis (mild), mucositis manifested by stomatitis, esophagitis, fatigue (asthenia), reddish-orange urine for 24-48 hrs, palmar-plantar erythrodysesthesia (PPE); HFS
Occasional (1%-10%):
Anorexia, diarrhea, hyperpigmentation of skin and nail beds, and phalangeal and dermal creases
Rare (Less Than 1%):
Fever, chills; ocular: conjunctivitis, excessive lacrimation

SPECIAL CONSIDERATIONS
Baseline Assessment
- Obtain patient's CBC with differential and platelet count before and periodically at 7-10 days then at 21 days during liposomal doxorubicin therapy.
- Obtain a baseline multiple gated acquisition scan or EKG before starting any liposomal doxorubicin-based therapy.
- Obtain liver function studies before administering each dose.
- Be aware that patients older than 70 years and children younger than 2 years of age are at increased risk for cardiotoxicity.

LIPOSOMAL DOXORUBICIN DOSE MODIFICATION FOR STOMATITIS

Toxicity Grade	Symptoms	Dose Adjustment
1	Painless ulcers, erythema, or mild soreness	Redose unless patient has experienced previous grade 3 or 4 toxicity. If so, delay up to 2 wks and decrease dose by 25%. Return to original dosing interval.
2	Painful erythema, edema, or ulcers, but can eat	Delay dosing up to 2 wks or until resolved to grade 0 to 1. If after 2 wks there is no resolution, liposomal doxorubicin should be discontinued. If resolved to grade 0 to 1 within 2 wks, and there was no prior grade 3 or 4 stomatitis, continue treatment at previous dose and return to original dosing interval. If patient experienced previous grade 3 or 4 toxicity, continue treatment with a 25% dose reduction and return to original dosing interval.
3	Painful erythema, edema, or ulcers, and cannot eat	Delay dosing up to 2 wks or until resolved to grade 0 to 1. Decrease dose by 25% and return to original dosing interval. If after 2 wks there is no resolution, liposomal doxorubicin should be discontinued.
4	Requires parenteral or enteral support	Delay dosing up to 2 wks or until resolved to grade 0 to 1. Decrease dose by 25% and return to liposomal doxorubicin original dosing interval. If after 2 wks there is no resolution, liposomal doxorubicin should be discontinued.

Intervention and Evaluation

- Be aware that before administration of Liposomal doxorubicin, the practitioner must know the EF of the patient. It should be at least 50% or per protocol; PPE can be doselimiting.
- Advise patient to avoid excessive use of hands and heat (sun, hot water in bathing, gardening).
- Instruct patient to wear gloves when doing dishes, handling hot pans, or placing hands in the oven or anywhere near heat.
- Advise patient to use sunblock whenever going outside; caution patients to NOT sit in the sun and to use sunscreen (SPF greater than 15).
- Instruct patient to avoid skin tape, tight clothing, and excess skin pressure and to wear shoes (low heal) that do not increase pressure on the plantar surface.
- Be aware that treatment may include bag balm, ice packs, and moisturizing lotions. Use Aquaphor, Bag Balm, Eucerin, Absorbase, or any other agents that patient feels improve skin moisturization; do not use perfumed moisturizers as they contain significant alcohol content that may dry the skin or cool baths.
- Monitor patient for signs and symptoms of stomatitis, including burning or erythema of the oral mucosa and difficulty swallowing. Be aware that stomatitis may lead to ulceration of mucous membranes within 2-3 days. Initiate a mouth care regimen as needed. Instruct patient on oral care and how to do a visual inspection of the oral cavity. An oral care regimen may include 1 tsp each of salt and baking soda in a glass of water to swish and spit after each meal and before bedtime.
- Examine patient's nail beds and skin for hyperpigmentation.
- Monitor patient's CBC with differential with platelets (delete hematologic status), liver and renal function test results, and serum uric acid levels.
- Assess patient's pattern of daily bowel activity and stool consistency. Instruct patient to report any signs of bleeding or changes in color of stool.
- Be aware that antiemetics are usually not necessary if liposomal doxorubicin is given as a single agent unless patient has had substantial emesis with a previous cycle of therapy.
- Monitor patient for signs and symptoms of hematologic toxicity, including excessive fatigue and weakness, ecchymosis, fever, signs of local infection, sore throat, and unusual bleeding from any site.

Education

- Educate patient on when to contact his or her health care provider: signs and symptoms of infection, fever greater than 38° C (greater than 101° F), chills, cough, nausea, or vomiting for greater than 24 hours, or diarrhea for greater than 24 hours.

- Evaluate skin to determine whether topical skin treatment is needed. Initiate a skin care regimen such as Aquaphor, Absorbase, Eucerin, or Bag Balm cream bid on palms of hands and soles of feet.
- Be aware that pyridoxine 150 mg 3 times daily or 200 mg twice daily have been used to decrease PPE.
- Monitor all areas of diaphoresis for any signs of erythema or skin changes: axilla, under breasts in women, groin, and inguinal areas.
- Warn patient to notify his or her health care provider if he or she experiences easy bruising, fever, signs of local infection, sore throat, or unusual bleeding from any site, or if nausea and vomiting persist after discharge.
- Urge patient receiving the lipid complex form of doxorubicin to avoid consuming alcohol during therapy because alcohol may cause GI irritation such as nausea and can have serious side effects on liver function.
- Caution patient not to receive vaccinations and to avoid contact with anyone who has recently received a live-virus vaccine.
- Advise patient regarding an oral hygiene program.
- Inform patient urine may turn a reddish-orange color for 48 hours after dosing.
- Inform patient that hair growth will resume 2-3 months after the last dose of doxorubicin, but new hair may have a different color and texture.
- Instruct patient to take no over-the-counter medications or herbal or vitamin supplements without checking with his or her health care provider.
- Instruct patient on local resources available and support groups related to their diagnosis.

EPIRUBICIN

BRAND NAMES
Ellence, Pharmorubicin

CLASS OF AGENT
Antitumor antibiotic, anthracycline

CLINICAL PHARMACOLOGY
Mechanism of Action
An anthracycline antibiotic for which the exact mechanism is unknown but it has been shown to generate cytotoxic free radicals. It is purported to complex with DNA and subsequently inhibit DNA, RNA, and protein synthesis. It also inhibits DNA helicase activity, preventing enzymatic separation of double-stranded DNA and interfering with replication and transcription. **Therapeutic Effect:** Produces antiproliferative and cytotoxic activity.

Absorption and Distribution
Epirubicin is widely distributed into tissues and has a volume of distribution of ~25 L/kg. Protein binding: 77%.
Half-life: The parent compound half-life is about 33 hrs. Its major metabolite (active), epirubicinol, has a half-life ranging from 20 to 31 hrs.

Metabolism and Excretion
Extensively and rapidly metabolized by the liver and is also metabolized by other organs and cells, including RBCs. It is metabolized to epirubicinol (active). Both the parent compound and epirubicinol are conjugated to the glucuronide. Inactive aglycones are formed as well. Epirubicin is primarily eliminated through biliary excretion. Epirubicin and its major metabolites are eliminated through biliary excretion and, to a lesser extent, by urinary excretion. Mass-balance data from one patient showed approximately 60% of the total radioactive dose in feces (34%) and urine (27%). Not removed by hemodialysis.

HOW SUPPLIED/AVAILABLE FORMS
Injection: 2-mg/mL single-use vials in 25 mL or 100 mL.

INDICATIONS AND DOSAGES
Breast Cancer
In combination with fluorouracil (5-FU) and cyclophosphamide, epirubicin is given as 100 mg/m^2 in repeated cycles of 3-4 wk
In combination with 5-FU and cyclophosphamide, epirubicin is given as 60 mg/m^2/dose on day 1 and 8 (total dose = 120 mg/m^2/cycle)
Dose Adjustment for Toxicities
If patient has a cycle nadir of ANC less than 250/mm^3 or platelet count less than 50,000/mm^3 or neutropenic fever, the day 1 dose should be reduced to 75% of the usual dose.
If patient has grade 3 or 4 nonhematologic toxicity, the day 1 dose should be reduced to 75%.

Day 1 chemotherapy should be delayed until ANC is greater than 1,500/mm³ or platelets are greater than 100,000/mm³ and nonhematologic toxicities have recovered to normal.

For patients receiving epirubicin on a day 1 and 8 schedule, the day 8 dose should be 75% of the day 1 dose if platelet counts are 75,000-100,000/mm³ and ANC is 1,000-1,499/mm³. If day 8 platelet counts are less than 75,000/mm³, ANC is less than 1,000/mm³, or grade 3/4 nonhematologic toxicity has occurred, the day 8 dose should be omitted.

Dosage Adjustment in Hepatic Dysfunction
In patients with elevated serum SGOT (AST) or serum total bilirubin concentrations, the following dose reductions were recommended in clinical trials, although few patients experienced hepatic impairment:
• Bilirubin 1.2-3 mg/dL or AST 2-4 × UNL: 50% of recommended starting dose.
• Bilirubin greater than 3 mg/dL or AST greater than 4 × UNL: 25% of recommended starting dose.

Dosage Adjustment in Renal Dysfunction
There are no definitive guidelines for renal dysfunction, but the package insert recommends that in patients with severe renal dysfunction (creatinine greater than 5 mg/dL), a lower starting dose be used.

UNLABELED USES
Treatment of lung or ovarian carcinoma, non-Hodgkin's lymphoma, sarcomas

PRECAUTIONS
Pregnancy Risk Category: D

CONTRAINDICATIONS
Baseline ANC less than 1,500/mm³, hypersensitivity to epirubicin, previous treatment with anthracyclines up to maximum cumulative dose, recent MI, severe hepatic impairment, severe myocardial insufficiency

DRUG PREPARATION/ADMINISTRATION/ SAFE HANDLING ISSUES
◀ ALERT ▶ The use of nitrile or latex gloves is recommended. If a spill or splash occurs, the area should be washed thoroughly with mild soap and water. Do not use antibacterial or waterless soap as either can increase

the risk of skin reactions. Splashes into the eyes should also be irrigated thoroughly with water or 0.9% NaCl.

A direct push injection is not recommended because of the risk of extravasation, which may occur even in the presence of adequate blood return upon needle aspiration.

The following administration method is intended to minimize the risk of thrombosis or perivenous extravasation, which could lead to severe cellulitis, vesication, or tissue necrosis. Epirubicin solution should be administered into the tubing of a freely flowing IV infusion. Patients receiving 100-120 mg/m² doses should generally have the drug infused over 15-20 min. For patients who require lower epirubicin starting doses due to organ dysfunction or who require dose modification, the epirubicin may be decreased in proportion to the infusion time, but should not be less than 3 min. Avoiding injections into small vessels or repeating injections into the same vein may minimize venous sclerosis.

STORAGE AND STABILITY
Store refrigerated at 2-8° C (36-46° F). Do not freeze. Protect from light. Epirubicin should be used within 24 hrs of the first penetration of the rubber stopper. Discard any unused solution.

INTERACTIONS
Drug
Taxanes (docetaxel, paclitaxel): Although coadministration of paclitaxel or docetaxel does not affect the pharmacokinetics of epirubicin when given immediately after the taxanes, it is recommended that the drugs by spaced by at least 24 hrs.
Cimetidine: Coadministration of cimetidine (400 mg bid for 7 days starting 5 days before chemotherapy) increased the mean area under the curve of epirubicin (100 mg/m²) by 50% and decreased its plasma clearance by 30%.
Blood dyscrasia-causing medications: May increase the patient's risk of developing leukopenia or thrombocytopenia.
Bone marrow depressants: May cause additive bone marrow suppression.
Calcium channel blockers: May increase the patient's risk of developing heart failure.
Drugs metabolized by cytochrome P450 enzymes: No systematic in vitro or in vivo evaluation has been performed to examine

the potential for inhibition or induction by epirubicin of oxidase cytochrome P450 isoenzymes.
Hepatotoxic medications: May increase the risk of hepatotoxicity.
Live-virus vaccines: May potentiate viral replication, increase vaccine side effects, and decrease the patient's antibody response to the vaccine.
Herbal
None known.

LAB EFFECTS/INTERFERENCE
None known.

Y-SITE COMPATIBLES
Amifostine, carboplatin, cisplatin, cyclophosphamide, cyclosporine, dexrazoxane, diphenhydramine, docetaxel, etoposide, gemcitabine, granisetron, hydrocortisone Na succinate, irinotecan, ifosfamide, mesna, mitomycin, ondansetron, oxaliplatin, paclitaxel, palonosetron, prochlorperazine, promethazine, tacrolimus, teniposide, thiotepa, vinblastine, vincristine, vinorelbine

INCOMPATIBLES
Acyclovir, allopurinol, aminophylline, amphotericin B conventional, amphotericin B liposomal (AmBisome), ampicillin, ampicillin-sulbactam, azithromycin, cefepime, cefoperazone, cefotetan, cefoxitin, ceftazidime, ceftriaxone, cefuroxime, dexamethasone, diazepam, fluorouracil, foscarnet, fosphenytoin, furosemide, ganciclovir, heparin, hydrocortisone, ketorolac, leucovorin, magnesium, meropenem, methohexital, methylprednisolone, nafcillin, pantoprazole, pemetrexed, pentobarbital, phenobarbital, phenytoin, piperacillin, piperacillin/tazobactam, K phosphates, Na bicarbonate, Na phosphates, sulfamethoxazole/trimethoprim, thiopental, ticarcillin, ticarcillin/clavulanate

SIDE EFFECTS
Serious Reactions
- The risk of cardiotoxicity (either acute, manifested as transient EKG abnormalities, or chronic, manifested as CHF) increases when the total cumulative dose exceeds 900 mg/m^2.
- Extravasation during administration may result in severe local tissue necrosis.
- Myelosuppression may cause hematologic toxicity, manifested principally as leukopenia and, to lesser extent, anemia and thrombocytopenia.

Other Side Effects
Frequent (10%-50%):
Alopecia, amenorrhea, anemia, cardiac arrhythmias, diarrhea, nausea, thrombocytopenia, vomiting
Occasional (1%-10%):
Conjunctivitis, diarrhea, fever, hot flashes, lethargy, pruritus, rash, stomatitis
Rare (Less Than 1%):
The cumulative risk of secondary acute myelogenous leukemia or myelodysplastic syndrome in patients who received adjuvant epirubicin therapy as a component of polychemotherapy regimens was approximately 0.27% at 3 years, 0.46% at 5 years, and 0.55% at 8 years.

SPECIAL CONSIDERATIONS
Baseline Assessment
- Assess patient's CBC with differential, platelets, electrolytes, BUN, and creatinine levels along with liver function tests, paying particular attention to the bilirubin level.
- Be aware that dose reductions are required in patients with elevated bilirubin levels.
- Be aware that baseline EKG or multiple gated acquisition (MUGA) scans are required before this therapy is initiated. An ejection fraction of greater than 50% is usually required or as protocol dictates.

Intervention and Evaluation
- Administer premedication with antiemetics as ordered.
- Assess results of MUGA scans or ECHO; do not administer until results are known and have been evaluated.
- Assess CBC with differential, platelet count, liver function tests (especially the bilirubin level), and electrolytes, BUN, and creatinine levels.
- Assess peripheral veins as epirubicin is a vesicant (black box warning); a central access device for drug delivery may be placed.
- Before peripheral administration, bring an extravasation kit to bedside and follow institutional protocol for implementation.
- Evaluate patient's nails on hands and feet as this agent can cause nail bed changes.
- Evaluate patient for alopecia with epirubicin.

Education
- Instruct patient to report any pain or burning upon delivery of the agent peripherally;

with this agent a central device is indicated for poor peripheral access because of the reported significant thrombophlebitis caused by epirubicin.

- Educate patient on signs and symptoms of neutropenia and when to contact his or her health care provider: fever greater than 38° C (greater than 101° F), shaking, chills cough, fatigue, petechiae, easy bruising, or bleeding from any site
- Advise patient to contact his or her health care provider if any rapid heart rate, palpitations, or dizziness is noted as this agent can cause cardiac changes.
- Make sure patient has a 24-hour number for the health care provider.
- Educate patient that total body alopecia will occur with epirubicin, but hair will regrow although it may be different in color and texture.
- Advise patient his or her urine will turn slightly orange for 24-48 hours and then will return to normal color.
- Instruct patient to take no over-the-counter medications or herbal or vitamin supplements without checking with his or her health care provider.
- Instruct patient on local resources available and support groups related to their diagnosis.

EPOETIN ALFA, ERYTHROPOIETIN

BRAND NAMES
Epogen, Procrit

CLASS OF AGENT
Colony-stimulating factor, growth factor, recombinant human erythropoietin

CLINICAL PHARMACOLOGY
Mechanism of Action
A glycoprotein that is produced in the kidneys and stimulates division and differentiation of erythroid progenitor cells in bone marrow. Epoetin alfa has the same biologic effects as endogenous erythropoietin and induces erythropoiesis and releases reticulocytes from bone marrow. **Therapeutic Effect:** Stimulates red cell production and improves anemia.
Absorption and Distribution
Well absorbed after subcutaneous administration. After administration, an increase in

reticulocyte count occurs within 10 days and increases in Hgb, Hct, and RBC counts are seen within 2-6 wks.
Half-life: IV administration 4-13 hrs. In patients with chronic renal failure, the half-life is 20% longer.
Metabolism and Excretion
No information.

HOW SUPPLIED/AVAILABLE FORMS
Injection: 2,000 units/mL; 3,000 units/mL; 4,000 units/mL; 10,000 units/mL; 20,000 units/mL; 40,000 units/mL.

INDICATIONS AND DOSAGES
Note: Before administration, iron stores should be evaluated: transferring should be at least 20% and ferritin at least 100 mcg/mL.
Treatment of Anemia in Chemotherapy Patients
IV, subcutaneous: 150 units/kg/dose 3 times/wk, or 40,000 units once wkly. If Hgb does not increase by 1 g/dL after the first 4 wks, increase dose to 60,000 units once wkly. Reduce dose by 25% if Hgb is greater than 12 g/dL or increases by more than 1 g/dL in any 2-wk period. Hold dose if Hgb is greater than 13 g/dL until Hgb falls to 12 g/dL, and restart at 25% below previous dose.
Pediatric patients (5-18 years of age): 600 units/kg once wkly (maximum 40,000 units). Increase to 900 units/kg if Hgb had not increased by 1 g/dL after the first 4 wks (maximum 60,000 units). Reduce dose by 25% if Hgb is >12 g/dL or increases by more than 1 g/dL in any 2-wk period. Hold dose if Hgb is greater than 13 g/dL until Hgb falls to 12 g/dL, and restart at 25% below previous dose.
Reduction of Allogenic Blood Transfusions in Elective Surgery
Subcutaneous: 300 units/kg/day 10 days before day of and 4 days after surgery. Alternative dose schedule is 600 units/kg once wkly (21, 14, and 7 days before surgery) plus a 4th dose on the day of surgery. Iron supplementation should be initiated before and during epoetin alfa therapy.
Chronic Renal Failure
IV bolus, subcutaneous: 50 to 100 units/kg 3 times/wk. Individually titrate upward monthly if Hgb dose not increase by 2 g/dL after 8 wks of therapy, and Hgb is less than 10-12 g/dL. Reduce dose by 25% if Hgb approaches 12 g/dL or increases by more

than 1 g/dL in any 2-wk period. Hold dose if Hgb is greater than 13 g/dL until Hgb falls to 12 g/dL, and restart at 25% below previous dose. For dialysis patients, the IV route is recommended. The pediatric patient starting dose is 50 units/kg 3 times/wk.

HIV Infection in Patients Treated with Zidovudine (AZT)

IV, subcutaneous: 100 units/kg 3 times/wk for 8 wks; may increase by 50-100 units/kg 3 times/wk. Evaluate response q4-8wk thereafter. Adjust dosage by 50-100 units/kg 3 times/wk. If dosages larger than 300 units/kg 3 times/wk are not eliciting a response, it is unlikely patient will respond.

UNLABELED USES

Prevention of anemia in patients donating blood before elective surgery or autologous transfusion.

PRECAUTIONS

Use epoetin alfa cautiously in patients with hemolytic anemia, a history of seizures, hypertension, liver disease, sickle cell anemia, hypercoagulable states, porphyria (an impairment of erythrocyte formation in bone marrow), and thrombotic events. Pure red cell aplasia (PRCA) and sudden severe anemia was reported postmarketing. If a patient suddenly develops a loss of response and experiences severe anemia and a low reticulocyte count, he or she should be evaluated for neutralizing antibodies. Do not switch to other erythropoietic proteins as they may cross-react.

Pregnancy Risk Category: C
Drug excretion into human breast milk is unknown. Caution should be used when administered to a nursing woman.

CONTRAINDICATIONS

History of sensitivity to mammalian cell-derived products or human albumin or uncontrolled hypertension

DRUG PREPARATION/ADMINISTRATION/ SAFE HANDLING ISSUES

◄ **ALERT** ► Patients receiving AZT who have serum erythropoietin levels greater than 500 mU are not likely to respond to therapy.
IV
• Avoid excessive agitation of vial; do not shake because it can cause foaming. Also, vigorous shaking may denature the medication, rendering it inactive.

• Reconstitution is not necessary.
• May be given as an IV bolus.
Subcutaneous
• Use one dose per vial; do not reenter vial. Discard unused portion.
• May be mixed in a syringe with bacteriostatic 0.9% NaCl with 0.9% benzyl alcohol or bacteriostatic saline at a 1:1 ratio. Benzyl alcohol acts as a local anesthetic and may reduce injection site discomfort.

STORAGE AND STABILITY

Store at 2-8° C (36-46° F). Do not freeze. Protect from light. Do not shake vials vigorously because doing so may denature the medication, rendering it inactive.

INTERACTIONS

Drug
Heparin: An increase in RBC volume may enhance blood clotting. Heparin dosage may need to be increased.
Herbal
None known.

LAB EFFECTS/INTERFERENCE

May increase BUN, serum phosphorus, serum K, serum creatinine, serum uric acid, and Na levels. May decrease bleeding time, iron concentration, and serum ferritin levels.

Y-SITE COMPATIBLES

None known.

INCOMPATIBLES

Do not mix with other medications.

SIDE EFFECTS

Serious Reactions
• Hypertensive encephalopathy, thrombosis, cerebrovascular accident, MI, and seizures have occurred rarely and may be fatal.
• Hyperkalemia occurs occasionally in patients with chronic renal failure, usually in those who do not conform to the medication regimen, dietary guidelines, and frequency of their dialysis regimen.
• PRCA and sudden severe anemia were reported postmarketing (see Precautions).
Other Side Effects
Frequent (10%-50%):
Diarrhea, dyspnea, edema, fever, headache, hypertension, hypotension, myalgia, paresthesia, peripheral edema

Occasional (1%-10%):
Asthenia, chest pain, dizziness, fatigue, injection site reaction, shortness of breath, trunk pain, vomiting
Rare (Less Than 1%):
CVA/TIA, MI, PRCA or severe anemia, seizure

SPECIAL CONSIDERATIONS
Baseline Assessment
- Assess patient's B/P before administering epoetin alfa. Because 80% of patients with chronic renal failure have a history of hypertension, expect that B/P will rise during early therapy.
- Monitor patient aggressively for increased B/P. Know that 25% of patients receiving epoetin alfa also require antihypertensive therapy and dietary restrictions.
- Assess patient's serum iron level. Keep in mind that transferrin saturation should be greater than 20%, and the serum ferritin level should be greater than 100 ng/mL before and during therapy.
- If patient is a Jehovah's Witness, ensure that he or she is informed that epoetin alfa contains albumin.
- Consider that all patients will eventually need supplemental iron therapy.
- Establish patient's CBC; especially note patient's Hct and Hgb levels.
Intervention and Evaluation
- Monitor patient's Hgb level and adjust dose accordingly but not more frequently than once monthly.
- Monitor patient's Hct level diligently. Reduce the dosage if patient's Hct level increases more than 4 points in 2 weeks.
- Assess patient's CBC routinely.
- Monitor patient's body temperature; especially in patients receiving chemotherapy and in patients with HIV infection treated with AZT.
- Monitor serum BUN, phosphorus, K, creatinine, and uric acid levels, especially in patients with chronic renal failure.
Education
- Educate patient on when to contact his or her health care provider: fever greater than 38° C (greater than 101° F), chills, cough, shortness of breath, palpitations, or severe headaches or weight gain of more than 4 pounds per wk.
- Stress to patient that frequent blood tests will be needed to determine correct dosage.

- Warn patient to report severe headache.
- Caution patient to avoid potentially hazardous activities during the first 90 days of therapy. There is an increased risk of seizure development in patients with chronic renal failure during the first 90 days of therapy.
- Educate patient on signs and symptoms of deep vein thrombosis and pulmonary embolus.
- Instruct patient to take no over-the-counter medications or herbal or vitamin supplements without checking with his or her health care provider.

ERLOTINIB
BRAND NAMES
Tarceva

CLASS OF AGENT
Antineoplastic agent, epidermal growth factor receptor (EGRF) inhibitor, tyrosine kinase inhibitor

CLINICAL PHARMACOLOGY
Mechanism of Action
The mechanism of action of erlotinib is not fully characterized. Erlotinib inhibits intracellular phosphorylation of tyrosine kinase associated with the EGFR. EGFRs are found on both normal and cancer cells and are involved with cell proliferation and survival. **Therapeutic Effect:** Inhibits the growth of cancer cells.
Absorption and Distribution
Absorption is approximately 60% without food and 100% with food. Peak plasma levels occur in 4 hrs. The time to steady state plasma concentration is 7-8 days. Protein bound: 93%. Volume of distribution: 232 L/kg.
Half-life: 36 hrs.
Metabolism and Excretion
Metabolized by cytochrome P450 (CYP) 3A4 and to lesser extent by CYP 1A2/1. Eliminated primarily via feces (83%).

HOW SUPPLIED/AVAILABLE FORMS
Tablets: 25 mg, 100 mg, 150 mg.

INDICATIONS AND DOSAGES
Non-Small Cell Lung Cancer
150 mg orally daily 1 hr before or 2 hrs after a meal as monotherapy after failure of at least one prior chemotherapy regimen. Continue until disease

progression or unacceptable toxicity occurs.

Pancreatic Cancer
100 mg orally daily 1 hr before or 2 hrs after a meal in combination with gemcitabine as first-line therapy. Continue until disease progression or unacceptable toxicity occurs.

Dose Adjustment for Toxicity
Decrease by 50-mg increments as necessary.

Dose Adjustment for Drug-Drug Interactions
Refer to Drug Interaction section: dosage adjustments may be considered.

Dosage Adjustment in Hepatic Dysfunction
No specific recommendations available. Dose reduction or interruption should be considered for severe changes in liver function.

Dosage Adjustment in Renal Dysfunction
No adjustments necessary.

UNLABELED USES
Breast cancer, colorectal cancer, ovarian cancer, renal cell carcinoma

PRECAUTIONS
Severe or persistent diarrhea, interstitial lung disease, grade 3 conjunctivitis and keratitis, and corneal ulcerations have been reported.

Pregnancy Risk Category: D
Use adequate contraceptive methods for at least 2 wks after erlotinib discontinuation. Drug excretion into breast milk is unknown/not recommended in nursing women.

CONTRAINDICATIONS
Hypersensitivity to erlotinib or any of its excipients

DRUG PREPARATION/ADMINISTRATION/SAFE HANDLING ISSUES
• Take orally on an empty stomach (1 hr before or 2 hrs after a meal).

STORAGE AND STABILITY
Store at 25° C (77° F) (excursions allowed 15-30° C; 59-86° F).

INTERACTIONS
Drug
CYP 3A4 inducers (aminoglutethimide, carbamazepine, nafcillin, nevirapine, phenobarbital, phenytoin, rifampin, rifabutin, rifapentine): May decrease the levels and effects of erlotinib. Avoid if possible. If

alternatives are not available, erlotinib doses greater than 150 mg should be considered and reduced when the CYP 3A4 inducer is discontinued.

CYP 3A4 inhibitors (ciprofloxacin, clarithromycin, diclofenac, doxycycline, erythromycin, imatinib, isoniazid, itraconazole, ketoconazole, nefazodone, nicardipine, propofol, protease inhibitors, quinidine, telithromycin, troleandomycin, verapamil, voriconazole): May increase the levels and effects of erlotinib. A decrease in the erlotinib dose should be considered if serious adverse effects occur.

Warfarin (coumarin-derivative anticoagulants): May raise international normalized ratio (INR) and increase risk of bleeding. Monitor INR or PT regularly.

Herbal
St John's Wort: May increase metabolism and decrease serum erlotinib concentration. Avoid use.

Food
Grapefruit inhibits CYP 3A4 enzymes and can potentially enhance erlotinib effects.

LAB EFFECTS/INTERFERENCE
May increase transaminases, bilirubin, and alkaline phosphatase.

SIDE EFFECTS
Serious Reactions
• If acute onset of new or progressive, unexplained symptoms such as dyspnea, cough, and fever occur, hold erlotinib and assess for interstitial lung disease (ILD). Rare occurrences of IDL have been reported and may be fatal.
• Severe uncontrolled diarrhea (median onset of diarrhea = 12 days) or severe skin reactions (median onset of rash = 8 days) may require a dose reduction or interruption. Decrease by 50-mg increments.
• Incidences of MI, cardiovascular accidents, and microangiopathic hemolytic anemia with thrombocytopenia have been reported in clinical trials.
• Overdosage in a single ingested dose of 1600 mg was reported without serious adverse events. Diarrhea, rash, and liver transaminase elevation may occur. Hold erlotinib and treat symptoms.

Other Side Effects
Frequent (10%-50%):
Anorexia, constipation, diarrhea, dry mouth, dyspnea, fatigue, rash

Occasional (1%-10%):
Abdominal pain, cough, dry skin, headache, hepatic enzyme elevations, infection, nausea, pruritus, stomatitis, vomiting

Rare (Less Than 1%):
Conjunctivitis, corneal ulcerations, GIbleeding (may be associated with warfarin or NSAID usage), interstitial lung disease, keratitis

SPECIAL CONSIDERATIONS

Baseline Assessment

- Assess patient's ability to be adherent with oral medications.
- Assess patient's history for any problems with constipation, diarrhea, oral ulcers, or any prior pulmonary disease.
- Obtain baseline skin assessment, with particular attention to any history of acne or other skin disorders.
- Evaluate patient for any history of ocular disorders.

Intervention and Evaluation

- Instruct patient to take erlotinib 1 hr before or 2 hrs after meals and take with a glass of water only. Make sure patient is aware water should be the only fluid to use for taking this medication. Erlotinib should be taken on an empty stomach.
- Assess patient for any signs or symptoms of diarrhea and initiate antidiarrheal drugs as necessary.
- Monitor for any changes in pulmonary function, new symptoms of shortness of breath, dyspnea upon exertion, or rhonchi on chest examination.
- Evaluate skin for rashes and eyes for dry eyes and conjunctivitis.

Education

- Instruct patient on how and when to take this medication: 1 hour before or 2 hours after meals and only with water. This agent should be taken on an empty stomach.
- Educate patient to maintain a drug diary and to bring medication and diary to each visit.
- Instruct patient on when to contact his or her health care provider: shortness of breath or any new symptoms.
- Remind patient to inform the health care provider before starting any and all new medications, including over-the-counter medications and herbal or vitamin supplements.

- Instruct patient on how to use loperamide for diarrheal symptoms.
- Instruct patient on a skin care regimen if an acneiform rash develops, applying moisturizers, not astringents, to the areas. Instruct patient that this is not like the acne he or she may have had as a teenager and must be treated differently. Patient may use any moisturizer of choice (Aquaphor, Eucerin, Absorbase, Bag Balm, or others). Encourage patients to avoid alcohol-containing products as these will dry the skin and can increase the drug reaction.
- Initiate a skin care regimen as soon as a rash develops; patient may require more than moisturizers such as topical or oral antibiotics for skin eruptions.
- Advise patient on what symptoms need to be reported immediately: diarrhea lasting greater than 24 hours, nausea lasting greater than 24 hours, the inability to take food or the medicine for greater than 24 hours, severe abdominal pain, fatigue, eye irritation, and dry eyes.
- Instruct patient on local resources available and support groups related to their diagnosis.
- Skin care for dermatologic reactions:
  - Wash thoroughly using a mild soap with the active agent pyrithione zinc, such as Head and Shoulders.
  - Use water-based creams such as Cetaphil or Vanicream; apply to ears and nose.
  - Avoid sun exposure use SPF 30 sunscreen.
  - Use hypoallergenic make-up.
  - Use nasal spray followed by Vaseline to reduce risk of nosebleeds.
  - Use 12% Lac-Hydrin or other exfoliating lotions during the dry phase.
  - Stay hydrated.
  - Apply a zinc barrier to the rectal area after washing to reduce irritation, use some type of baby wipe to reduce irritation from the toilet paper.
  - Clean all skin folds carefully and monitor for infection in groin and rectal areas.
  - Use plenty of water-soluble lubricant for intercourse, i.e., KY jelly.
  - Keep fingernails and toenails trimmed; apply liquid bandage for breaks.
  - Avoid artificial nails.

ESTRAMUSTINE PHOSPHATE

BRAND NAMES
Emcyt

CLASS OF AGENT
Antineoplastic agent, alkylating agent

CLINICAL PHARMACOLOGY
Mechanism of Action
A combination of estrogen and nitrogen mustard. It is an alkylating agent that acts more as a microtubule inhibitor in that it binds to microtubule-associated proteins, causing their disassembly. **Therapeutic Effect:** Impaired mitosis and consequently cell death by apoptosis.
Absorption and Distribution
Well absorbed from the GI tract (75%). Highly localized in prostatic tissue.
Half-life: 20 hrs.
Metabolism and Excretion
Rapidly dephosphorylated during absorption in peripheral circulation to estramustine, estradiol, and estrone. Oxidized in the liver. Major metabolite is estromustine. Primarily eliminated in feces by biliary system.

HOW SUPPLIED/AVAILABLE FORMS
Capsules: 140 mg.

INDICATIONS AND DOSAGES
Metastatic Prostatic Carcinoma
10-16 mg/kg/day orally in 3-4 divided doses
Dosage Adjustment in Hepatic Dysfunction
No recommendation available. Use with caution.
Dosage Adjustment in Renal Dysfunction
No adjustments required.

UNLABELED USES
No information available.

PRECAUTIONS
Pregnancy Risk Category: C
Use with caution in patients with CHF in case of possible edema and history of thrombosis, thrombophlebitis, or thromboembolic disorders and increase risk of thrombosis. Tolerance to glucose may decrease; monitor diabetic patients.

CONTRAINDICATIONS
Active thrombophlebitis or thromboembolic disorders except where actual tumor mass is the cause of thromboembolic event and benefits may outweigh the risks; hypersensitivity to estradiol or nitrogen mustard

DRUG PREPARATION/ADMINISTRATION/SAFE HANDLING ISSUES
• Take tablets with water on an empty stomach, 1 hr before or 2 hrs after meals.
• Do not take estramustine with calcium-rich products.
• Overdosage data are unavailable. In the event of overdosage, use of gastric lavage and symptomatic support should be initiated. Monitor hematologic and hepatic parameters.

STORAGE AND STABILITY
Refrigerate capsules. Capsules may be left out 24-48 hrs without affecting potency.

INTERACTIONS
Drug
Calcium-containing antacids: May impair estramustine absorption.
Hepatotoxic medications: May increase the risk of hepatotoxicity.
Herbal
None known.

LAB EFFECTS/INTERFERENCE
May increase blood glucose level and serum bilirubin, cortisol, lactate dehydrogenase, phospholipid, prolactin, AST (SGOT), Na, and triglyceride levels. May decrease urine pregnanediol level and serum antithrombin III, folate, and phosphate levels. May alter thyroid function test results.

SIDE EFFECTS
Serious Reactions
• Estramustine use may exacerbate CHF and increase the risk of pulmonary emboli, thrombophlebitis, and cerebrovascular accidents. Some protocols include prophylactic anticoagulation such as warfarin 2 mg/day or aspirin 325 mg/day.
Other Side Effects
Frequent (10%-50%):
Abdominal upset, breast tenderness or enlargement, diarrhea, dyspnea, flatulence, impotence, liver enzymes elevations, nausea, peripheral edema
Occasional (1%-10%):
Anorexia, CHF, dry skin, ecchymosis, hypertension, insomnia, leg cramps, leukopenia, MI, night sweats, thirst, thrombosis

Rare (Less Than 1%):
Allergic reactions, anxiety, burning throat, fatigue, flushing, glucose tolerance, gynecomastia, GI bleeding, headache, hoarseness, insomnia, rash, thinning hair, thirst, vomiting

SPECIAL CONSIDERATIONS
Baseline Assessment
- Assess patient for any history of deep vein thrombosis or thromboembolic disorders.
- Monitor for baseline complete blood count with differential, liver function tests, electrolytes, BUN, and creatinine. Coagulation status with platelet count, PT, partial thromboplastin time, and fibrinogen.
- Evaluate for any history of or concurrent hypertension.
- Monitor all current medications patient is receiving.

Intervention and Evaluation
- Assess laboratory data at each visit.
- Evaluate patient for any signs or symptoms of thrombophlebitis, deep vein thrombosis, chest pain, or hypertension.
- Monitor patient for evidence of edema and weight gain.
- Evaluate patient's ability to comply with an oral medication regimen.
- Assess patient for any evidence of tender or enlarged breasts.
- Monitor patient for symptoms of diarrhea and evaluate the need for antidiarrheal drugs.

Education
- Advise patient to take this agent 1 hour before or 2 hours after meals and to avoid taking this agent with milk or any calcium-based products.
- Instruct patient to maintain a drug diary and to bring medication bottles and diary to each appointment.
- Educate patient regarding signs and symptoms of lower extremity deep vein thrombosis: edema, erythema, or pain to touch in the area of the calf.
- Instruct patient on when to contact his or her health care provider: weight gain of more than 4 pounds in 1 week, diarrhea lasting greater than 24 hours, the inability to drink at least 1500 mL of fluid in 24 hours, chest pain, shortness of breath, bleeding from any site, swollen or painful breasts, headache, blurred vision, or weakness.
- Educate patient to not start any new medications, over-the-counter preparations or herbal or vitamin supplements without notifying the health care provider.

- Instruct patient on local resources available and support groups related to their diagnosis.

ETOPOSIDE, VP-16
BRAND NAMES
VePesid, Toposar

CLASS OF AGENT
Antineoplastic agent, podophyllotoxin derivative

CLINICAL PHARMACOLOGY
Mechanism of Action
An epipodophyllotoxin that induces single- and double-stranded breaks in DNA. Cell cycle-dependent and phase-specific agent; most effective in the S and G_2 phases of cell division. **Therapeutic Effect:** Inhibits or alters DNA synthesis.

Absorption and Distribution
Variably absorbed from the gastrointestinal tract. The bioavailability of oral (PO) etoposide is not affected by food for doses less than 200 mg. It is rapidly distributed, with low concentrations in CSF. Protein binding: 97%.
Half-life: 4-11 hrs.

Metabolism and Excretion
Metabolized in the liver. Primarily excreted in urine. Not removed by hemodialysis.

HOW SUPPLIED/AVAILABLE FORMS
Capsules (VePesid): 50 mg.
Injection (Toposar, VePesid): 20 mg/mL (may contain benzyl alcohol, polyethylene glycol, and/or ethanol 30.5% v/v); 5-mL, 7.5-mL, 10-mL, 25-mL vials.

INDICATIONS AND DOSAGES
Refer to individual disease protocols. Doses and schedules vary according to each protocol. Modifications are based on patient's response to therapy and tolerability.

Refractory Testicular Tumors
IV: 50-100 mg/m^2/day IV on days 1-5, or 100 mg/m^2/day IV on days 1, 3, and 5 (as combination therapy).

Small Cell Lung Carcinoma
PO: Twice the IV dose rounded to nearest 50 mg. Give once daily for doses less than 400 mg, in divided doses for dosages greater than 400 mg.
IV: 35 mg/m^2/day IV for 4 consecutive days up to 50 mg/m^2/day IV for 5 consecutive days (as combination therapy).

Dosage Adjustment in Renal Dysfunction
Dosage is modified based on Ccr.

Creatinine Clearance	Administer % of Dose
>50 mL/min	100
15-50 mL/min	75

UNLABELED USES
Treatment of leukemia, lymphoma, AIDS-associated Kaposi's sarcoma, bladder carcinoma, Ewing's sarcoma, Hodgkin's disease, non-Hodgkin's lymphoma

PRECAUTIONS
Use etoposide cautiously in patients with myelosuppression or hepatic or renal impairment.
Pregnancy Risk Category: D
Etoposide may cause fetal harm when administered during pregnancy, especially during the first trimester. Excretion into human breast milk is unknown/not recommended in nursing women.

CONTRAINDICATIONS
Hypersensitivity to etoposide or any component of the formulation. Certain formulations contain polysorbate 80.

DRUG PREPARATION/ADMINISTRATION/SAFE HANDLING ISSUES
◄ ALERT ► Etoposide dosage is individualized based on the patient's clinical response and tolerance of the drug's adverse effects. Treatment is repeated at 3- to 4-wk intervals.
◄ ALERT ► Because etoposide may be carcinogenic, mutagenic, or teratogenic, wear nitrile or latex, but not vinyl, gloves when handling the drug for IV use. If the drug comes in contact with the skin, wash the skin thoroughly with soap and water. Do not use waterless or antibacterial soap as either can increase the reaction from the agent. If the drug comes in contact with mucous membranes, flush the area with water.
PO
* Take once daily for dose less than 400 mg and in divided doses for dose greater than 400 mg.
* For doses less than 200 mg, take without regard to food.
IV (VePesid)
* Do not confuse etoposide (VePesid) with etoposide phosphate (Etopophos).
* Etoposide is considered an irritant.

* VePesid concentrate for injection normally is clear and yellow.
* Dilute with D5W or 0.9% NaCl to provide a final concentration of 0.2-0.4 mg/mL. Preparations with concentrations above 0.4 mg/mL may result in precipitation. Discard VePesid solution if crystallization occurs.
* Reconstituted VePesid solution is stable at room temperature for up to 96 hrs at 0.2 mg/mL and 48 hrs at 0.4 mg/mL.
* Infuse VePesid slowly, over 30-60 min. Rapid IV infusion may produce marked hypotension.
* Monitor patient receiving VePesid for an anaphylactic reaction manifested as back, chest, or throat pain; chills; diaphoresis; dyspnea; fever; lacrimation; and sneezing.

STORAGE AND STABILITY
* *PO:* Refrigerate gelatin capsules. Stable for 3 mos at room temperature. Do not freeze.
* *IV:* Store unopened vials at room temperature. Diluted solutions are stable for up to 48 hrs (plastic containers).

INTERACTIONS
Drug
Cytochrome P450 (CYP) 3A4-interacting drugs: Inducers (e.g., phenobarbital) may decrease etoposide levels; inhibitors (e.g., azole antifungals) may increase etoposide levels.
Bone marrow depressants: May increase myelosuppression.
Live-virus vaccines: May potentiate viral replication, increase vaccine side effects, and decrease the patient's antibody response to the vaccine.
Herbal
St John's Wort: May decrease etoposide levels. Avoid use.

LAB EFFECTS/INTERFERENCE
None known.

Y-SITE COMPATIBLES
Allopurinol, amifostine, carboplatin, cisplatin, cladribine, cyclophosphamide, cytarabine, daunorubicin, docetaxel, doxorubicin liposome (Doxil), fludarabine, gemcitabine, granisetron (Kytril), ifosfamide, melphalan, methotrexate, mitoxantrone, ondansetron (Zofran), oxaliplatin, palonosetron (Aloxi), pemetrexed, sargramostim (Leukine), topotecan, vinblastine, vincristine, vinorelbine

INCOMPATIBLES
Cefepime (Maxipime), filgrastim (Neupogen), idarubicin (Idamycin), lansoprazole (Prevacid), pantoprazole (Protonix)

SIDE EFFECTS
Serious Reactions
- Myelosuppression may result in hematologic toxicity, manifested as anemia, leukopenia (occurring 7-14 days after drug administration), thrombocytopenia (occurring 9-16 days after administration, and, to a lesser extent, pancytopenia. Do not treat if the ANC is less than 500/mm^3 or platelet count is less than 50,000/mm^3. Bone marrow recovery occurs by day 20.
- Hypotension may occur with rapid infusion. Slow infusion.

Other Side Effects
Frequent (10%-50%):
Alopecia, anorexia, myelosuppression, nausea and vomiting (mild to moderate)
Occasional (1%-10%):
Amenorrhea, diarrhea, hepatotoxicity, stomatitis, ovarian failure
Rare (Less Than 1%):
Anaphylaxis-like reaction, abdominal pain, aftertaste, asthenia, constipation, dysphagia, fatigue, hypotension (with rapid infusion), interstitial pneumonitis/pulmonary fibrosis, fever, malaise, optic neuritis, peripheral neuropathy, pigmentation, radiation recall dermatitis, rash, somnolence, urticaria

SPECIAL CONSIDERATIONS
Baseline Assessment
- Monitor patient's CBC with differential, platelets, electrolytes, BUN, and creatinine levels, and liver function test results before and frequently during etoposide therapy.
- Monitor vital signs before and after initial dose of etoposide.
- Assess for patient's normal bowel habits before dosing.
- Complete an oral inspection before dosing.
- Assess for neuropathy before initial and all subsequent doses.

Intervention and Evaluation
- Monitor patient's CBC with differential, platelets, electrolytes, BUN, and creatinine levels before each dose.
- Administer antiemetics, as ordered, to control nausea and vomiting.
- Monitor patient for possible allergic/hypersensitivity reactions with high doses: fever greater than 40° C (greater than

105° F), chills, erythema of the face and trunk, acidosis, decreased CO_2, shortness of breath and difficulty breathing, weight gain, and capillary leak syndrome.
- Assess patient's pattern of daily bowel activity and stool consistency.
- Monitor patient for signs and symptoms of hematologic toxicity, including excessive fatigue and weakness, ecchymosis, fever, signs of local infection, sore throat, and unusual bleeding from any site.
- Assess patient for signs and symptoms of paresthesia and peripheral neuropathy.
- Monitor patient for signs and symptoms of stomatitis.
- Perform oral assessment before each dose, and initiate an oral care regimen as per institutional protocol. An example is 1 tsp each of salt and baking soda in 1 glass of water to swish and spit after each meal and before bedtime.

Education
- Instruct patient to notify the physician if he or she experiences easy bruising, fever greater than 38° C (greater than 101° F) signs of local infection, sore throat, or unusual bleeding from any site.
- Instruct patient on signs and symptoms of neuropathy: numbness and tingling in hands or feet or difficulty walking.
- Instruct patient on an oral care regimen per institutional protocol.
- Educate patient on neutropenic precautions as necessary:
  Practice good handwashing technique.
  Avoid individuals who are ill.
  Wash and cook all foods well.
  Avoid crowds.
  Avoid fresh fruits and vegetables.
- Educate patient on thrombocytopenic precautions:
  Use of a soft bristle toothbrush.
  No flossing if platelet count is less than 50,000/mm^3.
  No IM injections.
  No rectal suppositories.
  No aerobic exercise.
- Instruct patient to contact his or her health care provider if nausea and vomiting continue for greater than 24 hours after dose completion, for any signs and symptoms or constipation or diarrhea or if unable to take in at least 1500 mL in 24 hours.
- Instruct patient to take oral etoposide with or without food.
- Urge patient to avoid receiving vaccinations and coming in contact with anyone

who has recently received a live-virus vaccine.

- Inform patient that alopecia is reversible but new hair growth may have a different color or texture.
- Instruct patient to take no over-the-counter medications or herbal or vitamin supplements without checking with his or her health care provider.
- Instruct patient on local resources available and support groups related to their diagnosis.

OTHER INFORMATION
Do not confuse VePesid with Pepcid or Versed.

ETOPOSIDE PHOSPHATE, VP-16
BRAND NAMES
Etopophos

CLASS OF AGENT
Antineoplastic agent, podophyllotoxin derivative

CLINICAL PHARMACOLOGY
Mechanism of Action
An epipodophyllotoxin that induces single- and double-stranded breaks in DNA. Cell cycle-dependent and phase-specific agent; most effective in the S and G_2 phases of cell division. **Therapeutic Effect:** Inhibits or alters DNA synthesis.
Absorption and Distribution
Protein binding: 97%.
Half-life: 4-11 hrs.
Metabolism and Excretion
Metabolized in the liver. Primarily excreted in urine. Not removed by hemodialysis.

HOW SUPPLIED/AVAILABLE FORMS
Lyophilized Powder for Injection (Water-soluble [Etopophos]): 100 mg.

INDICATIONS AND DOSAGES
Refer to individual disease protocols. Doses and schedules vary according to each protocol. Modifications are based on patient's response to therapy and tolerability.
Refractory Testicular Tumors
50-100 mg/m²/day IV on days 1-5, or 100 mg/m²/day IV on days 1, 3, and 5 (as combination therapy).

Small Cell Lung Carcinoma
35 mg/m²/day IV for 4 consecutive days up to 50 mg/m²/day IV for 5 consecutive days (as combination therapy).
Dosage Adjustment in Renal Dysfunction
Dosage is modified based on Ccr.

Creatinine Clearance	Administer % of Dose
>50 mL/min	100
15-50 mL/min	75

UNLABELED USES
Treatment of leukemia, lymphoma, AIDS-associated Kaposi's sarcoma, bladder carcinoma, Ewing's sarcoma, Hodgkin's disease, non-Hodgkin's lymphoma

PRECAUTIONS
Use etoposide cautiously in patients with myelosuppression or hepatic or renal impairment.
Pregnancy Risk Category: D
Etoposide may cause fetal harm during pregnancy, especially during the first trimester. Excretion into human breast milk is unknown/not recommended in nursing women.

CONTRAINDICATIONS
Hypersensitivity to etoposide or any component of the formulation

DRUG PREPARATION/ADMINISTRATION/ SAFE HANDLING ISSUES
◀ ALERT ▶ Etoposide dosage is individualized based on the patient's clinical response and tolerance of the drug's adverse effects. Treatment is repeated at 3- to 4-wk intervals.
◀ ALERT ▶ Because etoposide may be carcinogenic, mutagenic, or teratogenic, wear nitrile or latex, but not vinyl, gloves when handling the drug for IV use. If the drug comes in contact with the skin, wash the skin thoroughly with soap and water. Do not use waterless hand soap or any antibacterial soap as either can increase the reaction from the agent. If the drug comes in contact with mucous membranes, flush the area with water.
IV (Etopophos)
- Do not confuse etoposide (VePesid) with etoposide phosphate (Etopophos).
- Etoposide is considered an irritant.
- Reconstitute each 100 mg of Etopophos with 5-10 mL sterile water for injection,

D5W, 0.9% NaCl, bacteriostatic water for injection, or bacteriostatic 0.9% NaCl for injection to provide a concentration of 20 mg/mL or 10 mg/mL, respectively.
* Etopophos may be given without further dilution or may be further diluted with 0.9% NaCl or D5W to a concentration as low as 0.1 mg/mL.
* After reconstitution, Etopophos is stable for up to 24 hrs at room temperature or refrigerated.
* Administer Etopophos over 5-210 min, as appropriate.

STORAGE AND STABILITY
* Store unopened vials in refrigerator, 2-8° C (36-46° F).
* Diluted solutions are stable for up to 24 hrs at room temperature or refrigerated.

INTERACTIONS
Drug
Cytochrome (CYP) 344-interacting drugs: Inducers (e.g. phenobarbital) may decrease etoposide levels; inhibitors (e.g. azole antifungals) may increase etoposide levels
Bone marrow depressants: May increase myelosuppression.
Live-virus vaccines: May potentiate viral replication, increase vaccine side effects, and decrease the patient's antibody response to the vaccine.
Herbal
St John's Wort: May decrease etoposide levels. Avoid use.

LAB EFFECTS/INTERFERENCE
None known.

Y-SITE COMPATIBLES
Bleomycin, carboplatin (Paraplatin), carmustine, cisplatin (Platinol), cytarabine (Cytosar), dacarbazine (DTIC-Dome), dactinomycin, daunorubicin (Cerubidine), dexamethasone (Decadron), dexrazoxane, diphenhydramine (Benadryl), docetaxel, doxorubicin (Adriamycin), gemcitabine, granisetron (Kytril), ifosfamide, leucovorin, magnesium sulfate, mannitol, mesna, methotrexate, mitoxantrone (Novantrone), ondansetron (Zofran), oxaliplatin, paclitaxel, palonosetron (Aloxi), potassium chloride, rituximab, streptozocin, thiotepa, trastuzumab, vinblastine, vincristine, vinorelbine

INCOMPATIBLES
Allopurinol, amphotericin B conventional (Amphocin), cefepime (Maxipime), chlorpromazine (Thorazine), dantrolene, diazepam, droperidol, imipenem/cilastatin, methohexital, methylprednisolone succinate (Solu-Medrol), mitomycin, pantoprazole, phenytoin, prochlorperazine (Compazine)

SIDE EFFECTS
Serious Reactions
* Myelosuppression may result in hematologic toxicity, manifested as anemia, leukopenia (occurring 7-14 days after drug administration), thrombocytopenia (occurring 9-16 days after administration and, to a lesser extent, pancytopenia. Do not treat if the ANC is less than 500/mm^3 or the platelet count is less than 50,000/mm^3. Bone marrow recovery occurs by day 20.
* Hypotension or hypertension may occur with rapid infusion. Slow infusion.
Other Side Effects
Frequent (10%-50%):
Alopecia, anorexia, myelosuppression, nausea, and vomiting (mild to moderate)
Occasional (1%-10%):
Amenorrhea, diarrhea, hepatotoxicity, stomatitis, ovarian failure
Rare (Less Than 1%):
Anaphylaxis-like reaction, abdominal pain, aftertaste, asthenia, constipation, dysphagia, fatigue, hypotension (with rapid infusion), interstitial pneumonitis/pulmonary fibrosis, fever, malaise, optic neuritis, peripheral neuropathy, pigmentation, radiation recall dermatitis, rash, somnolence, urticaria

SPECIAL CONSIDERATIONS
Baseline Assessment
* Monitor patient's CBC with differential, platelets, electrolytes, BUN, and creatinine levels and liver function test results before and frequently during etoposide therapy.
* Administer antiemetics, as ordered, to control nausea and vomiting.
* Monitor vital signs before and after the initial dose of etoposide.
* Assess for patient's normal bowel habits before dosing.
* Complete an oral inspection before dosing.
* Assess for neuropathy before initial and all subsequent doses.

Intervention and Evaluation
- Monitor patient's CBC with differential, platelets, electrolytes, BUN, and creatinine levels before each dose.
- Monitor patient for allergic/hypersensitivity reactions with high doses: fever greater than 40° C or (greater than 105° F), chills, erythema of the face and trunk, acidosis, decreased CO_2, shortness of breath and difficulty breathing, weight gain, and capillary leak syndrome.
- Assess patient's pattern of daily bowel activity and stool consistency.
- Monitor patient for signs and symptoms of hematologic toxicity, including excessive fatigue and weakness, ecchymosis, fever, signs of local infection, sore throat, and unusual bleeding from any site.
- Assess patient for signs and symptoms of paresthesia and peripheral neuropathy.
- Monitor patient for signs and symptoms of stomatitis.
- Perform oral assessment before each dose, and initiate an oral care regimen as per institutional protocol. An example is 1 tsp each of salt and baking soda in 1 glass of water to swish and spit after each meal and before bedtime.

Education
- Instruct patient to notify the physician if he or she experiences easy bruising, fever greater than 38° C (greater than 101° F) signs of local infection, sore throat, or unusual bleeding from any site.
- Instruct patient on signs and symptoms of neuropathy: numbness and tingling in hands or feet or difficulty walking.
- Instruct patient on an oral care regimen per institutional protocol.
- Instruct patient to contact his or her health care provider if nausea and vomiting continue for greater than 24 hours after dose completion, for any signs and symptoms of constipation or diarrhea or if unable to take in at least 1500 mL in 24 hours.
- Educate patient on neutropenic precautions as necessary:
  Practice good handwashing technique.
  Avoid individuals who are ill.
  Wash and cook all foods well.
  Avoid crowds.
  Avoid fresh fruits and vegetables.
- Educate patient on thrombocytopenic precautions:
  Use of a soft bristle toothbrush.
  No flossing if platelet count is less than 50,000/mm³.

No IM injections.
No rectal suppositories.
No aerobic exercise.
- Instruct patient to take oral etoposide with or without food.
- Urge patient to avoid receiving vaccinations and coming in contact with anyone who has recently received a live-virus vaccine.
- Inform patient that alopecia is reversible but new hair growth may have a different color or texture.
- Instruct patient to take no over-the-counter medications or herbal or vitamin supplements without checking with his or her health care provider.
- Instruct patient on local resources available and support groups related to their diagnosis.

EXEMESTANE

BRAND NAMES
Aromasin

CLASS OF AGENT
Antineoplastic agent, aromatase inhibitor

CLINICAL PHARMACOLOGY
Mechanism of Action
In postmenopausal women, estrogen is produced by the adrenal gland in the form of androstenedione. Androstenedione is further converted in peripheral tissues to estrone and then to estradiol. Exemestane decreases estrogen levels by inhibiting aromatase, the enzyme that catalyzes the final step in estrogen production. Exemestane is an irreversible steroidal inactivator that binds to the active site of aromatase, resulting in aromatase deactivation. Exemestane has no effect on adrenal biosynthesis of corticosteroids or aldosterone and does not have partial estrogenic properties like tamoxifen. **Therapeutic Effect:** Deprives estrogen and inhibits the growth of hormone-dependent breast cancers that are stimulated by estrogens.

Absorption and Distribution
Rapidly absorbed (42%); absorption increases by 40% after a high-fat meal. Time to peak: 1.2 hrs. Distributed extensively into tissues. Protein binding: 90%. Maximal estrogen suppression occurs 2-3 days and persists for 4-5 days. *Half-life:* 24 hrs.

Metabolism and Excretion
Metabolized in the liver by cytochrome P450 (CYP) 3A4 via oxidation of the methylene group in position 6 and reduction of the 17-keto group to form inactive and less potent metabolites. Eliminated in urine (42%) and feces (42%). Excreted as unchanged drug (less than 1%).

HOW SUPPLIED/AVAILABLE FORMS
Tablets: 25 mg.

INDICATIONS AND DOSAGES
Postmenopausal Women with Early Breast Cancer Who Received 2-3 Years of Tamoxifen and Are Switched to Exemestane to Complete a Total of 5 Years of Hormonal Therapy; Postmenopausal Women with Advanced Breast Cancer Whose Disease Progressed Following Tamoxifen Therapy
25 mg orally daily after a meal; dose may increase to 50 mg for patients receiving potent CYP 3A4 inducer drugs such as rifampicin or phenytoin. Continue until tumor progression is evident in locally advanced or metastatic cancer. For patients with early breast cancer, continue treatment in the absence of recurrence or contralateral breast cancer until completion of 5 years of hormonal therapy.
Dosage Adjustment in Hepatic/Renal Dysfunction
No adjustments necessary.

UNLABELED USES
No information.

PRECAUTIONS
Pregnancy Risk Category: D
Exemestane is indicated for postmenopausal women. Drug excretion into human breast milk is unknown/not recommended in nursing women.

CONTRAINDICATIONS
Known hypersensitivity to exemestane or its excipients

DRUG PREPARATION/ADMINISTRATION/SAFE HANDLING ISSUES
• Give exemestane after a meal.
• Overdosage up to 800 mg daily resulted in no serious adverse events. Hold exemestane, give supportive care, and monitor vital signs frequently at close observation.

STORAGE AND STABILITY
Store at 25° C (77° F) (excursions allowed 15-30° C; 59-86° F).

INTERACTIONS
Drug
CYP 3A4 inducers (carbamazepine, nafcillin, nevirapine, phenobarbital, phenytoin, rifampin, rifabutin, rifapentine): May decrease serum concentrations and effectiveness of exemestane. Consider increasing dose to 50 mg daily and reduce dose back once CYP 3A4 drug is discontinued.
Herbal
St John's Wort: May increase metabolism and decrease serum exemestane concentration. Avoid use.

LAB EFFECTS/INTERFERENCE
May increase serum alkaline phosphatase, AST (SGOT), and ALT (SGPT) levels.

SIDE EFFECTS
Serious Reactions
• Cardiovascular events such as MI, angina, myocardial ischemia, cardiac failure, and stroke have been reported.
• Long-term exemestane use has been associated with decreased bone mineral density and clinical fractures. Calcium and vitamin D supplements or bisphosphonate therapy may be considered.
Other Side Effects
Frequent (10%-50%):
Arthralgia, fatigue, hot flashes, musculoskeletal pain (arm, leg, and back and osteoarthritis), dyspnea, nausea, pain
Occasional (1%-10%):
Abdominal pain, alopecia, anorexia, anxiety, asthenia, carpal tunnel syndrome, constipation, cough, depression, diaphoresis, diarrhea, dizziness, dyspnea, flu-like symptoms, fractures, headache, hepatic enzyme elevation, hypertension, increased appetite, infection, insomnia, osteoporosis, peripheral edema, pharyngitis, serum creatinine elevation, visual disturbances, vomiting
Rare (Less Than 1%):
Cardiac ischemic events (MI, angina, myocardial ischemia, or cardiac failure), neuropathy, endometrial hyperplasia, muscle cramps, stroke, thromboembolism, uterine polyps

SPECIAL CONSIDERATIONS
Baseline Assessment
- Obtain baseline CBC with differential, platelets, electrolytes, BUN, and creatinine levels, and liver function tests.
- Obtain baseline bone density scans.
- Assess patient's history for evidence of deep vein thrombosis.
- Review patient's history for any cardiac events.
- Monitor for history of hypertension.
- Assess patient's menopausal status.
- Obtain baseline visual acuity and any prior evidence of visual disturbances.

Intervention and Evaluation
- Assess laboratory data for any evidence of altered electrolyte, BUN, or creatinine levels and increasing liver function test results.
- Evaluate patient for any increasing symptoms of hypertension, angina, osteoarthritis, or visual changes.
- Administer premedications with antiemetic agents as ordered.
- Monitor for menopausal symptoms: hot flashes, insomnia, irritability, depression, and libido changes.
- Assess patient for any evidence of respiratory changes: increasing cough, shortness of breath, or dyspnea.
- Assess patient for the need to administer vitamin D or calcium supplementation.
- Plan for routine bone density scans, and assess need for bisphosphonate therapy.

Education
- Educate patient on dosing and timing of antiemetic medications.
- Instruct patient to take exemestane after a meal and at the same time each day.
- Educate patient on when to contact health care provider: fever greater than 38° C (greater than 101° F), chills, shortness of breath, chest pain, altered mental status, nausea lasting greater than 24 hours, or the inability to take in at least 1500 mL of fluid in 24 hours.
- Instruct patient on the need for bone density scans, and inform patient that osteoporosis is a risk with this agent.
- Educate patient on use of vitamin D and calcium supplements as ordered.
- Instruct patient on menopausal symptoms, hot flashes, night sweats, irritability, insomnia, and depression and to discuss these with his or her health care provider.

- Assess patient for changes in sexual function, vaginal dryness, and decreased libido. Make referrals as necessary to a gynecologist or psychosocial services.
- Monitor patient for any mental status changes, such as confusion, dizziness, or lightheadedness.
- Instruct patient not to take any over-the-counter medications, herbal therapy, or vitamin supplementation without first checking with his or her health care provider.
- Instruct patient on local resources available and support groups related to their diagnosis.

FILGRASTIM, GRANULOCYTE COLONY STIMULATING FACTOR

BRAND NAMES
Neupogen

CLASS OF AGENT
Granulocyte colony-stimulating factor (G-CSF)

CLINICAL PHARMACOLOGY
Mechanism of Action
A colony-stimulating factor that stimulates production of granulocyte within bone marrow. **Therapeutic Effect:** Increases ANC to fight off infection in patients with nonmyeloid malignancies who received chemotherapy. Decreases incidence of infection.

Absorption and Distribution
Readily absorbed after subcutaneous administration. Volume of distribution: 150 mL/kg. Renal clearance rate: 0.5-0.7 mL/min/kg.
Half-life: 3.5 hrs.

Metabolism and Excretion
No information.

HOW SUPPLIED/AVAILABLE FORMS
Injection (Vial): 300 mcg/mL, 480 mcg/1.6 mL.
Injection (Syringe): 300 mcg/0.5 mL, 480 mcg/0.8 mL.

INDICATIONS AND DOSAGES
Myelosuppression
IV infusion, subcutaneous injection: 5 mcg/kg/day. Doses may be increased in increments of 5 mcg/kg for each

chemotherapy cycle, according to the duration and severity of the ANC nadir.
Bone Marrow Transplant
IV infusion, subcutaneous continuous 24-hr infusion: 5-10 mcg/kg/day. Adjust dose daily during period of neutrophil recovery based on neutrophil response.
Mobilization of Progenitor Cells
IV infusion, subcutaneous injection: 10 mcg/kg/day beginning at least 4 days before the first leukapheresis and continuing until the last leukapheresis.
Chronic Neutropenia, Congenital Neutropenia
Subcutaneous: 6 mcg/kg/dose twice daily.
Idiopathic or Cyclic Neutropenia
Subcutaneous: 5 mcg/kg/dose once daily.
Dosage Adjustment in Hepatic/Renal Dysfunction
No adjustments required.

UNLABELED USES
Treatment of AIDS-related neutropenia, myelodysplastic syndrome, agranulocytosis, aplastic anemia, as component in dose-dense chemotherapy

PRECAUTIONS
Use filgrastim cautiously in patients with gout, malignancy with myeloid characteristics (because of the potential for G-CSF to act as a growth factor), preexisting cardiac conditions, and sickle cell disease.
Pregnancy Risk Category: C
Filgrastim should only be used in pregnant or nursing women if there is a clearly indicated benefit.

CONTRAINDICATIONS
Hypersensitivity to *Escherichia coli*–derived proteins, administration within 24 hrs before or after cytotoxic chemotherapy

DRUG PREPARATION/ADMINISTRATION/ SAFE HANDLING ISSUES
◀ ALERT ▶ Begin filgrastim therapy at least 24 hrs after last dose of chemotherapy; discontinue at least 24 hrs before the next dose of chemotherapy. Begin therapy at least 24 hrs after bone marrow infusion.
IV
- May be given as a short IV infusion (15-30 min), or by continuous IV infusion.
- Use single-dose vial. Do not reenter vial. Do not shake.
- Dilute with 10-50 mL of D5W to a concentration of 15 mcg/mL. Add 2 mL of 5% albumin to each 50 mL of D5W to provide a final concentration of 2 mg/mL. Do not dilute to a final concentration of less than 5 mcg/mL.
- For intermittent infusion (piggyback), infuse over 15-30 min. For continuous infusion, give single dose over 4-24 hrs.
- In all situations, flush IV line with D5W before and after administration. Do not dilute in saline because it may cause precipitation.
Subcutaneous:
- Remove vial from refrigeration before use and allow to warm to room temperature.
- Aspirate syringe before injecting drug to avoid intra-arterial administration.

STORAGE AND STABILITY
- Refrigerate vials in 2-8° C (36-46° F) and protect from light.
- Filgrastim is stable for up to 24 hrs at room temperature, provided vial contents are clear and contain no particulate matter. The drug remains stable if accidentally exposed to a freezing temperature.
- Do not dilute in NaCl as precipitation may occur.

INTERACTIONS
Drug
Lithium: May cause a greater-than-expected increase in WBC count.
Herbal
None known.

LAB EFFECTS/INTERFERENCE
May increase lactate dehydrogenase concentrations, leukocyte alkaline phosphatase scores, and serum alkaline phosphatase and uric acid levels.

Y-SITE COMPATIBLES
Bumetanide (Bumex), calcium gluconate, hydromorphone (Dilaudid), lorazepam (Ativan), morphine, potassium chloride

INCOMPATIBLES
Amphotericin conventional (Fungizone), cefepime (Maxipime), cefoperazone, cefotaxime (Claforan), cefoxitin (Mefoxin), ceftizoxime (Cefizox), ceftriaxone (Rocephin), ceftizoxime, cefuroxime (Zinacef), clindamycin (Cleocin), dactinomycin

(Cosmegen), etoposide (VePesid), fluoro-uracil, furosemide (Lasix), gentamicin, heparin, imipenem and cilastatin, mannitol, methylprednisolone (Solu-Medrol), metronidazole, mitomycin (Mutamycin), piperacillin, prochlorperazine (Compazine), thiotepa

SIDE EFFECTS
Serious Reactions
* Long-term administration occasionally produces chronic neutropenia and splenomegaly.
* Thrombocytopenia, MI, and arrhythmias occur rarely.
* Adult respiratory distress syndrome may occur in patients with sepsis.
Other Side Effects
Frequent (10%-50%):
Mild to severe bone pain that occurs more frequently with high-dose IV form and less frequently with low-dose subcutaneous form, alopecia, diarrhea, fever, fatigue, nausea, or vomiting
Occasional (1%-10%):
Anorexia, cough, dyspnea, headache, hematuria, rash, osteoporosis proteinuria, psoriasis
Rare (Less Than 1%):
Allergic reactions, adult respiratory distress syndrome, splenic rupture

SPECIAL CONSIDERATIONS
Baseline Assessment
* Obtain CBC with differential, platelets, electrolytes, BUN, and creatinine levels, and liver function tests.
* Assess patient for evidence of fatigue.
* Evaluate patient's history for cardiac problems, MI, hypertension, and any history of splenomegaly.
* Monitor patient for evidence of significant history of nausea and vomiting.
Intervention and Evaluation
* Monitor CBC with differential on a twice weekly basis at least and weekly liver function tests along with uric acid level.
* Obtain vital signs at each visit or every 4 hours if inpatient.
* Evaluate patient for any evidence of cardiac changes, such as chest pain or arrhythmias, or pulmonary changes, such as cough or shortness of breath.
* Assess for hypertension and the need for intervention.
* Monitor frequency of nausea and vomiting.
* Educate patient on self-injection techniques as needed and appropriate needle disposal procedures.

* Assess injection sites for evidence of erythema, edema, or infection.
* Evaluate for any skin rash as Sweet's syndrome is a rare side effect with this agent.
* Initiate neutropenic precautions as per institutional guidelines as necessary.
* Assess patient for frequency and severity of bone pain as analgesics may be required in some patients.
Education
* Instruct patient on when to contact his or her health care provider: fever greater than 38° C (greater than 101° F), cough, chills, shortness of breath, chest pain, palpitations, or severe bone pain.
* Educate patient on neutropenic precautions as necessary:
  Practice good handwashing technique.
  Avoid individuals who are ill.
  Wash and cook all foods well.
  Avoid crowds.
  Avoid fresh fruits and vegetables.
* Instruct patient to take no over-the-counter medications or herbal or vitamin supplements without checking with his or her health care provider.
* Instruct patient on local resources available and support groups related to their diagnosis.

FLOXURIDINE
BRAND NAMES
Prescription: FUDR

CLASS OF AGENT
Antineoplastic agent, fluoropyrimidine antimetabolite

CLINICAL PHARMACOLOGY
Mechanism of Action
Prodrug that is converted to active fluorouracil. Active fluorodeoxyuridine monophosphate binds to thymidylate synthase (TS), which is enhanced by reduced folate cofactors. TS is an essential enzyme in the formation of uridine, which is needed for the synthesis of both DNA and RNA. Floxuridine is cell cycle specific for S-phase cell division. **Therapeutic Effect:** Inhibition of DNA and RNA synthesis, leading to cell death.
Absorption and Distribution
Poorly absorbed by the oral route. After IV administration it primarily stays in the plasma. After intraarterial administration, a small amount crosses the blood-brain

barrier. Its active metabolites are localized intracellularly.

Half-life: After IV administration, the parent compound, floxuridine, has a plasma half-life of about 15 min. Pharmacokinetic data on intra-arterial infusion of floxuridine are not available.

Metabolism and Excretion

Rapidly and extensively metabolized in liver and tissues to the monophosphate derivative and fluorouracil. It is eliminated as the parent compound and as urea, fluorouracil, α-fluoro-β-ureidopropionic acid, dihydrofluorouracil, α-fluoro-β-guanidopropionic acid and α-fluoro-β-alanine in the urine. It is also eliminated through the lungs as carbon dioxide.

HOW SUPPLIED/AVAILABLE FORMS

Powder for Injection: 500 mg (FUDR).

INDICATIONS AND DOSAGES

Palliative Management of GIAdenocarcinoma Metastatic to Liver

Intrahepatic arterial infusion: The manufacturer recommends that floxuridine be administered by the intra-arterial route only. The adult dosage ranges from 0.1 to 0.6 mg/kg/day for 7-14 days for hepatic artery infusion. Most patients tolerate the lower dosage of 0.1 mg/kg/day for 7 days. Higher doses are associated with biliary sclerosis and fibrosis.

Dosage Adjustment in Hepatic Dysfunction

In patients with biliary obstruction, the drug should be discontinued until hepatic function normalizes.

Dosage Adjustment in Renal Dysfunction

No specific dose adjustment

UNLABELED USES

A variety of doses and schedules have been used in the treatment of solid tumors, particularly hepatic metastases from colorectal cancer. The most commonly used IV dose of floxuridine is 0.1-0.3 mg/kg/day for 7-14 days as a continuous infusion. The initial dose is usually 0.1-0.15 mg/kg/day because of the common occurrence of dose-limiting diarrhea and GI ulceration.

PRECAUTIONS

Use cautiously in patients who have received high-dose pelvic irradiation therapy or treatment with alkylating agents and those with impaired liver or kidney function.

Pregnancy Risk Category: D

CONTRAINDICATIONS

Poor nutritional state, depressed bone marrow function, or serious infection

DRUG PREPARATION/ADMINISTRATION/ SAFE HANDLING ISSUES

◀ ALERT ▶ Dosage is individualized, according to patient's clinical response and tolerance of adverse effects. When used in combination therapy, consult specific protocols for optimum dosage and sequence of drug administration.

• Give by continuous intra-arterial infusion via catheter inserted into the arterial blood supply of tumor.

• Reconstitute each 500-mg vial with 5 mL of sterile water for injection to provide a concentration of 100 mg/mL.

• Further dilute with D5W or 0.9% NaCl to the volume appropriate for the specific infusion apparatus used.

STORAGE AND STABILITY

• Floxuridine reconstituted with 5 mL of sterile water should be stored under refrigeration 2-8° C (36-46° F), which will be stable when stored at refrigeration temperature for 2 wks.

• When used in an implantable drug delivery pump with infusion times lasting between 4 and 12 day, there is less than 5% drug degradation.

• Floxuridine is stable in polypropylene infusion-pump syringes at 30° C (86° F) for 21 days when concentrations of 1-50 mg/mL in 0.9% NaCl are used.

INTERACTIONS

Drug

Bone marrow depressants: May increase risk of bone marrow depression.

Live-virus vaccines: May potentiate virus replication, increase vaccine side effects, and decrease the patient's antibody response to the vaccine.

Herbal

None known.

LAB EFFECTS/INTERFERENCE

May increase AST (SGOT), serum ALT (SGPT), alkaline phosphatase, lactate dehydrogenase, and bilirubin levels. Interferes with bromsulfophthalein test, PT, and sedimentation rate assays.

Y-SITE COMPATIBLES
Amifostine, aztreonam, calcium salts, cisplatin, filgrastim, granisetron, heparin Na, leucovorin, ondansetron, paclitaxel, piperacillin Na/tazobactam, sargramostim, vinorelbine

INCOMPATIBLES
Allopurinol (Zyloprim), cefepime

SIDE EFFECTS
Serious Reactions
Hepatic arterial infusion is associated with cirrhosis of the liver, extra-hepatic sclerosis of bile ducts, and acalculous cholecystitis.
Other Side Effects
Frequent (10%-50%):
Nausea, vomiting, diarrhea, anorexia, malaise, abdominal cramping, enteritis, rash, pruritus, and localized erythema
Occasional (1%-10%):
Duodenal ulcer, fever, gastritis, glossitis, pharyngitis, ataxia, blurred vision, vertigo, weakness, mental depression, lethargy, dacrycystitis (tear duct inflammation)
Rare (Less Than 1%):
Myocardial ischemia

SPECIAL CONSIDERATIONS
Baseline Assessment
- Be aware that this agent is usually given as a hepatic artery infusion and is NOT usually delivered intravenously.
- Obtain baseline CBC with differential, electrolytes, BUN, and creatinine levels, and liver function tests.
- Assess patient for any evidence of skin changes.
- Evaluate patient before initiation of therapy for dry eyes or conjunctivitis.
- Monitor patient before initiation of each dose for nausea, vomiting, diarrhea, or right upper quadrant pain.
Intervention and Evaluation
- Evaluate patient's laboratory data before initiating each dose via the infusion pump, paying particular attention to all liver function test results.
- Monitor patient for nausea, vomiting, weight loss, and diarrhea before reloading the hepatic infusion pump.
- Evaluate patient for any signs or symptoms of mucositis and stomatitis, and initiate an oral care regimen.
- Evaluate site of infusion device, hepatic arterial catheter, or infusion pump site.
- Premedicate patients as ordered with antiemetic agents, and make sure they are available for patient's home use if nausea continues.
- Assess patient for evidence of skin reactions, dryness, rashes, pruritus, and tear duct inflammation.
- Assess any patient older than 65 years of age for increased side effects, and monitor this patient more closely for any side effects and the need for dosage reduction.
Education
- Instruct patient on when to contact his or her health care provider: fever greater than 38° C (greater than 101° F), chills, cough, right upper quadrant pain, nausea lasting greater than 24 hours, diarrhea lasting greater than 24 hours, or the inability to take in at least 1500 mL in 24 hours.
- Educate patient on oral hygiene as per institutional protocol. An example is 1 tsp each of salt and baking soda dissolved in 1 glass of water to swish and spit at least 4 times/day.
- Instruct patient to contact the health care provider if mouth sores occur.
- Educate patient on side effects of this agent: nausea, vomiting, diarrhea, sore throat, and mucositis.
- Advise patient that anorexia may occur and to report the inability to take adequate hydration or nutritional supplements.
- Educate patient on neutropenic precautions as necessary:
    Practice good handwashing technique.
    Avoid individuals who are ill.
    Wash and cook all foods well.
    Avoid crowds.
    Avoid fresh fruits and vegetables.
- Advise patient to avoid any persons with infections, and instruct patient on good handwashing technique.
- Instruct patient to take no over-the-counter medications or herbal or vitamin supplements without checking with his or her health care provider.
- Instruct patient on local resources available and support groups related to their diagnosis.

FLUDARABINE
BRAND NAMES
Fludara

CLASS OF AGENT
Antineoplastic agent, antimetabolite

CLINICAL PHARMACOLOGY
Mechanism of Action
Fluorinated analog of adenine that inhibits DNA synthesis by inhibition of DNA polymerase and ribonucleotide reductase. **Therapeutic Effect:** Prevents DNA elongation and causes cell death.
Absorption and Distribution
Volume of distribution: 38-96 L/m²; it distributes and binds to tissue widely and extensively. Protein binding: 19%-29%.
Half-life: 9 hrs.
Metabolism and Excretion
Fludarabine phosphate is rapidly dephosphorylated to 2-fluorovidarabine, which subsequently enters tumor cells and is phosphorylated to the active triphosphate derivative. Fludarabine is excreted in urine (60% with 23% as 2-fluorovidarabine) within 24 hrs.

HOW SUPPLIED/AVAILABLE FORMS
Injection, Powder for Reconstitution: 50 mg.

INDICATIONS AND DOSAGES
Chronic Lymphocytic Leukemia That Has Not Responded to or Progressed While Patient is Receiving One Standard Alkylating Agent-Containing Regimen
25 mg/m²/day IV for 5 days every 28 days.
Non-Hodgkin's Lymphoma (Unlabeled)
Loading dose of 20 mg/m² IV followed by 30 mg/m²/day IV for 48 hrs.
Reduced-Intensity Conditioning Regimens Before Allogeneic Hematopoietic Stem Cell Transplantation (Unlabeled Use)
120-150 mg/m² IV administered in divided doses over 4-5 days.
Dosage Adjustment in Hepatic Dysfunction
No information available.
Dosage Adjustment in Renal Dysfunction
Creatinine clearance 30-70 mL/min: reduce dose by 20%.
Creatinine clearance less than 30 mL/min: not recommended.

UNLABELED USES
Treatment of non-Hodgkin's lymphoma and acute leukemias in pediatric patients, reduced-intensity conditioning regimens before allogeneic hematopoietic stem cell transplantation (generally administered in combination with busulfan and antithymocyte globulin or lymphocyte immune globulin or in combination with melphalan and alemtuzumab).

PRECAUTIONS
Use with caution in patients with renal insufficiency, fever, documented infection, or preexisting hematologic disorders (particularly granulocytopenia) or in patients with a preexisting CNS disorder (epilepsy), spasticity, or peripheral neuropathy. Life-threatening and sometimes fatal autoimmune hemolytic anemia has occurred. Severe myelosuppression (trilineage bone marrow hypoplasia/ aplasia) has been reported (rare); the duration of significant cytopenias in these patients may be prolonged (up to 1 year).
Pregnancy Risk Factor: D
Fludarabine may cause fetal harm when given during pregnancy. Excretion into human breast milk is unknown/not recommended in nursing women.

CONTRAINDICATIONS
Hypersensitivity to fludarabine or any component of the formulation or pregnancy

DRUG PREPARATION/ADMINISTRATION/ SAFE HANDLING ISSUES
◄ ALERT ► Because fludarabine may be carcinogenic, mutagenic, or teratogenic, wear nitrile or latex, but not vinyl, gloves when handling the drug. If the drug comes in contact with skin, wash the skin thoroughly with soap and water. Do not use waterless hand soap as it can increase the reaction from the agent. If the drug comes in contact with mucous membranes, flush the area with water.
- Reconstitute each 50-mg vial with 2 mL sterile water for injection to yield a 25 mg/mL solution.
- Further dilute the 25 mg/mL solution in 0.9% NaCl or D5W. Standard IV dilution is 100–125 mL of D5W or 0.9% NaCl.
- Administer IV over 30 min. Rapid IV infusion or continuous infusion has been used but may be associated with more toxicities.

STORAGE AND STABILITY
- Store intact vials under refrigeration (2-8° C [36-46° F]).
- Reconstituted solution is stable for 16 days at room temperature (22-25° C; 72-77° F) and under refrigeration (2-8° C; 36-46° F).
- Further dilution in 100 mL of D5W or 0.9% NaCl is stable for 48 hrs at room temperature or with refrigeration.
- Fludarabine contains no antimicrobial preservative and should be administered within 8 hrs of reconstitution.

INTERACTIONS
Drug
Pentostatin: Combined use with fludarabine may lead to severe, even fatal, pulmonary toxicity.
Herbal
No information available.

LAB EFFECTS/INTERFERENCE
No information available.

Y-SITE COMPATIBLES
Allopurinol, amifostine, amikacin, aminophylline, ampicillin, ampicillin/sulbactam, amsacrine, aztreonam, bleomycin, butorphanol, carboplatin, carmustine, cefazolin, cefepime, cefoperazone, cefotaxime, cefotetan, ceftazidime, ceftizoxime, ceftriaxone, cefuroxime, cimetidine, cisplatin, clindamycin, cotrimoxazole, cyclophosphamide, cytarabine, dacarbazine, dactinomycin, dexamethasone Na phosphate, diphenhydramine, doxorubicin, doxycycline, droperidol, etoposide, etoposide phosphate, famotidine, filgrastim, floxuridine, fluconazole, fluorouracil, furosemide, gemcitabine, gentamicin, granisetron, haloperidol, heparin, hydrocortisone Na phosphate, hydrocortisone Na succinate, hydromorphone, ifosfamide, imipenem/cilastatin, lorazepam, magnesium sulfate, mannitol, mechlorethamine, melphalan, meperidine, mesna, methotrexate, methylprednisolone Na succinate, metoclopramide, minocycline, mitoxantrone, morphine, multivitamins, nalbuphine, netilmicin, ondansetron, pentostatin, piperacillin, piperacillin/tazobactam, potassium chloride, promethazine, ranitidine, Na bicarbonate, teniposide, thiotepa, ticarcillin, ticarcillin/clavulanate, tobramycin, vancomycin, vinblastine, vincristine, vinorelbine, zidovudine

INCOMPATIBLES
Acyclovir, amphotericin B colloidal (Amphotec), chlorpromazine, daunorubicin, ganciclovir, hydroxyzine, pantoprazole, prochlorperazine edisylate, trastuzumab

SIDE EFFECTS
Serious Reactions
• There are clear dose-dependent toxic neurologic effects associated with fludarabine. Doses of 96 mg/m²/day for 5-7 days are associated with a syndrome characterized by delayed blindness, coma, and death. Symptoms have appeared from 21 to 60 days after the last dose. CNS toxicity has distinctive features of delayed onset and progressive encephalopathy, resulting in death. CNS toxicity is reported at an incidence rate of 36% at high doses (96 mg/m²/day for 5-7 days) and less than 0.2% for low doses (125 mg/m²/course).
• Postmarketing and/or case reports: acute renal failure; pulmonary toxicity (including interstitial pneumonitis, pulmonary fibrosis, pulmonary hemorrhage, respiratory failure, or adult respiratory distress syndrome) has been reported (may improve with steroid administration). Trilineage (bone marrow hypoplasia or bone marrow aplasia) has been reported and may require several mos for recovery.

Other Side Effects
Frequent (10%-50%):
Cardiovascular: Edema
CNS: Fatigue, somnolence (30%), chills, pain
Dermatologic: Rash
Hematologic: Myelosuppression, primarily leukopenia and thrombocytopenia, common, dose-limiting toxicity
Neuromuscular and skeletal: Paresthesia, myalgia, weakness
Occasional (1%-10%):
Cardiovascular: Congestive heart failure
CNS: Malaise, headache
Dermatologic: Alopecia
Endocrine and metabolic: Hyperglycemia
Gastrointestinal: Anorexia, stomatitis (1.5%), diarrhea (1.8%), mild nausea/vomiting (3%-10%)
Hematologic: Eosinophilia, hemolytic anemia; may be dose-limiting and possibly fatal in some patients
Rare (Less Than 1%):
Blurred vision, diplopia, increased risk for opportunistic infection due to decreased CD4 counts, metabolic acidosis, metallic taste, muscle weakness, paresthesia, photophobia (primarily in patients receiving high doses)
A syndrome characterized by cortical blindness, coma, and paralysis is seen in 36% of patients at doses greater than 96 mg/m² for 5-7 days and in less than 0.2% at doses less than 125 mg/m²/cycle (onset of neurologic symptoms may be delayed for 3-4 wks).

SPECIAL CONSIDERATIONS
Baseline Assessment
- Monitor CBC with differential, electrolytes, BUN, creatinine, calcium, phosphorus, and uric acid levels, and liver function tests.
- Evaluate patient for tumor lysis syndrome risk with large bulky nodal disease.
- Evaluate patient for any prior pulmonary disease.
- Assess patient for any prior renal disease.
- Assess patient for any evidence of prior neuromuscular symptoms, myalgias, or weakness.

Intervention and Evaluation
- Premedicate patient as ordered.
- Monitor laboratory data prior to each dose.
- Monitor for any evidence of altered mental status when delivering doses as part of a preparative regimen in stem cell transplantation.
- Evaluate patient for any evidence of symptoms of weakness, myalgias, or arthralgias.
- Monitor patient for any signs or symptoms of infection.
- Assess pulmonary function at each visit or every shift if inpatient.
- Monitor I&O and daily weight for inpatients or at each outpatient visit.
- Assess patient for symptoms of oliguria or decreased renal output.
- Encourage fluid in patients at risk for tumor lysis syndrome.
- Evaluate patient for symptoms of respiratory changes: cough, shortness of breath, or dyspnea upon exertion.
- Monitor for signs and symptoms of thrombocytopenia: easy bruising, bleeding, epistaxis, hematuria, hematemesis, or hematochezia.
- Monitor patient's laboratory data on a daily basis or at each clinic visit.

Education
- Instruct patient on when to contact his or her health care provider: fever greater than 38° C (greater than 101° F), chills, evidence of easy bruising, bleeding, epistaxis, shortness of breath, altered mental status, nausea lasting greater than 24 hours, diarrhea lasting greater than 24 hours, and the inability to take in at least 1500 mL of fluid in 24 hours.
- Instruct patient to report any new pulmonary symptoms such as productive cough, shortness of breath, and dyspnea upon exertion.
- Instruct patient to avoid individuals who are ill or who have received live virus vaccines.
- Educate patient on signs and symptoms of tumor lysis syndrome: flank pain, hematuria, and changes in the ability to pass urine.
- Educate patient on neutropenic precautions as necessary:
  Practice good handwashing technique.
  Avoid individuals who are ill.
  Wash and cook all foods well.
  Avoid crowds.
  Avoid fresh fruits and vegetables.
- Educate patient on thrombocytopenic precautions:
  Use of a soft bristle toothbrush.
  No flossing if platelet count is less than 50,000/mm^3.
  No IM injections.
  No rectal suppositories.
  No aerobic exercise.
- Advise patient to report any edema or significant weight gain of greater than or equal to 3 pounds in a 5-day period.
- Educate patient that fatigue and myalgias are frequent side effects of this agent.
- Instruct patient on local resources available and support groups related to their diagnosis.

FLUOROURACIL
BRAND NAMES
Adrucil, Efudex, Fluoroplex

CLASS OF AGENT
Antineoplastic agent, fluoropyrimidine antimetabolite

CLINICAL PHARMACOLOGY
Mechanism of Action
Fluorinated pyrimidine that acts as false antimetabolite. It is rapidly metabolized in tissues to active metabolites, fluorodeoxyuridine monophosphate (FdUMP) and fluorouridine triphosphate (FUTP). FdUMP blocks the methylation reaction of deoxyuridylic acid to thymidylic acid, creating a thymine deficiency, thus interfering with DNA synthesis. FUTP incorporates into cells and inhibits the formation of RNA. Both actions result in cell death, especially in cells that grow more rapidly and take up 5-fluorouracil (5-FU) rapidly. It is cell cycle specific with maximal effects in the S phase.

One mechanism of action of CMF (fluorouracil, methotrexate, and cyclophosphamide) therapy as adjuvant chemotherapy in early breast cancer may be due to ovarian suppression in premenopausal patients. The efficacy of the combination was observed only when permanent amenorrhea occurred in premenopausal patients. **Therapeutic Effect:** Inhibits DNA and RNA synthesis. Topical form destroys rapidly proliferating cells.

Absorption and Distribution
The oral absorption of 5-FU is incomplete and varies widely in patients from 0% to 80%. After topical administration, systemic absorption is minimal, ranging from 0.55% to 2.4% from solutions and from 0.5% and 5% from cream formulations. 5-FU is widely distributed to areas of body water. It is distributed into both tissue and extracellular fluid, including intestinal mucosa, bone marrow, liver, brain, cerebrospinal fluid, and neoplastic tissue. Significant quantities of 5-FU can enter the CNS.
Half-life: The elimination half-life of the parent compound, 5-FU, ranges from 6 to 22 min. After intrapericardial administration of 5-FU 200 mg to one patient, the elimination half-life was 169 min. The elimination half-life of the metabolites, FdUMP and FUTP, were 52.2 and 48 min after IV 5-FU bolus doses of 250 and 370 mg/m^2, respectively, in 20 patients with colorectal cancer.

Metabolism and Excretion
The liver is the primary site of 5-FU metabolism. It metabolizes 5-FU to dihyro-5-fluorouracil, which is potentially active. Other inactive metabolites include carbon monoxide urea and α-fluoro-β-alanine. The rate-limiting step in the metabolism of 5-FU is conversion to 5,6-dihydrofluorouracil by the enzyme dihydropyrimidine dehydrogenase (DPD). Individuals with a genetic DPD deficiency have altered 5-FU pharmacokinetic profiles and have experienced severe 5-FU-related toxicity.
A primary route is the excretion by the lungs as carbon dioxide. 5-FU is removed by hemodialysis. The liver is the primary site of metabolism (80%), but there is no evidence that patients with impaired liver function require dose reductions. The primary metabolites are dihydrofluorouracil and α-fluoro-β-alanine.

HOW SUPPLIED/AVAILABLE FORMS
Injection (Adrucil): 50 mg/mL. Sizes: 10 mL, 20 mL, 50 mL, 100 mL.
Topical Cream (Carac): 0.5% 30 g.
Topical Cream (Flurorplex): 1% 30 g.
Topical Cream (Efudex): 5% 25 g, 40 g.
Topical Solution (Flurorplex): 1% 30 mL.
Topical Solution (Efudex): 2%, 5% 10 mL.

INDICATIONS AND DOSAGES
Carcinoma of breast, colon, pancreas, rectum, and stomach; in combination with leucovorin or levamisole after surgical resection in patients with Duke's stage C colon cancer. Dosing varies widely. The doses provided below are taken from the ***NCCN guidelines for the treatment of colorectal cancer.

5-FU-Leucovorin
• Leucovorin 500 mg/m^2 given a 2-hour infusion and repeated wkly for 6 weeks.
• 5-FU 500 mg/m^2 given as an IV bolus 1 hour after the start of leucovorin and repeated weekly for 6 weeks.
• Leucovorin 20 mg/m^2 followed by 5-FU 425 mg/m^2 IV daily for 5 days, every 4-5 weeks for 6 cycles.
• Leucovorin 400 mg/m^2 daily for 5 days followed by 5-FU 370-400 mg/m^2 daily for 5 days every 28 days for 6 cycles.

FOLFOX 4
• Leucovorin 400 mg/m^2 IV over 2 hours, followed by bolus 5-FU 400 mg/m^2, then 600 mg/m^2 as a 22-hour infusion given for 2 consecutive days every 14 days for 12 cycles. Oxaliplatin 85 mg/m^2 over 2 hours on day 1, simultaneously with leucovorin.

FOLFOX 6
• Leucovorin 400 mg/m^2 IV over 2 hours on day 1 and 5-FU 400 mg/m^2 IV bolus on day 1, and then 2.4-3 g/m^2 IV over 46 hours as a continuous IV infusion

Multiple Actinic or Solar Keratoses
Topical (Efudex, Fluoroplex): Apply twice daily.
Topical (Carac): Apply once daily.

Basal Cell Carcinoma
Topical (Efudex): Apply twice daily.

Dosage Adjustment in Hepatic Dysfunction
In patients with serum bilirubin greater than 5 mg/dL, 5-FU should be avoided.

Dosage Adjustment in Renal Dysfunction
No adjustment is required.

Dosage Adjustment in Patients with Poor Nutritional Status
Lower doses of 5-FU should be used in patients with poor nutritional status. The total

daily dose in these patients should not exceed 400 mg.

UNLABELED USES
Parenteral: Treatment of bladder, cervical, endometrial, head and neck, liver, lung, ovarian, or prostate carcinomas; pericardial, peritoneal, or pleural effusions
Topical: Treatment of actinic cheilitis, radiodermatitis

PRECAUTIONS
Use 5-FU cautiously in patients with impaired hepatic or renal function, metastatic cell infiltration of bone marrow, or a history of high-dose pelvic irradiation.
Pregnancy Risk Category: D

CONTRAINDICATIONS
Major surgery within previous mo, myelosuppression, poor nutritional status, potentially serious infections
DPD deficiency: Both IV and topical 5-FU will call excessive toxicity and should be avoided.

DRUG PREPARATION/ADMINISTRATION/ SAFE HANDLING ISSUES
◄ ALERT ► Dosage of 5-FU is individualized based on the patient's clinical response, tolerance of the drug's adverse effects, and weight or BSA. When administering this drug in combination therapy, consult specific protocols for optimum dosage and sequence of drug administration.
◄ ALERT ► Give 5-FU by IV injection or IV infusion. Do not add this drug to other IV infusions. Because 5-FU may be carcinogenic, mutagenic, or teratogenic, handle the drug with extreme care during preparation and administration.
* The solution normally appears colorless to faint yellow. Slight discoloration does not adversely affect potency or safety.
* If a precipitate forms, redissolve the solution by heating it and shaking it vigorously, and then allow it to cool to body temperature.
* Administer IV push as undiluted. Inject it through a Y-tube or three-way stopcock of free-flowing solution.
* For IV infusion, further dilute with D5W or 0.9% NaCl.
* Give IV push slowly over 1-2 min.
◄ ALERT ► When accessing a vein for infusion, avoid areas overlying joints and

tendons, small veins, and swollen or edematous extremities.
* Administer the IV infusion over 30 min-24 hrs.
* Monitor patient for signs and symptoms of extravasation, including immediate pain and severe local tissue damage. If this occurs, follow your facility's protocol.

STORAGE AND STABILITY
* 5-FU solutions should be stored at 15-30° C (59-86° F) and protected from light.
* 5-FU solution (Roche) maintained 98%-100% potency over 48 hrs after dilution and storage in syringes and ethylene vinyl acetate infusion-pump reservoirs. Fluorouracil was diluted to 12 and 40 mg/mL with 0.9% NaCl or 5% dextrose injection and stored in 60-mL polypropylene syringes for 72 hrs. It was also diluted to 15 and 45 mg/mL with 0.9% NaCl and stored in ethylene vinyl acetate infusion pump reservoirs.
* The stability of aqueous 5-FU 50 mg/mL was studied in portable infusion pumps under simulated infusion conditions. The drug was found to be stable for 7 days at 37° C (99° F). However, at 25° C (77° F), a fine white precipitate was reported after 48-96 hrs in the extension tubing of the devices containing Roche brand 5-FU. Precipitate formation was also reported in all solutions adjusted to below pH 8.7. 5-FU 50 mg/mL was stable in polypropylene infusion pump syringes at 30° C (86° F) for 21 days.

INTERACTIONS
Drug
Bone marrow depressants: May increase the risk of myelosuppression.
Live virus vaccines: May potentiate virus replication, increase vaccine side effects, and decrease the patient's antibody response to the vaccine.
Leucovorin: Increases efficacy in certain tumor types with added toxicity.
Warfarin: May increase the anticoagulant effects of warfarin. Closely monitor PT or international normalized ratio.
Herbal
None known.

LAB EFFECTS/INTERFERENCE
May decrease serum albumin level. May increase excretion of 5-hydroxyindoleacetic

acid in urine. The topical form may cause eosinophilia, leukocytosis, thrombocytopenia, and toxic granulation.

Y-SITE COMPATIBLES
Amphotericin liposomal (AmBisome), bleomycin, carboplatin, cisplatin, cyclophosphamide, docetaxel, etoposide phosphate, fludarabine, gemcitabine, granisetron (Kytril), heparin, hydromorphone (Dilaudid), ifosfamide, leucovorin, melphalan, mitomycin, mitoxantrone, morphine, paclitaxel, palonosetron, pemetrexed, KCl, propofol (Diprivan), rituximab, sargramostim, teniposide, topotecan, vinblastine, vincristine

INCOMPATIBLES
Amphotericin B colloidal (Amphotec), doxorubicin, droperidol (Inapsine), epirubicin, filgrastim (Neupogen), gallium nitrate, lansoprazole, levofloxacin, ondansetron (Zofran), topotecan, vinorelbine (Navelbine)

SIDE EFFECTS
Serious Reactions
- The earliest sign of toxicity, which may occur 4-8 days after the start of therapy, is stomatitis (as evidenced by dry mouth, a burning sensation, mucosal erythema, and ulceration at the inner margin of lips).
- Hematologic toxicity may be manifested as leukopenia (generally within 9-14 days after drug administration, but possibly as late as the 25th day), thrombocytopenia (within 7-17 days after administration), pancytopenia, or agranulocytosis.
- The most common dermatologic toxicity is a pruritic rash on the extremities or, less frequently, the trunk. Palmar-plantar erythrodysesthesias are more common with continuous infusion than with bolus administration.

Other Side Effects
Frequent (10%-50%):
Parenteral: Stomatitis occurs frequently after fluorouracil-based regimens. Women had stomatitis more frequently than men (63% vs. 52%). Patients older than the age 65 had a higher incidence of stomatitis. Bone marrow suppression manifested by neutropenia or thrombocytopenia is dose related and appears after bolus doses of 425 mg/m^2.

Occasional (1%-10%):
Parenteral: Anorexia, diarrhea, minimal alopecia, fever, dry skin, skin fissures, scaling, erythema. Diarrhea is more frequent with high doses or those given by continuous infusions.
Topical: At the site of application, any of the following may occur: pruritus, hyperpigmentation, irritation, inflammation, burning, and photosensitivity

Rare (Less Than 1%):
Nausea, vomiting, anemia, esophagitis, proctitis, GI ulcer, confusion, headache, lacrimation, visual disturbances, angina, allergic reactions

SPECIAL CONSIDERATIONS
Baseline Assessment
- Monitor patient's CBC with differential, liver and renal function test results, and platelet count.
- Evaluate patient's oral hygiene.

Intervention and Evaluation
- Monitor CBC with differential and platelet count before each dose.
- Monitor liver function test results (total bilirubin, AST (SGOT), and ALT (SGPT) levels) along with renal function tests (creatinine and BUN levels) before each dose.
- Monitor patient for signs of GI bleeding, including bright red or tarry stools, intractable diarrhea, and rapidly falling WBC count.
- Assess patient for signs and symptoms of stomatitis, including difficulty swallowing, sore throat, and ulceration and erythema of the oral mucosa.
- Assess patient for signs and symptoms of diarrhea or constipation.
- Assess patient for any signs and symptoms of dehydration, orthostatic changes, or nausea and vomiting.
- Expect to discontinue 5-FU if intractable diarrhea, GI bleeding, or stomatitis occurs.
- Examine patient's skin for any signs and symptoms of skin reaction, erythema, or rash.
- Monitor patient for any changes on renal function or rising liver function test results.
- Consider testing for DPD deficiency if patient experiences unexpected severe toxicities. DPD deficiency is not a Food and Drug Administration–approved test but it is available through the University of Alabama at Birmingham.

Education
- Instruct patient to notify his or her health care provider for any signs or symptoms of fever greater than 38° C (greater than

101° F), or chills or other signs and symptoms of infection.

- Make sure patient has a thermometer and knows how to read it.
- Instruct patient to report any bleeding, easy bruising, chest pain, palpitations, or visual changes.
- Instruct patient to report any signs or symptoms of diarrhea or the inability to take at least 1500 mL of fluids in 24 hours.
- Instruct patient on the risk of hyperpigmentation and skin changes that may occur.
- Encourage patient to avoid overexposure to the sun or ultraviolet light and to wear protective clothing, sunglasses, and sunscreen (SPF greater than 15) when outdoors.
- Instruct patient in oral care regimen.
- Instruct patient on a skin care regimen as needed.
- Make sure patient has a 24-hour number for their health care provider.
- Instruct patient using topical 5-FU to apply the drug only to the affected area and not to cover it with an occlusive dressings. Advise patient to be careful when applying the drug near the eyes, mouth, and nose and to wash hands thoroughly after application. Inform patient that treated areas may be unsightly for several wks after therapy.
- Instruct patient to take no over-the-counter medications or herbal or vitamin supplements without checking with his or her health care provider.
- Instruct patient on local resources available and support groups related to their diagnosis.

OTHER INFORMATION
Do not confuse Efudex with Efidac.

FLUOXYMESTERONE

BRAND NAMES
Androxy, Halotestin

CLASS OF AGENT
Androgen

CLINICAL PHARMACOLOGY
Mechanism of Action
An androgen hormone that stimulates growth of male sex organs and maintenance of secondary sex characteristics.

Suppresses gonadotropin-releasing hormone, luteinizing hormone, and follicle-stimulating hormone.
Therapeutic Effect: Males: Stimulates spermatogenesis and virilism and accelerates linear growth rates in adolescence. Females: Inhibits growth of androgen-responsive tumors.

Absorption and Distribution
Rapidly absorbed from the GI tract.
Half-life: 9.2 hrs.

Metabolism and Excretion
Metabolized in liver. Excreted in urine.

HOW SUPPLIED/AVAILABLE FORMS
Tablets: 2 mg, 5 mg, 10 mg.

INDICATIONS AND DOSAGES
Males: Testosterone Replacement
5-20 mg orally daily. Hormone replacement: Start with full therapeutic dose and adjust thereafter. Delayed puberty: Start with lowest dose (2.5 mg) and titrate upwards for 4-6 mos.

Females: Palliative Breast Cancer Treatment in Postmenopausal Women
10-40 mg/day orally in divided doses.

Dosage Adjustment in Hepatic/Renal Dysfunction
No information available.

UNLABELED USES
Erythropoietin stimulation

PRECAUTIONS
Acute urethral obstruction and priapism may occur; both conditions may need immediate attention. Virilism in women is irreversible, and fluoxymesterone may need to be discontinued.

CONTRAINDICATIONS
Serious cardiac, renal, or hepatic dysfunction; men with carcinomas of the breast or prostate; hypersensitivity to fluoxymesterone or any component of the formulation, including tartrazine
Pregnancy Risk Category: X

DRUG PREPARATION/ADMINISTRATION/ SAFE HANDLING ISSUES
- Breast cancer: take in divided doses (e.g., 3 times daily or 4 times daily)
- Controlled Substance Schedule III

STORAGE AND STABILITY
Store at room temperature.

INTERACTIONS
Drug
Cyclosporine: May increase the risk of cyclosporine toxicity.
Hepatotoxic medications: May increase the risk of hepatotoxicity.
Insulin: May decrease blood glucose and decrease insulin requirements.
Oral anticoagulants: May increase the effects of these drugs.
Oxyphenbutazone: May increase oxyphenbutazone levels.
Herbal
Chaparral, comfrey, eucalyptus, germander, Jin Bu Huan, kava kava, pennyroyal, skullcap, valerian: May increase the risk of liver damage.

LAB EFFECTS/INTERFERENCE
May decrease levels of thyroxine-binding globulin, total thyroxine (T4) serum levels and increase resin uptake of triiodothyronine and T4. May increase alkaline phosphatase, SGOT (AST), bilirubin, calcium, K, Na, Hgb, hematocrit, and LDLs. May decrease HDLs.

SIDE EFFECTS
Serious Reactions
- Hepatic neoplasms, hepatocellular carcinoma, and peliosis hepatitis (liver and spleen replaced with blood-filled cysts) have been associated with prolonged use of high dosage of fluoxymesterone.
- Priapism may occur and requires immediate medical attention; it is indicative of excessive dosage and may require drug interruption.
- Virilism development in women is irreversible.
Other Side Effects
Frequent (10%-50%):
Females: amenorrhea, deepening voice, virilism (e.g., acne, decreased breast size, enlarged clitoris, and male pattern baldness)
Males: breast soreness, gynecomastia, priapism, urinary tract infections, virilism (e.g., acne and early pubic hair growth)
Occasional (1%-10%):
Anxiety, cholestatic hepatitis/jaundice (reversible with drug discontinuation), depression, decrease in libido, diarrhea, edema, electrolyte disturbance, generalized paresthesia, headache, liver enzyme level elevation, mild acne, nausea, stomach pain, vomiting
Males: Impotence, oligospermia, testicular atrophy

Rare (Less Than 1%):
Anaphylactoid reactions, hepatocellular neoplasms, peliosis hepatis

SPECIAL CONSIDERATIONS
Baseline Assessment
- Obtain a CBC with differential, platelets, electrolytes, BUN, creatinine, serum cholesterol, and triglyceride levels, and liver function tests.
- Assess for any history of GI upset, nausea, or dyspepsia.
- Evaluate for history of acne or dermatologic conditions.
Intervention and Evaluation
- Evaluate for nausea, vomiting, or dyspepsia with this agent.
- Monitor for electrolyte abnormalities.
- Assess for sexual alterations: For women these include amenorrhea, voice changes, changes in clitoral size, decreasing breast size, and libido changes. For men these include breast soreness or enlargement, priapism, or libido changes and impotence.
- Evaluate for increased feelings of anxiety in both men and women.
- Refer patients for counseling as appropriate.
- Provide emotional support to patient and family.
Education
- Instruct patient on when to contact his or her health care provider: nausea lasting greater than 24 hours, the inability to take in at least 1500 mL of fluid in 24 hour, headaches, significant anxiety, and dyspepsia.
- Instruct patient on sexual alterations that can occur with this agent: libido changes, priapism, impotence, breast changes in men and women, amenorrhea, and deepening voice in women.
- Advise patient to avoid any new over-the-counter medications or herbal or vitamin supplements without first checking with the health care provider.
- Instruct patient on local resources available and support groups related to their diagnosis.

FLUTAMIDE
BRAND NAMES
Eulexin

CLASS OF AGENT
Antiandrogen

CLINICAL PHARMACOLOGY
Mechanism of Action
A nonsteroidal antiandrogen hormone that inhibits androgen uptake and prevents androgen from binding to androgen receptors in target tissue. Used in conjunction with a luteinizing hormone-releasing hormone (LHRH) agonist analog to inhibit the stimulant effects of flutamide on serum testosterone levels. **Therapeutic Effect:** Decreases androgen effects and inhibits growth of prostate carcinoma.
Absorption and Distribution
Completely and rapidly absorbed from the GI tract. Food has no effect on the bioavailability of flutamide. Protein binding: 94%-96%.
Half-life: 8 hrs; 8-10 hrs (2-hydroxyflutamide).
Metabolism and Excretion
Rapidly and extensively metabolized in the liver to an active metabolite, 2-hydroxyflutamide. Excreted primarily in urine, and 4.2% excreted in the feces over 72 hrs. Not removed by hemodialysis.

HOW SUPPLIED/AVAILABLE FORMS
Capsules: 125 mg.

INDICATIONS AND DOSAGES
Prostatic Carcinoma (in Combination with LHRH Agonist)
250 mg orally every 8 hours without regard to meals. Alcohol should be avoided during administration as it may lead to excessive flushing.
Dosage Adjustment in Hepatic Dysfunction
Contraindicated in patients with severe hepatic impairment. No specific recommendations available.
Dosage Adjustment in Renal Dysfunction
Dose adjustments are not required in patients with chronic renal insufficiency. The elimination of the active metabolite was only slightly prolonged in patients with a Ccr less than 29 mL/min.

UNLABELED USES
Hirsutism (unlabeled): 250 mg orally daily

PRECAUTIONS
Hepatoxicity, including hepatic encephalopathy, jaundice, and acute hepatic failure, may be noted. Hepatic failure usually occurs within the first 3 mos of treatment and is reversible after discontinuation of therapy in some patients. Monitor for signs of liver function including hyperbilirubinuria, jaundice, right upper quadrant tenderness, nausea, vomiting, abdominal pain, fatigue, anorexia, and flu-like symptoms. Therapy should be discontinued if the patient experiences jaundice or increases in ALT (SGPT) 2 times ULN.
Use with caution in patients with glucose-6 phosphate dehydrogenase deficiency or Hgb M disease or in smokers as they have greater risk of developing toxicities associated with aniline exposure.
Pregnancy Risk Category: D

CONTRAINDICATIONS
Severe hepatic impairment and known hypersensitivity reaction to flutamide or any of its excipients.

DRUG PREPARATION/ADMINISTRATION/ SAFE HANDLING ISSUES
◀ ALERT ▶
- Discontinue flutamide therapy if jaundice develops or ALT 2 times ULN.
- Treatment with flutamide and goserelin acetate implant should start 8 wks before initiation of radiation therapy and continue during radiation therapy.
- Flutamide should be initiated with an LHRH agonist analog and continued until disease progression.
- Take capsules without regard to food.
- Overdose up to 1500 mg/day up to 36 wks resulted in no serious adverse effects. Adverse reactions included gynecomastia, breast tenderness, and increased AST (SGOT).

STORAGE AND STABILITY
Store at room temperature.

INTERACTIONS
Drug
Warfarin: May increase risk of bleeding. Monitor PT or international normalized ratio carefully.
Herbal
None known.

LAB EFFECTS/INTERFERENCE
May increase blood glucose level and serum estradiol, testosterone, bilirubin, creatinine, BUN, AST (SGOT), and ALT (SGPT) levels.

SIDE EFFECTS
Serious Reactions
- Hepatoxicity, including hepatic encephalopathy, jaundice, and acute hepatic failure, may be noted (see Precautions).
- Monitor methemoglobin levels in patients with glucose-6 phosphate dehydrogenase deficiency, Hgb M disease, or in smokers, as they have greater risk of developing toxicities associated with aniline exposure, including methemoglobinemia, hemolytic anemia, and cholestatic jaundice.

Other Side Effects
Frequent (10%-50%):
Asthenia, constipation, decreased libido, diarrhea, generalized pain, hot flashes, impotence
Occasional (1%-10%):
Anemia, anorexia, diaphoresis, dizziness, edema, flu-like syndromes, gynecomastia, headache, hematuria, insomnia, leukopenia, nausea, paresthesia, peripheral edema, photosensitivity, rash, urinary incontinence, vomiting
Rare (Less Than 1%):
Anxiety, confusion, depression, drowsiness, hepatitis, hypertension, jaundice, methemoglobinemia, nervousness, pulmonary symptoms, reduced sperm count, thrombocytopenia

SPECIAL CONSIDERATIONS
Baseline Assessment
- Assess CBC with differential, platelets, glucose, electrolytes, BUN, and creatinine levels and liver function tests.
- Evaluate patient for any history of diabetes and hypertension.
Intervention and Evaluation
- Monitor glucose and liver function test results at each provider visit.
- Assess patient's vital signs, evaluating for hypertension.
- Monitor patient for signs and symptoms of weight gain, peripheral edema, hot flashes, decreased libido, diarrhea, or pain.
- Assess skin for any evidence of rash, pruritus, or gynecomastia.
Education
- Advise patient to contact his or her health care provider if they experience pain, diarrhea, weight gain of greater than 2 kg per week, paresthesias, or changes in the color of urine or stool.
- Instruct patient on usual side effects, including hot flashes, decreased libido, and impotence.
- Advise patient to contact his or her health care provider for any signs or symptoms of altered mental status, headache, or a flu-like syndrome.
- Instruct patient to use sunscreen (at least SPF greater than 15) at all times when outside as this agent induces photosensitivity.
- Instruct patient to take no over-the-counter medications or herbal or vitamin supplements without checking with his or her health care provider.
- Instruct patient on local resources available and support groups related to their diagnosis.
- Advise patient to avoid alcohol during administration.

FULVESTRANT
BRAND NAMES
Faslodex

CLASS OF AGENT
Estrogen receptor antagonist

CLINICAL PHARMACOLOGY
Mechanism of Action
A pure estrogen antagonist that competes with endogenous estrogen at estrogen receptor binding sites. This results in downregulation of estrogen receptors on breast cancer cells. **Therapeutic Effect:** Inhibits tumor growth.
Absorption and Distribution
Extensively and rapidly distributed IM administration. Protein binding: 99%. Peak serum levels occur in 7-9 days.
Half-life: 40 days.
Metabolism and Excretion
Metabolized in the liver. Eliminated by the hepatobiliary route and excreted in feces (90%).

HOW SUPPLIED/AVAILABLE FORMS
Prefilled Syringe: 50 mg/mL in 2.5-mL and 5-mL syringes.

INDICATIONS AND DOSAGES
Postmenopausal Women with Hormone Receptor-Positive Advanced Breast Cancer with Disease Progression Following Prior Antiestrogen Therapy
250 mg given IM once monthly.
Dosage Adjustment in Hepatic Dysfunction
No dosage adjustments are needed for mild hepatic dysfunction. No information is

available for moderate to severe hepatic dysfunction.

UNLABELED USES
Endometriosis, dysfunctional uterine bleeding, and uterine fibroids

PRECAUTIONS
Pregnancy Risk Category: D

CONTRAINDICATIONS
Known hypersensitivity to fulvestrant or any component of its formulation. Known or suspected pregnancy.

DRUG PREPARATION/ADMINISTRATION/ SAFE HANDLING ISSUES
Administer IM slowly in the buttocks. Can be given either as one 250-mg IM injection or two separate, concurrent 125-mg injections.

STORAGE AND STABILITY
Store in refrigerator. Store in original container and protect from light.

INTERACTIONS
Drug
None known. Fulvestrant is not affected by the cytochrome P-450 enzyme system.
Herbal
Estrogen-containing herbals may decrease effect of fulvestrant.

LAB EFFECTS/INTERFERENCE
None known.

Y-SITE COMPATIBLES
No information.

INCOMPATIBLES
No information.

SIDE EFFECTS
Serious Reactions
Anemia, leukopenia, and thromboembolic phenomena occur rarely.
Other Side Effects
Frequent (10%-50%):
Asthenia, headache, hot flashes, nausea, pharyngitis, vasodilatation, vomiting
Occasional (1%-10%):
Abdominal pain, anorexia, anxiety, bone or back pain, constipation, depression, diaphoresis, diarrhea, dizziness, edema, fever, injection site pain, insomnia,

paresthesia, peripheral rash, vertigo, weight gain
Rare (Less Than 1%):
Hypersensitivity reactions, leukopenia, myalgia, thromboembolic events, vaginitis, vertigo

SPECIAL CONSIDERATIONS
Baseline Assessment
- Evaluate CBC with differential, platelets, partial thromboplastin time, PT, and fibrinogen level before initiating this therapy.
- Assess patient for any history of deep vein thrombosis or any other thromboembolic disorders such as a prior stroke or transient ischemic attack.
- Assess for any signs and symptoms of prior GI problems as this agent can induce nausea.

Intervention and Evaluation
- Monitor patient for menopausal-type symptoms: hot flashes, flushing, headache, night sweats, irritability, or evidence of depression.
- Evaluate injection sites for any evidence of phlebitis.
- Monitor for bone pain and treat as needed.
- Evaluate for weight gain, peripheral edema, diarrhea, and constipation.

Education
- Instruct patient to report any signs and symptoms of lower extremity edema, erythema, pain, or difficulty in walking.
- Instruct patient on when to contact his or her health care provider: severe headache, severe bone or back pain, nausea, diarrhea, or constipation lasting greater than 24 hours, or the inability to drink at least 1500 mL of fluid per 24 hours.
- Educate patient on the importance of compliance with this medication and to not stop this agent unless the health care provider is notified.
- Advise patient to avoid starting any new medications, either prescribed or over-the-counter, including herbal or vitamin supplements, without discussion with the health care provider.
- Instruct patient with potential for child-bearing (woman should be postmenopausal) to use contraceptive methods other than birth control pills; pregnancy should be avoided while a woman is receiving fulvestrant therapy.

GEFITINIB

BRAND NAMES
Iressa

CLASS OF AGENT
Antineoplastic agent, epidermal growth factor receptor (EGFR) inhibitor, tyrosine kinase inhibitor

CLINICAL PHARMACOLOGY
Mechanism of Action
Mechanism of action of gefitinib is not fully characterized. Gefitinib inhibits intracellular phosphorylation of tyrosine kinase associated with the EGFR. EGFRs are found on both normal and cancer cells and are involved with cell proliferation and survival. **Therapeutic Effect:** Inhibits the growth of cancer cells.
Absorption and Distribution
Slowly absorbed with a peak plasma level in 3-7 hr and a mean bioavailability of 60%. Bioavailability is not significantly affected by food. Steady state is achieved in 10 days. Protein binding: 90%.
Half-life: 48 hr.
Metabolism and Excretion
Undergoes extensive metabolism primarily via cytochrome P450 (CYP) 3A4 in the liver. Excreted in the feces (86%).

HOW SUPPLIED/AVAILABLE FORMS
Because of the lack of survival data and the availability of Food and Drug Administration-approved treatment alternatives, only patients who have previously taken gefitinib and are benefiting or have benefited from gefitinib or patients on clinical trials have access to gefitinib. (Contact: Iressa Access Program at Astra Zeneca toll-free at 1-800-601-8933 or via the Web at www.Iressa-access.com.)
Tablets: 250 mg.

INDICATIONS AND DOSAGES
Patients with non-Small Cell Lung Cancer Who Have Previously Taken Gefitinib and Are Benefiting or Have Benefited from Gefitinib
250 mg/day PO; increase to 500 mg/day for patients receiving drugs that may decrease gefitinib serum concentrations, such as rifampin and phenytoin.
Dosage Adjustment in Hepatic Dysfunction
In patients with liver metastasis and moderately to severely elevated liver biochemical abnormalities, gefitinib pharmacokinetics were similar to those in patients without liver abnormalities. However, it is recommended that medication be held if severe changes or elevations in liver transaminases occur.
Dosage Adjustment in Renal Dysfunction
No adjustments required.

UNLABELED USES
No information available.

PRECAUTIONS
Pregnancy Risk Category: D
Drug excretion into breast milk is unknown/not recommended in nursing women.

CONTRAINDICATIONS
Known hypersensitivity to gefitinib or its excipients.

DRUG PREPARATION/ADMINISTRATION/ SAFE HANDLING ISSUES
- Take tablets without regard to food.
- For patients with difficulty swallowing solids: disperse gefitinib tablets in one-half glass of drinking water (no other liquids should be used). Stir until tablet is dispersed (approximately 10 mins) and drink quickly. Rinse glass with more water and drink. Gefitinib may be administered via nasogastric tube.

STORAGE AND STABILITY
Store at room temperature (20-25° C [68-77° F]).

INTERACTIONS
Drug
CYP 3A4 inducers (phenytoin, ranitidine, rifampin): May decrease gefitinib blood concentration and effectiveness. Consider increasing gefitinib dose to 500 mg daily and monitoring for clinical response.
CYP 3A4 inhibitors (ciprofloxacin, clarithromycin, diclofenac, doxycycline, erythromycin, imatinib, isoniazid, itraconazole, ketoconazole, nefazodone, nicardipine, propofol, protease inhibitors, quinidine, verapamil): Increases gefitinib blood concentration. Monitor for gefitinib adverse affects.
Histamine H2-receptor antagonists (ranitidine, cimetidine): May reduce gefitinib plasma blood concentration and effectiveness.

Sodium bicarbonate: Increases gastric pH and may decrease gefitinib blood concentration and effectiveness.

Vinorelbine: May increase risk or severity of neutropenia.

Warfarin (coumarin-derivative anticoagulants): Increases the risk of bleeding. Monitor INR or PT regularly.

Herbal

St John's Wort: May decrease serum erlotinib concentration. Avoid use.

Food

Grapefruit inhibits CYP 3A4 enzymes and can potentially enhance gefitinib effects.

LAB EFFECTS/INTERFERENCE

May increase serum alkaline phosphatase, bilirubin, AST (SGOT), and ALT (SGPT) levels.

SIDE EFFECTS

Serious Reactions

- If acute onset of new or progressive, unexplained symptoms such as dyspnea, cough, and fever occur, hold gefitinib and assess for interstitial lung disease (ILD). Rare reports of ILD have been reported and may be fatal.
- Uncontrolled diarrhea or skin adverse reaction may be managed by holding therapy for 2 wks and reinitiating with a 250-mg daily dose.
- Onset of new eye symptoms such as pain may require drug interruption until symptoms resolve or medical evaluation and management are completed. Drug continuation or discontinuation may be determined at this time.

Other Side Effects

Frequent (10%-50%):

Acne, diarrhea, dry skin, nausea, rash, vomiting

Occasional (1%-10%):

Anorexia, asthenia, dyspnea, eye pain, peripheral edema, pruritus, weight loss

Rare (Less Than 1%):

Conjunctivitis, corneal membrane sloughing, interstitial lung disease, mouth ulceration, ocular ischemia/hemorrhage, pancreatitis, toxic epidermal necrolysis, erythema multiforme, allergic reactions, vesiculobullous rash

SPECIAL CONSIDERATIONS

Baseline Assessment

- Assess patient's ability to be compliant with oral medications.
- Assess patient's history for any problems with constipation, diarrhea, oral ulcers, or any prior pulmonary disease.
- Obtain baseline skin assessment with particular attention to any history of acne or other skin disorders.

Intervention and Evaluation

- Instruct patient that he or she they may take this drug with or without food but should be taken at the same time each day.
- Assess patient for any signs or symptoms of diarrhea and initiate antidiarrheal drugs as necessary.
- Monitor for any changes in pulmonary function, new symptoms of shortness of breath, dyspnea upon exertion, or rhonchi on chest examination.
- Evaluate for rashes on skin, dry eyes, and conjunctivitis.

Education

- Instruct patient on how and when to take this medication: with or without food, but at same time each day.
- Educate patient to maintain a drug diary and to bring medication and diary to each visit.
- Instruct patient on when to contact health care provider: shortness of breath, diarrhea greater than 4 stools over baseline, or any new significant symptoms.
- Remind patient to inform health care provider before starting any new medications, including OTC medications or herbal or vitamin supplements.
- Instruct patient on skin care regimen if acneiform rash occurs; apply moisturizers, not astringents, to the areas. Instruct patient this is not like acne he or she might have had as a teenager and must be treated differently. Patients may use any moisturizer of their choice (Aquaphor, Eucerin, Absorbase, Bag Balm, or other). Encourage patients to avoid alcohol-containing products as these will dry the skin and can increase the drug reaction.
- Initiate skin care regimen as soon as rash presents; patients may require more than moisturizers such as topical or oral antibiotics for skin eruptions.
- Advise patient what symptoms need to be reported immediately: diarrhea lasting greater than 24 hours, nausea lasting greater than 24 hours, the inability to take food or medicine for greater than 24 hours, severe abdominal pain, fatigue, and dry eyes.

- Provide patient with information on local resources and support groups available for his or her specific diagnosis.

GEMCITABINE HYDROCHLORIDE

BRAND NAMES
Gemzar

CLASS OF AGENT
Pyrimidine antimetabolite

CLINICAL PHARMACOLOGY
Mechanism of Action
Gemcitabine (2′,2′-difluorodeoxycytidine) is a pyrimidine antimetabolite structurally and pharmacologically similar to cytarabine. It differs from cytarabine only by substitution of geminal fluorines for the hydroxyl group at the 2′ position. Gemcitabine was specifically developed to extend the activity of cytarabine to nonhematologic malignancies. The cytotoxic effect of gemcitabine is attributed to a combination of two actions of the diphosphate and the triphosphate nucleosides, which inhibit ribonucleotide reductase, leading to inhibition of DNA synthesis. Gemcitabine exhibits cell phase specificity, primarily killing cells undergoing DNA synthesis (S phase) and also blocking the progression of cells through the G_1/S phase boundary. **Therapeutic Effect:** produces cell death in cells undergoing DNA synthesis.
Absorption and Distribution
Gemcitabine is given IV. After short infusions (less than 70 mins), the volume of distribution was 50 L/m^2, indicating that gemcitabine is not extensively distributed into tissues. With longer infusions, the volume of distribution rises to 370 L/m^2, reflecting slow equilibration of gemcitabine within the tissue compartment. Protein binding: less than 10%.
Half-life: The parent compound has a half-life with short infusion administration of 42-94 mins (influenced by gender and age of patient). Patients older than 65 have a half-life twice that of patients 48 or younger. Women also have a longer elimination half-life. The half-life for long infusion administration varies from 245 to 638 mins.
Metabolism and Excretion
Gemcitabine is metabolized intracellularly by deoxycytidine kinases to the active diphosphate (dFdCDP) and triphosphate (dFdCTP) nucleosides. Deoxycytidine kinase is the rate-limiting enzyme in activation of gemcitabine and is greater for gemcitabine than for cytidine deaminase (which can inactivate gemcitabine to difluorodeoxyuridine), and thus phosphorylation predominates over deamination. Peak levels of 2′,2′-difluorodeoxyuridine (dFdU) occur 5-15 mins after gemcitabine infusions and are proportional to the dose. Difluorodeoxyuridine has minimal antitumor activity but may contribute to gemcitabine toxicity. At 24 hrs after completion of gemcitabine 120-1000 mg/m^2 infusions plasma dFdU concentrations are independent of dose. The principle sites of deamination to dFdU are the liver, kidney, and, to some degree, plasma. dFdU is inactive.

Gemcitabine is excreted primarily in urine as its metabolite. After administration of a single 1000 mg/m^2/30 min infusion of radiolabeled drug, 92%-98% of the dose was recovered, almost entirely in the urine within 7 days. Gemcitabine (less than 10%) and the inactive uracil metabolite, dFdU, accounting for 99% of the excreted dose. The metabolite dFdU is also found in plasma.

HOW SUPPLIED/AVAILABLE FORMS
Powder for Reconstitution: 200-mg vial, 1-g vial.

INDICATIONS AND DOSAGES
Breast Cancer (in combination with Paclitaxel)
1250 mg/m^2 IV over 30 mins on days 1, 8. Repeat every 21 days.
Dosage Reduction Guidelines in Breast Cancer
Dosage adjustments should be based on granulocyte count and platelet count, as follows:

Absolute Granulocyte Counts (cells/mm³)		Platelet Count (cells/mm³)	% of Full Dose
1200	and	>75,000	100
1000-1199	or	50,000-75,000	75
700-999	and	>50,000	50
<700	or	<50,000	Hold

Non-Small Cell Lung Cancer (NSCLS) (in Combination with Cisplatin)

1000 mg/m^2 IV over 30 mins on days 1, 8, and 15, repeated every 28 days or 1250 mg/m^2 IV on days 1 and 8. Repeat every 21 days.

Dosage Reduction Guidelines in NSCLC Cancer

Dosage adjustments should be based on granulocyte count and platelet count, as follows:

Absolute Granulocyte Counts (cells/mm^3)		Platelet Count (cells/mm^3)	% of Full Dose
1000	and	>100,000	100
500-999	and	50,000-99,000	75
<500	or	<50,000	Hold

Ovarian Cancer (in combination with Carboplatin)

1000 mg/m^2 IV over 30 mins on days 1, 8. Repeat every 21 days.

Dosage Reduction Guidelines in Ovarian Cancer

Dosage adjustments should be based on granulocyte count and platelet count, as follows:

Absolute Granulocyte Counts (cells/mm^3)		Platelet Count (cells/mm^3)	% of Full Dose
>1500	and	>100,000	100
1000-1499	and/or	75,000-99,000	50
< 1000	and/or	<75,000	Hold

Pancreatic Cancer

1000 mg/m^2 IV over 30 mins once weekly for up to 7 wks or until toxicity necessitates decreasing dosage or withholding the dose, followed by 1 week of rest. Subsequent cycles should consist of once weekly dose for 3 consecutive wks of every 4 wks. For patients completing cycles at 1000 mg/m^2, increase dose to 1250 mg/m^2 as tolerated. Dose for next cycle may be increased to 1500 mg/m^2.

Dosage Reduction Guidelines in Pancreatic Cancer

Dosage adjustments should be based on granulocyte count and platelet count, as follows:

Absolute Granulocyte Counts (cells/mm^3)		Platelet Count (cells/mm^3)	% of Full Dose
>1,000	and	>100,000	100
500-999	or	50,000-99,000	75
<500	or	<50,000	Hold

Dosage Adjustment in Hepatic Dysfunction

One study suggested that starting doses be decreased to 800 mg/m^2 in patients with elevated bilirubin levels of 1.6-7 mg/dL and that doses in subsequent cycles be adjusted according to toxicities.

Dosage Adjustment in Renal Dysfunction

Has not been studied. Use with caution in patients with renal dysfunction.

UNLABELED USES

Treatment of biliary tract carcinoma, gallbladder carcinoma, Hodgkin's lymphoma, non-Hodgkin's lymphoma, ovarian carcinoma

PRECAUTIONS
Pregnancy Risk Category: D

CONTRAINDICATIONS

Known hypersensitivity to gemcitabine or any component of the formulation

DRUG PREPARATION/ADMINISTRATION/ SAFE HANDLING ISSUES

◀ ALERT ▶ Exercise caution in handling and preparing gemcitabine solutions. The use of gloves is recommended. If gemcitabine solution contacts the skin or mucosa, immediately wash the skin thoroughly with soap and water or rinse the mucosa with copious amounts of water.

◀ ALERT ▶ The recommended diluent for reconstitution of gemcitabine is 0.9% NaCl injection without preservatives. Because of solubility considerations, the maximum concentration for gemcitabine upon reconstitution is 40 mg/mL. Reconstitution at concentrations greater than 40 mg/mL may result in incomplete dissolution and should be avoided.

- To reconstitute, add 5 mL of 0.9% NaCl injection to the 200-mg vial or 25 mL of 0.9% NaCl injection to the 1000-mg vial.
- This mixture should be shaken to dissolve the powder completely.
- These dilutions will produce a gemcitabine concentration of 38 mg/mL, which accounts for the displacement volume of the lyophilized powder (0.26 mL for the 200-mg vial or 1.3 mL for the 1-g vial).
- The contents of these vials should be completely withdrawn to provide 200 and 1000 mg of gemcitabine, respectively.
- The calculated amount of drug may be administered as prepared or further diluted with 0.9% NaCl for injection to concentrations as low as 0.1 mg/mL.
- Gemcitabine may be infused over 30 mins (standard) or as a fixed dose infusion of 10 mg/m^2/min.

STORAGE AND STABILITY
- Unopened vials of gemcitabine are stable until the expiration date indicated on the package when stored at controlled room temperature 20-25° C (68-77° F).
- When prepared as directed, gemcitabine solutions are stable for 24 hrs at controlled room temperature (20-25° C [68-77° F]). Discard unused portion. Solutions of reconstituted gemcitabine should not be refrigerated, as crystallization may occur.
- The compatibility of gemcitabine with other drugs has not been studied.

INTERACTIONS
Drug
Bone marrow depressants: May increase the risk of myelosuppression.
Live-virus vaccines: May potentiate viral replication, increase vaccine side effects, and decrease the patient's antibody response to the vaccine.
Herbal
None known.

LAB EFFECTS/INTERFERENCE
May increase BUN, serum alkaline phosphatase, bilirubin, creatinine, AST (SGOT), and ALT (SGPT) levels. May decrease platelet and ANC levels.

Y-SITE COMPATIBLES
Bleomycin (Blenoxane), bumetanide (Bumex), calcium gluconate, cisplatin, cyclophosphamide, daunorubicin, dexamethasone (Decadron), dexrazoxane, diphenhydramine (Benadryl), dobutamine (Dobutrex), dopamine (Intropin), doxorubicin, floxuridine, granisetron (Kytril), heparin, hydrocortisone (Solu-Cortef), idarubicin, ifosfamide (IFEX), lorazepam (Ativan), mesna, mitoxantrone, paclitaxel, palonosetron, ondansetron (Zofran), potassium, rituximab (Rituxan), teniposide, topotecan (Hycamtin), trastuzumab (Herceptin), vinblastine, vincristine, vinorelbine (Navelbine)

INCOMPATIBLES
Acyclovir (Zovirax), amphotericin B conventional (Fungizone), amphotericin B liposomal (AmBisome), cefepime, cefoperazone (Cefobid), cefotaxime, chloramphenicol, dantrolene, diazepam, furosemide (Lasix), ganciclovir (Cytovene), imipenem and cilastatin (Primaxin), irinotecan (Camptosar), ketorolac, lansoprazole, methotrexate, methylprednisolone (Solu-Medrol), mitomycin (Mutamycin), piperacillin and tazobactam (Zosyn), nafcillin, pantoprazole, pemetrexed, phenytoin, prochlorperazine (Compazine), thiopental

SIDE EFFECTS
Serious Reactions
Severe myelosuppression, as evidenced by anemia, thrombocytopenia, leukopenia, is a common reaction.
Other Side Effects
Frequent (10%-50%):
Alopecia (mild), constipation, diarrhea, fever, dyspnea (mild to moderate), generalized pain, infection, nausea, paresthesia, peripheral edema, petechiae, rash (mild to moderate), stomatitis, somnolence, vomiting
Occasional (1%-10%):
Peripheral edema
Rare (Less Than 1%):
Bullous skin ulceration, cellulitis, diaphoresis, insomnia, malaise, rhinitis

SPECIAL CONSIDERATIONS
Baseline Assessment
- Assess patient's CBC with differential, platelet count, electrolyte, BUN, and creatinine levels, and liver function tests.
- Evaluate patient for any history of emesis and severity.
- Assess patient for any history of liver disease as dose reductions are required for elevated bilirubins.

Intervention and Evaluation

- Monitor patient's CBC with differential, platelet count, electrolyte, BUN, creatinine levels, and liver function tests, especially bilirubin level.
- Administer premedications as ordered.
- Evaluate skin for any evidence of rashes or skin changes.
- Assess patient for any signs and symptoms of diarrhea or stomatitis or paresthesias.
- Monitor for signs and symptoms of peripheral edema or significant weight gain; weigh patient before each dose.
- Although fever is common after gemcitabine administration (incidence of 41%), the incidence of infection is much less common (16%) and is associated with a flu-like syndrome. This reaction is usually mild and clinically manageable.

Education

- Instruct patient when to contact his or her health care provider: fever greater than 38° C (greater than 101° F), chills, nausea and vomiting lasting greater than 24 hours or diarrhea greater than 24 hours, or inability to take in at least 1500 mL of fluid in 24 hours.
- Educate patient on possibility of stomatitis or skin changes.
- Educate patient on possibility of weight gain or edema.
- Instruct patient to report any signs and symptoms of paresthesias: numbness or tingling in fingers or toes.
- Inform patient that he or she may experience fatigue with this agent and suggest ideas on how to manage this symptom: light exercise, taking naps, planning the day, and others.
- Advise patient to avoid all OTC medications, vitamins, and herbals without first checking with their health care provider.
- Provide patient with information on local resources and support groups available for his or her specific diagnosis.

GEMTUZUMAB OZOGAMICIN

BRAND NAMES
Mylotarg

CLASS OF AGENT
Antineoplastic agent

CLINICAL PHARMACOLOGY
Mechanism of Action
Composed of a recombinant humanized IgG4 κ antibody linked to an antitumor antibiotic, calicheamicin. Calicheamicin is isolated from *Micromonospora echinospora* subsp. *calichensis.* The agent binds to the CD33 antigen on the surface of leukemic blast cells, which is expressed in more than 80% of patients with acute myeloid leukemia (AML). The resulting formation is a complex that leads to the release of the cytotoxic antibiotic inside the myeloid cells. The antibiotic then binds to DNA, resulting in DNA double-strand breaks and cell death. CD33 is also expressed in normal myeloid colony-forming cells but not on pluripotent hematopoietic stem cells, and, therefore, myelosuppression is reversible. **Therapeutic Effect:** Inhibits colony formation of adult leukemic bone marrow cells.

Absorption and Distribution
Distributed in myeloid colony-forming cells that express CD33. The area under the curve of unconjugated calicheamicin increases by 30% after the second dose.
Half-life: Elimination half-life: 45 hrs after first infusion; 60 hrs after second infusion.

Metabolism and Excretion
Unknown.

HOW SUPPLIED/AVAILABLE FORMS
Powder for Injection: 5 mg.

INDICATIONS AND DOSAGES
Patients 60 Years Old or Older with CD33-Positive AML in First Relapse Who Are Not Candidates for Cytotoxic Chemotherapy
9 mg/m^2 IV infused over 2 hrs and repeated in 14 days for a total of two doses. Full recovery of myelosuppression is not needed before the second dose is administered.
Note: Premedicate with acetaminophen 650-1000 mg PO and diphenhydramine 50 mg PO to decrease acute infusion reactions. Methylprednisolone may also be used before gemtuzumab ozogamicin to reduce infusion-related symptoms. Consider hydration and allopurinol to prevent hyperuricemia. Consider leukoreduction with hydroxyurea or leukapheresis to reduce the risk of tumor lysis syndrome and serious pulmonary events (increased risk with WBC greater than 30,000/microliter).

Dosage Adjustment in Hepatic Dysfunction
Has not been studied in patients with
bilirubin level greater than 2 mg/dL.
Use extra caution.

Dosage Adjustment in Renal Dysfunction
Patients with renal dysfunction were not
studied according to the product insert.

UNLABELED USES
Acute promyelocytic leukemia as part of
initial combination therapy

PRECAUTIONS
• Neutropenia grade 3 or 4 occurred in
98% of patients, and it took approximately 40 days for recovery to ANC of
500/microliter. Grade 3 and 4 anemia
and thrombocytopenia occurred in
52% and 99% of patients, respectively.
• Hepatotoxicity, especially in the form of
veno-occlusive disease, may occur.
Symptoms include rapid weight gain,
right upper quadrant pain, hepatomegaly,
ascites, and elevations in bilirubin and or
liver enzyme levels. Patients who have
undergone hematopoietic stem cell transplant are at increased risk.
• Infusion-related reactions including
anaphylaxis might occur. Less severe
reactions may include symptoms such
as fever, chills, and less commonly
hypotension and dyspnea. Premedicate
before infusion. Vital signs should be
monitored during infusion and for 4 hrs
after infusion.
• Pulmonary events including dyspnea,
pulmonary infiltrates, pleural effusions,
noncardiogenic pulmonary edema, pulmonary insufficiency and hypoxia, and acute
respiratory distress syndrome have been
reported during postmarketing surveillance. Patients with symptomatic intrinsic
lung disease or WBC count greater than
30,000/microliter are at increased risk,
and leukoreduction with hydroxyurea or
leukapheresis should be considered.
• Tumor lysis syndrome may occur, and
hydration and allopurinol may be used to
prevent hyperuricemia.

Pregnancy Risk Category: D
Drug excretion into human breast milk is
unknown/not recommended in nursing
women.

CONTRAINDICATIONS
Known hypersensitivity to gemtuzumab
ozogamicin or any component for the
formulation (anti-CD33 antibody or
calicheamicin).

DRUG PREPARATION/ADMINISTRATION/
SAFE HANDLING ISSUES
◀ ALERT ▶ Give diphenhydramine 50 mg and
acetaminophen 650-1000 mg 1 hr before
administering gemtuzumab, as prescribed.
Follow with acetaminophen 650-1000 mg
every 4 hrs for two doses and then every
4 hrs as prescribed and as needed. Full
recovery from hematologic toxicities is not
a requirement for giving the second gemtuzumab dose.
◀ ALERT ▶ When handling this agent, use nitrile or latex gloves only. If a splash occurs,
wash with mild soap and water; do not use
waterless soap or any antibacterial soap as
either can enhance the skin reactions. If an
eye splash occurs, use copious amounts of
water or 0.9% NaCl to irrigate the eyes.
Irrigation should be done from inner to
outer canthus.
• Protect the drug from direct and
indirect sunlight and unshielded
fluorescent light during preparation
and administration.
• Prepare the drug in a biologic safety
hood with the fluorescent light off or
shielded.
• Before reconstitution, let the vials come
to room temperature.
• Using sterile syringes, reconstitute
each vial with 5 mL of sterile water for
injection to provide a concentration of
1 mg/mL.
• Gently swirl the vial; then inspect for
particulate matter or discoloration.
• After reconstitution, protect the solution
from light. The solution is stable for up
to 2 hrs at room temperature (total time
from reconstitution to end of administration should not exceed 20 hrs).
• Withdraw the desired volume from each
vial and inject into an IV bag containing
100 mL of 0.9% NaCl; place the IV bag
into an ultraviolet protectant bag.
• Administer the solution as soon as it has
been diluted in 100 mL of 0.9% NaCl.
The solution may appear hazy. Diluted
solution is stable at room temperature for
up to 16 hrs.
• Infuse the drug over 2 hrs, using a separate
peripheral or central line equipped with a
low protein-binding 1.2-micron filter.
• Do not give gemtuzumab by IV push
or bolus.

STORAGE AND STABILITY

- After reconstitution, protect the solution from light. The reconstituted vial is stable for up to 2 hrs at room temperature or under refrigeration. The diluted admixture is stable up to 16 hrs at room temperature. Total time from reconstitution to end of administration should not exceed 20 hrs.
- Store vials refrigerated at 2-8° C (36-46° F).

INTERACTIONS
Drug
None known.
Herbal
None known.

LAB EFFECTS/INTERFERENCE

May increase serum bilirubin, AST (SGOT), and ALT (SGPT) levels. May decrease blood Hgb and Hct levels, platelet count, WBC count, and serum magnesium and potassium levels. May increase or decrease serum calcium and glucose levels. May also increase prothrombin and partial thromboplastin times.

Y-SITE COMPATIBLES

None known.

INCOMPATIBLES

Do not mix gemtuzumab with any other medications, D5W, or any other electrolyte solutions.

SIDE EFFECTS
Serious Reactions

- Severe myelosuppression, characterized by neutropenia, anemia, and thrombocytopenia, occurs in 98% of all patients.
- Infection grade 3 or 4 occurred in 30% of patients.
- Veno-occlusive disease, infusion-related reactions including anaphylaxis, severe pulmonary events, and tumor lysis syndrome have all been reported.

Other Side Effects
Frequent (10%-50%):
(greater than 50%) Postinfusion symptom complex of fever, chills, nausea, and vomiting that resolves within 2-4 hrs with supportive therapy, myelosuppression
(44%-31%) Asthenia, diarrhea, abdominal pain, headache, stomatitis, dyspnea, epistaxis, hepatotoxicity
(25%-15%) Constipation, neutropenic

fever, nonspecific rash, herpes simplex infection, hypertension, hypotension, petechiae, peripheral edema, dizziness, insomnia, back pain, veno-occlusive disease (20% in patients after treatment of stem cell transplant), bleeding (at all sites)
(14%-10%) Pharyngitis, ecchymosis, dyspepsia, tachycardia, hematuria
Occasional (1%-10%):
Pruritus, hypercalcemia, hypoglycemia, hypomagnesemia, hypophosphatemia, myalgia, anxiety, depression, rhinitis, veno-occlusive disease (no treatment with stem cell transplant)
Rare (Less Than 1%):
Postmarketing surveillance: renal failure, renal failure due to tumor lysis syndrome, pulmonary events, pulmonary hemorrhage, GI hemorrhage

SPECIAL CONSIDERATIONS
Baseline Assessment

- Monitor the CBC with differential, liver function tests, electrolyte, BUN, magnesium, and creatinine levels.
- Assess for signs and symptoms of infection before drug administration.
- Assess for any allergies to prior agents received.
- Assess baseline vital signs and weight.

Intervention and Evaluation

- Monitor patient's blood chemistry values, CBC, and liver function studies.
- Premedicate patient as ordered with diphenhydramine 50 mg and acetaminophen 650 mg before dosing and every 4 hours two times and then prn.
- Evaluate patient's hydration status and check for any orthostatic changes.
- Assess patient for oral hygiene and the need to initiate an oral care regimen.
- Assess patient for signs and symptoms of infection and bleeding.
- Assess patient for diarrhea and the need for a bowel regimen.
- Monitor patient's B/P for evidence of hypertension or hypotension.

Education

- Instruct patient to continue acetaminophen as ordered to prevent fever, chills, and rigors from drug.
- Instruct patient on signs and symptoms of infection: fever greater than 38° C (greater than 101° F), shaking chills, cough, dyspnea, difficulty or pain upon urination.

- Make sure patient has a 24-hour number for his or her health care provider and knows what symptoms to call for.
- Inform patient that alopecia is not a usual side effect of this agent.
- Educate patient on neutropenic precautions as necessary:
  - Practice good handwashing technique.
  - Avoid individuals who are ill.
  - Wash and cook all foods well.
  - Avoid crowds.
  - Avoid fresh fruits and vegetables.
- Educate patient on thrombocytopenic precautions:
  - Use of a soft bristle toothbrush.
  - No flossing if platelet count is less than 50,000/mm³.
  - No IM injections.
  - No rectal suppositories.
  - No aerobic exercise.
- Instruct patient on an oral care regimen as necessary. An example is 1 tsp each of salt and baking soda dissolved in 1 glass of water to swish and spit at least 4 times/day with an evaluation by the provider to assess the need for any further medications.
- Urge patient not to receive vaccinations and to avoid contact with anyone who has recently received a live-virus vaccine.
- Instruct patient to notify his or her health care provider if he or she experiences easy bruising, sore throat, or unusual bleeding from any site.
- Provide patient with information on local resources and support groups available for his or her specific diagnosis.

GOSERELIN ACETATE

BRAND NAMES
Zoladex, Zoladex LA

CLASS OF AGENT
Luteinizing hormone-releasing hormone agonist (LHRH), gonadotropin-releasing hormone agonist (GnRH)

CLINICAL PHARMACOLOGY
Mechanism of Action
A potent LHRH agonist analog of the anterior pituitary gland; also known as a GnRH agonist. Circulating levels of luteinizing hormone, follicle-stimulating hormone, testosterone, and estradiol rise initially and then subside with continued therapy. **Therapeutic Effect:** In females, causes a reduction in ovarian size and function, a reduction in uterine and mammary gland size, and regression of sex hormone-responsive tumors. In males, produces pharmacologic castration and decreases the growth of abnormal prostate tissue.

Absorption and Distribution
Absorption is rapid. Time to peak concentrations: males: 12-15 days; females: 8-22 days. Protein binding: 27%. Volume of distribution: males: 44 L; females: 20 L. *Half-life:* Males: 4.2 hrs; females: 2.3 hrs.

Metabolism and Excretion
Undergoes metabolism by C-terminal amino acid hydrolysis, excreted mainly through urine (90%); unchanged drug (20%).

HOW SUPPLIED/AVAILABLE FORMS
Implant (Zoladex): 3.6 mg.
Implant (Zoladex LA): 10.8 mg.

INDICATIONS AND DOSAGES
Breast Cancer, Endometriosis, Endometrial Thinning, Prostate Cancer
3.6 mg every 28 days subcutaneously into abdominal wall below the navel line.
Prostate Cancer
10.8 mg every 12 wks subcutaneously into abdominal wall below the navel line.
Dosage Adjustment in Hepatic/Renal Dysfunction
No adjustments necessary.

UNLABELED USES
Dysfunctional uterine bleeding, precocious puberty, in vitro fertilization, uterine leiomyoma.

PRECAUTIONS
Pregnancy Risk Category: D (advanced breast cancer), **X** (endometriosis, endometrial thinning).
Goserelin may cause fetal harm when administered during pregnancy. Use nonhormonal contraception and for 12 wks after drug discontinuation. Excretion into human milk is unknown/not recommended in nursing women.

CONTRAINDICATIONS
Hypersensitivity to goserelin or any component of its formulation, LHRH or LHRH agonists, pregnancy

DRUG PREPARATION/ADMINISTRATION/ SAFE HANDLING ISSUES
- Prepare area on the anterior abdominal wall below navel.

- Remove syringe from foil pouch and check that at least a part of the goserelin implant is visible.
- Remove red plastic safety tab and needle cover.
- Do not try to expel any air bubbles.
- Administer subcutaneously. Hold syringe around the protective sleeve and pinch skin on the abdominal wall. With the bevel of needle facing up, insert needle at a 30- to 45-degree angle to the skin in one continuous deliberate motion until protective sleeve contacts the skin.
- If vessel is penetrated, blood will immediately be seen. Withdraw needle and inject elsewhere.
- Do not inject into muscle or peritoneum.

STORAGE AND STABILITY
Store at room temperature.

INTERACTIONS
Drug
None known.
Herbal
None known.

LAB EFFECTS/INTERFERENCE
May alter serum pituitary-gonadal function test results; normal functions usually restored in 12 wks after drug discontinuation. May cause changes in bone mineral density and lipid profile.

INCOMPATIBLES
Do not mix with any solution.

SIDE EFFECTS
Serious Reactions
- Arrhythmias, CHF, and hypertension occur rarely.
- Tumor flare may occur in the first few weeks after initiation of goserelin and is characterized by transient worsening of signs and symptoms. Ureteral obstruction and spinal cord compression have been observed. An immediate orchiectomy may be necessary if these events are severe.
- Hypercalcemia may occur in breast cancer and prostate cancer patients with bone metastases.
- Goserelin is rarely associated with pituitary apoplexy, which has presented as sudden headache, vomiting, visual changes, ophthalmoplegia, altered

mental status, and sometimes cardiovascular collapse.
Other Side Effects
Frequent (10%-50%):
Headache, hot flashes, depression, diaphoresis, decreased erection, lower urinary tract symptoms, sexual dysfunction, sweating
Occasional (1%-10%):
Pain, lethargy, dizziness, insomnia, anorexia, nausea, rash, upper respiratory tract infection, hirsutism, abdominal pain, edema, malaise, hypertension
Rare (Less Than 1%):
Pruritus, leg cramps, hypersensitivity reaction, urticaria

SPECIAL CONSIDERATIONS
Baseline Assessment
- Assess patient for any history of hypertension, cardiac dysfunction, arrhythmias, or depression.
- Evaluate baseline vital signs for hypertension.
- Assess for any history of urinary tract problems, urinary tract infection, or obstruction.
- Assess for any risk of spinal cord compression.
- Exclude pregnancy.
- Assess baseline bone mineral density, lipid profile, and patient's risk factors.
Intervention and Evaluation
- Monitor patient for any signs or symptoms of hot flashes, sexual dysfunction, or libido changes.
- Assess patient for any signs or symptoms of cardiac changes: tachycardia, arrhythmias, or chest pain.
- Monitor for hypertension at each visit and note changes in B/P.
- Evaluate patient's ability to comply with clinic visits for injections every 28 days or every 12 weeks.
- Assess patient for any evidence of hyperglycemia, polyuria, polydipsia, constipation, or diarrhea.
- Monitor for evidence of fever greater than 38° C or (greater than 101° F), chills, or gynecomastia, swelling, or tenderness of breasts.
Education
- Instruct patient on usual side effects of this agent: hot flashes, sexual dysfunction, and libido changes and to report significant symptoms to his or her health care provider.

- Educate patient on symptoms of hyperglycemia: polyuria, polydipsia, and polyphagia.
- Advise patient that constipation and urinary symptoms such as burning upon urination or difficulty passing urine may be a side effect of this agent.
- Inform patient that tenderness and swelling of the breasts can occur with this agent.
- Instruct female patients of the importance of nonhormonal contraceptive use while receiving therapy. Advise patients that one or more successive missed dose of goserelin may result in breakthrough bleeding or ovulation with the potential for pregnancy.
- Instruct patient to take no over-the-counter medications or herbal or vitamin supplements without checking with his or her health care provider.
- Provide patient with information on local resources and support groups available for his or her specific diagnosis.

HYDROXYUREA

BRAND NAMES
Droxia, Hydrea, Mylocel

CLASS OF AGENT
Antineoplastic agent, antimetabolite

CLINICAL PHARMACOLOGY
Mechanism of Action
A synthetic urea analog that inhibits DNA synthesis by acting as a ribonucleotide reductase inhibitor without interfering with RNA or protein synthesis. May also hold other cells of the cell cycle in the G_1 or pre-DNA synthesis stage where they are most susceptible to the effects of irradiation.
Therapeutic Effect: Inhibits DNA synthesis and interferes with the normal repair process of cancer cells damaged by irradiation.
Absorption and Distribution
Absorption rapid with peak plasma levels reached in 1-4 hrs after the dose. Bioavailability reported to be 78%. Widely distributed with a volume of distribution equal to total body water. Plasma to ascites fluid ratios range from 2:1 to 7.5:1. Concentrates in leukocytes and erythrocytes.
Half-life: 3-4 hrs.
Metabolism and Excretion
Metabolic pathways are not fully characterized. One minor pathway includes being de-

graded by urease found in intestinal bacteria. Excretion is nonlinear: saturable hepatic metabolism and first-order renal excretion.

HOW SUPPLIED/AVAILABLE FORMS
Capsules (Droxia): 200 mg, 300 mg, 400 mg.
Capsules (Hydrea): 500 mg.
Tablets (Mylocel): 1000 mg.

INDICATIONS AND DOSAGES
Melanoma, Ovarian Carcinoma
80 mg/kg PO every 3 days or 20-30 mg/kg/day daily.
Squamous Cell Carcinoma of the Head and Neck, Excluding Lips (in Combination with Radiation Therapy)
80 mg/kg PO every 3 days, start at least 7 days before radiation therapy.
Resistant Chronic Myelocytic Leukemia
20-30 mg/kg PO once daily.
Sickle cell anemia
Initially, 15 mg/kg PO once daily. May increase by 5 mg/kg/day every 12 wks. Maximum: 35 mg/kg/day.
Dosage Adjustment in Hepatic Dysfunction
No recommendations available.
Dosage Adjustment in Renal Dysfunction
No recommendations available. Use with caution because this drug is excreted through the kidneys.

UNLABELED USES
Treatment of cervical carcinoma, polycythemia vera; long-term suppression of HIV infection, essential thrombocythemia
HIV Infection (in Combination with Antiretroviral Agents)
500 mg PO bid.

PRECAUTIONS
- Gangrene and vasculitic ulcerations have been reported.
- Hydroxyurea may cause radiation recall in patients who have received radiation in the past. Treat with topical or oral anesthetics; if severe, hydroxyurea therapy may be interrupted for a few days.
- Serious cases of pancreatitis and peripheral neuropathy have been reported in HIV-positive patients treated with hydroxyurea and didanosine, with or without stavudine.
- Use with caution in elderly patients as they may have impaired renal function,

making them more at risk for toxicities. May require a lower dose.

Pregnancy Risk Category: D
Hydroxyurea is known to be a human carcinogen and may cause fetal harm when given to a pregnant woman. Hydroxyurea is excreted into human milk. Breast feeding is not recommended.

CONTRAINDICATIONS
WBC count less than 2500/mm^3 or platelet count less than 100,000/mm^3 or severe anemia.

DRUG PREPARATION/ADMINISTRATION/SAFE HANDLING ISSUES
◀ **ALERT** ▶ Wash hands before and after contact with the bottle or capsules.

- If capsule content is spilled, immediately wipe it up with a damp cloth and discard the cloth a closed container such as a plastic bag.
- Overdosage at several times the therapeutic dose has resulted in acute mucocutaneous toxicity: soreness, violet erythema, edema on palms and soles followed by scaling of hands and feet, severe generalized hyperpigmentation of skin, and stomatitis. Give supportive care.

STORAGE AND STABILITY
Store at room temperature.

INTERACTIONS
Drug
Bone marrow depressants: May increase myelosuppression.
Live virus vaccines: May potentiate viral replication, increase vaccine side effects, and decrease the patient's antibody response to the vaccine.
Herbal
None known.

LAB EFFECTS/INTERFERENCE
May increase BUN, serum creatinine, and uric acid levels.

SIDE EFFECTS
Serious Reactions
- Myelosuppression may cause hematologic toxicity (manifested as leukopenia and, to a lesser extent, as thrombocytopenia and anemia).
- Radiation recall has been reported.

- Pancreatitis, sometime fatal, has occurred in HIV-infected patients during concomitant therapy with didanosine, with or without stavudine.
- Severe cutaneous vasculitic toxicities, including vasculitic ulcerations and gangrene, have occurred in MDS patients receiving hydroxyurea. Patients with these reactions usually either had previously or were currently receiving interferon therapy.

Other Side Effects
Frequent (10%-50%):
Anemia, anorexia, constipation or diarrhea, leukopenia, nausea, vomiting
Occasional (1%-10%):
Chills, facial flushing, fever; malaise, rash (mild, reversible, itchy), stomatitis, thrombocytopenia
Rare (Less Than 1%):
Alopecia, atrophy of skin/nails, convulsions, disorientation, dizziness, drowsiness, dysuria, hallucinations, headache, hepatotoxicity, hyperpigmentation, pancreatitis, peripheral neuropathy, pulmonary reactions (acute: diffuse pulmonary infiltrates, fever, and dyspnea), secondary leukemia

SPECIAL CONSIDERATIONS
Baseline Assessment
- Monitor patient's CBC with differential, platelet count, electrolyte, BUN, creatinine, magnesium levels, and liver function tests.
- Assess patient for any history of constipation or diarrhea or gout.
- Review patient's history for any side effects of prior chemotherapy agents.
- Elderly patients with impaired renal function may require a lower dose and are more susceptible to toxicities.

Intervention and Evaluation
- Premedicate patient as ordered.
- Monitor patient for signs and symptoms of nausea, vomiting, anorexia, or bowel changes such as constipation or diarrhea.
- Assess patient for evidence of rashes or pruritus.
- Monitor vital signs for evidence of infection: fever greater than 38° C (greater than 101° F), chills, or rigors.
- Monitor for any signs of cutaneous vasculitic toxicities.
- Evaluate patient for any evidence of CNS alterations: headache, drowsiness, dizziness, or altered mental status.

CANCER DRUGS

- Initiate or adjust uricosuric medication as necessary according to serum uric acid levels.

Education

- Instruct patient when to contact his or her health care provider: signs or symptoms of infection, fever greater than 38° C (greater than 101° F), chills, cough, nausea or diarrhea lasting greater than 24 hours or the inability to drink at least 1500 mL in 24 hours.
- Educate patient on neutropenic precautions as necessary:
    Practice good handwashing technique.
    Avoid individuals who are ill.
    Wash and cook all foods well.
    Avoid crowds.
    Avoid fresh fruits and vegetables.
- Educate patient on thrombocytopenic precautions:
    Use of a soft bristle toothbrush.
    No flossing if platelet count is less than 50,000/mm³.
    No IM injections.
    No rectal suppositories.
    No aerobic exercise.
- Advise patient alopecia rarely occurs.
- Instruct patient to monitor for any skin changes, rash, pruritus, or dry scaly skin. Use moisturizers as needed.
- Teach patient to wash hands before and after contact with the bottle or capsule. People not taking hydroxyurea should not be exposed to it.
- If powder from a capsule is spilled, advise patient to wipe it up immediately with damp disposable towel and discard the towel in closed plastic container.
- Instruct patient to take no over-the-counter medications or herbal or vitamin supplements without checking with his or her health care provider.
- Provide patient with local resources and support groups available for his or her specific diagnosis.

IBRITUMOMAB TIUXETAN, IN-111 ZEVALIN, Y-90 ZEVALIN

BRAND NAMES
Zevalin

CLASS OF AGENT
Antineoplastic agent, monoclonal antibody, radiopharmaceutical

CLINICAL PHARMACOLOGY

Mechanism of Action
A radioimmunotherapeutic agent in which the targeting power of monoclonal antibodies (mAbs) is combined with the cancer-killing ability of radiation. Ibritumomab tiuxetan is an immunoconjugate resulting from a bond between the monoclonal antibody ibritumomab (murine IgG) and the chelator tiuxetan. This conjugate tightly binds yttrium-90 (Y-90) for radioimmunotherapy of B-cell non-Hodgkin's lymphoma and indium-111 (In-111) for imaging in this protocol. At 4 wks the median number of circulating B cells was zero; recovery began after 12 wks, and median level of B cells was within normal range (32-341 cells/mm³) by 9 mos after treatment. **Therapeutic Effect:** Targets the CD antigen (present on B cells in more than 90% of patients with B-cell non-Hodgkin's lymphoma), inducing cellular damage via formation of free radicals in the target and neighboring cells.

Absorption and Distribution
Tumor uptake is greater than that of normal tissue in non-Hodgkin's lymphoma. Binding to the tumor clears most of the dose.
Half-life: Y-90 ibritumomab: 30 hrs; indium-111 decays with a physical half-life of 67 hrs; yttrium-90 decays with a physical half-life of 64 hrs.

Metabolism and Excretion
Yttrium-90 radioactive decay is zirconium-90 (nonradioactive); indium-111 decays to cadmium-111 (nonradioactive). Ibritumomab tiuxetan is minimally excreted in urine. Over 7 days, a median of 7% of injected activity was excreted in urine.

HOW SUPPLIED/AVAILABLE FORMS
Injection: 3.2 mg of ibritumomab tiuxetan (In-111 Zevalin Kit and Y-90 Zevalin Kit)

INDICATIONS AND DOSAGES
Non-Hodgkin's Lymphoma (Including Rituximab-Refractory Non-Hodgkin's Lymphoma)
Indicated as a single course treatment. Regimen consists of two steps (see diagram showing overview of dosing schedule):
Step 1: Single infusion of 250 mg/m² rituximab preceding (within 4 hrs of completion) a fixed dose of 5 mCi (1.6 mg total antibody dose) of indium-111 ibritumomab administered IV push over 10 mins.

Step 2: Follows step 1 by 7-9 days and consists of a second infusion of 250 mg/m^2 rituximab preceding (within 4 hrs) a fixed dose of 0.4 mCi/kg of Y-90 ibritumomab administered IV push over 10 mins. Reduce dosage of ibritumomab to 0.3 mCi/kg in those with a platelet count is between 100,000 and 149,000 cells/mm^3. Maximal dosage: 32 mCi.

Dosage Adjustment in Hepatic and Renal Dysfunction
No information.

UNLABELED USES
No information.

PRECAUTIONS
Use cautiously in patients with prior radioimmunotherapy, mild thrombocytopenia, prior external beam radiation to 25% or more bone marrow, cardiovascular disease, hypertension, and hypotension. Severe and potentially fatal infusion reactions and cutaneous and mucocutaneous reactions have been reported.

Pregnancy Risk Category: D
Y-90 ibritumomab may cause fetal harm when administered to a pregnant woman. The manufacturer recommends the use of contraceptives for both male and female patients during and up to 12 mos after therapy. Excretion into human breast milk is unknown/not recommended in nursing women.

CONTRAINDICATIONS
Platelet count less than 100,000 cells/mm^3, neutrophil count less than 1500 cells/mm^3, history of failed stem cell collection, prior myeloablative therapies, hypocellular bone marrow, lymphoma marrow involvement of greater than 25%, or known hypersensitivity to murine proteins or any component of the product including rituximab. Y-90 ibritumomab should not be administered in patients with altered biodistribution of In-111 ibritumomab.

DRUG PREPARATION/ADMINISTRATION/ SAFE HANDLING ISSUES
◄ ALERT ► In-111 ibritumomab tiuxetan and Y-90 ibritumomab tiuxetan are radiopharmaceuticals and should be used only by physicians and other professionals qualified by training and experienced in the safe use and handling of radionuclides. This agent must be handled using strict radioactivity

guidelines. Proper aseptic technique and precautions should be used. Waterproof gloves should be utilized in the preparation and during the determination of radiochemical purity of In-111. Appropriate shielding should be used during radiolabeling, and use of a syringe shield is recommended during administration to the patient. Radiation safety precautions must be used to administer this agent. Patient must be placed in appropriate isolation after receipt of this agent. Contents of kits are not radioactive until during or after radiolabeling.

- For preparation of In-111 and Y-90 doses, refer to manufacturer's prescribing information (www.zevalin.com).
- For procedure to determine radiochemical purity, refer to manufacturer's specifications.
- Note that dose of rituximab is lower as part of the ibritumomab tiuxetan regimen compared with when it is used as a single agent.
- The first rituximab infusion is dosed at 250 mg/m^2. Administer at initial rate of 50 mg/hr. Increase rate in 50 mg/hr increments every 30 mins to a maximum of 400 mg/hr. If hypersensitivity or an infusion-related event occurs, the infusion should be temporarily slowed or stopped. The infusion can continue at half the previous rate upon symptom improvement.
- For the second rituximab infusion, the initial rate can start at 100 mg/hr (or 50 mg/hr for a documented infusion-related event with the first infusion). Increase by 100 mg/hr increments at 30-min intervals to a maximum of 400 mg/hr as tolerated.

STORAGE AND STABILITY
Store at 2-8° C (36-46° F). Do not freeze. Contents of kits are not radioactive.

INTERACTIONS
Drug
Anticoagulant agents (warfarin, heparin, low molecular weight heparins, thrombolytics): May increase potential for prolonged and severe thrombocytopenia and increase risk of bleeding.
Antiplatelet agents (NSAIDs, aspirin, clopidogrel, ticlopidine, glycoprotein IIb/IIIa antagonists): May increase potential for prolonged and severe thrombocytopenia and increase risk of bleeding.
Bone marrow depressants: May increase bone marrow depression

Live-virus vaccines: May potentiate virus replications, increase vaccine side effects, and decrease the patient's antibody response to vaccine

Herbal
Herbals with antiplatelet activity.

LAB EFFECTS/INTERFERENCE
May severely reduce Hgb and Hct values, platelet count, and WBC count.

Y-SITE COMPATIBLES
No information.

INCOMPATIBLES
Do not mix with any other medications.

SIDE EFFECTS
Serious Reactions
• Thrombocytopenia (95%), neutropenia (77%), and anemia (61%) may be severe

Overview of dosing schedule:

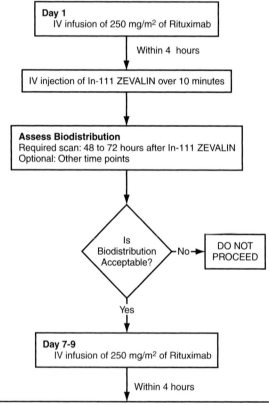

Overview from ibritumomab tiuxetan (Zevalin) prescribing information. Biogen Idec, September 2005.

and prolonged and may be followed by infection (29%). The median time to ANC nadir was 62 days, to platelet nadir was 53 days, and to Hgb nadir was 68 days. Hemorrhage and severe infections have occurred. Monitor up to 3 mos after therapy administration.

- Hypersensitivity reaction may be severe and potentially fatal; severe reactions usually occur during the first rituximab infusion 30-120 mins into the infusion.
- Erythema multiforme, Stevens-Johnson syndrome, toxic epidermal necrolysis, bullous dermatitis, and exfoliative dermatitis have been reported with a variable onset of days to 3-4 mos.

Other Side Effects

Frequent (10%-50%):
Abdominal pain, anemia, asthenia (loss of strength, energy), chills, dizziness, dyspnea, fever, headache, infection, mouth candidiasis, nausea, neutropenia, thrombocytopenia, vomiting

Occasional (1%-10%):
Angioedema, anorexia, arthralgia, back pain, bronchospasm, constipation, diarrhea, ecchymosis, flushing, hypotension, insomnia, myalgia, peripheral edema, pruritus rash, rhinitis

Rare (Less Than 1%):
Allergic reaction, apnea, arthritis, encephalopathy, GI hemorrhage, lung edema, melena, pulmonary embolus, tachycardia, subdural hematoma, tumor pain, urticaria, vaginal hemorrhage

SPECIAL CONSIDERATIONS

Baseline Assessment
- Monitor patient's baseline CBC with differential, electrolyte, BUN, and creatinine levels, and liver function tests.
- Premedicate as ordered for this agent with diphenhydramine and acetaminophen.
- Evaluate patient for any prior reactions to rituximab.
- Ensure patient does not object to receiving human-derived blood products (contains human-derived albumin).

Intervention and Evaluation
- Evaluate patient for any evidence of hypersensitivity reactions.
- Have an anaphylaxis kit available at bedside along with an oxygen setup and an Ambu bag. Should contain:
  Diphenhydramine 50 mg
  Hydrocortisone 50 mg
  Epinephrine 1:1000, administer 0.3 mL each time, and repeat as necessary

Syringes and needles
Alcohol wipes
- Monitor patient on a regular basis for any evidence of myelosuppression, paying particular attention to the platelet count (ANC nadir was 62 days, platelet nadir was 53 days, and Hgb nadir was 68 days).
- Assess need for hematologic support (granulocyte-colony-stimulating factor, erythropoietin, platelet transfusion, red blood cell transfusions).
- Assess for any evidence of GI toxicity. Nausea, vomiting, and abdominal pain were often reported within days of infusion. Diarrhea generally occurs days to weeks after infusion.
- Assess patient's family situation; if there are any young children in the household, this agent requires radiation precautions for 72 hours.

Education
- Instruct patient on possibility of allergic-type reactions and prevention strategies to be implemented.
- Instruct patient when to contact his or her health care provider: fever greater than 38° C (greater than 101° F), chills, cough, shortness of breath, easy bruising, bleeding, and fatigue (due to anemia).
- Educate patient on neutropenic precautions as necessary:
  Practice good handwashing technique.
  Avoid individuals who are ill.
  Wash and cook all foods well.
  Avoid crowds.
  Avoid fresh fruits and vegetables.
- Educate patient on thrombocytopenic precautions:
  Use of a soft bristle toothbrush.
  No flossing if platelet count is less than 50,000/mm^3.
  No IM injections.
  No rectal suppositories.
  No aerobic exercise.
- Educate patient on radiation safety precautions and the duration of time needed; instruct patient to avoid young children for 72 hours after dosing.
- Advise male and female patients that contraceptive methods should be used during treatment and for up to 12 months after therapy.
- Instruct patient to take no over-the-counter medications or herbal or vitamin supplements without checking with his or her health care provider.

• Provide patient with information on local resources and support groups available for his or her specific diagnosis.

IDARUBICIN

BRAND NAMES
Idamycin

CLASS OF AGENT
Antitumor antibiotic

CLINICAL PHARMACOLOGY
Mechanism of Action
An anthracycline antibiotic whose exact mechanism is unknown, but it has been shown to generate cytotoxic free radicals. It is purported to complex with DNA and subsequent inhibition of DNA, RNA, and protein synthesis and also inhibits DNA helicase activity, preventing enzymatic separation of double-stranded DNA and interfering with replication and transcription. Similar to daunorubicin, idarubicin exhibits inhibitory effects on DNA and RNA polymerase in vitro. Idarubicin has an affinity for DNA similar to that of the parent compound and somewhat higher efficacy than daunorubicin in stabilizing the DNA double helix against heat denaturation. Idarubicin has been as active as or more active than daunorubicin in inhibiting ^{3}H-thymidine uptake by DNA or RNA of mouse embryo fibroblasts. **Therapeutic Effect:** Produces antiproliferative and cytotoxic activity.

Absorption and Distribution
Although idarubicin is administered by the IV route in the United States, it is absorbed after oral administration; absorption is 25%-30%. Both the parent compound, idarubicin, and its major metabolite, idarubicinol, appear in nucleated blood and bone marrow cells more than 100 times the plasma concentrations. These levels are reached in a few minutes after injection. It is widely distributed in tissues and has a volume of distribution of about 64 L/kg. Intracellular concentrations of idarubicin and idarubicinol are reportedly up to 300 times the corresponding plasma concentrations. In some studies idarubicin has been reported to be retained in tissues and tumor cells in higher concentrations and for longer periods of time than daunorubicin, with a more favorable ratio of tumor-to-heart drug concentrations. It is highly protein bound: 94%.

Half-life: The elimination rate of idarubicin from plasma is slow with an estimated mean terminal half-life of 22 hrs (range 4-48 hrs) when used as a single agent and 20 hrs (range 7-38 hrs) when used in combination with cytarabine. The elimination of the primary active metabolite, idarubicinol, is considerably slower than that of the parent drug with an estimated mean terminal half-life that exceeds 45 hrs; hence, its plasma levels are sustained for a period longer than 8 days.

Metabolism and Excretion
Idarubicin is extensively and rapidly metabolized by the liver by aldoketoreductase and is also metabolized by other organs and cells, including red blood cells. It is metabolized to idarubicinol (active). Both the parent compound and idarubicinol are conjugated to the glucuronide forms. In addition, aglyclones (inactive) are formed.

After IV administration about 17% of idarubicin is eliminated in the bile through biliary excretion and 16% of the drug and its major metabolite appear in the urine. After oral administration, less drug (8% and 5%) appear in the bile and urine, respectively.

HOW SUPPLIED/AVAILABLE FORMS
Injection: 1 mg/mL in 5 mL, 10 mL, 20 mL single-use vials.

INDICATIONS AND DOSAGES
Acute Myeloid Leukemia
Several idarubicin-based regimens have been reported.
Induction: Idarubicin 12 mg/m^2/day for 3 days by slow IV injection (over 10-15 mins) plus with cytarabine 100 mg/m^2 IV continuous infusion over 7 days. *Consolidation:* Idarubicin 10-12 mg/m^2/day for 2 days.

Dosage Adjustment in Hepatic Dysfunction
It is known that in patients with hepatic impairment, the elimination half-life of idarubicin is substantially prolonged. Thus, the manufacturer recommends a dose reduction of idarubicin. However, currently, no specific guidelines exist. It is recommended that in patients with serum total bilirubin concentrations greater than 5 mg/dL that idarubicin should be held. In a number of phase III clinical trials, treatment was not given if bilirubin and/or creatinine serum levels exceeded 2 mg/100 mL. However, in one phase III trial, patients with bilirubin

levels between 2.6 and 5 mg/100 mL received the anthracycline with a 50% reduction in dose. Dose reduction of idarubicin should be considered if the bilirubin and/or creatinine levels are greater than the normal range.

Dosage Adjustment in Renal Dysfunction

Although there are no definitive guidelines for renal dysfunction, it is recommended that idarubicin be decreased by 25% in patients with serum creatinine levels greater than 2 mg/dL.

Dosage Adjustment for Severe Mucositis

The second course should be delayed in patients who experience severe mucositis, until recovery from this toxicity has occurred, and a dose reduction of 25% is recommended.

UNLABELED USES

Treatment of acute lymphoblastic leukemia, non-Hodgkin's lymphoma, pediatric acute lymphoblastic leukemia, breast cancer

PRECAUTIONS
Pregnancy Risk Category: D

CONTRAINDICATIONS

Baseline neutrophil count less than $1500/mm^3$, hypersensitivity to idarubicin, previous treatment with anthracyclines up to the maximum cumulative dose, recent MI, severe hepatic impairment, severe myocardial insufficiency

DRUG PREPARATION/ADMINISTRATION/ SAFE HANDLING ISSUES

◄ ALERT ► Idarubicin is a vesicant and great caution should be taken during drug administration. It is recommended that the drug be administered via the side port of a free-flowing central IV line.

The use of nitrile or latex gloves is recommended. If a spill or splash occurs, the area should be washed thoroughly with mild soap and water. Antibacterial or waterless soap should not be used as both can increase the risk of skin reactions. Splashes into the eyes should also be irrigated thoroughly with water or 0.9% NaCl.

STORAGE AND STABILITY

Store refrigerated at 2-8° C (36-46° F). Do not freeze. Protect from light. Discard unused portion.

INTERACTIONS
Drug

Blood dyscrasia-causing medications: May increase the patient's risk of developing leukopenia or thrombocytopenia.
Bone marrow depressants: May cause additive bone marrow suppression.
Calcium channel blockers: May increase the patient's risk of developing heart failure. Did not see in other references.
Cimetidine: May increase idarubicin serum concentration and toxicity. Did not see in other references.
Hepatotoxic medications: May increase the risk of hepatotoxicity. Did not see in other references.
Live-virus vaccines: May potentiate viral replication, increase vaccine side effects, and decrease the patient's antibody response to the vaccine.
Drugs metabolized by cytochrome P450 enzymes: Although no researchers have looked at the potential for inhibition or induction by idarubicin of oxidase cytochrome P450 isoenzymes, caution should be used in patients receiving agents metabolized by these enzymes.
Trastuzumab: May increase cardiotoxicity (like doxorubicin).
Herbal
None known.

LAB EFFECTS/INTERFERENCE
None known.

Y-SITE COMPATIBLES

Cisplatin, cladribine, cyclophosphamide, cytarabine, dactinomycin, filgrastim, gemcitabine, granisetron, melphalan, oxaliplatin, palonosetron, rituximab, vinorelbine

INCOMPATIBLES

Alkaline solutions, allopurinol sodium, ampicillin/sulbactam, ampicillin/sulbactam, amphotericin B liposomal (AmBisome), cefazolin, ceftazidime, clindamycin, dexamethasone, docetaxel, sodium phosphate, etoposide, furosemide, gentamicin, heparin sodium, hydrocortisone sodium succinate, imipenem/cilastatin, lorazepam, meperidine, methotrexate, mezlocillin, paclitaxel, pantoprazole, piperacillin sodium/tazobactam, sargramostim (sodium bicarbonate), teniposide, trastuzumab, vancomycin, vincristine, voriconazole

SIDE EFFECTS
Serious Reactions
- The risk of cardiotoxicity (either acute, manifested as transient EKG abnormalities, or chronic, manifested as CHF) increases when the total cumulative dose exceeds 900 mg/m^2.
- Extravasation during administration may result in severe local tissue necrosis.
- Myelosuppression may cause hematologic toxicity, manifested principally as leukopenia and, to lesser extent, anemia and thrombocytopenia.

Other Side Effects
Frequent (10%-50%):
Nausea, vomiting, alopecia, amenorrhea, cardiac arrhythmias, diarrhea, anemia, thrombocytopenia, stomatitis, GI hemorrhage

Occasional (1%-10%):
Diarrhea, hot flashes, elevations in renal function tests have been reported during therapy with idarubicin, particularly when given in combination with cytarabine
(2%-1%) Rash, pruritus, fever, lethargy, conjunctivitis

Rare (Less Than 1%):
Renal damage

SPECIAL CONSIDERATIONS
Baseline Assessment
- Assess patient's CBC with differential, platelet count, electrolyte, BUN and creatinine levels, and liver function tests, paying particular attention to the bilirubin level.
- Dose reductions are required in patients with elevated bilirubin levels.
- Baseline ECHO or MUGA scans are required before this therapy is initiated. An ejection fraction of greater than 50% is usually required or as protocol dictates.

Intervention and Evaluation
- Premedicate with antiemetics as ordered.
- Assess results of MUGA scans or ECHO; do not administer until results are known and have been evaluated.
- Assess CBC with differential, platelet count, liver function tests and in particular the bilirubin level, and electrolyte, BUN, and creatinine levels.
- Assess peripheral veins as idarubicin is a severe irritant; many centers treat it as a vesicant and a central access for drug delivery may be placed.
- Before peripheral administration, bring an extravasation kit to bedside and follow institutional protocol for implementation.
- Evaluate patient's nails on hands and feet as this agent can cause nail bed changes.

Education
- Instruct patient to report any pain or burning upon delivery of agent peripherally; with this agent if peripheral access is poor, a central device is indicated because of the reported significant thrombophlebitis that idarubicin can cause.
- Educate patient on signs and symptoms of neutropenia and when to contact his or her primary care provider: fever greater than 38° C (greater than 101° F), shaking, chills, cough, fatigue, petechiae, bruising, or bleeding from any site.
- Advise patient to contact his or her health care provider if any rapid heart rate, palpitations, or dizziness is noted as this agent can cause cardiac changes.
- Make sure patient has a 24-hour number for the health care provider.
- Educate patient that total body alopecia will occur with idarubicin, but hair will regrow though it may be different in color and texture.
- Advise patient that the urine will turn slightly orange for 24-48 hours and then will return to normal .
- Provide patient with local resources support groups available for his or her specific disease

IFOSFAMIDE
BRAND NAMES
Ifex

CLASS OF AGENT
Alkylating agent

CLINICAL PHARMACOLOGY
Mechanism of Action
An oxazaphosphorine analog of cyclophosphamide with alkylating activity. It is a pro-drug and must be activated by hepatic enzymes to 4-hydroxyifosfamide (4-OH-IF) and acrolein. The active metabolites alkylate DNA and RNA, thus inhibiting protein synthesis. Cross-linking with DNA and RNA strands prevents cell growth. Cell cycle

phase nonspecific. **Therapeutic Effect:**
Interferes with DNA and RNA function.
Absorption and Distribution
The bioavailability of oral ifosfamide is
92%-100%. Ifosfamide is also well absorbed
after subcutaneous injection with 90%-100%
bioavailability. It crosses the blood-brain
barrier (to a limited extent).
Half-life: Ifosfamide has a half-life of
7-15 hrs, although in 2001 Kerbusch
reported a range of 2.1-15.2 hrs in a
review of adult and pediatric data.
Metabolism and Excretion
The hepatic microsomal enzymes, cytochrome P450 (CYP) 2B1 and CYP 2B6, are
involved in ifosfamide metabolism. The
primary metabolites are 4-OH-IF (active),
aldoifosfamide (active), an acyclic tautomer,
in equilibrium with 4-OH-IF, which spontaneously splits into the alkylating agent ifos-
foramide mustard and acrolein, and dechlo-
roethylated and carboxy metabolites
(inactive), which account for 50% of the
urinary excretion of an IV administered dose
of ifosfamide in a 48-hr period. Chloroacet-
aldehyde is a by-product of carboxy metabolite formation and can deplete intracellular
glutathione stores, which makes it a potential
nephrotoxin. Urotoxicity (both bladder and
nephrotoxicity) is likely to be due to concentrations of both 4-OH-IF and acrolein. Ifosfamide is primarily excreted in urine. With a
dose of 1.6-2.4 g/m^2, between 12% and
18% is recovered in the urine compared with
70%-86% after doses of 5 g/m^2. Between
2.6% and 56% of unchanged drug in the
urine was reported in a review of published
adult and pediatric data. Ifosfamide is
removed by hemodialysis.

HOW SUPPLIED/AVAILABLE FORMS
Powder for Injection: 1 g, 3 g.

INDICATIONS AND DOSAGES
Germ Cell Testicular Carcinoma
700-2000 mg/m^2/day IV for 5 consecutive
days. Repeat every 3 wks or after recovery
from hematologic toxicity. Administer
with mesna.
**Dosage Adjustment
in Hepatic Dysfunction**
Ifosfamide is enzymatically metabolized
to cytotoxic compounds via hepatic
microsomes; therefore, it is theoretically
possible that higher doses would be
necessary in patients with hepatic disease.
However, because studies to establish

optimal dose schedules in patients with
compromised hepatic and/or renal function have not been performed, a recommended dose adjustment is not available.
Dosage Adjustment in Renal Dysfunction
Up to 50% of an IV administered dose of
ifosfamide is excreted as active metabolites. However, because studies to establish
optimal dose schedules in patients with
compromised hepatic and/or renal function
have not been performed, a recommended
dose adjustment is not available.

UNLABELED USES
Treatment of Ewing's sarcoma;
non-Hodgkin's lymphoma; and lung,
pancreatic, and soft-tissue carcinoma

PRECAUTIONS
Pregnancy Risk Category: D

CONTRAINDICATIONS
Pregnancy, severe myelosuppression

**DRUG PREPARATION/ADMINISTRATION/
SAFE HANDLING ISSUES**
◄ ALERT ► Use of latex or nitrile gloves is
recommended when preparing this agent.
If a splash occurs, wash area with mild
soap and water. Do not use antibacterial or
waterless soap as either can increase the
skin reaction. Eye splashes should be
rinsed with copious amounts of 0.9% NaCl
saline or water.

STORAGE AND STABILITY
• Ifosfamide vials should be stored at
controlled room temperature (20-25° C
[68-77° F]). They should be protected
from temperatures greater than 30° C
(greater than 86° F). Ifosfamide will
liquify at temperatures greater than 35° C.
• Further dilutions of ifosfamide to concentrations of 0.6-20 mg/mL in 5% dextrose
injection USP, 0.9% sodium chloride
injection USP, lactated Ringer's injection
USP, sterile water for injection USP are
stable when stored in large volume glass
bottles, Viaflex bags, or PAB bags. These
solutions should be refrigerated and used
within 24 hrs.
• Solutions of ifosfamide are compatible
with glass, polyvinyl chloride, and
polypropylene containers.
• When prepared according to manufacturer's directions, the resulting solution is
chemically and physically stable for 7 days

when stored at room temperature (30° C, 86° F) and 6 wks under refrigeration (2-8° C [36-46° F]).

INTERACTIONS
Drug
Aprepitant: Because aprepitant inhibits CYP 3A, concurrent use may lead to elevated ifosfamide plasma concentrations and enhance toxicity. If coadministered, monitor the patient for the following ifosfamide-related adverse effects: leukopenia, thrombocytopenia, CNS effects, urotoxicity, and urinary frequency.
Bone marrow depressants: May increase myelosuppression.
Live-virus vaccines: May potentiate viral replication, increase vaccine side effects, and decrease the patient's antibody response to the vaccine.
Warfarin: There have been three reports of increased bleeding in cancer patients given ifosfamide. The INR was increased by greater than 2-fold at 48 hrs after ifosfamide/mesna administration. *Clinical Management:* In patients receiving oral anticoagulant therapy with warfarin, the PT ratio or INR should be closely monitored for 3-4 days around the addition and withdrawal of treatment with ifosfamide and should be reassessed periodically during concurrent therapy. Adjustments of the warfarin dose may be necessary to maintain the desired level of anticoagulation.
Herbal
None known.
Food
Grapefruit inhibits CYP 3A4 enzymes and can potentially enhance ifosfamide effects.

LAB EFFECTS/INTERFERENCE
May increase BUN and serum bilirubin, creatinine, uric acid, AST (SGOT), and ALT (SGPT) levels.

Y-SITE COMPATIBLES
Granisetron hydrochloride, paclitaxel, palonosetron hydrochloride, propofol

INCOMPATIBLES
Cefepime (Maxipime), methotrexate

SIDE EFFECTS
Serious Reactions
- Hemorrhagic cystitis with hematuria and dysuria occurs frequently if a protective agent (mesna) is not used. Even with mesna, this reaction may still occur, especially with high doses of ifosfamide.
- Myelosuppression, characterized by leukopenia and, to a lesser extent, thrombocytopenia, occurs frequently.
- Pulmonary toxicity, hepatotoxicity, nephrotoxicity, cardiotoxicity, and CNS toxicity (manifested as confusion, hallucinations, somnolence, and coma) may require discontinuation of therapy. These reactions are dose-related (doses greater than 10 g/m^2)

Other Side Effects
Frequent (10%-50%):
Alopecia, confusion, somnolence, hallucinations, infection, cardiac arrhythmias (doses greater than 6 g/m^2), hemorrhagic cystitis (40%-50% incidence without concurrent mesna), nausea, vomiting

Occasional (1%-10%):
Dizziness, seizures, disorientation, fever, malaise, stomatitis, Fanconi's syndrome (fever, polyuria, polydipsia, muscle weakness, joint pain, hyperaminoaciduria, phosphate reabsorption impairment, and renal tubule damage), hemorrhagic cystitis (3.3% incidence with concurrent mesna)

Rare (Less Than 1%):
Cerebral edema and seizures, serum inappropriate antidiuretic hormone syndrome (hyponatremia and seizures), encephalopathy (associated with renal or hepatic dysfunction)

SPECIAL CONSIDERATIONS
Baseline Assessment
- Assess patient for any prior chemotherapeutic agents and his or her reaction, especially nausea and vomiting.
- Evaluate CBC with differential, platelet count, liver function tests, and electrolyte, BUN, and creatinine levels.
- Assess patient for any history of bladder problems: dysuria, frequency, urgency, burning, history of urinary tract infections (UTIs), or bleeding from the bladder.
- Check urinalysis before starting agent to determine whether any microscopic hematuria is present.

Intervention and Evaluation
- Assess CBC with differential, platelet count, liver function tests, and electrolyte, BUN and creatinine levels before each dose.
- Premedicate with antiemetics as ordered.

- Prehydrate as ordered per institutional protocol.
- Do not start this agent until mesna has been ordered and delivered. Mesna is the agent that inactivates acrolein, the active metabolite of ifosfamide acrolein.
- Make sure patient voids every 2 hours during the day and every 4 hours at night.
- Monitor strict intake and output and patient's weight daily.
- Check dipstick of urine for blood with each void or send urine for daily urinalysis per institutional protocol.

Education
- Instruct patient to report any signs and symptoms of fever greater than 38° C (greater than 101° F), any signs and symptoms of urinary tract bleeding, any change in color of urine, any symptoms of a UTI, frequency, urgency, or burning upon urination.
- Instruct patient to drink at least 2 L of fluid per day and void every 2 hours during the day and every 4 hours during the night for the first 24 hours after discharge from the inpatient setting or if receiving this agent as an outpatient to continue this regimen until 24 hours after the last dose of ifosfamide.
- Instruct patient to contact his or her health care provider if he or she is unable to take at least 1500 mL of fluid in 24 hours.
- Instruct patient to contact his or her health care provider with symptoms of nausea lasting greater than 24 hours or diarrhea lasting greater than 24 hours.
- Continue antiemetics as ordered.
- Take colony-stimulating factor (CSF) as ordered (granulocyte-CSF, granulocyte-macrophage-CSF, or pegylated GCSF). Make sure patient knows how to administer injections if the agent is administered daily.
- Instruct patient to avoid pregnancy while receiving this agent.
- Advise patient to avoid all vaccinations during this chemotherapy program.
- Educate patient on neutropenic precautions as necessary:
  Practice good handwashing technique.
  Avoid individuals who are ill.
  Wash and cook all foods well.
  Avoid crowds.
  Avoid fresh fruits and vegetables.
- Educate patient on thrombocytopenic precautions:

  Use of a soft bristle toothbrush.
  No flossing if platelet count is less than 50,000/mm^3.
  No IM injections.
  No rectal suppositories.
  No aerobic exercise.
- Advise patient that he or she may become neutropenic after receipt of ifosfamide and to avoid crowds and any individuals with signs or symptoms of infection.
- Instruct patient to take no over-the-counter medications or herbal or vitamin supplements without checking with his or her health care provider.
- Provide patient with local resources and support groups available for his or her specific diagnosis.

IMATINIB MESYLATE

BRAND NAMES
Gleevec

CLASS OF AGENT
Antineoplastic agent, tyrosine kinase inhibitor

CLINICAL PHARMACOLOGY
Mechanism of Action
Inhibits BCR-ABL tyrosine kinase, a constitutive abnormal enzyme created by the Philadelphia chromosome abnormality found in patients with chronic myeloid leukemia (CML). Imatinib also inhibits receptor tyrosine kinases for platelet-derived growth factor (PDGF) and stem cell factor, c-Kit. **Therapeutic Effect:** Suppresses tumor growth and promotes apoptosis in BCR-ABL cells during the three stages of CML: blast crisis, accelerated phase, and chronic phase. Inhibits GI stromal tumor (GIST) cells that express the activating c-Kit mutation.

Absorption and Distribution
Well absorbed after oral administration with a bioavailability of 98%. Time to peak plasma concentration is 2-4 hrs postdose. Protein binding: 95%.
Half-life: 18 hrs (imatinib) and 48 hrs (active metabolite).

Metabolism and Excretion
Metabolized in the liver by cytochrome P450 (CYP) 3A4 (major) and CYP 1A2, CYP 2D6, CYP 2C9, and CYP 2C19 (minor). The main active metabolite is an *N*-desmethylpiperazine derivative with in vitro potency similar to that of imatinib.

Imatinib is eliminated mainly in the feces as metabolites with 25% excreted as unchanged drug; 81% of the dose (81%) is eliminated within 7 days, 68% in feces and 13% in urine.

HOW SUPPLIED/AVAILABLE FORMS
Tablets: 100 mg, 400 mg.

INDICATIONS AND DOSAGES
Administer with food. Treatment may be continued until disease progression or unacceptable toxicity occurs. The dose may need to be increased by 50% if imatinib is taken concurrently with rifampin or phenytoin.

CML Ph$^+$
400 mg/day PO for patients in chronic phase CML; 600 mg/day PO for patients in accelerated phase or blast crisis. May increase dosage from 400 to 600 mg/day for patients in chronic phase or from 600 to 800 mg/day (given as 400 mg PO bid) for patients in accelerated phase or blast crisis in the absence of a severe drug reaction or severe thrombocytopenia or neutropenia in the following circumstances: progression of the disease, failure to achieve a satisfactory hematologic response after 3 mos or more of treatment, or loss of a previously achieved hematologic response.
Pediatrics: For children over 3 years of age with Ph$^+$ chronic phase CML recurrent after stem cell transplant or for those resistant to interferon-alpha therapy, the recommended monotherapy dosage is 260 mg/m^2/day. The dose can be administered once daily or divided into 2 doses.

GIST c-Kit$^+$ Metastatic or Unresectable Tumors
GIST dosage is 400-600 mg PO daily.

Dermatofibrosarcoma Protuberans (DFSP)
DFSP dosage is 800 mg PO daily.

Myelodysplastic/Myeloproliferative Diseases (MDS/MPD)
MDS/MPD dosage is 400 mg PO daily.

Aggressive Systemic Mastocytosis (ASM)
ASM without or unknown c-Kit mutation status dosage is 400 mg PO daily.
ASM associated with eosinophilia dosage is 100 mg PO daily.

Hypereosinophilic Syndrome/Chronic Eosinophilic Leukemia (HES/CEL)
HES/CEL dosage is 400 mg PO daily.
HES/CEL with FIP1L1-PDGFR alpha fusion kinase starting dosage is 100 mg PO daily.

Relapsed or Refractory ALL Ph$^+$
ALL Ph$^+$ dosage is 600 mg PO daily.

Dosage Adjustment in Hepatic Dysfunction or Other Nonhematologic Adverse Reactions
If elevations of total bilirubin greater than 3 $\times$ the ULN or ALT (SGPT)/AST (SGOT) greater than 5 $\times$ ULN occur, withhold until total bilirubin is less than 1.5 $\times$ ULN or ALT/AST is less than 2.5 $\times$ ULN. Resume adult treatment at a reduced dose: If initial dose was 400 mg, then reduce dose to 300 mg. If initial dose was 600 mg/day, then reduce dose to 400 mg/day.

Dosage Adjustment in Neutropenia and Thrombocytopenia
Chronic phase CML (initial dose 400 mg/day in adults) or GIST (initial dose 400 or 600 mg/day): If the ANC is less than 1.0 $\times$ 10^9/L and/or platelet count is less than 50 $\times$ 10^9/L, discontinue until ANC is 1.5 $\times$ 10^9/L and platelet count is 75 $\times$ 10^9/L; resume treatment at original initial dose of 400 or 600 mg/day. If depression in neutrophil count or platelet count recurs, withhold until recovery, and reinstitute treatment at a reduced dose: If initial dose was 400 mg/day, then reduce dose to 300 mg/day. If initial dose was 600 mg/day, then reduce dose to 400 mg/day.
Accelerated phase or blast crisis (initial dose 600 mg/day in adults): If ANC is less than 0.5 $\times$ 10^9/L and/or platelet count is less than 10 $\times$ 10^9/L, check whether cytopenia is related to leukemia (bone marrow aspirate). If it is unrelated to leukemia, reduce dose of imatinib to 400 mg/day. If cytopenia persists for an additional 2 wks, further reduce dose to 300 mg/day. If cytopenia persists for 4 wks and is still unrelated to leukemia, stop treatment until ANC is 1.0 $\times$ 10^9/L and platelet count is 20 $\times$ 10^9/L; then resume treatment at 300 mg/day or 50% of original dose.

UNLABELED USES
Philadelphia chromosome-positive acute lymphocytic leukemia

PRECAUTIONS
Severe fluid retention and severe hepatotoxicity occur rarely. Interrupt treatment until event resolves. Severe congestive heart failure and left ventricular dysfunction occur occasionally. Monitor, assess, and treat any patients with signs or symptoms consistent with cardiac failure.

Pregnancy Risk Category: D
Drug excretion into human breast milk is unknown/not recommended in nursing women.

CONTRAINDICATIONS
Known hypersensitivity to imatinib or its excipients.

DRUG PREPARATION/ADMINISTRATION/ SAFE HANDLING ISSUES
• Give oral daily dosing of 800 mg/day and above in divided doses (400 mg PO bid). Use 400-mg tablets to reduce iron exposure.
• Take with food and a large glass of water to minimize nausea and GI upset.
• For patients who are unable to swallow, disperse tablet in water or apple juice and stir with a spoon. Suspension should be consumed immediately after complete disintegration of tablet.
• Overdosage of repeated doses of 1600 mg have been reported. Symptoms resolved within 1 week. Observe patient and give supportive treatments where appropriate.

STORAGE AND STABILITY
Store at room temperature.

INTERACTIONS
Drug
CYP 3A4 inducers (carbamazepine, dexamethasone, phenobarbital, phenytoin, rifampicin): Decrease imatinib plasma concentration. Monitor clinical response; may need to increase imatinib dose by 50%.
CYP 3A4 inhibitors (clarithromycin, erythromycin, itraconazole, ketoconazole): Increase imatinib plasma concentration.
CYP 3A4 substrates (cyclosporine, pimozide, dihydropyridine calcium channel blockers, simvastatin, triazolobenzodiazepines): Imatinib may act as a inhibitor of CYP 3A4 thereby altering the levels and effects of drugs known as CYP 3A4 substrates.
Warfarin: Increases the effect of warfarin. Monitor PT or INR. May require therapy change to low-molecular-weight heparin.
Acetaminophen (Tylenol): May increase risk of liver toxicity.
Live-virus vaccines: May potentiate viral replication, increase vaccine side effects, and decrease the patient's antibody response to the vaccine.
Herbal
St John's Wort: Decreases imatinib serum concentration. Avoid use.

Food
Grapefruit inhibits CYP 3A4 enzymes and can potentially enhance the effects of imatinib.

LAB EFFECTS/INTERFERENCE
May increase bilirubin, AST (SGOT), and ALT (SGPT) levels. May decrease platelet count, WBC count, and serum potassium level.

SIDE EFFECTS
Serious Reactions
• Severe fluid retention (manifested as pleural effusion, pericardial effusion, pulmonary edema, and ascites) and severe hepatotoxicity occur rarely. Interrupt treatment until event resolves.
• Neutropenia and thrombocytopenia are expected responses.
• May cause severe congestive heart failure and left ventricular dysfunction. Monitor carefully and evaluate and treat any patients with signs or symptoms consistent with cardiac failure.
Other Side Effects
Frequent (10%-50%):
Abdominal pain, anorexia, arthralgia, constipation, cough, diarrhea, dizziness, dyspepsia, fatigue, fever, fluid retention (periorbital and lower extremities), headache, musculoskeletal pain, muscle cramps, myalgia, myelosuppression, nausea (moderate emetic potential), night sweats, pruritus, rash, vomiting, weight increase
Occasional (1%-10%):
Asthenia, depression, epistaxis, insomnia, hepatotoxicity, nasopharyngitis, petechiae, pharyngolaryngeal pain, upper respiratory tract infection
Rare (Less Than 1%):
Cardiac failure, cardiac tamponade, cerebral edema, erythema multiforme, flushing, hemorrhage, hypertension, hypotension, increased intracranial pressure, skin pigmentation changes, Stevens-Johnson syndrome, tachycardia, ulcer

SPECIAL CONSIDERATIONS
Baseline Assessment
• Assess patient for any history of cardiac dysfunction, edema, or liver disease.
• Monitor patient for CBC with differential, platelet count, electrolyte, BUN, and creatinine levels, and liver function tests.

Intervention and Evaluation

- Monitor CBC with differential, platelet count, electrolyte, BUN, and creatinine levels and liver function tests at each visit.
- Premedicate patient as ordered.
- Assess patient for signs and symptoms of weight gain, nausea, vomiting, diarrhea, or evidence of fluid retention. Order diuretics or reduce imatinib dose as appropriate.
- Assess patient for any signs or symptoms of infection or thrombocytopenia.
- Evaluate for any signs or symptoms of abdominal pain, cough, myalgias, or arthralgias.
- Consider use of 400-mg tablets for all daily doses equal to 800 mg/day to limit iron exposure and improve patient convenience.

Education

- Instruct patient on when to contact his or her health care provider: fever greater than 38° C (greater than 101° F), infection, nausea, vomiting, diarrhea, weight gain, or orbital swelling.
- Advise patient to report ant difficulty tolerating the pills and to take with an 8-ounce glass of water.
- Inform patient on signs and symptoms of thrombocytopenia: easy bruising, bleeding, or epistaxis.
- Educate patient to report any signs or symptoms of pulmonary changes: cough, shortness of breath, or dyspnea.
- Advise patient of risk of rashes and to report any significant rashes to his or her health care provider.
- Remind patient to inform the health care provider before starting any and all new medications, including OTC medications and herbal or vitamin supplements.
- Provide patient with information on local resources and support groups available for his or her specific diagnosis.

INTERFERON ALFA-2A AND-2B

BRAND NAMES

Intron-A (interferon alfa-2b), Roferon-A (interferon alfa-2a)

CLASS OF AGENT

Interferon

CLINICAL PHARMACOLOGY

Mechanism of Action

A biologic response modifier that suppresses cell proliferation, inhibits viral replication in virus-infected cells, and modulates the host immune response by increasing the phagocytic action of macrophages and augmenting the specific cytotoxicity of lymphocytes for target cells. **Therapeutic Effect:** Prevents rapid growth of malignant cells; inhibits hepatitis virus.

Absorption and Distribution

Well absorbed after IM and subcutaneous administration.

Half-life: 2-3 hrs (interferon alfa-2b; IM, IV, and subcutaneous); 3.7-8.5 hrs (interferon alfa-2a; subcutaneous).

Metabolism and Excretion

Undergoes proteolytic degradation during reabsorption in kidneys. Not removed by hemodialysis or peritoneal dialysis.

HOW SUPPLIED/AVAILABLE FORMS

Interferon Alfa-2b (Intron-A)

Powder for Injection: 5, 10, 18, 25, and 50 million international units per single-dose vial.

Solution for Injection Multidose Pens: 18, 30, and 60 million international units per pen.

Solution for Injection: 3, 5, and 10 million international units per single-dose vial; 18 and 25 million IU per multidose vial.

Interferon Alfa-2a (Roferon-A)

Prefilled Syringes (Single-Use): 3, 6, and 9 million international units per syringe.

INDICATIONS AND DOSAGES

Hairy Cell Leukemia

Interferon Alfa-2b: IM, Subcutaneous

2 million international units/m^2/dose 3 times/wk for up to 6 mos. If severe adverse reactions occur, reduce dose by 50% or temporarily discontinue drug and resume at 50% dose.

Interferon Alfa-2a: Subcutaneous

Induce with 3 million international units daily for 16-24 wks. Maintenance dose is 3 million international units 3 times/wk. Reduce dose by 50% or temporarily interrupt therapy if severe adverse reactions occur. Doses higher than 3 million international units are not recommended for hairy cell leukemia. If there is no response within 6 mos, then discontinue treatment. The optimal duration of treatment for this disease has not been determined.

Malignant Melanoma

Interferon Alfa-2b: IV

Initially, 20 million international units/m^2/dose IV over 20 mins for 5 consecutive days/wk for 4 wks.

Maintenance dose is 10 million international units/m^2/dose IM or subcutaneous 3 times/wk for 48 wks. Hold the dose for severe adverse reactions, including ANC greater than 250 mm^3 but less than 500 mm^3 or ALT (SGPT)/AST (SGOT) greater than 5-10 × ULN. Restart at 50% of original dose.

Follicular Lymphoma
Interferon Alfa-2b: Subcutaneous
5 million international units 3 times/wk for up to 18 mos in conjunction with chemotherapy and after completion of chemotherapy. Discontinue interferon therapy if AST is greater than 5 × ULN or serum creatinine level is greater than 2 mg/dL. Interrupt therapy if ANC is less than 1000/mm^3 or platelet count is less than 50,000/mm^3. Reduce dose by 50% (2.5 million international units 3 times/wk) for ANC greater than 1000/mm^3 but less than 1500/mm^3. Increase dose to 5 million international units 3 times/wk when ANC recovers to greater than 1500/mm^3.

Ph$^+$ Chronic Myelogenous Leukemia—Chronic Phase
Interferon Alfa-2a: Subcutaneous
9 million international units daily. May initiate therapy with a titration of 3 million international units daily for 3 days to 6 million international units daily for 3 days to 9 million international units daily to improve short-term tolerance. Continue until treatment progression.

Condyloma Acuminatum
Interferon Alfa-2b: Intralesional
1 million international units per lesion for a maximum of 5 lesions per course. Inject a course 3 times/wk on alternate days for 3 wks. Additional courses may be administered at 12-16 wks.

AIDS-Related Kaposi's Sarcoma
Interferon Alfa-2b: IM, Subcutaneous
30 million international units/m^2/dose 3 times/wk until disease progression or maximal response has been achieved after 16 wks. If severe adverse reactions occur, reduce dose by 50% or temporarily discontinue drug and resume at 50% dose.

Chronic Hepatitis C
Interferon Alfa-2b: IM, Subcutaneous
3 million international units 3 times/wk for up to 6 mos. For patients who tolerate therapy and whose ALT (SGPT) level normalizes within 16 wks, therapy may be extended for up to 18-24 mos.

Interferon Alfa-2a: Subcutaneous
3 million international units 3 times/wk for 12 mos. or as an alternative, induce with 6 million international units 3 times/wk for the first 3 mos followed by 3 million international units 3 times/wk for 9 mos. Patients who do not respond within 3 mos are not likely to respond. If severe adverse reactions occur, reduce dose by 50% or temporarily discontinue drug and resume at 100% dose. Retreatment may be considered for those who have a relapse. Retreat with 3 million international units 3 times/wk or 6 million international units 3 times/wk for 6-12 mos.

Chronic Hepatitis B
Interferon alfa-2b: IM, Subcutaneous
30-35 million international units weekly, either as 5 million international units/day or 10 million international units 3 times/wk.

Dosage Adjustment in Hepatic Dysfunction
Discontinue therapy if AST greater than 5 × ULN.

Dosage Adjustment in Renal Dysfunction
Use with caution in patients with Ccr less than 50 mL/min.

UNLABELED USES
Treatment of bladder, cervical, or renal carcinoma; chronic myelocytic leukemia; laryngeal papillomatosis; multiple myeloma; mycosis fungoides; non-Hodgkin's lymphoma, essential thrombocythemia

PRECAUTIONS
Use with caution in patients with a history of pulmonary disease, diabetes mellitus, coagulation disorders, a history of cardiovascular disease; severe myelosuppression; or preexisting depression and suicidal behavior.
Pregnancy Risk Category: C, X
(for the Rebetron (ribavirin/interferon alfa) regimen). Nursing women should discontinue nursing while receiving interferon therapy.

CONTRAINDICATIONS
Known hypersensitivity reaction to interferon alfa or any component of the injection. Pregnant women or men with pregnant female partners and patients with autoimmune hepatitis should not use Rebetron.

DRUG PREPARATION/ADMINISTRATION/ SAFE HANDLING ISSUES
◄ ALERT ►
- Administer at night when possible to reduce adverse effects.
- Acetaminophen may be administered before injection to reduce certain adverse reactions (e.g., chills and fever).
- Intralesional injections should be administered with a tuberculin syringe and a 25- to 30-gauge needle. Inject in the center of the base of the wart and at an angle almost parallel to the plane of the skin (similar to purified protein derivative tests). Do not go beneath the lesion too deeply or too superficially as this may result in possible leakage, and the drug will not penetrate the dermal core.
- Intron-A Powder for Injection: Reconstitute using sterile water for injection. Follow the manufacturer's recommendations for the required diluent volume corresponding to the vial size. Swirl gently. This preparation does not contain preservative, and any remaining drug should be discarded.
- Intron-A IV Infusion: Withdraw the dose volume and inject into a 100-mL 0.9% NaCl bag. The final concentration of interferon should be not less than 10 million international units/100 mL.
- Intron-A Multidose Pens: Each pen delivers 3-12 doses, depending on the individual dose. Pens include a dial mechanism and are for subcutaneous injections only. Use a new needle for each dose; needles are provided in the packaging.
- Do not administer IM if platelet count is less than 50,000/mm^3, but rather subcutaneously.

STORAGE AND STABILITY
- Store at 2-8° C (35-46° F). Do not shake or freeze. Protect from light.
- After reconstitution, the solution should be used immediately but may be stored up to 24 hrs refrigerated.

INTERACTIONS
Drug
Bone marrow depressants: May increase myelosuppression. Monitor blood counts.
Angiotensin-converting enzyme inhibitors (enalapril): May increase risk of granulocytopenia and thrombocytopenia. Monitor blood counts.

Interkeukin-2: Concomitant use with interferon alfa-2a (Roferon) may increase risk of renal failure.
Theophylline: Decreases theophylline clearance, resulting in a 100% increase of serum levels. May require decreasing theophylline dose.
Zidovudine: May increase risk of neutropenia. Monitor blood counts.
Herbal
None known.

LAB EFFECTS/INTERFERENCE
May increase PT, aPTT, and serum LDH, triglyceride, bilirubin, alkaline phosphatase, AST (SGOT), and ALT (SGPT) levels. May decrease blood HGB level, Hct, and leukocyte and platelet counts.

Y-SITE COMPATIBLES
No information available. It is recommended that interferon not be administered concurrently in the same IV line with other cytotoxic agents.

INCOMPATIBLES
No information available. Do not mix with other medications for Y-site administration.

SIDE EFFECTS
Serious Reactions
- Hypersensitivity reactions occur rarely.
- Pulmonary infiltrates, pneumonitis, and pneumonia have been observed. Monitor patients with a history of pulmonary diseases carefully.
- Rare cases of autoimmune diseases including thrombocytopenia, vasculitis, Raynaud's syndrome, rheumatoid arthritis, lupus erythematosus, and rhabdomyolysis have been reported.
- Depression and suicidal behavior including suicidal ideation, suicidal attempts, and completed suicides have been reported.
- Severe cytopenias including aplastic anemia have been reported. Discontinue therapy in patients with ANC less than 500/mm^3 or platelet count less than 25,000/mm^3.
- Hypothyroidism and hyperthyroidism have occurred with interferon therapy.
- Decrease in or loss of vision and other ophthalmic complications have been reported.
- Cardiovascular events including hypotension, arrhythmia tachycardia, and

rarely, cardiomyopathy and MI have been reported.
* Diabetes and hyperglycemia may occur.

Other Side Effects
Frequent (10%-50%):
Alopecia (mild), anorexia, chills, depression, diarrhea, dry mouth, dyspepsia, fatigue, fever, flu-like symptoms, headache, myalgia, nausea, rash, rigors, thirst
Occasional (1%-10%):
Altered taste, anxiety, dermatitis, diaphoresis, dizziness, dry skin, eye complications, hyperthyroidism or hypothyroidism, paresthesia, pruritus, vision decrease, vision loss
Rare (Less Than 1%):
Back pain, cardiomyopathy, confusion, exacerbation of sarcoidosis and psoriasis, eye pain, flushing, gingivitis, leg cramps, MI, nervousness, tremor

SPECIAL CONSIDERATIONS
Baseline Assessment
* Monitor baseline CBC with differential, platelet count, electrolyte, BUN, creatinine, and LDH levels, and liver function tests.
* Obtain baseline weight.
* Assess patient's history of diabetes, thyroid disorders, and autoimmune diseases.
* Obtain baseline vital signs to assess for hypotension.
* Evaluate patient for any evidence of eye disease or visual disturbances.
* Assess patient for any evidence of skin reactions.

Intervention and Evaluation
* Monitor CBC with differential, platelet count, electrolyte, BUN, creatinine, and LDH levels, and liver function tests at each visit.
* Administer premedication as required.
* Instruct patient on self-injection techniques, safe handling of drug, and appropriate needle disposal procedures.
* Monitor for any evidence of hypersensitivity reaction and have anaphylaxis kit available at bedside for initial dosing along with an oxygen setup and an Ambu bag. The anaphylaxis kit should contain the following:
    Hydrocortisone 50 mg
    Diphenhydramine 50 mg
    Epinephrine 1:1000 (1 mg/1 mL), use only 0.3 mL/dose and repeat as necessary
    Syringes
    Needle to draw up epinephrine

2 by 2 gauze pad to break ampule of epinephrine
    Alcohol wipes
* Assess patient for any evidence of hypotension, bradycardia, chest pain, tachycardia, or diaphoresis.
* Evaluate patient for tolerance of agent, assess for a flu-like syndrome: fever, chills, malaise and pain.
* Monitor patient for evidence of weight gain, edema, visual disturbances, or insomnia.
* Assess patient for any evidence of dermatologic changes, rash, pruritus, or skin reactions.
* Monitor patient for evidence of neurologic changes: confusion, dizziness, weakness, irritability, or increasing lethargy.

Education
* Instruct patient on when to contact his or her health care provider: fever greater than 38° C (greater than 101° F), chills, shortness of breath, palpitations, chest pain, nausea or vomiting lasting greater than 24 hours, diarrhea lasting greater than 24 hours, or the inability to take in at least 1500 mL of fluid in 24 hours.
* Instruct patients to not change interferon brands without first consulting with the health care provider, as a change of dose may be required.
* Monitor patient's ability to self-inject.
* Educate patient on appropriate safe handling and disposal procedures; make sure patient has a needle box for disposal.
* Instruct patient on expected side effects of a flu-like syndrome, lethargy, insomnia, and irritability, and make sure patient is aware that he or she should contact the health care provider if these become problematic.
* Educate patient on when and how to take this medication; many patients will have fewer symptoms if they inject at night.
* Inform patient that acetaminophen may be taken for the flu-like symptoms as directed by the health care provider.
* Advise patient that weight gain and edema may occur and that these should be reported to his or her health care provider at the regular follow-up visit unless these symptoms are severe and troublesome and then patient should contact the provider immediately.
* Instruct patient to take no over-the-counter medications or herbal or vitamin

supplements without checking with his or her health care provider.

- Provide patient with information on local resources and support groups available for his or her specific diagnosis.

IRINOTECAN

BRAND NAMES
Camptosar

CLASS OF AGENT
Antineoplastic agent, Camptothecin analogue

CLINICAL PHARMACOLOGY
Mechanism of Action
Irinotecan is a DNA topoisomerase inhibitor that inhibits the action of intracellular topoisomerase I and DNA, preventing the repair of single-strand DNA breaks, thus causing lethal damage to DNA during DNA replication. Both cytotoxic and inhibitory concentrations between 2 and 10 mg/L have been observed in plasma. **Therapeutic Effect:** Kills cancer cells.

Absorption and Distribution
Irinotecan is currently administered by the IV route. The volume of distribution is large (110 L/m^2) and widely variable, suggesting extensive cellular distribution. Salivary levels of both irinotecan and its active metabolite, SN-38, parallel serum concentrations, making salivary monitoring a feasible alternative.

Protein binding: 95% (SN-38).

Half-life: The elimination half-life for irinotecan ranges from 5 to 14 hrs. The half-life of the lactone form is about 6 hrs; the half life of total SN-38 ranges from 10 to 22 hrs.

Metabolism and Excretion
About 20% of irinotecan is excreted unchanged in the urine. Only small amounts of SN-38 and SN-38 glucuronide have been recovered (0.25%-3%) in the urine. Biliary excretion accounts for about 25% of the drug. Both irinotecan and SN-38 undergo enterohepatic recirculation. Metabolism to the active metabolite, SN-38, is mediated by hepatic carboxylesterase enzymes and occurs primarily in the liver after IV administration. The inhibitory concentration of the active metabolite, SN-38, ranges between 0.3 and 3.6 mg/L. Peak concentrations are achieved at the end of a 30- to 90-min infusion. The active form (SN-38) and lactone forms appear in the circulation about 1 hr after the end of the infusion.

In plasma, both irinotecan and its active metabolite, SN-38, exist in the closed (lactone) ring and open ring carboxylate forms. Only the closed lactone ring forms of each compound are active as topoisomerase I inhibitors. Conversion of the closed lactone ring forms of both SN-38 and irinotecan to the open carboxylate forms occurs via a reversible and pH-dependent hydrolysis; a dynamic equilibrium exists in vivo, with an acidic pH favoring the lactone form and basic pH favoring formation of the inactive, open ring configuration. Although irinotecan itself has cytotoxic properties, SN-38 is responsible for the majority of in vivo antitumor activity of the drug. SN-38 is metabolized to SN-38 glucuronide (inactive). SN-38 is conjugated to form a glucuronide metabolite by the enzyme UDP-glucuronosyl transferase 1A1 (UGT1A1). Genetic polymorphisms exist in the enzyme UGT1A1, leading to reduced activity of UGT1A1 in individuals with the UGT1A1*28 genetic polymorphism. The homozygous UGT1A1*28 allele exists in approximately 10% of the North American population. In a prospective study, patients who were homozygous for the UGT1A1*28 allele had a greater exposure to SN-38 than patients with the wild-type UGT1A1 allele. This test is commercially available for screening patients with this homozygous allele.

HOW SUPPLIED/AVAILABLE FORMS
Injection: 20 mg/mL. Sizes: 2 mL, 5 mL

INDICATIONS AND DOSAGES
Carcinoma of the Colon or Rectum That Has Progressed or Recurred after Treatment with 5-Fluorouracil
Initially, 125 mg/m^2 IV once weekly for 4 wks, followed by a rest period of 2 wks. Additional courses may be repeated every 6 wks. Dosage may be adjusted in 25-50 mg/m^2 increments to as high as 150 mg/m^2 or as low as 50 mg/m^2.

Dosage Adjustment in Hepatic Dysfunction
The influence of hepatic dysfunction on the pharmacokinetics of irinotecan and its metabolites is not known. It has been reported that patients with modestly elevated baseline serum total bilirubin levels (1-2 mg/dL) had a significantly higher incidence of first-cycle grade 3 or 4

neutropenia than those with bilirubin levels that were less than 1 mg/dL (50% [19 of 38] versus 17.7% [47 of 226]; $P < 0.001$). Patients with abnormal glucuronidation of bilirubin, such as those with Gilbert's syndrome, may also be at greater risk of myelosuppression when receiving therapy with irinotecan HCl. An association between baseline bilirubin elevations and an increased risk of late diarrhea has not been observed in studies of the weekly dosage schedule.

Dosage Adjustment in Renal Dysfunction
The effect of renal dysfunction on the pharmacokinetics and toxicity of irinotecan and its metabolites has not been studied.

Dose Adjustment Based on UGT Gene Profile
Patients who are homozygous for the UGT1A1 gene or UGT1A1*28 allele should be monitored very closely for myelosuppression and diarrhea. Such patients should receive a lower dose of irinotecan, but no specific guidelines have been developed.

UNLABELED USES
Lung cancer, pancreatic cancer, recurrent malignant glioma

PRECAUTIONS
- Use irinotecan cautiously in patients who have previously received abdominal or pelvic irradiation because they are at increased risk for myelosuppression.
- Use cautiously in patients older than 65 years of age.
- Patients with the UGT1A1*28 genetic polymorphism should receive a lower dose of irinotecan.

Pregnancy Risk Category:
C (first trimester), **D** (second and third trimesters)

CONTRAINDICATIONS
Known hypersensitivity

DRUG PREPARATION/ADMINISTRATION/ SAFE HANDLING ISSUES
◂ ALERT ▸ Begin a new irinotecan course when the patient's granulocyte count recovers to at least 1500/mm³, platelet count recovers to at least 100,000/mm³, and treatment-related diarrhea fully resolves.
◂ ALERT ▸ Use nitrile or latex gloves to mix this agent. If a splash occurs, wash with mild soap and water. Do not use antibacterial soap or waterless soap as either may

increase the skin reaction. If an eye splash occurs, irrigate with copious amounts of water or 0.9% NaCl.
- Administer all doses by IV infusion over 90 mins.
- Assess patient for signs and symptoms of extravasation. If extravasation occurs, flush the site with sterile water and apply warm heat.

STORAGE AND STABILITY
- Store vials at room temperature, and protect them from light.
- Dilute the drug in D5W (the preferred diluent) or 0.9% NaCl to a concentration of 0.12-2.8 mg/mL.
- If the solution is reconstituted in D5W, it remains stable for up to 24 hrs at room temperature or 48 hrs if refrigerated. However, because the drug contains no preservative, it should be used within 6 hrs if kept at room temperature or within 24 hrs if refrigerated.
- Do not refrigerate the solution if it is diluted with 0.9% NaCl.

INTERACTIONS
Drug
Antineoplastics that cause diarrhea: May increase the risk of irinotecan-induced diarrhea.
Dexamethasone: Concomitant use with dexamethasone as an antiemetic may enhance hyperglycemia.
Laxatives: Should be avoided during irinotecan therapy as they may exacerbate the risk of diarrhea.
Systemic diuretics: Should be avoided because of the risk of worsening dehydration in patients who develop diarrhea.
Ketoconazole: May decrease metabolism of irinotecan or its metabolites. Use is contraindicated and should be discontinued at least 1 week before irinotecan therapy.
CYP 2B6 and CYP 3A4 inhibitors: May decrease metabolism of irinotecan or its metabolites.
CYP 2B6 and CYP 3A4 inducers: May increase metabolism of irinotecan or its metabolites.
Herbal
St John's Wort: May increase metabolism of irinotecan or its metabolites. Use is contraindicated and should be discontinued at least 2 wks before irinotecan therapy.

LAB EFFECTS/INTERFERENCE
May increase serum alkaline phosphatase and AST (SGOT) levels.

Y-SITE COMPATIBLES
Docetaxel, epirubicin, oxaliplatin, paclitaxel, palonosetron, rituximab, vinorelbine

INCOMPATIBLES
Gemcitabine (Gemzar), pemetrexed, trastuzumab

SIDE EFFECTS
Serious Reactions
- Myelosuppression characterized as neutropenia occurs in 97% of patients; severe neutropenia, a neutrophil count less than 500/mm³ occurs in 78% of patients.
- Thrombocytopenia, anemia, and sepsis are common reactions.
- Early and late forms of diarrhea appear to be mediated by different mechanisms. Early diarrhea occurs within 24 hrs of administration and is association with excess cholinergic effects but is rarely severe. Patients experiencing increased salivation, miosis, lacrimation, diaphoresis, and flushing may benefit from the prophylactic or rescue use of atropine 0.25-1 mg IV or subcutaneously.
- Late diarrhea can occur after 24 hrs of administration and can be prolonged and life-threatening. It appears to be mediated by direct toxic effects of SN-38 to the gut mucosa. It must be treated promptly with loperamide. At the first episode of poorly formed or loose stools, loperamide 4 mg initially followed by 2 mg every 2 hrs should be given until the patient is free of diarrhea for 12 hrs. Fluid and electrolyte therapy should be given in patients with evidence of dehydration. The subsequent dose of irinotecan should be decreased by 50 mg/m².

Other Side Effects
Frequent (10%-50%):
Alopecia, vomiting, diarrhea, constipation, fatigue, fever, asthenia, skeletal pain, abdominal pain, dyspnea, anorexia, headache, stomatitis, rash, eosinophilia, hepatic enzyme elevation, nausea
Occasional (1%-10%):
Cardiac arrhythmias
Rare (Less Than 1%):
Pancreatitis

SPECIAL CONSIDERATIONS
Baseline Assessment
- Assess patient's CBC with differential, serum electrolyte, BUN, and creatinine levels, and hydration status before giving each dose of irinotecan.
- Assess patient for any history of nausea and vomiting if patient has received prior chemotherapy.
- Assess patient for an usual number of bowel movements per day as this agent can cause diarrhea.
- Premedicate patient with antiemetics on the day of irinotecan treatment, as prescribed, at least 30 mins before irinotecan administration.

Intervention and Evaluation
- Monitor patient's CBC with differential, electrolyte, BUN, creatinine, and magnesium levels, and liver function tests before each dose.
- Assess patient for early signs and symptoms of diarrhea, usually preceded by abdominal cramping and complaints of diaphoresis. This agent can induce both early and late diarrhea. Early diarrhea is treated with atropine as it is cholinergically mediated. The usual atropine dose is 0.4 mg IV or subcutaneous.
- Late diarrhea occurring greater than 24 hours after dosing is treated initially with 4 mg of loperamide and then 2 mg every 2 hours during the day and 4 mg every 4 hours at night until patient is diarrhea free for 12 hours.
- Assess patient's hydration status, weight, and intake and output.
- Assess patient for signs and symptoms of an inability to take at least 1500 mL of fluid in 24 hours and nausea lasting greater than 24 hours after dosing.
- Monitor infusion site for signs and symptoms of inflammation.
- Examine patient's skin for evidence of rash.
- Offer patient and family emotional support.

Education
- Instruct patient on when to contact his or her health care provider: fever greater than 38° C (greater than 101° F), chills, sore throat, nausea lasting greater than 24 hours, diarrhea lasting greater than 24 hours, and the inability to drink at least 1500 mL of fluid in 24 hours.
- Teach patient how to recognize signs and symptoms of electrolyte depletion and

dehydration and to notify the health care provider if they occur. Intractable diarrhea or nausea lasting greater than 24 hours can lead to significant electrolyte depletion. Monitor for feelings of dizziness, lightheadedness, faintness, or passing out.

- Advise patient to use an antiemetic and/or antidiarrheal regimen if prescribed, and make sure the patient knows how to take the medications.
- Inform patient that hair loss is reversible, but that new hair may have a different color or texture.
- Instruct patient to use contraception while receiving this agent.
- Urge patient to avoid receiving live-vaccinations and contact with crowds, people with known infections, and anyone who has recently received a live-virus vaccine.
- Instruct patient to take no over-the-counter medications or herbal or vitamin supplements without checking with his or her health care provider.
- Provide patient with information on local resources and support groups available for his or her specific diagnosis.

LENALIDOMIDE
BRAND NAMES
Revlimid

CLASS OF AGENT
Angiogenesis inhibitor, immunosuppressant agent, tumor necrosis factor-blocking agent

CLINICAL PHARMACOLOGY
Mechanism of Action
An immunomodulator whose exact mechanism is unknown. Lenalidomide possesses antiangiogenic and immunosuppressive properties. Several proposed mechanisms include reducing angiogenic-promoting factors, inhibiting the secretion of proinflammatory cytokines, and increasing the secretion of anti-inflammatory cytokines in peripheral blood mononuclear cells.
Therapeutic Effect: Reduce RBC transfusion dependence in patients with myelodysplastic syndrome (MDS) with RBC transfusion-dependent anemia.
Absorption and Distribution
Rapidly absorbed with a mean time to peak plasma concentration from 0.6 to 1.5 hrs postdose. Protein binding: 30%.
Half-life: 3 hrs.

Metabolism and Excretion
Metabolism is unknown. Lenalidomide is excreted via kidneys actively or partially actively with two thirds as unchanged drug.

HOW SUPPLIED/AVAILABLE FORMS
Capsules: 5 mg, 10 mg.
Available only through prescribers and pharmacies registered with the RevAssist Program. Informed consent and compliance with mandatory patient registry and surveys are required for both male and female patients. (Contact: Celgene Customer Care Center toll-free at 1-888-423-5436.)

INDICATIONS AND DOSAGES
MDS with Deletion 5q
10 mg PO daily.
Dosage Adjustment in Thrombocytopenia
If Thrombocytopenia Develops WITHIN 4 Wks of Initiation at 10 mg Daily

If Baseline ≥100,000/Microliter	Recommended Course
When platelets Fall to <50,000/microliter	Interrupt Revlimid treatment
Return to ≥50,000/microliter	Resume Revlimid at 5 mg daily

If Baseline <100,000/Microliter	Recommended Course
When platelets Fall to 50% of the baseline value	Interrupt Revlimid treatment
If baseline ≥60,000/microliter and returns to ≥50,000/microliter	Resume Revlimid at 5 mg daily
If baseline <60,000/microliter and returns to ≥30,000/microliter	Resume Revlimid at 5 mg daily

If Thrombocytopenia Develops AFTER 4 Weeks of Initiation at 10 mg Daily

When Platelets	Recommended Course
<30,000/microliter or <50,000/microliter and platelet transfusions	Interrupt Revlimid treatment
Return to ≥30,000/microliter (without hemostatic failure)	Resume Revlimid at 5 mg daily

Patients who experience thrombocytopenia at 5 mg daily should have their dosage adjusted as follows:

If Thrombocytopenia Develops DURING Treatment at 5 mg Daily

When Platelets	Recommended Course
<30,000/microliter or <50,000/microliter and platelet transfusions	Interrupt Revlimid treatment
Return to ≥30,000/microliter (without hemostatic failure)	Resume Revlimid at 5 mg every other daily

From FDA Center for Drug Evaluation and Research. Revlimid (lenalidomide) information label. Updated 6/26/2006. Available at www.fda.gov/cder/drug/infopage/lenalidomide/default.htm

Patients who experience neutropenia at 5 mg daily should have their dosage adjusted as follows:

If Neutropenia Develops During Treatment at 5 mg Daily

When Neutrophils	Recommended Course
<500/microliter for ≥7 days or <500/microliter associated with fever (38.5° C)	Interrupt lenalidomide treatment
Return to ≥500/microliter	Resume lenalidomide at 5 mg every other day

From FDA Center for Drug Evaluation and Research. Revlimid (lenalidomide) information label. Updated 6/26/2006. Available at www.fda.gov/cder/drug/infopage/lenalidomide/default.htm

Dosage Adjustment for Neutropenia

Patients who experience neutropenia at an initial dose of 10 mg should have their dosage adjusted as follows:

If Neutropenia Develops WITHIN 4 wks of Initiation at 10 mg Daily

If Baseline ANC ≥ 1000/Microliter	Recommended Course
When neutrophils Fall to <750/microliter	Interrupt lenalidomide treatment
Return to ≥1000/microliter	Resume lenalidomide at 5 mg daily

If Baseline ANC <1000/Microliter	
When neutrophils Fall to <500/microliter	Interrupt lenalidomide treatment
Return to ≥500/microliter	Resume lenalidomide at 5 mg daily

If Neutropenia Develops AFTER 4 wks of Initiation at 10 mg Daily

When Neutrophils	Recommended Course
<500/microliter for ≥7 days or <500/microliter associated with fever (≥38.5° C)	Interrupt lenalidomide treatment
Return to ≥500/microliter	Resume lenalidomide at 5 mg daily

Patients with Multiple Myeloma Who Received at Least One Prior Treatment or Combination Therapy with Dexamethasone

25 mg PO once daily for days 1-21 of a 28-day treatment cycle combined with dexamethasone. Dexamethasone recommended dose is 40 mg/day on daavys 1-4, 9-12, and 17-20 of each 28-day treatment cycle for the first four cycles then 40 mg/day on days 1-4 of each 28-day treatment cycle thereafter.

Dosage Adjustment in Thrombocytopenia

When Platelets	Recommended Course
Fall to <30,000/microliter	Interrupt lenalidomide treatment, follow CBC weekly
Return to ≥30,000/microliter	Restart lenalidomide at 15 mg daily
For each subsequent drop <30,000/microliter	Interrupt lenalidomide treatment
Return to ≥30,000/microliter	Resume lenalidomide at 5 mg less than the previous dose; do not dose below 5 mg daily

Dosage Adjustment in Neutropenia

When Neutrophils	Recommended Course
Fall to <1000/microliter	Interrupt lenalidomide treatment, add granulocyte-colony-stimulating factor, follow CBC weekly
Return to ≥1000/microliter and neutropenia is the only toxicity	Resume lenalidomide at 25 mg daily
Return to ≥1000/microliter and if other toxicity	Resume lenalidomide at 15 mg daily
For each subsequent drop <1000/microliter	Interrupt lenalidomide treatment
Return to ≥1000/microliter	Resume lenalidomide at 5 mg less than the previous dose; do not dose below 5 mg daily

From FDA Center for Drug Evaluation and Research. Revlimid (lenalidomide) information label. Updated 6/26/2006. Available at www.fda.gov/cder/drug/infopage/lenalidomide/default.htm

Dosage Adjustment in Hepatic Dysfunction
No information available. Patients had AST (SGOT) or ALT (SGPT) less than 3 × the UNL and serum direct bilirubin less than 2 mg/dL were enrolled in one study.

Dosage Adjustment in Renal Dysfunction
No information available. In one study patients had creatinine levels less than 2.5 mg/dL. Lenalidomide should be used with caution because it is excreted renally. The pharmacokinetics in patients with MDS who also have renal dysfunction has not been determined. In patients with multiple myeloma, mild renal function resulted in an area under the curve 56% greater than that in those with normal renal function.

UNLABELED USES
Multiple myeloma

PRECAUTIONS
• Neutropenia grade 3 or 4 occurred in up to 48% of patients with a median onset of 42 days and median time to recovery of 17 days.
• Thrombocytopenia grade 3 or 4 occurred in up to 54% of patients with a median onset of 28 days and median time to recovery of 22 days. CBCs should be monitored weekly for first 8 weeks and monthly thereafter. Use of blood support products or growth factors and dose interruption or reduction should be considered.
• Deep vein thrombosis (DVT) and pulmonary embolism risks increase significantly. Use of prophylactic anticoagulants and antiplatelet therapy has not been studied.

CONTRAINDICATIONS
Pregnant women or women capable of becoming pregnant (unless there are no treatment alternatives and patient takes precaution to avoid pregnancy); patients who cannot adhere to the RevAssist program; hypersensitivity to lenalidomide or any of its excipient ingredients

Pregnancy Risk Category: X
Lenalidomide may cause severe birth defects or death to an unborn baby. Excretion into human breast milk is unknown/not recommended in nursing women.

DRUG PREPARATION/ADMINISTRATION/ SAFE HANDLING ISSUES
• Swallow capsule whole with water once daily.
• Do not break, chew, or open capsules.

STORAGE AND STABILITY
Store at room temperature.

INTERACTIONS
Drug
Lenalidomide: does not affect the cytochrome P450 pathway.
Medications that decrease effectiveness of hormonal contraceptives (such as carbamazepine, protease inhibitors, rifampin): May decrease the effectiveness of the contraceptive; female patients must use two other methods of contraception.
Warfarin: no drug interaction.
Herbal
None known.

LAB EFFECTS/INTERFERENCE
Decreases neutrophil and platelet counts, Hgb, and Hct.

SIDE EFFECTS
Serious Reactions
• Severe neutropenia and thrombocytopenia were seen in 80% of patients in one study. Dose interruption or reduction and use of growth factors and blood support products should be considered.

- DVT and pulmonary embolism have been reported. Instruct patients on signs and symptoms including shortness of breath, chest pain, or arm/leg swelling and to seek medical attention.

Other Side Effects
Frequent (10%-50%):
Abdominal pain, anemia, arthralgia, asthenia, back pain, constipation, cough, diarrhea, dizziness, dry skin, dyspnea, edema, epistaxis, fatigue, headache, muscle cramp, nausea, neutropenia, pharyngitis, pruritus, rash, thrombocytopenia, upper respiratory infection
Occasional (1%-10%):
Acquired hypothyroidism, anorexia, chest pain, depression, diaphoresis, dry mouth, dysuria, ecchymosis, erythema, hypokalemia, hypomagnesemia, hypertension, insomnia, night sweats, palpitations, peripheral neuropathy, rhinitis, rigors
Rare (Less Than 1%):
Hypersensitivity reaction, thromboembolic events

SPECIAL CONSIDERATIONS
Baseline Assessment
- Obtain CBC with differential, platelet count, electrolyte, BUN, creatinine, and magnesium levels, liver function tests, and thyroid function tests.
- Assess patient for history of DVT.
- Evaluate patient for any history of pulmonary disease.
- Assess patient for prior allergic reactions as this agent may induce hypersensitivity.
- Obtain a baseline EKG to evaluate for any evidence of arrhythmias.
- Perform a pregnancy test 10-14 days and a second test 24 hours before initiation of lenalidomide.

Intervention and Evaluation
- Perform pregnancy tests weekly during the first month and monthly thereafter in women with regular menstrual cycles. If menstrual cycles are irregular, the pregnancy testing should occur every 2 weeks. Two effective contraceptive methods must be used for at least 1 month before beginning therapy, during therapy, and for 1 month after discontinuation of lenalidomide therapy unless the woman has been postmenopausal for 24 months or has had a hysterectomy. Male patients must use latex condoms when having sexual intercourse with women of childbearing potential, even if they have undergone successful vasectomy.
- Assess CBC with differential, platelet count, and electrolyte, BUN, creatinine, and magnesium levels at each visit.
- Monitor patient for neutropenia, thrombocytopenia, and any respiratory changes.
- Evaluate patient for any skin changes, including rash, pruritus, or desquamation, and initiate skin care as necessary.
- Monitor patient for evidence of neutropenia, and initiate neutropenic precautions as needed.
- Assess patient for evidence of thrombocytopenia, including epistaxis, petechiae, and bleeding, and initiate bleeding precautions as needed.
- Evaluate patient for any evidence of arrhythmias or palpitations and need for serial EKGs.
- Monitor patient for evidence of thrombosis; assess vascular access device if patient has one in place, as there is an increased risk of thrombosis with this agent.
- Assess patient for evidence of constipation or diarrhea and initiate bowel program as needed.
- Monitor for signs and symptoms of hypothyroidism.

Education
- Advise patient on when to contact his or her health care provider: fever greater than 38° C (greater than 101° F), chills, cough, shortness of breath, upper respiratory symptoms, epistaxis, diarrhea lasting greater than 24 hours, nausea lasting greater than 24 hours, or inability to take in at least 1500 mL in 24 hours.
- Instruct patient to report any evidence of neuropathy: numbness or tingling in fingers and toes.
- Educate patient on neutropenic precautions as necessary:
    Practice good handwashing technique.
    Avoid individuals who are ill.
    Wash and cook all foods well.
    Avoid crowds.
    Avoid fresh fruits and vegetables.
- Educate patient on thrombocytopenic precautions:
    Use of a soft bristle toothbrush.
    No flossing if platelet count is less than 50,000/mm^3.
    No IM injections.
    No rectal suppositories.
    No aerobic exercise.
- Instruct patient on possibility of thrombus formation and to report any evidence of swelling, erythema, or pain in lower extremities or in arm with vascular access device.

- Reinforce contraception information at each visit. Female patients must use two effective contraceptive methods for at least 1 month before beginning therapy, during therapy, and for 1 month after discontinuation of therapy. Male patients must use latex condoms when having sexual intercourse with women of childbearing potential, even if they have undergone successful vasectomy.
- Instruct patient to avoid all OTC medications and herbal and vitamin supplements without first checking with his or her health care provider.
- Inform patient that he or she should not give blood and that male patients should not donate sperm.
- Keep medication out of reach of children.
- Provide patient with information on local resources and support groups available for his or her specific diagnosis.

LETROZOLE

BRAND NAMES
Femara

CLASS OF AGENT
Antineoplastic agent, aromatase inhibitor

CLINICAL PHARMACOLOGY
Mechanism of Action
In postmenopausal women, estrogen is produced by the adrenal gland in the form of androstenedione. Androstenedione is further converted in peripheral tissues to estrone and then to estradiol. Hormone-responsive tumor cells may be stimulated by estrogen. Letrozole decreases the level of circulating estrogen by inhibiting aromatase, an enzyme that catalyzes the final step in estrogen production. Letrozole is a nonsteroidal, pure antiestrogen and does not have any estrogenic properties like tamoxifen. Maximal suppression is achieved within 2-3 days. Glucocorticoid, mineralocorticoid, luteinizing hormone, and follicle-stimulating hormone levels are not affected by letrozole. **Therapeutic Effect:** Deprive estrogen and inhibit the growth of hormone-dependent breast cancers that are stimulated by estrogens.
Absorption and Distribution
Rapidly and completely absorbed in the GI tract. Steady-state plasma concentration reached in 2-6 wks. Weakly protein bound.

Volume of distribution: 1.9 L/kg.
Half-life: 48 hrs.
Metabolism and Excretion
Metabolized in the liver to an inactive carbinol metabolite by cytochrome P450 (CYP) 3A4 and CYP 2C19. Eliminated primarily by the kidneys (90%). Unknown whether removed by hemodialysis.

HOW SUPPLIED/AVAILABLE FORMS
Tablets: 2.5 mg.

INDICATIONS AND DOSAGES
- First-line adjuvant therapy in postmenopausal women with hormone receptor-positive or receptor-unknown early breast cancer.
- First-line treatment in advanced or metastatic cancer after failure of prior antiestrogen therapy.
- Adjuvant therapy for early breast cancer after 5 years of tamoxifen, 2.5 mg PO daily. Continue until tumor progression is evident in locally advanced or metastatic cancer. Optimal duration of treatment is under evaluation in the adjuvant early breast cancer therapy setting.
Dosage Adjustment in Hepatic Dysfunction
- No adjustments necessary for mild to moderate hepatic impairment.
- For severe hepatic dysfunction or cirrhosis (Child-Pugh class C: total bilirubin 2-11 × UNL with minimal to severe ascites, etc.): letrozole 2.5 mg every other day.
Dosage Adjustment in Renal Dysfunction
No adjustments necessary if creatinine clearance greater than 10 mL/min.

UNLABELED USES
No information.

PRECAUTIONS
Pregnancy Risk Category: D
Letrozole is indicated for postmenopausal women. Drug excretion into breast milk is unknown/not recommended in nursing women.

CONTRAINDICATIONS
Known hypersensitivity to letrozole or any of its excipients

DRUG PREPARATION/ADMINISTRATION/ SAFE HANDLING ISSUES
Take PO without regard to food.

STORAGE AND STABILITY
Store at room temperature.

INTERACTIONS
Drug
Estrogen (premarin, estradiol): May counteract therapeutic effects of letrozole.
Tamoxifen: Coadministration of letrozole and tamoxifen resulted in a reduction of letrozole plasma levels of 38% on average. Therapeutic effect of letrozole therapy is not impaired if letrozole is administered immediately after tamoxifen
Herbal
None known.

LAB EFFECTS/INTERFERENCE
May increase serum calcium, cholesterol, GGT, AST (SGOT), and ALT (SGPT) levels.

SIDE EFFECTS
Serious Reactions
Overdosage in a single ingested dose of 62.5 mg was reported without serious adverse events. Induce emesis if situation is safe and appropriate. Give supportive care and monitor vital signs frequently.
Other Side Effects
Frequent (10%-50%):
Arthralgia, fatigue, hot flashes, headache, musculoskeletal pain (back, arm, and leg), nausea (low emetic potential)
Occasional (1%-10%):
Abdominal pain, anorexia, asthenia, cardiovascular events, cerebrovascular events, chest pain, constipation, cough, diarrhea, dizziness, dyspepsia, dyspnea, rash, hypertension, osteoporosis, peripheral edema, somnolence, thromboembolic events, vomiting, weight gain/loss
Rare (Less Than 1%):
Blurred vision, increased hepatic enzyme, pruritus

SPECIAL CONSIDERATIONS
Baseline Assessment
- Obtain CBC with differential, platelet count, electrolyte, BUN, creatinine, cholesterol and triglyceride levels, and liver function tests.
- Assess patient for menopausal status.
- Obtain baseline weight.
- Monitor patient for a history of osteoporosis in the family.
- Obtain a baseline bone density scan to assess for any evidence of osteoporosis.
- Evaluate patient for any history of hypertension.
- Assess patient for any history of deep vein thrombosis or evidence of thromboembolism.
- Assess cardiac history for any evidence of angina or myocardial disease or past MI.

Intervention and Evaluation
- Monitor laboratory data as needed per baseline alterations, and perform routine evaluation of liver transaminases, cholesterol, and triglycerides.
- Evaluate patient's ability to comply with oral medication regimen.
- Assess patient for increasing evidence of menopausal symptoms of hot flashes, night sweats, insomnia symptoms, arthralgia, or headaches.
- Monitor B/P for evidence of hypertension.
- Evaluate for evidence of paresthesias, weakness, chest pain, or leg pains.
- Examine patient for evidence of peripheral edema, weight gain, or skin rashes.

Education
- Educate patient on when to contact his or her health care provider: fever greater than 38° C (greater than 101° F), significant headaches, chest pain, evidence of weakness or paresthesias, arthralgias, myalgias, peripheral edema, and weight gain of greater than 2 kg/week.
- Instruct patient on side effects of menopausal symptoms such as night sweats, insomnia, and hot flashes that may occur with this agent.
- Instruct patient to take no over-the-counter medications or herbal or vitamin supplements without checking with his or her health care provider.
- Instruct patient the changes in skin integrity presenting as rashes or pruritus may occur.
- Instruct patient on the risk associated with osteopenia and the need for bone density studies on an annual basis.
- Provide patient with information local resources and support groups available for his or her specific diagnosis.

LEUCOVORIN
BRAND NAMES
Wellcovorin

CLASS OF AGENT
Cytoprotectant antidote for dihydrofolate reductase inhibitors; fluoropyrimidine-potentiating agent

CLINICAL PHARMACOLOGY
Mechanism of Action
Leucovorin is a reduced form of folic acid. It is an antidote to methotrexate

that may limit the action of methotrexate on normal cells by competing with methotrexate for the same transport processes into the cells. In combination with fluorouracil, leucovorin enhances the binding of fluorouracil to the enzyme thymidylate synthase. **Therapeutic Effect:** As a cytoprotectant, it reverses toxic effects of folic acid antagonists and reverses folic acid deficiency. As a potentiating agent, leucovorin will enhance the cytotoxic effects of the fluoropyrimidine drug, 5-fluorouracil. It does not enhance the efficacy of capecitabine while increasing toxicity.

Absorption and Distribution
Readily absorbed from the GI tract, but the extent of absorption is dose related. After administration of a 25-mg oral tablet, absorption is 97%. However, absorption is only 31% for a 200-mg dose. Leucovorin transport into cells occurs through active transport. It competes with methotrexate for transport. It is primarily concentrated in the liver and is metabolized in the liver and intestinal mucosa to active metabolite.
Half-life: 6.2 hrs after 25 mg PO.

Metabolism and Excretion
Leucovorin is rapidly converted by the enzyme dihydrofolate reductase to 5-methyltetrahydrofolic acid, which is the normal plasma folate. This conversion takes place more rapidly and more completely when leucovorin is given PO rather than injected. Leucovorin is metabolized to 5-methyltetrahydrofolic acid (active), L-formyltetrahydrofolate (active), and D-formyltetrahydrofolate (inactive). The inactive isomer D-formyltetrahydrofolate is largely eliminated unchanged in the urine, whereas the active isomer L-formyltetrahydrofolate undergoes both urinary excretion and extensive hepatic metabolism.

HOW SUPPLIED/AVAILABLE FORMS
Tablets: 5 mg, 10 mg, 15 mg, 25 mg.
Injection: 10 mg/mL vial, 50mL vial.
Powder for Injection: 50 mg, 100 mg, 200 mg, 350 mg.

INDICATIONS AND DOSAGES
Conventional Rescue Dosage in High-Dose Methotrexate Therapy
PO, IV, IM: 10 mg/m² IM or IV one time, then PO every 6 hrs until the serum methotrexate level is less than 10^{-8} M. If 24-hr serum creatinine level increases by $\geq$50% over baseline or methotrexate level exceeds $5\text{-}10^{-6}$ M or 48-hr level exceeds $5\text{-}10^{-7}$ M, increase to 100 mg/m² IV every 3 hrs until methotrexate level is less than 10^{-8} M. Individual protocols may vary.

Folic Acid Antagonist Overdose
PO: 2-15 mg/day for 3 days or 5 mg every 3 days.

Megaloblastic Anemia
IM: 3-6 mg/day.

Megaloblastic Anemia Due to Folate Deficiency
IM: 1 mg/day.

Prevention of Hematologic Toxicity (for Toxoplasmosis), with Sulfadiazine
PO, IV: 5-10 mg/day, repeat every 3 days.

Prevention of Hematologic Toxicity with Pyrimethamine, PCP
PO, IV: 25 mg once weekly.

Combination with Fluorouracil-Based Regimens for Colorectal Cancer
IV: 200-500 mg/m² IV (refer to regimen protocol for dosing and schedule).

Dosage Adjustment in Hepatic Dysfunction
No adjustment necessary.

Dosage Adjustment in Renal Dysfunction
In patients with renal insufficiency, methotrexate excretion may be delayed, and high leucovorin doses (higher than those recommended for oral use) or prolonged administration is recommended and must be given IV. If there is evidence of acute renal failure (i.e., serum methotrexate level greater than or equal to 50 Micrometer at 24 hrs or greater than or equal to 5 Micrometer at 48 hrs or a 100% or greater increase in serum creatinine levels at 24 hrs is seen after methotrexate administration), the recommended dosage of leucovorin is 150 mg IV every 3 hrs until the serum methotrexate level decreases to less than 1 Micrometer. Then 15 mg is recommended IV every 3 hrs until the methotrexate level is less than 0.1 Micrometer (1×10^{-8} M).

UNLABELED USES
Treatment of Ewing's sarcoma, gestational trophoblastic neoplasms, or non-Hodgkin's lymphoma; treatment adjunct for head and neck carcinoma

PRECAUTIONS
• Use leucovorin cautiously in patients with bronchial asthma or a history of allergies.
• Use leucovorin with 5-fluorouracil cautiously in patients with GI toxicities.

Pregnancy Risk Category: C

CONTRAINDICATIONS
Pernicious anemia, other megaloblastic anemias due to vitamin B_{12} deficiency

DRUG PREPARATION/ADMINISTRATION/ SAFE HANDLING ISSUES
◀ ALERT ▶ For rescue therapy in chemotherapy, refer to specific protocol being used for optimal dosage and sequence of leucovorin administration.
PO
• Scored tablets may be crushed.
IV
• The injection solution normally appears clear and yellowish.
• Reconstitute each 50-mg with 5 mL of sterile water for injection or bacteriostatic water for injection (containing benzyl alcohol) to provide a concentration of 10 mg/mL. Reconstitute doses greater than 10 mg/m² with sterile water for injection.
• Further dilute with D5W or 0.9% NaCl.
• Use the solution immediately if reconstituted with sterile water for injection and within 7 days if reconstituted with bacteriostatic water for injection.
• Do not exceed an infusion rate of 160 mg/min (because of the calcium content of the drug).

STORAGE AND STABILITY
IV/Tablets
Store vials for parenteral use or oral tablets at room temperature.

INTERACTIONS
Drug
Anticonvulsants: May decrease the effects of anticonvulsants.
Chemotherapeutic agents: May increase the effects and toxicity of these drugs when taken in combination.
Sulfamethoxazole/trimethoprim (SMX/ TMP): May decrease efficacy of SMX/TMP treatment of *Pneumocystis carinii pneumonia* infections in HIV-infected patients.
Herbal
None known.

LAB EFFECTS/INTERFERENCE
None known.

Y-SITE COMPATIBLES
Cisplatin (Platinol AQ), cyclophosphamide (Cytoxan), doxorubicin, etoposide (VePesid), 5-fluorouracil (0.8 mg/mL), gemcitabine (Gemzar), granisetron (Kytril), heparin, methotrexate, metoclopramide (Reglan), mitomycin (Mutamycin), palonosetron, piperacillin/tazobactam (Zosyn), vinblastine (Velban), vincristine (Oncovin), vitamin B complex with C

INCOMPATIBLES
Amphotericin B colloidal (Amphotec), amphotericin B liposomal (AmBisome), carboplatin, doxorubicin HCl, droperidol (Inapsine), epirubicin, foscarnet (Foscavir), gallium nitrate, lansoprazole, pantoprazole, sodium bicarbonate, vincristine sulfate, vinorelbine tartrate

SIDE EFFECTS
Serious Reactions
• Excessive dosage may negate chemotherapeutic effects of folic acid antagonists.
• Anaphylaxis occurs rarely.
• Diarrhea may cause rapid clinical deterioration.
Other Side Effects
Frequent (10%-50%):
When combined with chemotherapeutic agents: diarrhea, stomatitis, nausea, vomiting, lethargy or malaise or fatigue, alopecia, anorexia
Occasional (1%-10%):
Urticaria, dermatitis
Rare (Less Than 1%):
Hypersensitivity reactions, seizures and/or syncope

SPECIAL CONSIDERATIONS
Baseline Assessment
For treatment of accidental overdosage of folic acid antagonists, give leucovorin as soon as possible (preferably within 1 hr), as prescribed.
Intervention and Evaluation
• Monitor patient for vomiting, which may require a change from oral to parenteral therapy.
• Observe elderly and debilitated patients closely because of the risk of severe toxicities.
• Assess patient's CBC and BUN and serum creatinine levels to determine renal function (important in leucovorin rescue).
• Assess electrolyte levels and liver function test results of patients receiving chemotherapeutic agents in combination with leucovorin.

Education
- Encourage patient with folic acid deficiency to eat foods high in folic acid, including dried beans, meat proteins, and green leafy vegetables.
- Urge patient to notify his or her health care provider physician if he or she experiences an allergic reaction or vomiting.
- Instruct patient to take no over-the-counter medications or herbal or vitamin supplements without checking with his or her health care provider.

OTHER INFORMATION
Do not confuse Wellcovorin with Wellbutrin or Wellferon.

LEUPROLIDE ACETATE
BRAND NAMES
Eligard, Lupron, Lupron Depot, Lupron Depot Ped, Viadur

CLASS OF AGENT
Luteinizing hormone-releasing hormone agonist (LHRH), gonadotropin-releasing hormone agonist (GnRH)

CLINICAL PHARMACOLOGY
Mechanism of Action
A potent LHRH agonist analog of the anterior pituitary gland, also known as a GnRH agonist. Circulating levels of luteinizing hormone, follicle-stimulating hormone, testosterone, and estradiol rise initially, and then subside with continued therapy. **Therapeutic Effect:** In females, causes a reduction in ovarian size and function, a reduction in uterine and mammary gland size, and regression of sex hormone-responsive tumors. In males, produces pharmacologic castration and decreases the growth of abnormal prostate tissue.
Absorption and Distribution
Rapidly and well absorbed after subcutaneous/IM administration with a time to peak concentration occurring 4-5 hrs postdose. Volume of distribution: 27 L. Protein binding: 43%-49%.
Half-life: 3-4 hrs.
Metabolism and Excretion
Metabolized primarily by peptidase and not by cytochrome P450 enzymes into inactive metabolites. Urine excretion with less than 5% unchanged drug.

HOW SUPPLIED/AVAILABLE FORMS
Implant (Viadur): 72 mg.
Depot (Eligard): 7.5 mg, 22.5 mg, 30 mg, 45 mg.
Depot (Lupron Depot): 3.75 mg, 7.5 mg, 11.25 mg, 22.5 mg, 30 mg.
Depot (Lupron Depot-Ped): 7.5 mg, 11.25 mg, 15 mg.
Multidose Vial Solution 2.8 mL (Lupron): 5 mg/mL.

INDICATIONS AND DOSAGES
Advanced Prostatic Carcinoma
Intramuscular (Lupron Depot): 7.5 mg every month or 22.5 mg every 3 mos or 30 mg every 4 mos.
Subcutaneous (Eligard): 7.5 mg every month or 22.5 mg every 3 mos or 30 mg every 4 mos or 45 mg every 6 mos.
Subcutaneous (Lupron): 1 mg daily.
Subcutaneous (Viadur): 72 mg implanted every 12 mos.
Endometriosis
Intramuscular (Lupron Depot): 3.75 mg every month or 11.25 mg every 3 mos. Recommended duration of 6 mos.
Uterine Leiomyomata (Fibroids)
Intramuscular (with iron [Lupron Depot]): 3.75 mg every month or 11.25 mg as a single injection. Recommended duration of 3 mos.
Dosage Adjustment in Hepatic/Renal Dysfunction
No recommendations available.

UNLABELED USES
In vitro fertilization

CONTRAINDICATIONS
Hypersensitivity to leuprolide or any component of its formulation, LHRH or LHRH agonists, pregnancy, undiagnosed vaginal bleeding
Pregnancy Risk Category: X
Leuprolide may cause fetal harm when administered during pregnancy. Use nonhormonal contraception. Excretion into human milk is unknown/not recommended in nursing women. Eligard is indicated for prostate cancer and has not been studied in women or children.

DRUG PREPARATION/ADMINISTRATION/ SAFE HANDLING ISSUES
- Eligard should be brought to room temperature before administration. Use within 30 mins after mixing.

- Refer to manufacturer's package inserts for instructions on use of syringe devices and single-use kits.

STORAGE AND STABILITY
- Store Lupron and Viadur in original packaging at room temperature 20-25° C (68-77° F).
- Refrigerate leuprolide multidose vials in original packaging at 2-8° C (35-46° F). Patient may store current vial at room temperature of 20-25° C (68-77° F).
- Refrigerate Eligard in original packaging at 2-8° C (68-77° F).

INTERACTIONS
Drug
None known. Leuprolide is metabolized primarily by peptidase and not by cytochrome P450.
Herbal
None known.

LAB EFFECTS/INTERFERENCE
May alter serum pituitary-gonadal function test results; normal functions are usually restored in 12 wks after drug discontinuation. May cause changes in bone mineral density and lipid profile.

INCOMPATIBLES
No information available.

SIDE EFFECTS
Serious Reactions
- Signs and symptoms of metastatic prostatic carcinoma (such as bone pain, dysuria or hematuria, and weakness or paresthesia of the lower extremities) may worsen 1-2 wks after the initial dose but then subside with continued therapy. Uretal obstruction and spinal cord compression have been reported.
- Pulmonary embolism and MI occur rarely.
- Anaphylaxis and asthmatic events have been reported in postmarketing surveillance.

Other Side Effects
Frequent (10%-50%):
Fatigue, headache, hot flashes (ranging from mild flushing to diaphoresis), malaise
Females: amenorrhea, spotting
Occasional (1%-10%):
Angina, arrhythmias; asthenia, blurred vision, constipation, dizziness, dry mouth, edema, injection site (burning, itching, or swelling), nausea, insomnia, palpitations, weight gain/loss
Females: altered mood, decreased libido, deepening voice, hirsutism, increased breast tenderness/changes, vaginal dryness, vaginitis
Males: decreased testicle size, gynecomastia, impotence
Rare (Less Than 1%):
Appetite decrease, backache, depression, flatulence, joint pain, taste/smell disturbance, myalgia, thrombophlebitis, tremor, vertigo

SPECIAL CONSIDERATIONS
Baseline Assessment
- Assess for any risk of spinal cord compression and uretal obstruction before initiating therapy.
- Obtain baseline CBC with differential, platelet count, electrolyte, BUN, and creatinine levels, and liver function tests.
- Assess patient for any history of deep vein thrombosis or thrombophlebitis.
- Evaluate females for menopausal status.
- Assess for any history of cardiac disease, palpitations, or chest pain in both men and women.
- Assess for history of depression or neuromuscular disease.
- Obtain baseline assessment of current disease status especially in men with prostate cancer as this agent can induce increased bone pain.
- Assess patient's ability to do self-injection or ability to have family member inject.
- Evaluate patient for any history of dermatologic conditions.

Intervention and Evaluation
- Monitor laboratory parameters at each follow-up visit, especially for elevated liver function test results and thrombocytopenia.
- Instruct patient on self-injection techniques, and assess patient's ability to comply with drug delivery; assess for evidence of injection site reactions at each visit.
- Evaluate for menopausal symptoms in women: hot flashes, night sweats, irritability, insomnia, and libido changes.
- Evaluate men for evidence of breast tenderness, gynecomastia, libido changes, and impotence.
- Assess pulmonary and cardiac status at each visit, evaluating for signs or symptoms of cardiac or pulmonary changes.
- Monitor for evidence of nausea or diarrhea and intervene as necessary.

- Assess for evidence of rashes, skin reactions, weight gain, and/or peripheral edema.
- Evaluate patient for any evidence of neurologic disease or mood changes, depression, nervousness, irritability, asthenia, paresthesias, and insomnia not associated with menopausal symptoms.
- Provide support for patient to assist in coping with symptoms associated with this agent.
- Make appropriate psychologic referrals as necessary to deal with the side effects of this agent.

Education
- Advise patient on when to contact his or her health care provider: fever greater than 38° C (greater than 101° F), chills, infections, nausea lasting greater than 24 hours, diarrhea lasting greater than 24 hours, the inability to take in at least 1500 mL in 24 hours, chest pain, difficulty breathing, or evidence of increased bone pain.
- Instruct women on side effects of vaginal bleeding or discharge, menopausal symptoms of hot flashes, night sweats, irritability, insomnia, and libido changes, voice changes, peripheral edema, or weight gain.
- Instruct men on side effects of gynecomastia, loss of libido, impotence, irritability, insomnia, and bone pain.
- Instruct patient that mood changes may be a result of this agent, and assist patient in coping with the changes.
- Advise patient to avoid all OTC medications or herbal or vitamin supplements without first checking with the health care provider as some of these can interfere with the effectiveness of this agent.
- Provide patient with information on local resources and support groups available for his or her specific diagnosis.

LOMUSTINE, CCNU

BRAND NAMES
CeeNU

CLASS OF AGENT
Antineoplastic agent, alkylating agent

CLINICAL PHARMACOLOGY
Mechanism of Action
An alkylating agent and nitrosourea that inhibits DNA and RNA protein synthesis by cross-linking with DNA and RNA strands, preventing cell division. Not cross-resistant with other alkylators. As a nitrosourea, it may also inhibit key enzymatic processes by carbamoylation of amino acids. Cell cycle phase nonspecific. **Therapeutic Effect:** Interferes with DNA and RNA function.

Absorption and Distribution
Rapidly and completely absorbed on oral administration. Highly lipid soluble with tissue levels comparable to plasma levels 15 mins after IV administration. Crosses the blood-brain barrier easily.
Half-life: 16-48 hrs (metabolites).

Metabolism and Excretion
Metabolized by the hepatic microsomal enzyme oxidation system. Metabolites are primarily excreted in the urine 24 hrs after oral administration.

HOW SUPPLIED/AVAILABLE FORMS
Capsules: 10 mg, 40 mg, 100 mg.

INDICATIONS AND DOSAGES
Hodgkin's Disease, Brain Tumors
Initial dose 100-130 mg/m^2 PO as single dose depending on bone marrow function. Repeat dose at intervals of at least 6 wks but not until circulating blood elements have returned to acceptable levels. Adjust dose based on hematologic response to previous dose.

Dosage Adjustment Based on Hematologic Responses from Preceding dose

NADIR AFTER PRIOR DOSE		% of Prior Dose to be Given
Leukocytes	Platelets	
>4000	>100,000	100
3000-3999	75,000-99,999	100
2000-2999	25,000-74,999	70
<2000	<25,000	50

Lomustine (CeeNU) Prescribing Information, Bristol-Myers Squibb, February 2006.

Dosage Adjustment in Hepatic Dysfunction
No information available.

Dosage Adjustment in Renal Dysfunction
No information available. Consider reduced dose.

UNLABELED USES
Breast, GI, lung, or renal carcinoma, malignant melanoma, multiple myeloma

PRECAUTIONS
Thrombocytopenia and leukopenia may be delayed and severe and lead to major bleeding and serious infections.

Pregnancy Risk Category: D
Drug excretion into breast milk is unknown/
not recommended in nursing women.

CONTRAINDICATIONS
Hypersensitivity to lomustine, other nitrosoureas, mannitol, or any of its excipients

DRUG PREPARATION/ADMINISTRATION/
SAFE HANDLING ISSUES
◀ ALERT ▶ Dosage adjustment should be
made on the basis of nadir count. Do not
administer unless platelet count is greater
than 100,000/mm^3 and leukocyte count is
greater than 4000/mm^3.
• Because the incidence of nausea is high,
premedicate with antiemetics as necessary and administer dose at bedtime on
an empty stomach.
• Lomustine is considered a hazardous
agent. Wash hands before and after contact with the bottle or capsules.
• If capsule content is spilled, immediately
wipe it up with a damp cloth and discard
the cloth in a closed container such as a
plastic bag.
• Symptoms of overdose should be
treated with symptomatic and
supportive care.

STORAGE AND STABILITY
Store at room temperature. Avoid excess heat
greater than 40° C (greater than 104° F).

INTERACTIONS
Drug
Bone marrow depressants: May increase
myelosuppression.
Cimetidine: May increase myelosuppression
Live virus vaccines: May potentiate viral
replication, increase vaccine side effects,
and decrease the patient's antibody response
to the vaccine.
Herbal
None known.

LAB EFFECTS/INTERFERENCE
May increase transaminase, alkaline
phosphatase, and bilirubin levels.

SIDE EFFECTS
Serious Reactions
• Myelosuppression may be cumulative
and manifested principally as leukopenia,
mild anemia, and thrombocytopenia.
Leukopenia occurs about 5-6 wks after a
dose, thrombocytopenia about 4 wks after

a dose; both persist for 1-2 wks.
• Pulmonary toxicity characterized by
pulmonary infiltrates and/or fibrosis has
been reported with long-term therapy
and with cumulative doses greater than
1100 mg/m^2. Lung fibrosis may be
slowly progressive and has been known
to be fatal.
• Acute leukemia and bone marrow
dysplasia have occurred with long-term
nitrosourea therapy.
Other Side Effects
Frequent (10%-50%):
Nausea, vomiting (occurring 45 mins-6 hrs
after dosing and lasting 12-24 hrs); anorexia
(often follows for 2-3 days), thrombocytopenia, leukopenia
Occasional (1%-10%):
Darkening of skin, diarrhea, elevated transaminase, pruritus, rash, nephrotoxicity
(cumulative doses greater than 1200 mg/m^2)
Rare (Less Than 1%):
Alopecia, neurotoxicity (ataxia, confusion, dysarthria, lethargy, and slurred
speech), stomatitis, optic atrophy, visual
disturbances (blindness), pulmonary
fibrosis/toxicity

SPECIAL CONSIDERATIONS
Baseline Assessment
• Obtain CBC with differential, platelet
count, electrolyte, BUN, and creatinine
levels, and liver function tests.
• Assess for history of neurologic disorders,
hepatic impairment, or dermatologic
conditions.
• Obtain baseline pulmonary function.
Intervention and Evaluation
• Assess CBC with differential, platelet
count, electrolyte, BUN, and creatinine
levels, and liver function tests at each visit.
• Monitor for signs and symptoms of neutropenia, anemia, and thrombocytopenia.
• Evaluate patient for any evidence of neurotoxicity, confusion, disorientation, and
aphasia.
• Premedicate with antiemetics as ordered.
• Monitor for evidence of skin changes,
rash, hyperpigmentation, or pruritus.
• Assess patient for any evidence of renal
disease, decreased urine output, any
evidence of blood in urine, and painful
urination.
• Evaluate for evidence of infection, fatigue,
or bleeding and implementation of neutropenic precautions.
• Assess for changes in pulmonary function.

Education

- Instruct patient on when to contact his or her health care provider: fever greater than 38° C (greater than 101° F), chills, cough, evidence of easy bruising, or bleeding.
- Advise patient and caregiver to assess for evidence of neurotoxicity, including confusion, disorientation, or slurred speech, and to contact the health care provider if it occurs.
- Advise patient that alopecia will occur and when hair returns it may have a different color or texture.
- Instruct patient on neutropenic precautions:
   Practice good handwashing technique.
   Avoid raw foods and salad bars.
   Avoid crowds and persons with colds or flu-like symptoms
- Advise patient on thrombocytopenic precautions: use of soft toothbrush, no flossing when platelet count is less than 50,000/mm³, use of electric razors only when platelet count is less than 50,000/mm³, and no straining activities.
- Teach patient to wash hands before and after contact with the bottle or capsule. People not taking lomustine should not be exposed to it.
- If powder from a capsule is spilled, advise patient to wipe it up immediately with a damp disposable towel and discard the towel in a closed plastic container.
- Instruct patient to avoid OTC medications or herbal or vitamin supplements without first checking with health care providers.
- Provide patient with information on local resources and support groups available for his or her specific diagnosis.

MECHLORETHAMINE HYDROCHLORIDE

BRAND NAMES
Mustargen

CLASS OF AGENT
Antineoplastic agent, alkylating agent

CLINICAL PHARMACOLOGY
Mechanism of Action
A bifunctional alkylating agent that undergoes intramolecular cyclization of one of its 2-chloroethyl side chains, with release of a chloride ion, to form a highly reactive ethylenimonium ion. In tissues, the ionic form of mechlorethamine reacts with guanine and other base residues in the DNA chain; this results in DNA interstrand and DNA protein cross-links. **Therapeutic Effect:** Cross-links strands of DNA and RNA and inhibits protein synthesis.

Absorption and Distribution
Incompletely absorbed after intracavitary administration, probably due to rapid deactivation by body fluids.
Half-life: 10 mins.

Metabolism and Excretion
Once mechlorethamine is diluted in water or body fluids, chemical transformation occurs to the highly reactive, electrophilic, ethylenimonium derivative. Because this form reacts rapidly with cellular components, the active drug is no longer present in the blood within minutes of administration. Less than 1% excreted in urine. Not removed by hemodialysis.

HOW SUPPLIED/AVAILABLE FORMS
Powder for Injection: 10 mg (Mustargen).

INDICATIONS AND DOSAGES
Bronchiogenic Carcinoma, Hodgkin's Disease, Chronic Lymphocytic Leukemia, Chronic Myelocytic Leukemia, Lymphosarcoma, Mycosis Fungoides, Polycythemia Vera
In the MOPP (mechlorethamine, vincristine [oncovorin], procarbazine, and prednisone) chemotherapy regimen: 6 mg/m² IV days 1 and 8.
Malignant Effusions
Intracavitary: 0.4 mg/kg injection.
Intrapericardial: 0.2 mg/kg injection.
After injection, change the position of the patient every 5-10 mins for 1 hr for a more uniform distribution of the drug.
Dosage Adjustment in Hepatic and Renal Dysfunction
None.

UNLABELED USES
Chronic lymphocytic leukemia

PRECAUTIONS
Use cautiously in patients with chronic lymphatic leukemia, hyperuricemia (especially in the treatment of lymphoma), leukopenia, thrombocytopenia, or anemia.

Pregnancy Risk Category: D

CONTRAINDICATIONS
Presence of known infectious diseases, previous anaphylactic reactions to mechlorethamine

DRUG PREPARATION/ADMINISTRATION/ SAFE HANDLING ISSUES
◀ ALERT ▶ **The dosage of** this drug is individualized according to clinical response and the patient's tolerance to adverse effects. When used in combination therapy, consult specific protocols for optimum drug dosage and sequence of drug administration.

◀ ALERT ▶ Mechlorethamine may be carcinogenic, mutagenic, or teratogenic. Handle with extreme care during preparation and administration.

◀ ALERT ▶ Do not use if foci of acute and chronic superlative inflammation are present.

• Initially dissolve the drug to 1 mg/mL with 0.9% NaCl or sterile water for injection.
• Further dilute to 50 mL of 0.9 NaCl. The solution should be prepared immediately before use because of spontaneous decomposition.
• Protective gloves should be used throughout the preparation and administration of topical mechlorethamine. When preparing this agent, use nitrile or latex gloves only. If a skin exposure occurs, wash the area with mild soap and water; do not use waterless or antibacterial soap as either can increase the skin reaction. If an eye splash occurs, irrigate with copious amounts of water or 0.9% NaCl, irrigating from inner to outer canthus.
• Mechlorethamine is given preferably at night in case sedation for side effects is required.
• Alternate courses of mechlorethamine with other chemotherapy or radiation therapy.
• Repeat doses should be held until hematologic recovery occurs.

STORAGE AND STABILITY
In dry form, the drug is a light yellow-brown and is stable at temperatures up to 40° C (up to 104° F). Solutions of mechlorethamine hydrochloride decompose on standing and should be prepared immediately before use. Mechlorethamine hydrochloride is even less stable in neutral or alkaline solutions than in the acidic reconstituted solution. Do not use if the solution is discolored or if water droplets form within the vial before reconstitution. If neutralization of the remaining mechlorethamine solutions or equipment exposed to the drug is desired, an aqueous solution containing equal volumes of sodium thiosulfate (5%) and sodium bicarbonate (5%) for 45 mins may be used. Neutralize any unused injection solution by mixing with an equal volume of sodium thiosulfate/sodium bicarbonate solution. Allow the mixture to stand for 45 mins. Treat vials that have contained mechlorethamine the same way with thiosulfate/bicarbonate solution before disposal.

INTERACTIONS
Drug
Live virus vaccines: May decrease patient's antibody response to vaccine, increase vaccine side effects, and potentiate viral replication.
Herbal
None known.

LAB EFFECTS/INTERFERENCE
May increase isocitric acid dehydrogenase and uric acid levels. May decrease cholinesterase level.

Y-SITE COMPATIBILITY
Amifostine, granisetron hydrochloride, fludarabine, melphalan, ondansetron, palonosetron, sargramostim, teniposide, vinorelbine

INCOMPATIBLES
Allopurinol, cefepime HCl, pantoprazole

SIDE EFFECTS
Serious Reactions
• Leukopenia, immunosuppression, infection, and thrombocytopenia may occur.
• Hepatotoxicity has been reported.
• Secondary leukemia and amyloidosis may occur.

Other Side Effects
Frequent (10%-50%):
Atopic dermatitis, nausea, vomiting, allergic dermatitis with topical administration, azoospermia or oligospermia, gonadal hormone deficiency, amenorrhea
Occasional (1%-10%):
Diarrhea, loss of appetite, metallic taste, drowsiness, headache, weakness, myelosuppression, hyperuricemia in patients with lymphoma, secondary leukemia

Rare (Less Than 1%):
Hepatotoxicity, peptic ulcer, peripheral neuropathy, ototoxicity, cardiotoxicity, dermatologic skin reactions including erythema multiforme, facial angioedema, maculopapular skin eruption

SPECIAL CONSIDERATIONS
Baseline Assessment
- Obtain CBC with differential, electrolyte, BUN, and creatinine levels, and liver function tests before dosing with this agent.
- Evaluate patient's history of nausea and vomiting as this agent is highly emetogenic.
- Be aware that this agent is a vesicant and the extravasation kit must be available before administration.
- Assess patient's peripheral veins and if access is poor, evaluate patient for a central venous access device.
- Assess patient's skin for any evidence of history of dermatologic problems.

Intervention and Evaluation
- Evaluate CBC with differential, electrolyte, BUN, and creatinine levels, and all liver function tests before each dose.
- Premedicate with antiemetics as ordered.
- Assess patient's access before each dose for consideration of placement of a vascular access device.
- Obtain the extravasation kit before administering this agent.
- Monitor patient for any evidence of significant nausea, vomiting, or diarrhea after discharge home.
- Assess patient's skin for any evidence of dermatologic reactions before each dose.
- Evaluate patient for any evidence of infection or evidence of thrombocytopenia or anemia.
- Monitor patient for increasing fatigue with each dose.
- Evaluate patient for any evidence of hepatic toxicity, right upper quadrant pain, pruritus, jaundice, or icterus.

Education
- Instruct patient that this drug is a vesicant and to report any signs of pain or burning upon drug administration; educate patient on side effects of extravasation, skin sloughing, and necrosis.
- Educate patient on antiemetics needed for this agent and to take the doses of antiemetics as ordered.

- Instruct patient on when to contact his or her health care provider: fever greater than 38° C (greater than 101° F), chills, cough, shortness of breath, any evidence of easy bruising, bleeding, increasing fatigue, nausea lasting greater than 24 hours, diarrhea lasting greater than greater than 24 hours, or the inability to take in at least 1500 mL in 24 hours.
- Advise patient to report any increasing abdominal pain or fullness, changes in color of urine or stool, increasing pruritus, or jaundice.
- Instruct patient that skin reactions in the form of dermatitis, rashes, or pruritus may occur and to use a moisturizer and notify the heath care provider.
- Educate patient on neutropenic precautions as necessary:
  Practice good handwashing technique.
  Avoid individuals who are ill.
  Wash and cook all foods well.
  Avoid crowds.
  Avoid fresh fruits and vegetables.
- Educate patient on thrombocytopenic precautions:
  Use of a soft bristle toothbrush.
  No flossing if platelet count is less than 50,000/mm^3.
  No IM injections.
  No rectal suppositories.
  No aerobic exercise.
- Provide patient with information on local resources and support groups available for his or her specific diagnosis.

MEDROXYPROGESTER-ONE ACETATE
BRAND NAMES
Depo-Provera, Depo-Provera Contraceptive, Depo-Subcutaneous Provera 104, Provera

CLASS OF AGENT
Progestin, contraceptive

CLINICAL PHARMACOLOGY
Mechanism of Action
A hormone that transforms the endometrium from proliferative to secretory. Inhibits secretion of pituitary gonadotropins. **Therapeutic Effect:** Prevents follicular maturation and ovulation and causes endometrial thinning.
Absorption and Distribution
Oral administration is rapid with maximum concentrations obtained 2-4 hrs after

administration. Bioavailability is variable, but usually low. Medroxyprogesterone is slowly absorbed after IM administration. Protein binding: 90%.

Half-life: Oral: 12-17 hrs; IM: 50 days; subcutaneous: 40 days.

Metabolism and Excretion
Extensively metabolized in the liver by cytochrome P450 enzymes, resulting in more than 10 metabolites. Primarily excreted in urine as glucuronide conjugates.

HOW SUPPLIED/AVAILABLE FORMS
Tablets (Provera): 2.5 mg, 5 mg, 10 mg.
Injection (Depo-Subcutaneous Provera 104): 104 mg/0.65 mL.
Injection (Depo-Provera Contraceptive): 150 mg/mL.
Injection (Depo-Provera): 400 mg/mL.

INDICATIONS AND DOSAGES
Endometrial Carcinoma, Renal Carcinoma
Initially, 400-1000 mg IM; repeat at 1-week intervals. If improvement occurs and disease is stabilized, begin maintenance with as little as 400 mg monthly.

Endometrial Hyperplasia
2.5-10 mg/day PO for 12-14 days.

Endometriosis-Associated Pain
104 mg subcutaneously every 12-14 wks (every 3 mos).

Secondary Amenorrhea
5-10 mg/day PO for 5-10 days. Withdrawal bleeding usually occurs 3-7 days after therapy ends.

Abnormal Uterine Bleeding
5-10 mg/day PO for 5-10 days, beginning on calculated day 16 or day 21 of the menstrual cycle.

Prevention of Pregnancy
IM: 150 mg every 3 mos.
Subcutaneous: 104 mg every 12-14 wks (every 3 mos). If given for more than 14 weeks, pregnancy should be ruled out before next injection.

Dosage Adjustment in Hepatic Dysfunction
For mild or moderate dysfunction, a lower dose or less frequent administration should be considered. Medroxyprogesterone is contraindicated in severe hepatic dysfunction.

Dosage Adjustment in Renal Dysfunction
No information available.

UNLABELED USES
Hormone replacement therapy in estrogen-treated menopausal women

PRECAUTIONS
Use with caution in patients with cardiovascular diseases because thrombotic events and edema have been reported. Prolonged use may result in decreased bone mineral densities.

CONTRAINDICATIONS
Estrogen-dependent neoplasm; history of or active thrombotic disorders, thrombophlebitis, thromboembolic disorders, or cerebrovascular disease; hypersensitivity to progestins; known or suspected pregnancy; severe hepatic dysfunction; undiagnosed abnormal genital bleeding

Pregnancy Risk Category: X
Medroxyprogesterone has been known to cause minor birth defects in children whose mothers had taken this drug during the first trimester of pregnancy. Medroxyprogesterone is known to enter human breast milk and is compatible with breast-feeding.

DRUG PREPARATION/ADMINISTRATION/ SAFE HANDLING ISSUES
◀ **ALERT** ▶ Shake suspension vigorously before administration.
• Administer IM injections in the gluteal or deltoid muscle.
• Administer subcutaneous injections in the upper thigh or abdomen.
• Contraceptive indications: Administer first dose during the first 5 days of menstrual period, or within the first 5 days postpartum if patient is not breast-feeding, or at the sixth week postpartum if patient is breast-feeding exclusively.

STORAGE AND STABILITY
Store at room temperature.

INTERACTIONS
Drug
Aminoglutethimide: May decrease concentration of medroxyprogesterone.
Cytochrome P450 3A4 inhibitors: May increase levels of medroxyprogesterone
Herbal
None known.

LAB EFFECTS/INTERFERENCE
Plasma and urinary progesterone, estradiol, pregnanediol, testosterone, and cortisol

levels may decrease; gonadotropin levels are decreased; sex hormone-binding globulin concentrations are decreased; protein-bound iodine and butanol-extractable protein-bound iodine may increase; triiodotyronine uptake values may decrease; coagulation test values for prothrombin (factor II) and factors VII, VIII, IX, and X may increase; sulfobromophthalein and other liver function test values may increase; lipid metabolism values may alter and are inconsistent.

SIDE EFFECTS
Serious Reactions
- Thrombophlebitis, pulmonary or cerebral embolism, and retinal thrombosis occur rarely.
- Sudden partial or complete loss of vision or sudden onset of proptosis, diplopia, or migraine has been reported.

Other Side Effects
Frequent (10%-50%):
Acne, decreased libido, transient menstrual abnormalities (including spotting, a change in menstrual flow or cervical secretions, and amenorrhea) at initiation of therapy, weight gain

Occasional (1%-10%):
Abdominal pain, alopecia, asthenia, bloating, breast pain/tenderness, depression, dizziness, edema, fatigue, glucose tolerance decreased, headache, injection site reaction, insomnia, leg cramps, nausea, nervousness, ocular disorders, pelvic pain, rash, vaginitis

Rare (Less Than 1%):
Anaphylaxis, appetite changes, asthma, chest pain, chills, convulsions, dermatologic changes, diaphoresis, drowsiness, dry skin, dyspareunia, dyspnea, excessive thirst, fever, galactorrhea, GI disturbances, genitourinary infections, hoarseness, increased libido, jaundice, osteoporotic fractures, paresthesia, pulmonary embolus, syncope, tachycardia, thrombotic events

SPECIAL CONSIDERATIONS
Baseline Assessment
- Monitor CBC with differential, platelet count, electrolyte, BUN, and creatinine levels and liver function tests; evaluate thyroid function and coagulation parameters.
- Assess for menopausal status and smoking status.
- Evaluate for history of deep vein thrombosis and depression.
- Assess for baseline bone density scan.
- Assess baseline weight.

Intervention and Evaluation
- Assess laboratory data as needed, and check glucose as this agent can cause hyperglycemia.
- Monitor patient for injection site reaction.
- Assess patient for menopausal symptoms, amenorrhea, weight loss or gain, night sweats, irritability, and insomnia.
- Evaluate patient for sexual alteration, decreased libido, and vaginal dryness, and refer for appropriate counseling as necessary.
- Monitor patient for side effects of arthralgias, asthenia, dizziness, edema, or nausea.
- Evaluate for evidence of deep vein thrombosis, leg pain or swelling, or tenderness on palpation.

Education
- Instruct patient when to contact his or her health care provider: lower extremity swelling or pain upon walking, polyphagia, polydipsia, or polyuria.
- Educate patient on usual side effects: menstrual irregularities, weight gain, abdominal pain, asthenia, dizziness, and headache.
- Instruct patient on need for bone density scans at regular intervals because of the risk of osteoporosis.
- Advise patient of menopausal side effects of night sweats, irritability, insomnia vaginal dryness, and depression.
- Instruct patient to avoid all OTC medications and herbal and vitamin supplements without first checking with the health care provider.
- Provide patient with information on local resources and support groups available for his or her specific diagnosis.

MEGESTROL
BRAND NAMES
Megace, Megace ES

CLASS OF AGENT
Antineoplastic agent, appetite stimulant, progestin

CLINICAL PHARMACOLOGY
Mechanism of Action
The exact anticancer mechanism of action is unknown. Studies suggest that megestrol suppresses the release of luteinizing hormone from the anterior pituitary

gland, resulting in decreased ovarian estrogen secretion. Another study suggests that it produces a local effect on cancer cells by converting stroma into decidual tissue. **Therapeutic Effect:** Reduces estrogen and inhibits the growth of hormone-dependent cancers that are stimulated by estrogens. Increases appetite by an unknown mechanism.

Absorption and Distribution
Absorption from the GI tract is rapid and variable. Time to peak concentration ranges from 1 to 3 hrs.
Half-life: 13-105 hrs (mean 34 hrs).

Metabolism and Excretion
Megestrol is metabolized in the liver to free steroids and glucuronide conjugates, which are excreted in urine (56%-78%) and feces (8%-30%) and to a lesser extent through respiration within 10 days. Dialysis is not likely to be effective.

HOW SUPPLIED/AVAILABLE FORMS
Tablets: 20 mg, 40 mg.
Suspension: 40 mg/mL (Megace), 625 mg/5 mL (Megace ES).

INDICATIONS AND DOSAGES
Palliative Treatment of Advanced Breast Cancer
160 mg/day PO in four equally divided doses at least for 2 mos to determine efficacy.
Palliative Treatment of Advanced Endometrial Carcinoma
40-320 mg/day PO in divided doses for at least 2 mos to determine efficacy.
Anorexia, Cachexia, Weight Loss
400-800 mg (10-20 mL/day) PO daily (Megace) or 625 mg/5 mL PO daily (Megace ES).
Dosage Adjustment in Hepatic Dysfunction
No information available.
Dosage Adjustment in Renal Dysfunction
No information available. Drug is excreted primarily through the kidneys.

UNLABELED USES
Treatment of hormone-dependent or advanced prostate carcinoma

PRECAUTIONS
Use with caution in patients with a history of thromboembolic disease including thrombophlebitis and pulmonary embolism. Megestrol may also cause new-onset diabetes and exacerbate preexisting diabetes and overt Cushing's syndrome. In patients receiving or being withdrawn from chronic megestrol acetate therapy, adrenal insufficiency has been observed. Watch for symptoms of hypoadrenalism (e.g., hypotension, nausea, vomiting, dizziness, or weakness)

Pregnancy Risk Category:
X (as appetite stimulant), D (for carcinomas) Nursing should be discontinued while patient is receiving megestrol acetate therapy.

CONTRAINDICATIONS
Known hypersensitivity to megestrol or any of its excipients. Pregnancy for appetite stimulant indication.

DRUG PREPARATION/ADMINISTRATION/ SAFE HANDLING ISSUES
• Give PO without regard to food.
• Suspension is a lemon-lime flavor. Megace suspension is compatible with water, apple and orange juice.
• Shake suspension before use.
• Overdose as high as 1600 mg/day has not resulted in serious unexpected side effects.

STORAGE AND STABILITY
Store at room temperature 25° C (77° F) with excursions to 15-30° C (59-86° F).

INTERACTIONS
Drug
None known.
Herbal
None known.

LAB EFFECTS/INTERFERENCE
May increase blood glucose level.

SIDE EFFECTS
Serious Reactions
Thrombophlebitis and pulmonary embolism occur rarely.
Other Side Effects
Frequent (10%-50%):
Diarrhea, weight gain secondary to increased appetite
Occasional (1%-10%):
Asthenia, backache, breakthrough menstrual bleeding, breast tenderness, carpal tunnel syndrome, decreased libido, dyspnea, edema, flatulence, headache, hyperglycemia, hypertension, hot flashes, impotence, lethargy, malaise, mood changes, nausea, rash, sweating, tumor flare, vaginal dryness

Rare (Less Than 1%):
Glucose intolerance, pulmonary embolism, thrombophlebitis

SPECIAL CONSIDERATIONS
Baseline Assessment
* Obtain baseline assessment of CBC with differential, platelet count, electrolyte, BUN, creatinine, glucose, cholesterol, and triglyceride levels, liver function tests, and coagulation parameters as needed.
* Assess patient for any history of diabetes, deep vein thrombosis (DVT), MI, or CHF.
* Obtain baseline EKG as needed per history.
* Assess baseline weight.
* Assess patient employment history for evidence of repetitive hand movement and any history of carpal tunnel syndrome.
* Assess patient for compliance in taking an oral regimen.

Intervention and Evaluation
* Monitor CBC with differential, platelet count, liver function tests, and glucose level at each visit.
* Evaluate for any evidence of thrombophlebitis, DVT, or chest pain.
* Assess vital signs for evidence of hypertension, change in respiratory status or edema, or decreased saturation as this agent can increase the risk of DVT and pulmonary embolisms.
* Monitor weight at each visit for evidence of significant weight gain, which can occur with this agent.
* Evaluate patient for any new side effects since last visit, which could include breast enlargement, tenderness, headaches, backaches, or carpal tunnel syndrome.
* Assess for alterations in sexual function, decreasing libido, and vaginal dryness in women or impotence in men, and make appropriate referrals as needed to a gynecologist or urologist.
* Evaluate at each visit for patient compliance in taking the medication as ordered.
* Assess patient for any evidence of increasing alopecia.

Education
* Instruct patient on when to contact his or her health care provider: fever greater than 38° C (greater than 101° F), chest pain, shortness of breath or symptoms of elevated glucose, polyuria, polyphagia, polydipsia, diarrhea lasting greater than 24 hours, nausea lasting greater than 24 hours, or the inability to take in at least 1500 mL of fluid in 24 hours.
* Educate patient on signs and symptoms of DVT: swelling, erythema, or pain in the extremities.
* Instruct patient there may be changes in his or her sexual functioning, menopausal symptoms of hot flashes, night sweats, and vaginal dryness in women, and impotence in men.
* Educate patient breast changes may occur in both men and women as manifested by enlargement and tenderness.
* Instruct patient on how to take medication and not skip doses and to contact health care provider if unable to take the medication as ordered.
* Educate patient to avoid OTC medications or herbal or vitamin supplements without first checking with the health care provider.
* Provide patient with information on local resources and support groups available for his or her specific diagnosis.

MELPHALAN
BRAND NAMES
Alkeran

CLASS OF AGENT
Antineoplastic agent, alkylating agent

CLINICAL PHARMACOLOGY
Mechanism of Action
A phenylalanine derivative of nitrogen mustard that acts as an alkylating agent. It cross-links with strands of DNA and RNA, producing cell death, and is cell cycle phase nonspecific. **Therapeutic Effect:** Disrupts nucleic acid function.

Absorption and Distribution
Oral absorption is variable and incomplete with a bioavailability that is unpredictable. Food affects absorption. Steady-state volume of distribution: 0.5 L/kg. Penetration into CNS is low. Protein binding: 60%-90%.
Half-life: 1.5 hrs.

Metabolism and Excretion
Metabolized by chemical hydrolysis to monohydroxymelphalan and dihydroxymelphalan. Eliminated primarily through feces (20%-50%) and urine (10%-15%) (unchanged drug). Not removed by hemodialysis.

HOW SUPPLIED/AVAILABLE FORMS
Tablets: 2 mg.
Powder for Injection: 50 mg.

INDICATIONS AND DOSAGES
Ovarian Carcinoma
0.2 mg/kg/day PO for 5 successive days.
Repeat at 4- to 6-week intervals.
Multiple Myeloma
PO: Initially, 6 mg daily, adjusted as indicated or 0.15 mg/kg/day for 7 days or 0.25 mg/kg/day for 4 days. After 2-3 wks of treatment, the drug should be held for up to 4 wks to allow for recovery of myelosuppression. Maintenance therapy of 1-3 mg orally daily or 0.05 mg/kg/day or less may be implemented when WBC count and platelet levels rises.
IV: 16 mg/m^2/dose every 2 weeks for 4 doses and then repeated monthly according to protocol.
Dosage Adjustment in Hepatic Dysfunction
No adjustments required.
Dosage Adjustment in Renal Dysfunction
BUN greater than 30 mg/dL or serum creatinine greater than 1.5 mg/dL: decrease melphalan IV dosage by 50% due to increased risk of myelosuppression.

UNLABELED USES
Treatment of breast carcinoma, neuroblastoma, rhabdomyosarcoma, testicular carcinoma, part of myeloablative therapy for stem cell transplants

PRECAUTIONS
Melphalan causes suppression of ovarian function in premenopausal women. Amenorrhea may occur. Reversible and irreversible testicular suppression have been noted.
Pregnancy Risk Category: D
Melphalan may cause fetal harm when administered during pregnancy. Excretion of drug into human breast milk is unknown/not recommended in nursing women.

CONTRAINDICATIONS
Pregnancy, severe myelosuppression, prior resistance to melphalan

DRUG PREPARATION/ADMINISTRATION/ SAFE HANDLING ISSUES
◄ ALERT ► Because melphalan has been shown to be carcinogenic, mutagenic, or teratogenic, wear nitrile or latex, but not vinyl, gloves when handling the drug for IV use. If the drug comes in contact with skin, wash the skin thoroughly with soap and water. Do not use waterless hand soap or any antibacterial soap as either can increase the reaction from the agent. If the drug comes in contact with mucous membranes, flush the area with water.
• Oral melphalan should be administered on an empty stomach (1 hr before meals or 2 hrs after meals).
• IV: melphalan is reconstituted with 10 mL of supplied diluent. Shake vial vigorously until solution becomes clear. Concentration is 5 mg/mL.
• Further dilute melphalan dose into 0.9% NaCl to a concentration no greater than 0.45 mg/mL.
• Administer diluted product over minimum of 15 mins.
• Complete administration within 60 mins of reconstitution. Diluted solutions are unstable.

STORAGE AND STABILITY
• Store IV vials at room temperature. Protect from light.
• Refrigerate tablets. Protect from light.
• Precipitate forms if reconstituted solution is stored at 5° C (41° F). Do not refrigerate reconstituted product.
• Diluted solutions are unstable. The citrate derivative of melphalan has been detected at as few as 30 mins after reconstitution.

INTERACTIONS
Drug
Bone marrow depressants: May increase myelosuppression.
Carmustine: May reduce the threshold for carmustine lung toxicity.
Cimetidine and other H2 blockers: May decrease oral melphalan bioavailability.
Cisplatin and nephrotoxic drugs: May increase risk of renal toxicity and decrease melphalan clearance.
Cyclosporine: May increase cyclosporine toxicity, especially nephrotoxicity.
Live virus vaccines: May potentiate viral replication, increase vaccine side effects, and decrease the patient's antibody response to the vaccine.
Nalidixic acid: May increase risk for severe hemorrhagic necrotic enterocolitis.

Herbal
None known.

LAB EFFECTS/INTERFERENCE
May increase serum uric acid level and liver enzymes.

Y-SITE COMPATIBLES
Bleomycin, carboplatin, carmustine, cisplatin, cyclophosphamide, cytarabine, dacarbazine, dactinomycin, daunorubicin, doxorubicin, etoposide, filgrastim, floxuridine, fludarabine, fluorouracil, granisetron, idarubicin, ifosfamide, mechlorethamine, mesna, methotrexate, mitomycin, mitoxantrone, ondansetron, palonosetron, streptozocin, teniposide, vinblastine, vincristine, vinorelbine

INCOMPATIBLES
Amphotericin B conventional, chlorpromazine, pantoprazole

SIDE EFFECTS
Serious Reactions
• Myelosuppression is the most common side effect and may be manifested principally as leukopenia and thrombocytopenia and to a lesser extent as anemia, pancytopenia, and agranulocytosis. Leukopenia may occur as early as 5 days after drug initiation. Myelosuppression is more prominent with IV dosing than with oral dosing.
• WBC and platelet counts nadirs occur in 14-21 days after treatment and return to normal levels 28-35 days or longer after therapy, but leukopenia and thrombocytopenia may last more than 6 wks after the drug is discontinued. Irreversible bone marrow failure has been reported.
• Hypersensitivity reactions have been reported primarily with IV melphalan and may also occur with oral melphalan.
• Secondary malignancies have been reported in patients with cancer treated with alkylating agents.
Other Side Effects
Frequent (10%-50%):
Myelosuppression, nausea, vomiting (may be severe with large IV doses)
Occasional (1%-10%):
Diarrhea, stomatitis, rash, pruritus, alopecia, elevated liver enzyme levels, hepatitis, hypersensitivity reactions, jaundice
Rare (Less Than 1%):
Hepatic veno-occlusive disease, pulmonary fibrosis, interstitial pneumonitis, vasculitis, hemolytic anemia

SPECIAL CONSIDERATIONS
Baseline Assessment
• Monitor patients for CBC with differential and platelet count, electrolyte, BUN, creatinine and uric acid levels, and liver function tests.
• Dose reductions are required for creatinine greater than 1.5 mg or BUN greater than 30 mg/dL.
• Evaluate patient for history of gout and kidney stones.
• Review patient's current medication list.
• Assess patient's ability to comply with oral medications.
Intervention and Evaluation
• Premedicate patient for nausea and vomiting as ordered.
• Assess patient for signs and symptoms of stomatitis, diarrhea, nausea, or mucositis before each dose.
• Initiate an oral care regimen per institutional guidelines. An example is 1 tsp each of salt and baking soda dissolved in 1 glass of water to swish and spit at least 4 times/day.
• Monitor patient for any changes in renal function, decreased urine output, or a change in urine color, maintain accurate intake and output, and weigh patient at each visit.
• Monitor patient for any signs or symptoms of peripheral edema.
• Assess cardiac and pulmonary status at each visit, evaluating for any signs of pulmonary edema or tachycardia due to edema.
• Monitor skin for any evidence of rash or pruritic areas and initiate skin care as needed; may use topical moisturizers as needed.
• If you do not see any myelosuppression after oral doses, consider that there may be malabsorption or low bioavailability.
Education
• Instruct patient on when to contact his or her health care provider: fever greater than 38° C (greater than 101° F), chills, cough, shortness of breath, fatigue, easy bruising, bleeding, petechiae, ecchymoses, and nausea or diarrhea lasting greater than 24 hours.
• Instruct patient to take oral melphalan on an empty stomach (1 hours before meals or 2 hours after meals).
• Educate patient on need for oral care and give example of requested care.

- Instruct patient alopecia usually occurs with IV dosing and hair may take 4-6 months to recover but may be of different color and texture.
- Educate patient on neutropenic precautions as necessary:
  Practice good handwashing technique.
  Avoid individuals who are ill.
  Wash and cook all foods well.
  Avoid crowds.
  Avoid fresh fruits and vegetables.
- Educate patient on thrombocytopenic precautions:
  Use of a soft bristle toothbrush.
  No flossing if platelet count is less than 50,000/mm³.
  No IM injections.
  No rectal suppositories.
  No aerobic exercise.
- Advise patient that pruritus and rashes can occur with this agent and to call the health care provider if these are significant.
- Instruct patient to let health care provider know if he or she is starting any new medications.
- Instruct patient to take no over-the-counter medications or herbal or vitamin supplements without checking with his or her health care provider.
- Educate patient on local resources available and support groups related to their particular diagnosis.

MERCAPTOPURINE, 6-MP

BRAND NAMES
Purinethol

CLASS OF AGENT
Antimetabolite

CLINICAL PHARMACOLOGY
Mechanism of Action
An analog of purine bases adenine and hypoxanthine that is incorporated into RNA and DNA, blocks purine synthesis, and inhibits DNA and RNA synthesis. **Therapeutic Effect:** Causes death of cancer cells.
Absorption and Distribution
Absorption is approximately 50% and variable. Protein binding: 19%. Volume of distribution exceeds that of total body water. Cerebrospinal fluid penetration is poor. *Half-life:* IV: 47 mins (adults); 21 mins (pediatrics).

Metabolism and Excretion
Metabolism occurs through two major pathways. Thiol methylation is catalyzed by polymorphic enzyme thiopurine *S*-methyltransferase (TPMT) to form the inactive metabolite methyl-6-MP. TPMT is highly variable, and individuals may be TPMT deficient or have low or intermediate TPMT activity. Metabolism through oxidation is catalyzed by xanthine oxidase (XO) to form 6-thiouric acid. XO is inhibited by allopurinol. Urine excretion: 46% (parent compound and metabolites) in 24 hrs.

HOW SUPPLIED/AVAILABLE FORMS
Tablets: 50 mg.

INDICATIONS AND DOSAGES
Acute Lymphatic (Lymphocytic or Lymphoblastic) Leukemia
2.5-5 mg/kg PO once a day as induction dose (100-200 mg usual adult dose). If no response is seen in 4 wks, dose may be increased to 5 mg/kg/day. Maintenance dose is 1.5-2.5 mg/kg/day. Doses are usually rounded to nearest 25 mg.
Reduce mercaptopurine dose by 75% (25% of usual dose) if given concurrently with allopurinol.
Dosage Adjustment in Hepatic/Renal Dysfunction
No recommendations available. Initiate at lower end of dosing range to reduce drug accumulation.

UNLABELED USES
Irritable bowel syndrome, Crohn's disease, ulcerative colitis

PRECAUTIONS
Pregnancy Risk Category: D
Patients who are TPMT deficient or demonstrate low/intermediate TPMT activity will require dose reductions and have a higher risk for myelosuppression. If patient shows clinical or laboratory evidence of severe toxicity, TPMT genotyping or phenotyping should be considered.

CONTRAINDICATIONS
Hypersensitivity to mercaptopurine or any of its excipients, patients whose disease has demonstrated prior resistance to the mercaptopurine or thioguanine, patients with preexisting severe myelosuppression or hepatic disease, and pregnant patients

DRUG PREPARATION/ADMINISTRATION/ SAFE HANDLING ISSUES

Take on an empty stomach (1 hrs before or 2 hrs after meals) and at the same time daily.

STORAGE AND STABILITY

Store at room temperature.

INTERACTIONS

Drug

Allopurinol: Increase the effects and toxicity of mercaptopurine by inhibiting xanthine oxidase. Reduce mercaptopurine dose by 75%.
Bone marrow depressants: May increase the risk of myelosuppression.
Doxorubicin and hepatotoxic drugs: Increases risk for hepatotoxicity.
Live virus vaccines: May potentiate viral replication, increase vaccine side effects, and decrease the patient's antibody response to the vaccine.
Olsalazine, mesalazine, sulfasalazine: Inhibits TPMT and increases risk of mercaptopurine effect/toxicity. Avoid concurrent use if possible.
Warfarin: May decrease the effects of warfarin. Monitor INR or PT.

Herbal

None known.

LAB EFFECTS/INTERFERENCE

May increase bilirubin, AST, alkaline phosphatase, and uric acid levels.

SIDE EFFECTS

Serious Reactions

- Myelosuppression and gastroenteritis may occur.
- Hepatic toxicity (intrahepatic cholestasis, hepatic necrosis) is common and characterized by hyperbilirubinemia, increased alkaline phosphatase and AST levels, jaundice, ascites, and encephalopathy. It usually occurs within 2 mos of therapy but may occur within 1 week or be delayed for up to 8 years and is more frequent at doses greater than 2.5 mg/kg/day.

Other Side Effects

Frequent (10%-50%):

Intrahepatic cholestasis, myelosuppression (leading to leukopenia, thrombocytopenia, anemia)

Occasional (1%-10%):

Abdominal pain, anorexia, diarrhea, drug fever, hyperpigmentation, hyperuricemia, mucositis, nausea, rash, stomatitis, radiation recall, vomiting

Rare (Less Than 1%):

Alopecia, hepatic necrosis, oligospermia

SPECIAL CONSIDERATIONS

Baseline Assessment

- Obtain CBC with differential, platelet count, electrolyte, BUN, creatinine, and uric acid levels and liver function tests.
- Assess patient for history of abnormal liver function tests and gout.
- Evaluate patient for any history of dermatologic conditions.

Intervention and Evaluation

- Assess laboratory parameters listed above at each visit.
- Evaluate the need for chronic antiemetics before taking this agent; many patients have low-grade nausea while receiving this drug.
- Evaluate for compliance with this medication as nausea increases the risk of noncompliance.
- Monitor patient for evidence of signs or symptoms of neutropenia, thrombocytopenia, anemia, nausea, vomiting, GI symptoms, and diarrhea.
- Evaluate patient for any evidence of right upper quadrant pain, jaundice, and changes in color of urine or stool.
- Assess skin for evidence of rashes, pruritus, and desquamation.
- Monitor for evidence of mucositis, and initiate an oral care regimen as necessary. An example is 1 tsp each of salt and baking soda dissolved in 1 glass of water to swish and spit at least 4 times/day. Discourage patient from flossing if the platelet count is less than 50,000/mm^3, and avoid commercial mouthwashes if the patient is neutropenic and has mucositis as they contain alcohol and that increases oral pain.

Education

- Advise patient on when to contact his or her health care provider: fever greater than 38° C (greater than 101° F), chills, cough, shortness of breath, signs of infection, significant right upper quadrant pain, evidence of bleeding from any orifice, nausea lasting greater than 24 hours, diarrhea lasting greater than 24 hours, or the inability to drink at least 1500 mL of fluid in 24 hours.
- Instruct patient on the importance of taking this agent as ordered and not skipping doses.

- Educate patient on the use of antiemetics as necessary to decrease nausea, which may be caused by this agent.
- Have patient monitor for rashes, desquamation, or increasing pruritus, and encourage the use of moisturizing creams.
- Instruct patient to report any evidence of pain in lower extremities especially feet, as this may be evidence of gout.
- Instruct patient on an oral care regimen.
- Educate patient on neutropenic precautions as necessary:
  Practice good handwashing technique.
  Avoid individuals who are ill.
  Wash and cook all foods well.
  Avoid crowds.
  Avoid fresh fruits and vegetables.
- Educate patient on thrombocytopenic precautions:
  Use of a soft bristle toothbrush.
  No flossing if platelet count is less than 50,000/mm³.
  No IM injections.
  No rectal suppositories.
  No aerobic exercise.
- Avoid individuals who have recently been vaccinated with live vaccines, especially young children.
- Educate patient to avoid all OTC medications or herbal and vitamin supplements without first checking with his or her health care provider.
- Provide patient with information on local resources and support groups available for his or her specific diagnosis.

MESNA

BRAND NAMES
Mesnex

CLASS OF AGENT
Cytoprotectant

CLINICAL PHARMACOLOGY
Mechanism of Action
Cytoprotectant of urinary system used for preventing hemorrhagic cystitis caused by cyclophosphamide or ifosfamide. Mesna is a thiol compound that inactivates acrolein and prevents urothelial toxicity without affecting the cytostatic activity of the other metabolites. Mesna protects the urinary endothelium in the ureter or bladder by inactivating the acrolein metabolite. The mesna-metabolite complex is soluble and is excreted in the urine. Mesna is selective

in the urinary tract due to rapid plasma dimerization to inactive dimesna in the blood. Dimesna is distributed poorly outside the vascular circulation because it is poorly lipophilic.

Absorption and Distribution
Bioavailability after oral administration of mesna is about 50% (range is 45%-79%). After oral or IV administration, mesna is rapidly converted in plasma water to chemically inert dimesna, which is inactive. It distributes to the renal parenchyma where glutathione converts dimesna back to active mesna. After IV and oral administration, the time to peak urinary concentration of thiols is about 1 and 3 hrs, respectively. Both mesna and dimesna are very water soluble; mesna distribution is in plasma water. It does not cross the blood-brain barrier. It is moderately protein bound (69%-75%)
Half-life: After IV administration, the plasma half-life of mesna is 18-70 mins.

Metabolism and Excretion
After IV administration approximately 31% and 28% of the dose were excreted in urine within 4 hrs as mesna and dimesna, respectively. After oral administration, about 25% of free mesna and 25% dimesna are excreted in the urine. The remaining 25% is excreted as free thiols.

HOW SUPPLIED/AVAILABLE FORMS
Injection Solution: 1 g multidose (100 mg/mL) vial.
Tablets: 400 mg scored tablets, containing 10 blister packs per card.

INDICATIONS AND DOSAGES
To Protect the Urinary System from Hemorrhagic Cystitis Caused by Ifosfamide or Cyclophosphamide
IV Dose Only Schedule
It is recommended that IV bolus injections be equal to 20% of the ifosfamide dosage (w/w) at the time of ifosfamide administration and 4 and 8 hrs after each dose of ifosfamide. The total daily dose of mesna is 60% of the ifosfamide dose.
IV Dosing Schedule for Mesna

	0 hrs	4 hrs	8 hrs
Ifosfamide	1.2 g/m²	—	—
Mesna injection	240 mg/m²	240 mg/m²	240 mg/m²

IV and Oral Dosing
A fractionated dosing schedule of three IV bolus injections or a single bolus injection followed by two oral mesna tablets is recommended for prophylaxis of ifosfamide-induced hemorrhagic cystitis. When both IV and oral mesna are used, the recommended regimen is an IV bolus dose equal to 20% of the ifosfamide dosage (w/w) at the time of ifosfamide administration followed by mesna tablets equal to 40% of the ifosfamide dose given PO 2 and 6 hrs after each dose of ifosfamide. The total daily dose of mesna is 100% of the ifosfamide dose.

IV and Oral Dosing Schedule for Mesna

	0 hrs	2 hrs	6 hrs
Ifosfamide	1.2 g/m^2	—	—
Mesna injection	240 mg/m^2	—	—
Mesna tablet	—	480 mg/m^2	480 mg/m^2

Patients who have emesis within 2 hrs of taking oral mesna should repeat the dose or be changed to IV mesna. This dosing schedule is repeated on each day that ifosfamide is administered. If the dosage of ifosfamide is adjusted, the ratio of mesna to ifosfamide should be maintained.

Subcutaneous Administration
For prevention of ifosfamide-induced hemorrhagic cystitis, the administration of ifosfamide via the subcutaneous route is a safe alternative to IV and PO routes. The initial dose of mesna is 20% of the ifosfamide dose (30 mins before ifosfamide), with a continuous infusion of 40% of the ifosfamide dose over 8 hrs. Minimal adverse effects were noted in 12 patients, with one episode of microscopic hematuria in one patient.

Dosage Adjustment in Hepatic and Renal Dysfunction
Dosage adjustments not required.

UNLABELED USES
To protect the urinary system from hemorrhagic cystitis caused by cyclophosphamide and as a prophylactic agent to decrease the incidence of hemorrhagic cystitis in bone marrow transplantation patients receiving high-dose cyclophosphamide; cytoprotectant for neurotoxicity from cisplatin or taxanes. It has been used in a limited number of patients receiving cyclophosphamide for immunologically mediated disorders (e.g., systemic lupus erythematosus [SLE], polyarteritis, Wegener's granulomatosis, and dermatomyositis).

PRECAUTIONS
Pregnancy Risk Category: B
Drug excretion into human breast milk is unknown/not recommended in nursing women.

CONTRAINDICATIONS
Avoid in patients with hypersensitivity to mesna/other thiol compounds.

DRUG PREPARATION/ADMINISTRATION/SAFE HANDLING ISSUES
◀ ALERT ▶ Mesna dosage is individualized on the basis of the patient's chemotherapy doses. When administering this drug, consult specific protocols for optimum dosage and sequence of drug administration.
◀ ALERT ▶ Mesna is not considered hazardous.

STORAGE AND STABILITY
IV
- Store vials at room temperature.
- The reconstituted solution is stable for up to 24 hrs at room temperature or up to 48 hrs if refrigerated.
- Protect the reconstituted solution from prolonged exposure to sunlight; discard any unused portions.
- After entry into the vial, mesna vials may be stored and used for up to 8 days. Mesna is stable in standard polypropylene syringes for 9 days at temperatures ranging from 5 to 35° C. Furthermore, no detectable changes were observed in mesna concentrations when they were further diluted to 1:5 or 1:2 and stored at room temperature for 1 week.
- Under refrigeration, IV mesna for oral use was stable for 24 hrs when mixed with six carbonated beverages, two juices, or milk at dilutions of 1:2, 1:10, or 1:100.

PO
- Store tablets at room temperature.

INTERACTIONS
Drug
None.

Herbal
None.

LAB EFFECTS/INTERFERENCE
False-positive results of sodium nitroprusside tests for urinary ketone determinations. This reaction presumably occurs because the sulfonate group contained in mesna interacts with the sodium nitroprusside reagent.

Y-SITE COMPATIBLES
Carboplatin, cladribine, cyclophosphamide (admixture compatible), dactinomycin, docetaxel, doxorubicin, doxorubicin liposomal (Doxil), epirubicin, etoposide, filgrastim, fludarabine, gallium nitrate, gemcitabine, granisetron hydrochloride, hydroxyzine, ifosfamide (admixture and syringe compatible), melphalan, methotrexate, mitoxantrone, ondansetron, oxaliplatin, paclitaxel, pemetrexed, rituximab, sargramostim, teniposide, thiotepa, trastuzumab, vinorelbine

INCOMPATIBLES
Amphotericin B colloidal (Amphotec), lansoprazole

SIDE EFFECTS
Serious Reactions
- Hypersensitivity reactions, ranging from mild allergic reactions to systemic anaphylactic reactions, have been reported in patients receiving mesna. Patients with autoimmune disorders (e.g., rheumatoid arthritis, SLE, and nephritis) may be at increased risk of developing hypersensitivity reactions to mesna.
- Each 400-mg Mesnex tablet contains 59.3 mg of lactose; thus, patients with a history of lactose intolerance may be sensitive to this formulation of the drug.

Other Side Effects
Frequent (10%-50%):
No information.
Occasional (1%-10%):
Coughing, diarrhea, flushing, nausea, vomiting
Rare (Less Than 1%):
No information.

SPECIAL CONSIDERATIONS
Baseline Assessment
- Assure that mesna orders are written concurrently with all ifosfamide orders or with any high dose cyclophosphamide orders. Mesna should be ordered with bone marrow transplant regimens using cyclophosphamide.
- Identify any patient who may have had an allergic reaction to this agent.
- Obtain baseline B/P as this agent may induce hypotension.

Intervention and Evaluation
- Evaluate patient's ability to take this agent PO and comply with an oral regimen if this is planned.
- Assess patient for evidence of anaphylaxis or allergic reaction.
- Evaluate patient for evidence of side effects such as nausea, diarrhea, headache, dizziness, anorexia, conjunctivitis, arthralgias, and somnolence.
- Assess patient for hypotension, increasing fatigue, and injection site reactions.

Education
- Educate patient on when to contact his or her health care provider: fever greater than 38° C (greater than 101° F), chills, headache, somnolence, arthralgias and myalgias, nausea lasting greater than 24 hours, diarrhea lasting greater than 24 hours, or the inability to take in at least 1500 mL of fluid in 24 hours.
- Instruct patient on how to take this agent if it is being administered PO, and make sure patient recognizes the importance of taking this agent on time and reporting any missed doses to the health care provider.
- Instruct patient to take no over-the-counter medications or herbal or vitamin supplements without checking with his or her health care provider.
- Educate patient to report any injection site reactions as this agent can induce phlebitis in some patients.

METHOTREXATE

BRAND NAMES
Apo-Methotrexate [Canada], Ledertrexate [Australia], Methoblastin [Australia], Rheumatrex, Trexall, Folex (US), Mexate, Mexate-AQ

CLASS OF AGENT
Antineoplastic antimetabolite, antipsoriatic agent, disease-modifying antirheumatic drug

CLINICAL PHARMACOLOGY
Mechanism of Action
An antimetabolite that competes with dihydrofolate reductase, an enzyme

necessary for purine metabolism, which results in the inhibition of DNA, RNA, and protein synthesis. **Therapeutic Effect:** Causes death of cancer cells.

Absorption and Distribution

Methotrexate is variably absorbed from the GI tract. In doses less than 30 mg/m^2, methotrexate is almost completely absorbed. Peak absorption occurs within 1-2 hrs of oral administration. At doses greater than 80 mg/m^2, absorption is incomplete, and serum concentrations are only 10% of that achieved after IV administration. Absorption is 30%-40% with doses of 0.1 mg/kg. This suggests that the oral absorption of methotrexate is a saturable process. After IM administration, it is completely absorbed. Methotrexate is distributed in intracellular cytoplasm and into third spaces, such as the intrathecal, pleural, and peritoneal cavities. These spaces act a reservoir for methotrexate and impede the clearance of the drug, which can increase the risk of toxic side effects (mucositis and myelosuppression). Control of third space effusions is recommended before use of methotrexate. Protein binding: 50%-70%.

Half-life: After IV administration, methotrexate serum concentrations decline in three phases: an initial distribution half-life of 45 mins, a second half-life of 2-4 hrs (representing renal clearance), and a terminal half life ranging from 8 to 15 hrs (representing release of intracellular methotrexate into the peripheral bloodstream). The terminal half-life begins when the serum concentration falls to 0.1 Micrometer (1×10^{-7} M). Cytotoxic effects correlate with serum concentrations of 0.1 Micrometer or greater.

Metabolism and Excretion

Except when high doses are given (greater than 250 mg), methotrexate undergoes little metabolism. Methotrexate is metabolized intracellularly in the liver by aldehyde oxidase. After high doses are given IV, about 10% of the drug is excreted in the urine as an inactive metabolite, 7-hydroxymethotrexate, which is very water insoluble, especially in acidic urine, and can crystallize in the renal tubules, leading to renal failure. After oral administration, up to 35% of the drug is excreted as metabolites. About 90% of methotrexate is excreted unchanged primarily in urine. Nearly 50% of methotrexate is excreted unchanged in the urine within 6 hrs of IV administration, 90% within 24 hrs, and 95% in 30 hrs.

Methotrexate clearance is directly related to renal function and is approximately 60% greater than glomerular filtration rate (or about 1.6 times creatinine clearance). In patients with normal renal function, methotrexate clearance is approximately 110 mL/min/m^2, of which 103 mL/min/m^2 is due to renal clearance. Methotrexate is removed by hemodialysis but not by peritoneal dialysis. Hemodialysis may be indicated in patients who develop renal failure during methotrexate therapy.

HOW SUPPLIED/AVAILABLE FORMS

Tablets (Rheumatrex): 2.5 mg.
Tablets (Trexall): 5 mg, 7.5 mg, 10 mg, 15 mg.
Injection Solution (Available as Preserved Multidose Vials and as Preservative-Free Single-Use Vials): 25 mg/mL
Injection Lyophilized Powder (Preservative-Free): 20-mg vial, 25-mg vial, 50-mg vial, 100-mg vial, 250-mg vial, 1-g vial.

INDICATIONS AND DOSAGES

Nonhematologic Cancers: Trophoblastic Neoplasms, Osteogenic Sarcoma, Choriocarcinoma, Chorioadenoma Destruens, Hydatidiform Mole, Head and Neck Cancer, Breast Cancer; Hematologic Cancers: Acute Lymphocytic Leukemia, Burkitt's Lymphoma, Lymphosarcoma, Mycosis Fungoides

IV: Low: 10-50 mg/m^2; med: 100-250 mg/m^2; high: 250 mg/m^2 and above with leucovorin.
Intrathecal: 10-15 mg/m^2
IM: 25 mg/m^2
Note: Leucovorin must be given after methotrexate for rescue in patients who have received doses greater than 250 mg/m^2 or in those patients at risk for developing severe toxicity from methotrexate (e.g., patients with renal dysfunction).
PO: Oral dosing of methotrexate is primarily reserved for rheumatic disorders or psoriasis. The usual dosing regimens are 7.5-20 mg given once weekly. There are also regimens using oral methotrexate for the treatment of trophoblastic tumors, choriocarcinoma, adult acute lymphoblastic leukemia, Burkitt's lymphoma, and other non-Hodgkin's lymphomas. The reader is referred to other clinical oncology literature for recommended doses for these diseases.

Dosage Adjustment in Renal Impairment

Methotrexate should be administered to patients with adequate renal function to clear the drug from the body. It should not be administered until a recent creatinine clearance value is evaluated. Although there are several formulas to estimate CCr, the most commonly used and most economical is the simple Cockroft-Gault formula:

$$CCr \text{ (mL/min) [Adult]} = \frac{(140 - age) \times (weight \text{ in kg}) \times (0.85 \text{ if female})}{Serum\ creatinine \text{ (mg/dL)} \times 72}$$

Other formulas such as Jeliffe or modified Jeliffe may also be used. These are shown in Appendix 1. Methotrexate should not be administered if the serum creatinine is greater than 1.5 mg/dL of if the creatinine clearance is less than 50 mL/min. Patients receiving high-dose methotrexate regimens over 4-6 hrs with estimated creatinine clearance less than 70 mL/min will exhibit higher 24-hr methotrexate concentrations than those with normal renal function. With intermediate degrees of renal function (between 50 and 75 mL/min), careful monitoring of serum methotrexate concentrations is required to determine the duration of leucovorin for methotrexate rescue therapy.

MONITORING GUIDELINES
- In those receiving high-dose methotrexate, urine pH should be higher than 7.0 before and during therapy along with adequate fluid input of approximately 3000 mL/m^2).
- Methotrexate concentrations must always be monitored for the following conditions:
    Patients receiving high-dose methotrexate (greater than 250 mg/m^2) with leucovorin rescue
    Patients with moderate or worse renal dysfunction, regardless of the methotrexate dose
    Patients who have experienced excessive toxicity with prior methotrexate therapy
- Cerebrospinal fluid methotrexate concentrations must be monitored in patients receiving intrathecal therapy at intervals of less than 7 days.

High-Dose Methotrexate
Most high dose regimens require at least 72 hrs of leucovorin rescue. The goal of monitoring is to assure that the drug is appropriately excreted from the body. Monitoring allows one to identify patients with delayed methotrexate clearance who will need prolonged leucovorin rescue. Leucovorin should be continued until the serum methotrexate levels are less than 0.05 Micrometer or 5×10^{-8} M. If leucovorin is discontinued

too soon, the patient will be exposed to toxic levels of methotrexate.

After high doses of methotrexate are infused over 4-6 hrs, serum concentrations will approach 1000 Micrometer (1×10^{-4} M) at the end of the infusion but fall quickly to about 1 micromolar (1×10^{-6} M) at 24 hrs. If methotrexate serum concentrations exceed 10 Micrometer (1×10^{-5} M) at 24 hrs or 1 Micrometer (1×10^{-6} M) at 48 hrs after drug administration, the patient is at risk for excessive toxicity and will require either a higher dose of leucovorin or a longer duration of leucovorin rescue. Although the standard is to obtain 24 and 48 serum oncentrations, we prefer monitoring serum concentrations at 12, 24, 48, and 72 hrs after methotrexate administration. This allows us to determine high-risk patients earlier and make adjustments in leucovorin rescue more quickly.

UNLABELED USES
Treatment of acute myelocytic leukemia; bladder, cervical, ovarian, prostatic, renal, and testicular carcinomas; psoriatic arthritis; systemic dermatomyositis

PRECAUTIONS
Use methotrexate cautiously in patients with ascites, pleural effusion, myelosuppression, peptic ulcer disease, moderate or worse renal dysfunction or ulcerative colitis.
Pregnancy Risk Category: D, X (for patients with psoriasis or rheumatoid arthritis)

CONTRAINDICATIONS
Preexisting myelosuppression, severe hepatic or renal impairment

DRUG PREPARATION/ADMINISTRATION/ SAFE HANDLING ISSUES
◄ ALERT ► Because methotrexate may be carcinogenic, mutagenic, or teratogenic, it must be handled with extreme care during preparation and administration. Gloves should be worn when preparing the solution. If methotrexate powder or solution comes in contact with skin, the exposed area should be washed immediately and thoroughly with soap and water.
◄ ALERT ► Be aware that the drug may be given IM, IV, intra-arterially, or intrathecally.
- Reconstitute each 5-mg vial with 2 mL of sterile water for injection or 0.9% NaCl to provide a concentration of 2.5 mg/mL up to a maximum of 25 mg/mL.

- The solution may be further diluted with D5W or 0.9% NaCl.
- For intrathecal use, dilute with preservative-free 0.9% NaCl to provide a concentration of 1-2 mg/mL.
- Give IV push at 10 mg/min.
- Give IV infusion over 30 mins-4 hrs.

STORAGE AND STABILITY
- Store vials and tablets at room temperature and protect from light.
- Reconstituted solution is stable for up to 24 hrs at room temperature and under refrigeration. Stability varies per formulation and concentration. Please refer to detailed reference.

INTERACTIONS
Drug
Cyclosporin, salicylates (aspirin), penicillins, probenecid, procarbazine, and sulfonamides: May decrease the renal excretion of methotrexate, leading to enhanced bone marrow suppression and mucositis. These drugs should be avoided for 3 days before and 3 days after the administration of methotrexate.
Phenytoin: May increase phenytoin elimination.
Warfarin: May increase INR in patients receiving warfarin therapy. Monitor INR or PT.
Asparaginase: Concurrent use with methotrexate may result in decreased methotrexate antineoplastic activity.
Nephrotoxic agents (aminoglycosides or amphotericin B): May decrease renal function and the renal clearance of methotrexate. Avoid these drugs 24 hrs before or after methotrexate therapy.
Herbal
None known.

LAB EFFECTS/INTERFERENCE
May increase serum uric acid and AST (SGOT) levels.

Y-SITE COMPATIBILITIES
Allopurinol, amifostine, amphotericin B lipid colloid (Amphotec), asparaginase, bleomycin sulfate, cimetidine, cisplatin (Platinol AQ), cyclophosphamide (Cytoxan), cytarabine, dactinomycin, daunorubicin (DaunoXome), diphenhydramine, doxorubicin (Adriamycin), doxorubicin liposome (Doxil), etoposide (VePesid), etoposide phosphate (Etopophos), famotidine, filgrastim, fludarabine, granisetron (Kytril), leucovorin, melphalan, mesna, mitomycin (Mutamycin), ondansetron (Zofran), paclitaxel (Taxol), palonosetron, ranitidine, sargramostim, teniposide, thiotepa, trastuzumab, vinblastine (Velban), vincristine (Oncovin), vinorelbine (Navelbine)

INCOMPATIBILITIES
Chlorpromazine (Thorazine), dexamethasone, droperidol (Inapsine), fluorouracil, gemcitabine (Gemzar), idarubicin (Idamycin), ifosfamide, levofloxacin, midazolam (Versed), nalbuphine (Nubain), pantoprazole, prednisolone, promethazine, propofol, vancomycin

SIDE EFFECTS
Serious Reactions
- GI toxicity may produce gingivitis, glossitis, pharyngitis, stomatitis, enteritis, and hematemesis.
- Hepatotoxicity is more likely to occur with frequent small doses than with large intermittent doses.
- Pulmonary toxicity may be characterized by interstitial pneumonitis.
- Hematologic toxicity, which may develop rapidly from marked myelosuppression, may be manifested as leukopenia, thrombocytopenia, anemia, and hemorrhage.
- Dermatologic toxicity may produce a rash, pruritus, urticaria, pigmentation, photosensitivity, petechiae, ecchymosis, and pustules.
- Severe nephrotoxicity may produce azotemia, hematuria, and renal failure.

Other Side Effects
Frequent (10%-50%):
Nausea, vomiting, stomatitis
Occasional (1%-10%):
Burning and erythema at psoriatic site (in patients with psoriasis)
Rare (Less Than 1%):
Diarrhea, rash, dermatitis, pruritus, alopecia, dizziness, anorexia, malaise, headache, drowsiness, blurred vision

SPECIAL CONSIDERATIONS
Baseline Assessment
- Determine whether patient with psoriasis or rheumatoid arthritis is pregnant before initiating methotrexate therapy because the drug has a pregnancy risk category of X in these patients. It is category D for patients with malignancy.
- Evaluate diagnostic test results, including renal and liver function tests, CBC with differential levels, and platelet count, before and periodically during methotrexate therapy. Creatinine clearance should be

greater than 50 mL/min (adults) unless specified if recommended in a protocol.

- Give antiemetics, if ordered, to prevent or treat nausea and vomiting.

Intervention and Evaluation

- Monitor methotrexate serum concentrations for 1) all patients receiving high-dose methotrexate, 2) patients with moderate renal dysfunction, and 3) patients who have had excessive toxicity from prior methotrexate therapy.
- Monitor patient's complete blood count with differential, electrolytes, BUN, creatine, chest radiographs, liver and renal function test results, serum uric acid level, urinalysis results, platelet count, and WBC count with differential.
- Monitor patient for signs and symptoms of hematologic toxicity, including excessive fatigue and weakness, ecchymosis, fever, signs of local infection, sore throat, and unusual bleeding from any site.
- Examine patient's skin for evidence of dermatologic toxicity.
- As prescribed, administer IV fluids to keep patient well hydrated and medication, such as sodium bicarbonate, to alkalinize the urine in patients receiving high-dose methotrexate.
- Avoid giving IM injections, taking rectal temperatures, and performing traumatic procedures that may cause bleeding.
- Apply pressure to the IV site for 5 full mins after administration has been completed.

Education

- Urge patient to avoid receiving live virus vaccinations and contact with crowds and those with known infections.
- Educate patient on neutropenic precautions as necessary:
    Practice good handwashing technique.
    Avoid individuals who are ill.
    Wash and cook all foods well.
    Avoid crowds.
    Avoid fresh fruits and vegetables.
- Educate patient on thrombocytopenic precautions:
    Use of a soft bristle toothbrush.
    No flossing if platelet count is less than 50,000/mm³.
    No IM injections.
    No rectal suppositories.
    No aerobic exercise.
- Urge patient to avoid alcohol, salicylates, and overexposure to sun or ultraviolet light during methotrexate therapy.

- Teach both male and female patients contraceptive methods to use during therapy and for a certain period afterward.
- For patients who are discharged from the hospital before the completion of leucovorin therapy, instruct them to take the oral leucovorin doses as directed.
- Advise patient to avoid platelet-inhibiting drugs such as nonsteroidal agents (ibuprofen, indomethacin, and aspirin) as these will inhibit methotrexate renal clearance and worsen the toxic effects.
- Warn patient to report easy bruising, fever, signs of local infection, sore throat, and unusual bleeding from any site.
- Teach patient to maintain fastidious oral hygiene.
- Inform patient that alopecia is reversible, but that new hair may have a different color or texture.
- Caution patient to notify his or her health care provider if nausea and vomiting continue at home.

MITOMYCIN

BRAND NAMES
Mutamycin

CLASS OF AGENT
Antitumor antibiotic alkylating agent

CLINICAL PHARMACOLOGY
Mechanism of Action
An antineoplastic antibiotic grown from *Streptomyces caespitosus*. Its mechanism of action is thought to be an inhibition of DNA synthesis, a degradation of preformed DNA, nuclear lysis, and formation of giant cells. Mitomycin occurs as a bluish-grey lyophilized powder. It is an alkylating agent that requires activation by reduction of its quinone group and loss of the methoxy group.
Therapeutic effect: Cross-links strands of DNA and RNA. Inhibits protein synthesis.
Absorption and Distribution
The drug is administered IV and intravesically. Systemic absorption from bladder instillation is low.
Volume of distribution ranges from 11 to 49 L/m², indicating tissue distribution. Animal studies have revealed high concentrations of mitomycin in kidney, tongue, muscle, heart, and lung tissues 5 mins after a single IV dose of 4 mg/kg. No drug was detected in the brain.

Half-life: 23-78 mins.
Metabolism and Excretion
Mitomycin is metabolized rapidly in the liver. Metabolites are unknown. Renal excretion as unchanged drug is less than 10%. Because metabolic pathways are saturated at relatively low doses, the percentage of a dose excreted in urine increases with increasing dose.

HOW SUPPLIED/AVAILABLE FORMS
Powder for Injection: 5 mg; 20 mg; 40 mg.

INDICATIONS AND DOSAGES
Adenocarcinoma of the Stomach or Pancreas
Single doses of 10-20 mg/m^2 IV may be administered at 6- to 8-week intervals via a functioning IV catheter
Intravesical mitomycin (unlabeled):
20-40 mg in 40 mL of sterile water instilled into the bladder for 3 hrs after transurethral resection decreased the recurrence rate of superficial bladder cancer in a controlled trial. This procedure may be repeated up to 3 times/wk for up to 20 procedures. Other protocols have used weekly intravesical instillation of 30-60 mg in 20-60 mL of sterile water for injection for six doses and then monthly for 1 year.
Dosage Adjustment Based on Hematologic Status
Hematologic recovery should dictate mitomycin dosing; the manufacturer recommends the following dosage adjustment based on hematologic nadir:

Leukocytes	Platelets	Percentage of Prior Dose
>4000	>100,000	100
3000-3999	75,000-99,999	100
2000-2999	25,000-74,999	70
<2000	<25,000	50

Dosage Adjustment in Hepatic Dysfunction
No adjustments required.
Dosage Adjustment in Renal Dysfunction
The manufacturer recommends that mitomycin not be used in patients with a serum creatinine level greater than 1.7 mg/dL. Mitomycin clearance may be reduced in renal insufficiency and mitomycin is nephrotoxic. Others have recommended that patients with severe renal failure (glomerular filtration rate

[GFR] less than 10 mL/min) should receive 75% of the usual dose given at the normal dosage interval and no dose adjustments be made for patients with GFR >10 mL/min.

UNLABELED USES
Leukemia, chronic lymphocytic, palliative treatment, bladder cancer, breast cancer, colorectal cancer

PRECAUTIONS
Use cautiously in patients with chronic lymphocytic leukemia, hyperuricemia (especially in the treatment of lymphoma), leukopenia, thrombocytopenia, or anemia.
Pregnancy Risk Category: D

CONTRAINDICATIONS
Presence of known infectious diseases, previous anaphylactic reactions to mitomycin, coagulation disorders, thrombocytopenia, or increase in bleeding tendency due to other causes.

DRUG PREPARATION/ADMINISTRATION/ SAFE HANDLING ISSUES
◄ ALERT ► The dosage of this drug is individualized according to clinical response and the patient's tolerance to adverse effects. When used in combination therapy, consult specific protocols for optimum drug dosage and sequence of drug administration.
◄ ALERT ► Mitomycin may be carcinogenic, mutagenic, or teratogenic. Handle with extreme care during preparation and administration. When preparing this agent, use nitrile or latex gloves only. If a splash occurs, wash with mild soap and water; do not use waterless or antibacterial soap as either can increase the skin reaction. If an eye splash occurs, irrigate with copious amounts of water or 0.9% NaCl, irrigating from inner to outer canthus.
• Add sterile water for injection to mitomycin to make a final concentration of 0.5 mg/mL.
• Shake to dissolve. If product does not dissolve immediately, allow to stand at room temperature until solution is obtained.
• Dilute solution further in various IV fluids to a final concentration of 20-40 mcg/mL.

STORAGE AND STABILITY
• Mitomycin is stable for the lot life indicated on the package at room temperature.

- Although solutions reconstituted with sterile water for injection to a final concentration of 0.5 mg/mL will remain stable for 14 days refrigerated or 7 days at room temperature, the manufacturer recommends that the reconstituted drugs in sterile water for injection should be used within 24 hrs. Protect from light. Mitomycin C was not stable in either glass or plastic when dissolved in 5% dextrose injection.

INTERACTIONS
Drug
Live virus vaccines: May decrease patient's antibody response to vaccine, increase vaccine side effects, and potentiate viral replication.
Vincristine: When given after mitomycin may increase the incidence of bronchospasm.
Herbal
None known.

LAB EFFECTS/INTERFERENCE
May increase isocitric acid dehydrogenase and uric acid levels. May decrease cholinesterase level.

Y-SITE COMPATIBLES
Allopurinol, amifostine, bleomycin sulfate, cisplatin, cyclophosphamide, doxorubicin HCl, droperidol, fluorouracil, furosemide, granisetron HCl, heparin sodium, leucovorin calcium, melphalan HCl, methotrexate sodium, metoclopramide HCl, ondansetron HCl, oxaliplatin, paclitaxel, palonosetron, teniposide, thiotepa, trastuzumab, vinblastine sulfate, vincristine sulfate

INCOMPATIBLES
Aztreonam, cefepime HCl, etoposide, filgrastim, gemcitabine, pantoprazole, piperacillin sodium/tazobactam sodium, sargramostim, topotecan, vinorelbine tartrate

SIDE EFFECTS
Serious Reactions
- Drug extravasation often leads to local skin necrosis.
- Leukopenia, immunosuppression, infection, and thrombocytopenia may occur.
- Hepatotoxicity has been reported. Veno-occlusive disease of the liver clinically characterized by the development of hepatomegaly, ascites, and jaundice in association with altered liver function tests has been reported to occur after both standard and high-dose mitomycin therapy.
- Hemolytic uremic syndrome, consisting primarily of microangiopathic hemolytic anemia, thrombocytopenia, and irreversible renal failure, has been reported. The syndrome may occur at any time during systemic therapy with mitomycin as a single agent or in combination with other cytotoxic drugs; however, most cases occur at doses greater than or equal to 60 mg of mitomycin.
- Pulmonary toxicity has occurred infrequently but can be severe and may be life threatening. Dyspnea with a nonproductive cough and radiographic evidence of pulmonary infiltrates may be indicative of mitomycin-induced pulmonary toxicity.

Other Side Effects
Frequent (10%-50%):
Myelosuppression (especially thrombocytopenia), dermatitis, nausea, vomiting
Occasional (1%-10%):
Diarrhea, loss of appetite, metallic taste, drowsiness, headache, weakness
Rare (Less Than 1%):
Allergic reaction, hepatotoxicity, peptic ulcer, peripheral neuropathy

SPECIAL CONSIDERATIONS
Baseline Assessment
- Obtain CBC with differential, electrolyte, BUN, and creatinine levels, and liver function tests before dosing with this agent.
- Evaluate patient's history of nausea and vomiting as this agent is highly emetogenic.
- Be aware that this agent is a vesicant and the extravasation kit must be available before administration.
- Assess patient's peripheral veins and if access is poor, evaluate patient for a central venous access device.
- Assess patient's skin for any evidence of history of dermatologic problems.
Intervention and Evaluation
- Evaluate CBC with differential, electrolyte, BUN, and creatinine levels, and all liver function tests before each dose.
- Premedicate with antiemetics as ordered.
- Assess patient's access before each dose for consideration of placement of a vascular access device.
- Obtain the extravasation kit before administering this agent.

Mitotane 189

CANCER DRUGS

• Monitor patient for any evidence of significant nausea, vomiting or diarrhea after discharge home.
• Assess patient's skin for any evidence of dermatologic reactions before each dose.
• Evaluate patient for any evidence of infection, thrombocytopenia, or anemia.
• Monitor patient for increasing fatigue with each dose.
• Evaluate patient for any evidence of hepatic toxicity, right upper quadrant pain, pruritus, jaundice, or icterus.

Education
• Instruct patient this drug is a vesicant and to report any signs of pain or burning upon drug administration; educate patient on the side effects of extravasation, skin sloughing, and necrosis.
• Educate patient on antiemetics needed for this agent and to take the doses of antiemetics as ordered.
• Instruct patient on when to contact his or her health care provider: fever greater than (38° C) (greater than 101° F), chills, cough, shortness of breath, any evidence of easy bruising, bleeding, increasing fatigue, nausea lasting greater than 24 hours, diarrhea lasting greater than 24 hours, or the inability to take in at least 1500 mL of fluid in 24 hours.
• Advise the patient to report any increasing abdominal pain or fullness, change in color of urine or stool, increasing pruritus or jaundice
• Instruct patient skin reactions may occur in the forms of dermatitis, rashes or pruritus and to use a moisturizer if these occur and notify their heath care provider.
• Educate patient on neutropenic precautions as necessary:
  Practice good handwashing technique.
  Avoid individuals who are ill.
  Wash and cook all foods well.
  Avoid crowds.
  Avoid fresh fruits and vegetables.
• Educate patient on thrombocytopenic precautions:
  Use of a soft bristle toothbrush.
  No flossing if platelet count is less than 50,000/mm^3.
  No IM injections.
  No rectal suppositories.
  No aerobic exercise.
• Instruct patient to take no over-the-counter medications or herbal or vitamin supplements without checking with his or her health care provider.

• Provide patient with information on local resources and support groups available for his or her specific diagnosis

MITOTANE
BRAND NAMES
Lysodren

CLASS OF AGENT
Antineoplastic agent

CLINICAL PHARMACOLOGY
Mechanism of Action
An agent that inhibits adrenal activity by causing necrosis and atrophy of the adrenal cortex. Modifies peripheral metabolism of steroids as well. The biochemical mechanism is unknown. **Therapeutic Effect:** Suppresses functional and nonfunctional adrenocortical neoplasms by a direct cytotoxic effect.
Absorption and Distribution
Oral absorption is approximately 40%. Mitotane is distributed in most tissues of the body with fat tissues as the primary site. Blood levels are undetectable after 6-9 wks in most patients.
Half-life: 18-159 days.
Metabolism and Excretion
Approximately 10% is recovered in the urine as water-soluble metabolites. Excretion through bile ranges from 1% to 10%.

HOW SUPPLIED/AVAILABLE FORMS
Tablets: 500 mg.

INDICATIONS AND DOSAGES
Adrenocortical Carcinomas
Initially, 2-6 g/day PO in 3-4 divided doses. Increase by 2-4 g/day every 3-7 days up to usual dose of 9-10 g/day or to maximum tolerated dose. Range: 2-16 g/day. If after 3 mos at the maximum tolerated dose there is no clinical benefit then mitotane treatment is generally considered a clinical failure; however, 10% of patients require more than 3 mos of therapy. Continue therapy as long as there is a clinical benefit.
Dosage Adjustment in Hepatic/Renal Dysfunction
No information available. Use with caution.

UNLABELED USES
Treatment of Cushing's syndrome

PRECAUTIONS
Pregnancy Risk Category: C
Drug should be given only if the potential benefit justifies the potential risk to the fetus. Drug excretion into human breast milk is unknown/not recommended in nursing women.

CONTRAINDICATIONS
Known hypersensitivity to mitotane or any of its excipients.

DRUG PREPARATION/ADMINISTRATION/ SAFE HANDLING ISSUES
- Take in 3-4 divided doses.
- Mitotane is considered a hazardous agent. Wash hands before and after contact with the bottle or tablets.
- Do not crush or chew on a tablet. If a tablet is accidentally crushed, immediately wipe it up with a damp cloth and discard the cloth in a closed container such as a plastic bag.
- Symptoms of overdose should be treated with symptomatic and supportive care.

STORAGE AND STABILITY
Store at room temperature.

INTERACTIONS
Drug
CNS depressants: May increase CNS depression.
Warfarin (coumarin-type anticoagulants): May increase metabolism of warfarin. Monitor PT or INR. Adjust dose as needed.
Spironolactone: May decrease effectiveness of mitotane. Avoid concomitant use if possible.
Herbal
None known.

LAB EFFECTS/INTERFERENCE
May decrease levels of plasma cortisol, urinary 17-hydroxycorticosteroids, and protein-bound iodine.

SIDE EFFECTS
Serious Reactions
- Brain damage and functional impairment may occur with long-term, high-dose therapy.
- Adrenal insufficiency may develop. Mitotane should be interrupted after shock or severe trauma and exogenous steroids should be administered.

Other Side Effects
Frequent (10%-50%):
Anorexia, nausea, vomiting, diarrhea, lethargy, somnolence, adrenocortical insufficiency, dizziness, vertigo, maculopapular rash
Occasional (1%-10%):
Blurred or double vision, retinopathy, hearing loss, excessive salivation, urine abnormalities (hematuria, cystitis, albuminuria), hypertension, orthostatic hypotension, flushing, wheezing, dyspnea
Rare (Less Than 1%):
Generalized aching, fever, lowered protein-bound iodine level

SPECIAL CONSIDERATIONS
Baseline Assessment
- Obtain CBC with differential, electrolyte, BUN, and creatinine levels, and liver function tests.
- Note that it has been suggested that steroid replacement therapy be started along with initiation of mitotane therapy. Exogenous steroid metabolism may be modified and higher doses than normal for replacement may be required.
- Monitor baseline vital signs and oxygen saturation.
- Evaluate patient for history of hypertension or orthostatic hypotension.
- Assess patient for history of hearing loss, visual difficulties, or adrenal insufficiency.
- Evaluate patient for any evidence of pulmonary disease.
Intervention and Evaluation
- Evaluate laboratory data as needed at each visit.
- Monitor patient for side effects of nausea, lethargy, somnolence, visual deficits, auditory changes, or rashes.
- Monitor vital signs, evaluating B/P and checking for orthostatic changes and any evidence of hypertension. Sometimes mineralocorticoid replacement is required for orthostatic changes.
- Assess patient's pulmonary status at each visit.
- Evaluate for chronic nausea, which may be caused by this agent.
- Assess for evidence of diarrhea, lethargy, dizziness, and evidence of urinary changes.
- Perform complete behavioral and neurologic assessments at each visit as prolonged use of this agent may cause brain damage.

Education

- Instruct patient on when to contact his or her health care provider: fever greater than 38° C (greater than 101° F), chills, rigors, nausea lasting greater than 24 hours, diarrhea lasting greater than 24 hours, and the inability to drink at least 1500 mL of fluid in 24 hours.
- Educate patient on potential side effects of lethargy, somnolence, wheezing, myalgias, or achiness.
- Instruct patient to use caution when driving or operating machinery.
- Instruct patient to report to any visual or auditory changes.
- Educate patient on signs or symptoms of urinary tract abnormalities: frequency, urgency, burning, or pain upon urination.
- Encourage patient to drink at least 2 L of fluid per day.
- Teach patient to wash hands before and after contact with the bottle or tablet. People not taking mitotane should not be exposed to it.
- Instruct patient to avoid any OTC medications or herbal or vitamin supplements without first checking with the health care provider.
- Provide patient with information on local resources and support groups available for his or her specific diagnosis.

MITOXANTRONE HYDROCHLORIDE

BRAND NAMES
Novantrone

CLASS OF AGENT
Antineoplastic agent, anthracenedione

CLINICAL PHARMACOLOGY
Mechanism of Action
An anthracenedione that intercalates with DNA through hydrogen bonding and causes cross-links and strand breaks. Interferes with RNA and also acts as a topoisomerase II inhibitor, resulting in DNA repair damage. Mitoxantrone inhibits B-cell, T-cell, and macrophage proliferation and impairs antigen presentation.
Therapeutic Effect: Causes cell death throughout the entire cell cycle.
Absorption and Distribution
Protein binding: 78%. Binding is not affected by the presence of phenytoin, doxorubicin, methotrexate, prednisone, prednisolone, heparin, or aspirin. Widely distributed with a steady-state volume of distribution greater than 1000 L/m^2 as per the manufacturer.
Half-life: $t_{1/2}$ α: 6-12 mins; $t_{1/2}$ β 1.1-3.1 hrs; $t_{1/2}$ γ = 23-215 hrs.
Metabolism and Excretion
Metabolized in the liver into inactive metabolites, monocarboxylic and dicarboxylic acid derivatives and their glucuronide conjugates. The metabolic pathway is unknown. Mitoxanthrone is primarily eliminated in feces by the biliary system (25%). Urine excretion is 11%, consisting of 65% unchanged drug. It is not removed by hemodialysis.

HOW SUPPLIED/AVAILABLE FORMS
Injection: 2 mg/mL as 10-mL, 12.5-mL, 15-mL multidose vials.

INDICATIONS AND DOSAGES
Please refer to protocols for individual diseases as doses and schedules vary.
Acute Nonlymphocytic Leukemia (ANLL; Including Myelogenous, Promyelocytic, Monocytic, and Erythroid Acute Leukemias)
In Combination with Cytarabine:
Induction phase: mitoxantrone 12 mg/m^2/day IV for days 1-3.
Secondary induction: mitoxantrone 12 mg/m^2/day IV for days 1-2.
Consolidation phase: mitoxantrone 12 mg/m^2/day IV for days 1-2 usually 6 wks after the final induction course. Second consolidation therapy is administered 4 wks after the first consolidation course.
Hormone-Refractory Prostate Cancer
12-14 mg/m^2 IV every 21 days.
Multiple Sclerosis: Secondary (Chronic) Progressive, Progressive Relapsing, Worsening Relapsing-Remitting
12 mg/m^2/dose IV every 3 mos. Maximum lifetime dose is 140 mg/m^2.
Dosage Adjustment in Hepatic Dysfunction
No recommendations available. Consider dosage reduction as clearance is reduced with hepatic impairment. For severe hepatic dysfunction (total bilirubin level greater than 3.4 mg/dL), the area under the curve is more than 3 times greater than that of patients with normal function. Patients with multiple sclerosis who have hepatic dysfunction should not be treated with mitoxantrone.

Dosage Adjustment in Renal Dysfunction
No adjustments required.

UNLABELED USES
Treatment of breast cancer, ovarian cancer, hepatic carcinoma, non-Hodgkin's lymphoma

PRECAUTIONS
Use with caution in patients with preexisting myelosuppression and patients with severe hepatic dysfunction. Mitoxantrone may increase the risk of development of cardiac toxicity, which can be fatal in some patients, and secondary acute myelogenous leukemia (AML).
Pregnancy Risk Category: D
Mitoxantrone may cause fetal harm when given during pregnancy. Mitoxantrone is excreted into human breast milk in significant concentrations, and breast-feeding is not recommended during mitoxantrone therapy.

CONTRAINDICATIONS
Hypersensitivity to mitoxantrone or any component of the formulation. For patients with multiple sclerosis: baseline left ventricular ejection fraction (LVEF) less than 50% or a clinically significant decrease in LVEF, cumulative lifetime mitoxantrone dose is 140 mg/m^2 or hepatic impairment.

DRUG PREPARATION/ADMINISTRATION/ SAFE HANDLING ISSUES
◀ ALERT ▶ Because mitoxantrone may be carcinogenic, mutagenic, or teratogenic, wear nitrile or latex, but not vinyl, gloves when handling the drug. If the drug comes in contact with skin, wash the skin thoroughly with soap and water. Do not use the waterless hand soap or any antibacterial soap as either can increase the reaction from the agent. If the drug comes in contact with mucous membranes, flush the area with water.
◀ ALERT ▶ Do not administer when ANC is less than 1500 cells/mm^3 (except for ANLL).
• Mitoxantrone is considered an irritant and may cause tissue necrosis. If extravasation symptoms occur, such as blue skin discoloration, burning, pain, pruritus, erythema, and swelling ulceration, discontinue at that site and start at another vein. Use intermittent ice packs and elevate affected extremity. Examine area frequently.

• Dilute dose into at least 50 mL of 0.9% NaCl, D5W, or dextrose 5% in 0.9% NaCl.
• Infuse over 10-30 mins (no less than 3 mins).

STORAGE AND STABILITY
• Store intact vials at room temperature.
• Punctured multidose vials are stable for 7 days at 15-25° C (59-77° F) or 14 days under refrigeration. Contains no preservatives.

INTERACTIONS
Drug
Does not inhibit cytochrome P450 (CYP) 1A2, 2A6, 2C9, 2C19, 2D6, 2E1, or 3A4.
Bone marrow depressants: May increase myelosuppression.
Live virus vaccines: May potentiate viral replication, increase vaccine side effects, and decrease the patient's antibody response to the vaccine.
Herbal
None known.

LAB EFFECTS/INTERFERENCE
May increase serum bilirubin, AST (SGOT), ALT (SGPT), and uric acid levels.

Y-SITE COMPATIBLES
Allopurinol (Aloprim), carboplatin, carmustine, cisplatin, cladribine, cyclophosphamide, cytarabine, dexrazoxane, docetaxel, etoposide (VePesid), filgrastim, fludarabine, gemcitabine (Gemzar), granisetron (Kytril), ifosfamide, leucovorin, melphalan, mesna, methotrexate, ondansetron (Zofran), oxaliplatin, palonosetron, potassium chloride, rituximab, sargramostim, trastuzumab, vinorelbine

INCOMPATIBLES
Amphotericin B colloidal (Amphotec), amphotericin B conventional, amphotericin B liposomal (AmBisome), ampicillin, ampicillin/sulbactam, azithromycin, aztreonam, cefazolin, cefepime, cefoperazone, cefotaxime, cefoxitin, ceftazidime, ceftriaxone, cefuroxime, clindamycin, dantrolene, dexamethasone, diazepam, digoxin, doxorubicin, foscarnet, fosphenytoin, furosemide, heparin, lansoprazole, methylprednisolone, nafcillin, nitroprusside, paclitaxel (Taxol), pantoprazole, pemetrexed, phenytoin, piperacillin/tazobactam (Zosyn), propofol, sodium phosphates, ticarcillin, ticarcillin/clavulanate, voriconazole

SIDE EFFECTS
Serious Reactions
- Myelosuppression may be severe. The nadir occurs in 10 days with recovery in 21 days. Do not administer when ANC is less than 1500 cells/mm³ (except for ANLL).
- Cardiac toxicity, such as decreases in LVEF and irreversible CHF can occur. CHF can occur during therapy or months to years after termination of therapy. Cardiac toxicity is more common in patients with prior treatment with anthracyclines, prior mediastinal radiation, or with preexisting cardiovascular disease.
- Development of secondary AML occurs rarely.

Other Side Effects
Frequent (10%-50%):
Abdominal discomfort, alopecia (mild hair thinning), anorexia, cough, diarrhea, fever, headache, nausea (mild to moderate), stomatitis, vomiting
Occasional (1%-10%):
Anemia, arrhythmias, bruising, conjunctivitis, constipation, decreased LVEF, ecchymosis, abnormal EKG, edema, elevated liver enzymes, fungal infection, menstrual disorder, myelosuppression, nail bed changes, jaundice, upper respiratory infection, urine blue-green color (1-2 days), urinary tract infection
Rare (Less Than 1%):
Anaphylactoid reaction

SPECIAL CONSIDERATIONS
Baseline Assessment
- Obtain CBC with differential, platelet count, electrolyte, BUN, and creatinine levels, and liver function tests.
- Assess patient for any history of renal disease or GI bleeding.
- Evaluate for history of use of other chemotherapeutic agents and any difficulty with emesis.
- Obtain a baseline MUGA scan or echocardiogram to asses for ejection fraction (EF) before dosing; EF should be greater than 50% or per protocol.
- Monitor for evidence of cardiac history, CHF, or arrhythmias.
- Assess allergy history.
- Obtain a pregnancy test for women of childbearing potential.

Intervention and Evaluation
- Assess laboratory parameters before each dose.
- Assess MUGA scan or echocardiogram before dosing; avoid dosing if EF is less than 50%.
- Perform a pregnancy test for female patients of childbearing potential with multiple sclerosis before every dose.
- Vital signs before each dose along with oxygen saturation.
- Assess need to do an EKG before dosing if any arrhythmia is detected.
- Premedicate as ordered.
- Monitor for evidence of anaphylaxis.
- Assess patient for evidence of myelosuppression, anemia, neutropenia, and thrombocytopenia.
- Educate patient on neutropenic precautions as necessary:
  Practice good handwashing technique.
  Avoid individuals who are ill.
  Wash and cook all foods well.
  Avoid crowds.
  Avoid fresh fruits and vegetables.
- Educate patient on thrombocytopenic precautions:
  Use of a soft bristle toothbrush.
  No flossing if platelet count is less than 50,000/mm³.
  No IM injections.
  No rectal suppositories.
  No aerobic exercise.
- Initiate oral care regimen if oral ulcers are present.
- Monitor patient for upper respiratory infections and urinary tract infections.
- Assess patient for evidence of pulmonary changes.

Education
- Instruct patient on when to contact his or her health care provider: fever greater than 38° C (greater than 101° F), chills, cough, shortness of breath, nausea lasting greater than 24 hours, diarrhea lasting greater than 24 hours, or the inability to drink at least 1500 mL of fluid in 24 hours.
- Educate patient the urine will change color for 24-48 hours.
- Advise patient that alopecia will occur and when hair recovers it may have a different color and consistency.
- Instruct patient in neutropenic precautions as needed:
  Practice good handwashing technique.
  Cook all foods.
  Avoid fresh fruits or vegetables.
  Avoid fresh flowers.
  Avoid all persons with infection and crowds.

- Instruct patient on thrombocytopenic precautions:
  Use soft toothbrush.
  Avoid flossing.
  Avoid straight razors; use electric razors only.
  Avoid shaving legs (women).
  Avoid heavy lifting and strenuous activities.
- Educate patient that menstrual irregularities and amenorrhea are usual for this agent.
- Instruct patient on the usual side effects: nausea, fatigue, mouth sores, constipation, and diarrhea.
- If mouth sores occur, initiate an oral care regimen. An example is 1 tsp each of salt and baking soda dissolved in 1 glass of water to swish and spit at least 4 times/day.
- Advise patient to avoid all OTC preparations or herbal or vitamin supplements without first checking with the health care provider.
- Provide patient with information on local resources and support groups available for his or her specific diagnosis.

NELARABINE

BRAND NAMES
Arranon

CLASS OF AGENT
Antineoplastic agent, antimetabolite

CLINICAL PHARMACOLOGY
Mechanism of Action
A prodrug of deoxyguanosine analog 9-β-D-arabinofuranosylguanine (ara-G), which is subsequently converted to ara-GTP. Ara-GTP accumulation in leukemic blasts results in incorporation into deoxyribonucleic acid. **Therapeutic Effect:** Inhibits DNA synthesis and causes cell death.

Absorption and Distribution
Extensively distributed throughout the body. Apparent steady-state volumes of distribution were 197 ± 216 and 33 ± 9.3 L/m^2 for adult and pediatric patients.
Half-life: Nelarabine = 30 mins; ara-G = 3 hrs; ara-GTP = unknown (too long to calculate)

Metabolism and Excretion
Primary metabolism is through O-demethylation by adenosine deaminase to form ara-G, which undergoes hydrolysis to form guanine. Some nelarabine is hydrolyzed to form methylguanine, which is O-demethylated to form guanine. Guanine is N-deaminated to form xanthine, which is oxidized to uric acid. Nelarabine and ara-G are eliminated by kidneys with $6.6 \pm 4.7\%$ and $27 \pm 15\%$ of administered dose, respectively.

HOW SUPPLIED/AVAILABLE FORMS
Solution for Injection: 250 mg (5 mg/mL) vials.

INDICATIONS AND DOSAGES
T-Cell Acute Lymphoblastic Leukemia and T-Cell Lymphoblastic Lymphoma That Has Not Responded to or Relapse after Two Prior Therapies
1500 mg/m^2/dose IV on days 1, 3, and 5 repeated every 3 wks

Dosage Adjustment for Neurologic Events
Discontinue nelarabine for neurologic events of National Cancer Institute Common Toxicity Criteria grade 2 or higher. Full recovery has not always occurred with discontinuation of therapy.

Dosage Adjustment in Hepatic Dysfunction
Has not been evaluated in patients with hepatic dysfunction. Use with caution.

Dosage Adjustment in Renal Dysfunction
No adjustments required for CrCl greater than or equal to 50 mL/min. No recommendations available for CrCl less than 50 mL/min; monitor for toxicities. The kidney excretes 5%-10% of nelarabine, whereas 20%-30% of ara-G is excreted. The mean clearance of ara-G was 15%-40% lower in patients with mild and moderate renal impairment, respectively, compared with patients with normal renal function.

UNLABELED USES
No information.

PRECAUTIONS
Neurotoxicity is the dose-limiting toxicity and includes somnolence, confusion, convulsions, ataxia, paraesthesias, hypoesthesia, coma, status epilepticus, craniospinal demyelination, or ascending neuropathy similar in presentation to Guillain-Barré syndrome. Neuropathies have ranged from numbness and paresthesias to motor weakness and paralysis. Patients are at risk for tumor lysis

syndrome and should receive IV hydration and/or allopurinol. Seizures have occurred.

Pregnancy Risk Category: D
Nelarabine may cause fetal harm when administered during pregnancy. Drug excretion into breast milk is unknown/ not recommended in nursing women.

CONTRAINDICATIONS
Hypersensitivity to nelarabine or any component of the formulation

DRUG PREPARATION/ADMINISTRATION/ SAFE HANDLING ISSUES
◀ ALERT ▶ Because nelarabine may be carcinogenic, mutagenic, or teratogenic, wear nitrile or latex, but not vinyl, gloves when handling the drug. If the drug comes in contact with skin, wash the skin thoroughly with soap and water. Do not use waterless hand soap or any antibacterial soap as either can increase the reaction from the agent. If the drug comes in contact with mucous membranes, flush the area with water.

- Nelarabine is not diluted before administration.
- Draw up dose and transfer to an empty polyvinyl chloride (PVC) infusion bag or glass container.
- Infuse over 2 hrs for adults and 1 hr for children.

STORAGE AND STABILITY
- Store intact vials at room temperature of 20° C (77° F); excursions permitted to 15-30° C (59-86° F).
- Drug is stable in PVC infusion bags and glass containers for up to 8 hrs at 30° C (86° F).

INTERACTIONS
Drug
Nelarabine: does not inhibit cytochrome P450 (CYP) enzymes 1A2, 2A6, 2B6, 2C8, 2C9, 2C19, 2D6, or 3A4 in vitro.
Herbal
No information.

LAB EFFECTS/INTERFERENCE
May decrease WBC and platelet counts and increase uric acid levels.

Y-SITE COMPATIBLES
None known.

INCOMPATIBLES
None known.

SIDE EFFECTS
Serious Reactions
- Severe neurotoxicity, such as coma, status epilepticus, craniospinal demyelination, or ascending neuropathy similar to presentation to Guillain-Barré syndrome, has been reported. Discontinue drug if neurologic events of grade 2 or higher occur. Full recovery has not always occurred with discontinuation of therapy.
- Patients are at risk for tumor lysis syndrome and should receive IV hydration and/or allopurinol.
- Myelosuppression is expected with nelarabine.

Other Side Effects
Frequent (10%-50%):
CNS: Dizziness, somnolence, headache, hypoesthesia, paresthesia, peripheral neurologic disorders (neuropathy, peripheral neuropathy, motor neuropathy, sensory neuropathy)
General: Asthenia, fatigue, fever, peripheral edema, edema, pain
GI: Diarrhea, constipation, nausea, vomiting
Hematologic: Anemia, thrombocytopenia, neutropenia febrile neutropenia
Respiratory: Cough, dyspnea, pleural effusion
Occasional (1%-10%):
Cardiovascular: Hypotension, tachycardia
CNS: Amnesia, ataxia, balance disorder, depressed level of consciousness, dysgeusia, paresthesia, sensory loss, tremor
General: Abnormal gait, chest pain, non-cardiac chest pain, rigors
GI: Abdominal pain, abdominal distension, stomatitis
Infections: Infection, pneumonia, sinusitis
Metabolism: Anorexia, dehydration, hyperglycemia
Musculoskeletal: Arthralgia, back pain, muscular weakness, myalgia
Respiratory: Epistaxis, wheezing
Vascular: Petechiae
Rare (Less Than 1%):
Aphasia, convulsion, hemiparesis, loss of consciousness, cerebral hemorrhage, intracranial hemorrhage, leukoencephalopathy, metabolic encephalopathy, abnormal coordination, burning sensation, disturbance in attention, dysarthria, hyporeflexia, nystagmus, peroneal nerve palsy, sciatica

SPECIAL CONSIDERATIONS
Baseline Assessment
- Assess CBC with differential, platelet count, electrolyte, magnesium, phosphorus,

calcium, BUN, creatinine, glucose, and uric acid levels and liver function tests.
- Assess patient for any evidence or history of seizure disorder, peripheral neuropathy, respiratory disorders, or cardiac problems.
- Evaluate patient for evidence of muscle weakness, arthralgias, or myalgias before initiation of therapy.
- Assess patient for history of GI problems, nausea, vomiting, or diarrhea.

Intervention and Evaluation
- Monitor laboratory data before each dosing, paying particular attention to the CBC with differential, electrolyte, BUN, creatinine, and glucose levels and tumor lysis laboratory data as tumor lysis syndrome has been reported with this agent.
- Monitor patient for any changes in neurologic, cardiac, or respiratory status.
- Evaluate patient for evidence of seizures or neurologic changes such as an ascending myelopathy as Guillain-Barré syndrome has been reported with this agent.
- Assess patient for any evidence of nausea, vomiting, or diarrhea, and initiate therapy as ordered.
- Monitor patient for evidence of hyperglycemia.
- Monitor vital signs, looking for evidence of decreased oxygen saturation or evidence of tachycardia or arrhythmias.
- Monitor for evidence of neutropenia and thrombocytopenia.
- Initiate neutropenic and thrombocytopenic precautions as needed per institutional guidelines.

Education
- Instruct patient on when to contact his or her health care provider: fever greater than 38° C (greater than 101° F), cough, shortness of breath, chills, evidence of numbness or tingling in fingers and toes, seizure activity, weakness, palpitations, nausea lasting greater than 24 hours, diarrhea lasting greater than 24 hours, or the inability to take in at least 1500 mL of fluid in 24 hours.
- Educate patient on neutropenic precautions:
  Practice good handwashing techniques.
  Avoid raw fruits and vegetables.
  Avoid crowds.
  Avoid contact with individuals who are ill.
  Wash and cook all foods well.
- Instruct patient on thrombocytopenic precautions:

Do not use rectal suppositories.
Use a soft toothbrush.
Avoid flossing teeth if platelet count is less than 50,000/mm³.
Avoid strenuous and aerobic exercise.
No IM injections.
- Instruct patient on the use of antinausea and antidiarrheal medications as necessary.
- Instruct patient to avoid all OTC medications and herbal and vitamin supplements without first checking with the health care provider.
- Provide patient with information on local resources and support groups available for his or her specific diagnosis.

NILUTAMIDE

BRAND NAMES
Nilandron

CLASS OF AGENT
Antineoplastic agent, antiandrogen

CLINICAL PHARMACOLOGY
Mechanism of Action
Used as a complement to surgical/chemical castration, nilutamide is a non-steroidal, antiandrogen hormone that competitively inhibits androgen action by binding to androgen receptors in target tissue. Nilutamide does not affect mineralocorticoid, glucocorticoid, progesterone, or estrogen levels.
Therapeutic Effect: Decreases growth of abnormal prostate tissue.
Absorption and Distribution
Completely and rapidly absorbed. Steady state is reached within 2-4 wks for most patients. Protein binding: 80%.
Half-life: 38-59 hrs.
Metabolism and Excretion
Extensively metabolized in the liver into five metabolites. Eliminated in urine (62%) during the first 120 mins. Fecal elimination 1.4%-7%).

HOW SUPPLIED/AVAILABLE FORMS
Tablets: 150 mg.

INDICATIONS AND DOSAGES
Metastatic Prostate Cancer in Combination with Surgical Castration
300 mg PO daily for 30 days, then 150 mg PO daily. Begin on day of, or day after, surgical castration.

Dosage Adjustment in Hepatic Dysfunction

Discontinue nilutamide pending diagnostic workup if marked increases of liver enzymes or sign/symptoms of liver damage occur.

Dosage Adjustment in Renal Dysfunction

No information available.

UNLABELED USES

No information.

PRECAUTIONS

Pregnancy Risk Category: C

Nilutamide is indicated for men only.

CONTRAINDICATIONS

Severe hepatic impairment, severe respiratory insufficiency, known hypersensitivity to nilutamide or its excipients

DRUG PREPARATION/ADMINISTRATION/ SAFE HANDLING ISSUES

- Take tablets without regard to food.
- Begin nilutamide on day of, or day after, surgical castration.
- Overdosage: dose tolerance studies of repeated doses of 600 and 900 mg/day resulted in GI disorders, nausea, vomiting, malaise, headache, dizziness, and transient hepatic enzyme elevations. One case of a single ingestion of 13 g did not result in serious adverse events. Supportive care including frequent monitoring of vital signs, pulmonary symptoms, and liver function tests under close observation is indicated. Therapy may include gastric lavage and/or activated charcoal. Emesis induction should be considered if situation is safe and appropriate. Dialysis is unlikely to be of benefit.

STORAGE AND STABILITY

Store at 25° C (77° F) (excursions allowed 15-30° C [(59-86° F]).

INTERACTIONS

Drug

Alcohol: Disulfiram reaction in 5% of patients.

Phenytoin and theophylline: May decrease phenytoin/theophylline elimination and lead to toxicity. May need to adjust phenytoin/theophylline dose.

Warfarin: May increase warfarin effect. Monitor prothrombin time or international normalized ratio; may need to adjust warfarin dose

Herbal

None known.

LAB EFFECTS/INTERFERENCE

May increase serum bilirubin, creatinine, AST (SGOT), and ALT (SGPT) levels.

SIDE EFFECTS

Serious Reactions

- Interstitial pneumonitis occurs rarely. Symptoms include dyspnea, cough, chest pain, and fever and in most cases occurred within the first 3 months of treatment. X-rays showed alveolointerstitial changes. If symptoms occur, nilutamide should be discontinued until it can be determined whether they are drug related. Routine x-rays and baseline pulmonary function tests should be done before nilutamide treatment is initiated.
- Cases of aplastic anemia without certain causal relationship with nilutamide have been reported in postmarketing surveillance.
- Visual disturbances have been reported if there is a delay of seconds to minutes in recovering vision when passing from a lighted area to a dark area. Wearing tinted glasses during the day may help alleviate this side effect. Use caution when driving at night or through tunnels.

Other Side Effects

Frequent (10%-50%):

Alcohol intolerance, asthenia, constipation, diminished sexual function, generalized pain, gynecomastia, hepatic enzyme elevation, hot flashes, impaired adaptation to dark, insomnia, mild nausea, peripheral edema

Occasional (1%-10%):

Abnormal vision, anorexia, chest pain, decreased libido, depression, dizziness, dyspnea, flu-like symptoms, headache, hypertension, pneumonia, rash, sweating, upper respiratory infection, urinary tract infections

Rare (Less Than 1%):

Angina, body hair loss, diarrhea, dry mouth, GI disorders, heart failure, interstitial pneumonitis, malaise, syncope

SPECIAL CONSIDERATIONS

Baseline Assessment

- Assess baseline CBC with differential, platelet count, electrolyte, BUN, and creatinine levels, and liver function tests.
- Assess alcohol history as this agent can induce intolerance.

- Evaluate patient for any evidence of visual changes or disturbances.
- Assess for evidence of hypertension, cardiac history, or urinary tract infections.
- Evaluate pulmonary status and smoking history for evidence of chronic obstructive pulmonary disease as this agent rarely induces interstitial pneumonitis.
- Obtain baseline weight, assess for any evidence of edema.

Intervention and Evaluation
- Monitor vital signs at each visit, assessing for evidence of hypertension.
- Assess pulmonary status and any evidence of changes.
- Evaluate for any evidence of visual changes or disturbances.
- Assess patient for evidence of sexual dysfunction, impotence, or gynecomastia.
- Evaluate patient for night sweats, mood changes, insomnia, irritability, and depression and make appropriate referrals.
- Assess pain for evidence of increasing pain in areas of abdomen or back.
- Monitor weight at each visit, and assess patient for evidence of peripheral edema.

Education
- Instruct patient on when to contact his or her health care provider: fever greater than 38° C (greater than 101° F), chills, respiratory changes, nausea lasting greater than 24 hrs, or the inability to take in at least 1500 mL of fluid in 24 hrs.
- Educate patient on usual side effects of this agent: alcohol intolerance and visual changes. Encourage patient not to drive at night and to wear tinted glasses during the day when driving to help adjust from lighted to darker areas.
- Encourage patient to report changes in sexual function, such as impotence, gynecomastia, and hot flashes.
- Encourage patient to drink at least 2 L of fluid per day as this agent has been associated with increased risk of urinary tract infections and cause constipation.
- Encourage patient to monitor weight gain and assess for any evidence of increasing peripheral edema.
- Instruct patient to not take any over-the-counter medications or herbal or vitamin supplements without first checking with his or her health care provider as they can affect the efficacy of this agent.
- Provide patient with information on local resources and support groups available for his or her specific diagnosis.

OPRELVEKIN (INTERLEUKIN-11, IL-11)

BRAND NAMES
Neumega

CLASS OF AGENT
Thrombopoietic growth factor, human interleukin-11

CLINICAL PHARMACOLOGY
Mechanism of Action
A recombinant thrombopoietic growth factor that stimulates the proliferation of hematopoietic stem cells and megakaryocyte progenitors and induces megakaryocytic maturation, which leads to production of blood platelets. **Therapeutic Effect:** Increases platelet production to prevent severe thrombocytopenia and to reduce the need for platelet transfusions.

Absorption and Distribution
Absolute bioavailability: 80% or more. Volume of distribution: 112-152 mL/kg. *Half-life:* Single subcutaneous infusion: 6.9-8.1 hrs. Single IV infusion: 1.8-2.4 hrs.

Metabolism and Excretion
There are few data on metabolism. Oprelvekin is excreted extensively through the urine. Total body clearance: 2.2-2.7 mL/min/kg; clearance decreases with age and is about 1.2-1.6 times faster in children than in adults.

HOW SUPPLIED/AVAILABLE FORMS
Injection: 5 mg powder for reconstitution

INDICATIONS AND DOSAGES
Prevention of Thrombocytopenia
50 mcg/kg subcutaneously once daily. Continue for 14-21 days or until platelet count reaches 50,000 cells/mm^3 after its nadir. Discontinue the drug at least 2 days before the start of the next chemotherapy cycle. *Pediatrics:* A safe and effective dose of oprelvekin in children has not been established. According to package insert, oprelvekin should not be administered to pediatric patients, particularly those younger than 12 years of age, other than in a clinical trial setting.

Dosage Adjustment in Hepatic Dysfunction
No adjustments required.

Dosage Adjustment in Renal Dysfunction
Not provided by manufacturer; however, clearance of oprelvekin in patients with severe renal impairment (CrCl less than

15 mL/min) was approximately 40% of the value of normal subjects.

PRECAUTIONS
Use oprelvekin cautiously in patients with or susceptible to developing left ventricular dysfunction or CHF and in those with a history of atrial arrhythmia or heart failure. Oprelvekin may cause severe fluid retention; therefore, use cautiously in patients with conditions in which plasma volume expansion may be detrimental (hypertension and preexisting fluid collections, including pericardial/pleural effusions or ascites). In addition, patients should not receive oprelvekin after myeloablative chemotherapy.
Pregnancy Risk Category: C
Drug excretion into human breast milk is unknown/not recommended in nursing women.

CONTRAINDICATIONS
Hypersensitivity to oprelvekin or any component of its formulation

DRUG PREPARATION/ADMINISTRATION/ SAFE HANDLING ISSUES
- Add 1 mL of sterile water for injection to provide concentration of 5 mg/mL oprelvekin. Inject along inside surface of vial, and swirl contents gently to avoid excessive agitation.
- Discard unused portion.
- Give single injection in the abdomen, thigh, hip, or upper arm.
- Begin oprelvekin administration 6-24 hrs after completion of chemotherapy dose.

STORAGE AND STABILITY
- Store in refrigerator. Do not freeze. Once reconstituted, use within 3 hrs.

INTERACTIONS
Drug
Diuretics: May increase the risk of hypokalemia.
Herbal
None known.

LAB EFFECTS/INTERFERENCE
Dilutional anemia appears within 3 days of initiation of therapy and resolves in about 1 wk after cessation of oprelvekin.

Y-SITE COMPATIBLES
Do not mix with other drugs.

SIDE EFFECTS
Serious Reactions
- Severe fluid retention may exacerbate conditions such as cardiac dysfunction, CHF, hypertension, and ascites.
- Anaphylaxis is rarely reported.
Other Side Effects
Frequent (10%-50%):
Atrial arrhythmias, dizziness, dyspnea, fatigue, fever, fluid retention, insomnia, headache, nausea, palpitations, peripheral edema, rash, tachycardia, vomiting
Occasional (1%-10%):
Pleural effusions, syncope, weight gain
Rare (Less Than 1%):
Anaphylaxis

SPECIAL CONSIDERATIONS
Baseline Assessment
- Assess CBC with differential, electrolyte, BUN, creatinine, and magnesium levels, and liver function tests.
- Obtain baseline EKG to assess arrhythmias.
- Assess baseline B/P for any evidence of hypotension.
- Monitor weight.
Intervention and Evaluation
- Assess laboratory data before each dose, paying particular attention to electrolyte levels.
- Evaluate vital signs for evidence of hypotension before each dose.
- Assess EKG before each high dose for evidence of arrhythmias.
- Premedicate for nausea as ordered.
- Monitor for evidence of neutropenia, and initiate neutropenic precautions as needed.
- Weigh patient before each dose to assess for fluid retention, and assess for evidence of pulmonary edema.
- Monitor patient for evidence of thrombocytopenia, and initiate thrombocytopenic precautions as needed.
- Avoid the use of all steroids as these will reverse the activity of this agent.
Education
- Instruct patient on when to contact his or her health care provider: fever greater than 38° C (greater than 101° F), chills, shortness of breath, weight gain of greater than 2 kg per day, nausea lasting greater than 24 hours, diarrhea lasting greater than 24 hours, or the inability to take in at least 1500 mL of fluid in 24 hours.
- Educate patient on the possibility of weight gain, changes in respiratory functions,

cough, shortness of breath, and dyspnea upon exertion.

* Instruct patient on neutropenic precautions: Practice good handwashing techniques. Avoid crowds and persons who are ill. Avoid fresh fruits and vegetables. Cook all food well. Avoid crowds.
* Advise patient on thrombocytopenic precautions:
  Use a soft toothbrush.
  Avoid flossing if platelets are less than 50,000/mm³.
  Avoid heavy lifting or strenuous activities.
  Use an electric razor, not a straight razor.
  No IM injections.
* Instruct patient to report any signs of rapid heart rate, palpitations, lightheadedness, or feeling faint.
* Educate patient to avoid all OTC medications and herbal and vitamin supplements without first checking with his or her health care provider.
* Provide patient with information on local resources and support groups available for his or her specific diagnosis.

OXALIPLATIN

BRAND NAMES
Eloxatin

CLASS OF AGENT
Antineoplastic agent, alkylating agent

CLINICAL PHARMACOLOGY
Mechanism of Action
A platinum-containing complex that cross-links with DNA strands, preventing cell division. Cell cycle phase nonspecific. Although the exact mechanism of oxaliplatin is unknown, its cytotoxic action results from inhibition of DNA synthesis. Oxaliplatin forms DNA intrastrand adducts by cross-linking of activated platinum species and either adjacent guanine residues or adjacent guanine-adenine bases. **Therapeutic Effect:** Inhibits DNA replication.
Absorption and Distribution
Oxaliplatin is administered IV only. It is rapidly distributed and has a volume of distribution of ultrafilterable platinum of 440 L after a single 2-hour infusion of 85 mg/m² oxaliplatin.
Protein binding: 70%-90%.

Half-life: Ultrafilterable platinum concentrations fall in a triexponential manner. It has α and β half-lives (0.43 hour and 16.8 hours, respectively) and a long terminal γ half-life (391 hours).
Metabolism and Excretion
Oxaliplatin is rapidly and extensively biotransformed nonenzymatically to 17 different platinum-containing derivatives. In vitro data have demonstrated 30% biotransformation after 1 hour (based on total platinum) and no unchanged oxaliplatin after 2 hours. In vitro studies indicate no cytochrome P450-mediated metabolism. Oxaliplatin is excreted in the urine. Its renal clearance ranges from 9.3 to 17 L/hour and correlates with glomerular filtration rate.

HOW SUPPLIED/AVAILABLE FORMS
Solution for Injection: 5 mg/mL as 10-mL vials, 20-mL vials.

INDICATIONS AND DOSAGES
Oxaliplatin in combination with infusional 5-fluorouracil (FU)/leucovorin (LV) is indicated for adjuvant treatment of stage III colon cancer in patients who have undergone complete resection of the primary tumor. The indication is based on an improvement in disease-free survival with no demonstrated benefit in overall survival after a median follow-up of 4 years.
Oxaliplatin in combination with infusional 5-FU/LV is indicated for the treatment of advanced carcinoma of the colon or rectum.
Day 1: Oxaliplatin 85 mg/m² in 250-500 mL D5W and LV 200 mg/m², both given simultaneously over more than 2 hours in separate bags using a Y-line, followed by 5-FU 400 mg/m² IV bolus given over 2-4 minutes, followed by 5-FU 600 mg/m² in 500 mL D5W as a 22-hour continuous IV infusion. *Day 2:* Leucovorin 200 mg/m² IV infusion given over more than 2 hours, followed by 5-FU 400 mg/m² IV bolus given over 2-4 minutes, followed by 5-FU 600 mg/m² in 500 mL D5W as a 22-hour continuous IV infusion.
Dosage Adjustment in Hepatic Dysfunction
No adjustments required.
Dosage Adjustment in Renal Dysfunction
The safety and effectiveness of oxaliplatin/ 5-FU/LV has not been evaluated in patients with renal impairment. However, because the primary route of elimination is

renal, caution should be used in patients with mild to severe renal impairment.

Dosage Adjustment for Elderly Patients
Age has no significant effect on the clearance of ultrafiltrable platinum. In a randomized study, adverse events, including grade 3 or 4, were similar among patients younger than and older than 65 years of age. However, a higher incidence of diarrhea, dehydration, leukopenia, syncope, hypokalemia, and fatigue was seen in patients older than 65 years of age.

Dosage Adjustment for Neurotoxicity
Grade 2 neurosensory events that do not resolve. Consider reducing the dose to 65 mg/m^2. Grade 3 neurosensory events: discontinue oxaliplatin.

Dosage Adjustment for GI Events (Abdominal Pain, Diarrhea, Mucositis, or Emesis)
Grade 3 or 4: Decrease the oxaliplatin dose to 65mg/m^2 and infusional fluorouracil by 20% (300 mg/m^2 bolus) or 500 mg/m^2 as a 22-hr continuous IV infusion).

Dosage Adjustment for Hematologic Events
Grade 3 or 4 neutropenia or thrombocytopenia: decrease the oxaliplatin dose to 65 mg/m^2 and infusional 5-FU by 20% (300 mg/m^2 bolus) or 500 mg/m^2 as a 22-hour continuous IV infusion).

UNLABELED USES
Ovarian cancer, metastatic pancreatic cancer

PRECAUTIONS
Use oxaliplatin cautiously in patients with peripheral neuropathy (past or present), impaired renal function, or infection; in pregnant or immunosuppressed patients; and in those who have previously been treated with other antineoplastic drugs or radiation.
Pregnancy Risk Category: D

CONTRAINDICATIONS
History of allergy to platinum compounds

DRUG PREPARATION/ADMINISTRATION/ SAFE HANDLING ISSUES
◀ **ALERT** ▶ Because oxaliplatin may be mutagenic, teratogenic, and carcinogenic, wear nitrile or latex gloves during drug preparation and administration. If the solution comes in contact with skin, wash the skin immediately with mild soap and water. Do not use antibacterial soap or waterless soap as either of these agents can enhance skin toxicity to the area. If an eye splash occurs, use copious amounts of water or 0.9% NaCl to irrigate the eye. Do not use aluminum needles or administration sets that may come in contact with the drug because they may cause degradation of platinum compounds.
◀ **ALERT** ▶ Do not allow patient to suck on ice chips or drink or touch glasses of cold liquids during the infusion because this can precipitate or exacerbate acute neuropathy.
* Never reconstitute oxaliplatin with sodium chloride or other chloride-containing solutions.
* Reconstitute each 50-mg vial with 10 mL of sterile water for injection or D5W (100-mg vial with 20 mL). Further dilute with 150-500 mL D5W.
* Administer the drug at the prescribed infusion rate or according to protocol. Usual infusions last 2 hours. Prolonging infusions to 6 hrs may mitigate acute toxicities.

STORAGE AND STABILITY
* After reconstitution, the solution is stable for up to 6 hours at room temperature and up to 24 hours in the refrigerator.

INTERACTIONS
Drug
Live-virus vaccines: May potentiate viral replication, increase vaccine side effects, and decrease patient's antibody response to the vaccine.
Nephrotic medications: May decrease the clearance of oxaliplatin.
Herbal
None known.

LAB EFFECTS/INTERFERENCE
May alter serum bilirubin, AST (SGOT), and ALT (SGPT) levels. May decrease blood Hgb and Hct levels and platelet count.

Y-SITE COMPATIBLES
Amifostine, bleomycin, carboplatin, dactinomycin, daunorubicin, dexamethasone, dexrazoxane, docetaxel, dolasetron, doxorubicin, epirubicin, etoposide, fludarabine, gemcitabine, granisetron, idarubicin, ifosfamide, irinotecan, leucovorin, mesna, mitomycin, mitoxantrone, ondansetron, paclitaxel, palonosetron, pemetrexed, teniposide, thiotepa, vinblastine, vincristine, vinorelbine

INCOMPATIBLES

Cefepime, cefoperazone, dantrolene, diazepam
Note: Do not infuse oxaliplatin with alkaline medications. Do not reconstitute or make the final dilution of oxaliplatin with chloride-containing solutions.

SIDE EFFECTS
Serious Reactions

- Cold sensitivity reactions can occur during IV infusions. These are manifested as laryngeal or pharyngeal dysesthesia characterized by dysphagia, shortness of breath, or bronchospasm and are triggered by cold climate conditions. Patients should be in a warm room during infusion. Ice chips that might be prescribed to prevent fluorouracil-induced mucositis may precipitate this reaction and should be avoided.
- Peripheral or sensory neuropathy can occur, sometimes precipitated or exacerbated by drinking or holding a glass of cold liquid during the IV infusion.
- Pulmonary fibrosis, characterized by a nonproductive cough, dyspnea, crackles, and radiologic pulmonary infiltrates, may require drug discontinuation.
- Hypersensitivity reaction (rash, urticaria, or pruritus) occurs rarely.

Other Side Effects
Frequent (10%-50%):
Peripheral or sensory neuropathy (usually occurs in hands, feet, perioral area, and throat but may present as jaw spasm, abnormal tongue sensation, eye pain, chest pressure, or difficulty walking, swallowing, or writing), nausea (occurs in 64%), fatigue, diarrhea, vomiting, constipation, abdominal pain, fever, anorexia, hypocalcemia, hypomagnesemia, hypokalemia, stomatitis, earache, insomnia, cough, difficulty breathing, backache, edema
Occasional (1%-10%):
Dyspepsia, dizziness, rhinitis, flushing, alopecia
Rare (Less Than 1%):
Hypersensitivity

SPECIAL CONSIDERATIONS
Baseline Assessment

- Assess patient's CBCs with differential, platelet count, and electrolyte, BUN, creatinine, and magnesium levels before each dose, paying particular attention to the electrolyte levels; potassium and magnesium levels may be low with this agent.

- Assess patient for any signs or symptoms of peripheral neuropathy.
- Ensure that patient does not suck on ice or drink or touch a glass of cold liquid during the IV infusion because this can precipitate or exacerbate neurotoxicity, which may occur within hours or days of a dose and may continue for a period of time, usually 14 days but can be longer.

Intervention and Evaluation

- Evaluate patient's CBC with differential, platelets, liver function tests, and electrolyte, BUN, and creatinine levels before each dose; monitor potassium and magnesium levels closely.
- Premedicate with antiemetics as ordered.
- Assess patient for signs and symptoms of peripheral neuropathy before each dose.
- Assess patient for any signs and symptoms of diarrhea or GI changes such as bright red or tarry stools before each dose.
- Evaluate oral cavity for signs and symptoms of stomatitis, mucositis, and ulceration before each dose.
- Evaluate patient's hydration status before each dose.
- Assess whether patient had nausea and, if so, its duration after completing the last dose.

Education

- Instruct patient to report any signs and symptoms of fever greater than 38° C (greater than 101° F), chills, petechiae, bruising, bleeding, cough, sore throat, nausea lasting greater than 24 hours, or diarrhea lasting greater than 24 hours. Make sure patient has a 24-hour number to contact health care provider.
- Advise patient to report any signs or symptoms of peripheral neuropathy: numbness in fingers and toes, weakness, or fatigue.
- Educate patient to use gloves when removing food from freezer as cold can trigger neuropathy; instruct patient to not drink through a straw and to avoid cold beverages for at least 24 hours after dosing.
- Instruct patient to inspect his or her oral cavity daily, and make sure an oral care regimen is started. The oral hygiene regimen should be completed after meals and before bedtime. Instruct patient to swish and spit with 1 tsp of salt and 1 tsp of baking soda in a 8-ounce glass of water. If any mouth sores are noted, instruct patient to contact his or her health care provider.

- Urge patient not to receive vaccinations during therapy and to avoid contact with anyone who has recently received a live-virus vaccine.
- Instruct patient to take no over-the-counter medications or herbal or vitamin supplements without checking with his or her health care provider.
- Educate patient on local resources available and support groups related to their particular diagnosis.

PACLITAXEL
BRAND NAMES
Onxol, Taxol

CLASS OF AGENT
Antineoplastic agent, taxane

CLINICAL PHARMACOLOGY
Mechanism of Action
An antimitotic agent that promotes microtubule assembly and prevents depolymerization. Blocks cells in the late G_2 phase and M phase of the cell cycle. **Therapeutic Effect:** Inhibits cellular mitosis and replication.
Absorption and Distribution
Does not readily cross the blood-brain barrier. Protein binding: 89%-98%.
Half-life: 1.3-8.6 hours.
Metabolism and Excretion
Metabolized primarily via cytochrome P450 (CYP) 2C8/9 and 3A4 (substrate: major) in the liver to active metabolites. Eliminated by bile. Not removed by hemodialysis.

HOW SUPPLIED/AVAILABLE FORMS
Injection: 6 mg/mL.

INDICATIONS AND DOSAGES
Breast Cancer, Kaposi's Sarcoma, Non–Small Cell Lung Cancer, Ovarian Cancer
Refer to individual disease protocols. Doses and schedules vary according to each protocol. Modifications are based on patient's clinical response and tolerability.
Every 3 weeks: 135-200 mg/m² over 3 hours or 24 hours.
Every 2 weeks: 100 mg/m² over 3 hours.
Every week: 50-80 mg/m² over 1 hour.
Every week intraperitoneal: 60-65 mg/m².
Dosage Adjustment in Hepatic Dysfunction
Based on initial dose of 135 mg/m² over 24-hour infusion and 175 mg/m² over 3-hour infusion. Data to make recommendations for other regimens are unavailable.

Liver Function Parameters	24-Hour Infusion
Total bilirubin ≤1.5 + AST <2× ULN	Total dose 135 mg/m²
Total bilirubin ≤1.5 + AST 2-10× ULN	Total dose 100 mg/m²
Total bilirubin 1.6-7.5 + AST <10× ULN	Total dose 50 mg/m²
Total bilirubin >7.5 + AST ≥10× ULN	Avoid use
	3-Hour Infusion
Total bilirubin ≤1.25× ULN + AST <10× ULN	Total dose 175 mg/m²
Total bilirubin 1.26-2× ULN + AST <10× ULN	Total dose 135 mg/m²
Total bilirubin 2.01-5× ULN + AST <10× ULN	Total dose 90 mg/m²
Total bilirubin >5× ULN + AST ≥10× ULN	Avoid use

Dosage Adjustment in Severe Neutropenia (ANC less than 500 cells/mm³ for 1 Wk or Longer) or Severe Peripheral Neuropathy
Reduce dose by 20%.

UNLABELED USES
Treatment of upper GI tract adenocarcinoma, head and neck cancer, hormone-refractory prostate cancer, non-Hodgkin's lymphoma, small cell lung cancer, transitional cell cancer of urothelium.

PRECAUTIONS
Severe hypersensitivity reactions have been reported. Use paclitaxel cautiously in patients with hepatic impairment, peripheral neuropathy, or severe neutropenia.avw
Pregnancy Risk Category: D

CONTRAINDICATIONS
Baseline neutrophil count less than 1500 cells/mm³ in solid tumor patients; baseline neutrophil count less than 1000 cells/mm³ in Kaposi's sarcoma patients; hypersensitivity to paclitaxel, Cremophor EL (polyoxyethylated castor oil), or any component of the formulation

DRUG PREPARATION/ADMINISTRATION/ SAFE HANDLING ISSUES
◀ ALERT ▶ Because paclitaxel may be carcinogenic, mutagenic, or teratogenic, wear nitrile or latex, but not vinyl, gloves when handling the drug. If the drug comes in contact with skin, wash the skin thoroughly with soap and water. Do not use waterless hand soap or any antibacterial soap as

either can increase the reaction from the agent. If the drug comes in contact with mucous membranes, flush the area with water.

◄ **ALERT** ▶ Premedicate patient with dexamethasone 20 mg PO 12 and 6 hours before or 20 mg IV 30 minutes before, diphenhydramine 50 mg or equivalent IV 30-60 minutes before, and a histamine H_2 antagonist such as cimetidine 300 mg or ranitidine 50 mg IV 30-60 minutes before dosing.

• Paclitaxel is considered an irritant.
• Dilute with 0.9% NaCl or D5W to a final concentration of 0.3-1.2 mg/mL.
• Dispense in either glass or Excel/PAB containers. Use non-polyvinyl chloride tubing (e.g., polyethylene) to minimized leaching of di-(2-ethylhexyl) phthalate from polyvinyl chloride infusion bags or administration sets.
• Administer through an in-line filter not greater than 0.22 micron.
• When administered as a sequential infusion, give paclitaxel before platinum derivatives (e.g., cisplatin and carboplatin) to limit myelosuppression.
• Monitor patient's vital signs during the infusion, especially during the first hour.
• Discontinue paclitaxel administration and notify physician if patient experiences a severe hypersensitivity reaction.

STORAGE AND STABILITY

• Store intact vials at room temperature and protect from light.
• If refrigerated, product may precipitate. The product is not harmed if it returns to solution after warming to room temperature.
• Reconstituted solution is stable at room temperature for up to 27 hours.

INTERACTIONS
Drug

Bone marrow depressants: May increase myelosuppression.
CYP 2C8 inducers (carbamazepine, phenytoin, phenobarbital, rifampin): May decrease the levels/effects of paclitaxel.
CYP 2C8 inhibitors (ethinyl estradiol, fluconazole, ketoconazole, sulfonamides, testosterone, tretinoin): May increase the levels/effects of paclitaxel.
CYP 3A4 inducers (carbamazepine, phenytoin, phenobarbital, rifampin): May decrease the levels/effects of paclitaxel.

CYP 3A4 inhibitors (ciprofloxacin, clarithromycin, doxycycline, erythromycin, isoniazid, protease inhibitors, verapamil): May increase the levels/ effects of paclitaxel
Live-virus vaccines: May potentiate viral replication, increase vaccine side effects, and decrease patient's antibody response to the vaccine.
Platinum derivatives (cisplatin and carboplatin): When administered as a sequential infusion, give paclitaxel before platinum derivatives to limit myelosuppression.

Herbal
St John's Wort: May decrease paclitaxel serum concentrations. Avoid use.

Food
Grapefruit inhibits CYP 3A4 enzymes and can potentially enhance paclitaxel effects.

LAB EFFECTS/INTERFERENCE
May elevate serum alkaline phosphatase, bilirubin, AST (SGOT), and ALT (SGPT) levels. Decreases blood Hgb and Hct levels and platelet, RBC, and WBC counts.

Y-SITE COMPATIBLES
Allopurinol, bleomycin, busulfan, calcium chloride, carboplatin (Paraplatin), carmustine, chlorpromazine (Thorazine), cisplatin (Platinol AQ), cladribine, cyclophosphamide (Cytoxan), cytarabine (Cytosar), dacarbazine (DTIC-Dome), dactinomycin, daunorubicin, dexamethasone (Decadron), dexrazoxane, diphenhydramine (Benadryl), doxorubicin (Adriamycin), doxorubicin liposomal (Doxil), etoposide (VePesid), etoposide phosphate (Etopophos), famotidine (Pepcid), floxuridine, fludarabine, fluorouracil, furosemide (Lasix), gemcitabine (Gemzar), granisetron (Kytril), hydrocortisone sodium succinate (Solu-Cortef), hydromorphone (Dilaudid), hydroxyzine (Vistaril), ifosfamide (Ifex), irinotecan, leucovorin, lorazepam (Ativan), magnesium sulfate, mannitol, methotrexate, methylprednisolone sodium succinate (Solu-Medrol), metoclopramide (Reglan), mitomycin, mitoxantrone (Novantrone), morphine, ondansetron (Zofran), oxaliplatin, palonosetron, pemetrexed, phenytoin, prochlorperazine (Compazine), palonosetron (Aloxi), potassium chloride, propranolol, rituximab, streptozocin, thiotepa, topotecan, vinblastine (Velban), vincristine (Oncovin), vinorelbine

INCOMPATIBLES

Amiodarone, amphotericin B (Fungizone), amphotericin B conventional (Amphocin), amphotericin B complex (Abelcet), chlorpromazine (Thorazine), diazepam, digoxin, doxorubicin liposomal (Doxil), hydroxyzine (Vistaril), idarubicin, indomethacin, labetalol, methylprednisolone sodium succinate (Solu-Medrol), mitoxantrone (Novantrone), phenytoin, propranolol

SIDE EFFECTS
Serious Reactions

- Neutropenic nadir occurs at approximately day 11 of paclitaxel therapy.
- Anemia and leukopenia are common reactions. Thrombocytopenia occurs occasionally.
- A severe hypersensitivity reaction, including dyspnea, severe hypotension, angioedema, and generalized urticaria, occurs rarely. Occurrence usually is within the first 15 minutes of infusion of the first or second dose and may vary per individual. Premedication and prolonged infusion (greater than 6 hours) may minimize the effect. Use diphenhydramine 50-100 mg IV, hydrocortisone succinate 100 mg IV, epinephrine 1:1000 (1 mg/mL) 0.3 mL IV, albuterol inhaler 2-4 puffs, and oxygen as necessary. Rechallenge of paclitaxel is not recommended for severe reactions. However, for patients with limited treatment options, several variations of paclitaxel desensitization protocols described in the literature have successfully been used.

Other Side Effects
Frequent (10%-50%):

Allergic reactions, alopecia, arthralgia, bradycardia during infusion, diarrhea, elevated liver enzymes, hypotension, mild to moderate nausea and vomiting, myalgia, mucositis, myelosuppression, peripheral neuropathy

Occasional (1%-10%):
Myocardial infarction, phlebitis

Rare (Less Than 1%):
Ataxia, atrial fibrillation, enterocolitis, hepatic encephalopathy, intestinal obstruction, interstitial pneumonia, ototoxicity, pancreatitis, paralytic ileus, pruritus, pulmonary fibrosis, radiation recall, rash, seizure, Stevens-Johnson syndrome, toxic epidermal necrolysis, visual disturbances

SPECIAL CONSIDERATIONS
Baseline Assessment

- Record baseline vital signs.
- Assess patient's blood counts, particularly neutrophil and platelet counts, before each course of paclitaxel therapy or as clinically indicated.

Intervention and Evaluation

- Monitor patient's CBC with differential, electrolytes, BUN creatinine liver function tests, platelet count, and vital signs.
- Monitor patient for signs and symptoms of hematologic toxicity, including excessive fatigue and weakness, ecchymosis, fever, signs of local infection, sore throat, and unusual bleeding.
- Have anaphylaxis kit available at bedside along with an oxygen setup and an Ambu bag before administration of this agent. The anaphylaxis kit should include the following:
    Diphenhydramine 50 mg
    Hydrocortisone 50 mg
    Epinephrine 1:1000
    Draw up the syringe, but only inject 0.3cc each time. Do not administer entire dose all at once.
    Albuterol inhaler
    Syringes and needles
    Alcohol wipes
    2-by-2 gauze pads to break ampule
- Monitor patient for and report diarrhea.
- Educate patient on neutropenic precautions as necessary:
    Practice good handwashing technique.
    Avoid individuals who are ill.
    Wash and cook all foods well.
    Avoid crowds.
    Avoid fresh fruits and vegetables.
- Educate patient on thrombocytopenic precautions:
    Use of a soft bristle toothbrush.
    No flossing if platelet count is less than 50,000/mm^3.
    No IM injections.
    No rectal suppositories.
    No aerobic exercise.
- Apply pressure to the IV site for a full 5 minutes after administration.
- Offer emotional support to patient and family.

Education

- Warn patient to immediately notify his or her health care provider if he or she experiences signs of infection, including fever and flu-like symptoms.
- Caution patient to notify his or her health care provider if nausea and vomiting continue at home.
- Teach patient to recognize the signs and symptoms of peripheral neuropathy.
- Urge patient not to receive vaccinations and to avoid contact with crowds and people with known infections.

- Warn patient to avoid pregnancy during paclitaxel therapy. Teach patient various contraception methods.
- Inform patient that alopecia is reversible but that new hair growth may have a different color or texture.
- Instruct patient to take no over-the-counter medications or herbal or vitamin supplements without checking with his or her health care provider.
- Educate patient on local resources available and support groups related to their particular diagnosis.

PACLITAXEL PROTEIN-BOUND PARTICLES

BRAND NAMES
Abraxane

CLASS OF AGENT
Antineoplastic agent, taxane

CLINICAL PHARMACOLOGY
Mechanism of Action
An antimitotic agent in the taxoid family that promotes microtubule assembly and prevents depolymerization. Blocks cells in the late G_2 phase and M phase of the cell cycle. **Therapeutic Effect:** Inhibits cellular mitosis and replication.
Absorption and Distribution
Distributed extensively in extravascular and or tissue sites. Does not readily cross the blood-brain barrier. Protein binding: 89%-98%. Volume of distribution: 632 L/m^2.
Half-life: 27 hours.
Metabolism and Excretion
Metabolized primarily via cytochrome P450 (CYP) 2C8/9 and 3A4 (substrate: major) in the liver to active metabolites. Eliminated by urine (4% unchanged) and feces (20%).

HOW SUPPLIED/AVAILABLE FORMS
Powder for Injection: 100 mg.

INDICATIONS AND DOSAGES
Breast Cancer after Failure of Combination Chemotherapy for Metastatic Disease or Relapse within 6 Months of Adjuvant Chemotherapy
Prior therapy should have included an anthracycline unless clinically contraindicated.
Weekly: 100-120 mg/m^2 IV over 30 mins.
Every 3 weeks: 260 mg/m^2 IV over 30 mins.

Dosage Adjustment for Neutropenia
No dosage recommendations available for weekly dosing. Neutrophils less than 500 cells/mm^3 for 1 week or longer
- Decrease dose to 220 mg/m^2.
- Decrease dose to 180 mg/m^2 with subsequent severe neutropenia.
Dosage Adjustment for Neuropathy
No dosage recommendations available for weekly dosing.
Grade 3 neuropathy:
- Hold for Grade 3 neuropathy. Resume with dose reduction for all subsequent doses when symptoms resolve to grade 1 or 2.
- First event, decrease dose to 220 mg/m^2.
- Recurrent event, decrease dose to 180 mg/m^2.
- No current recommendations for grade 4 neuropathy.
Dosage Adjustment in Hepatic/Renal Dysfunction
No recommendations available. Not studied in patients with total bilirubin greater than 1.5 mg/dL or renal insufficiency.

UNLABELED USES
Anal cancer; head and neck cancer

PRECAUTIONS
The dose of protein-bound paclitaxel is different from that of Cremophor-based paclitaxel. Do not interchange paclitaxel albumin-bound for Cremophor-based paclitaxel formulation. Use paclitaxel cautiously in patients with hepatic impairment, peripheral neuropathy, or severe neutropenia.
Pregnancy Risk Category: D

CONTRAINDICATIONS
Hypersensitivity to paclitaxel or any component of the formulation. Patients with ANC less than 1500 cell/mm^3: withhold treatment until ANC recovers to more than 1500 cell/mm^3 and platelets count recovers to more than 100,000 cells/mm^3.

DRUG PREPARATION/ADMINISTRATION/SAFE HANDLING ISSUES
◄ ALERT ► Because paclitaxel may be carcinogenic, mutagenic, or teratogenic, wear nitrile or latex, but not vinyl, gloves when handling the drug. If the drug comes in contact with skin, wash the skin thoroughly with soap and water. Do not use waterless hand soap or any antibacterial soap as either can increase the reaction from the agent. If the

drug comes in contact with mucous membranes, flush the area with water.
• Paclitaxel is considered an irritant.
• Do not substitute with or for other paclitaxel formulations.
• Dilute with 0.9% NaCl to a final concentration of 5 mg/mL. Slowly inject 20 mL of 0.9% NaCl directed at the vial wall. Do not inject directly into the lyophilized cake as this results in foaming.
• Gently swirl or invert the vial slowly. Do not shake.
• Dissolution may take 15 mins or longer.
• Inject the appropriate amount of drug into an empty polyvinyl chloride bag. Do not use an in-line filter.
• When administered as a sequential infusion, give paclitaxel protein-bound before platinum derivatives (e.g., cisplatin and carboplatin) to limit myelosuppression.
• Premedication is not necessary to prevent hypersensitivity reactions.

STORAGE AND STABILITY
• Store intact vials at room temperature of 20-25° C (68-77° F).
• The reconstituted solution is stable at refrigerated or room temperature for up to 8 hours if protected from bright light (ambient light okay) as there are no preservatives in the formulation.

INTERACTIONS
Drug
Bone marrow depressants: May increase myelosuppression.
CYP 2C8 inducers (carbamazepine, phenytoin, phenobarbital, rifampin): May decrease the levels/effects of paclitaxel.
CYP 2C8 inhibitors (fluconazole, ketoconazole, sulfonamides, testosterone, tretinoin): May increase the levels/effects of paclitaxel.
CYP 3A4 inducers (carbamazepine, phenytoin, phenobarbital, rifampin): May decrease the levels/effects of paclitaxel.
CYP 3A4 inhibitors (ciprofloxacin, clarithromycin, doxycycline, erythromycin, isoniazid, protease inhibitors, verapamil): May increase the levels/effects of paclitaxel
Live-virus vaccines: May potentiate virus replication, increase vaccine side effects, and decrease patient's antibody response to the vaccine.
Herbal
St John's Wort: May decrease the levels/effects of paclitaxel. Avoid use.

Food
Grapefruit inhibits CYP 3A4 enzymes and can potentially enhance paclitaxel effects.

LAB EFFECTS/INTERFERENCE
May elevate serum alkaline phosphatase, bilirubin, AST (SGOT), and ALT (SGPT) levels. Decreases blood Hgb and Hct levels and platelet, RBC, and WBC counts.

Y-SITE COMPATIBLES
None known.

INCOMPATIBLES
None known.

SIDE EFFECTS
Serious Reactions
• Neutropenic nadir occurs at approximately day 11 of paclitaxel therapy. Anemia and leukopenia are common reactions. Thrombocytopenia occurs occasionally.
Other Side Effects
Frequent (10%-50%):
Alopecia, anemia, arthralgia, diarrhea, dyspnea, EKG abnormalities, elevated liver enzymes, infections, mild to moderate nausea and vomiting, myalgia, myelosuppression, peripheral neuropathy (less with weekly dosing), visual disturbances
Occasional (1%-10%):
bleeding, edema, febrile neutropenia, hypersensitivity reaction (less common than Cremophor-based paclitaxel), hypotension, increased serum creatinine, mucositis, phlebitis
Rare (Less Than 1%):
Bradycardia, injection site reactions, pneumothorax

SPECIAL CONSIDERATIONS
Baseline Assessment
• Record baseline vital signs. Monitor patient's vital signs before and after the first dose infusion. For the first dose, a nurse should be present or readily available at bedside to monitor for any allergic or hypersensitivity reactions.
• Assess patient's blood counts, particularly neutrophil and platelet counts, before each course of paclitaxel therapy or as clinically indicated. Monitor liver function tests before initial dosing, and if elevated dose reduction must be completed before administration.
• Monitor electrolytes, BUN, creatinine and liver function tests.

- Ensure that patient does not object to receiving human-derived blood products (contains human-derived albumin).

Intervention and Evaluation

- No premedications are required to avoid hypersensitivity reactions.
- Monitor patient's CBC with WBC differential, platelet count, liver function test results, and vital signs.
- Monitor patient for signs and symptoms of hematologic toxicity, including excessive fatigue and weakness, ecchymosis, epistaxis, gingival bleeding, petechiae, fever, any sign of local infection, sore throat, and unusual bleeding.
- Evaluate for any peripheral neuropathy.
- Assess patient's response to the drug and any signs or symptoms of allergic reaction.
- Monitor patient for and report diarrhea.
- Avoid giving patient IM injections, taking rectal temperatures, giving rectal suppositories, and performing procedures that may induce bleeding.
- Apply pressure to the IV site for a full 5 minutes after completion of any invasive procedure.
- Provide emotional support to patient, family, and significant others.

Education

- Instruct patient to immediately notify his or her health care provider if he or she experiences signs of infection or bleeding including fever and flu-like symptoms, epistaxis, petechiae, easy bruising, or bleeding.
- Caution patient to notify his or her health care provider if nausea and voavmiting continue for greater than 24 hours after therapy completion.
- Instruct patient regarding the signs and symptoms of peripheral neuropathy: numbness tingling, and burning of hands and feet. Describe the "stocking glove" effects of this agent. Usually the symptoms will proceed from distal to proximal and will recede proximal to distal. Instruct patient to notify all providers of the symptoms and severity before each drug administration.
- Educate patient not to receive vaccinations and to avoid contact with crowds and people with known infections while receiving therapy.
- Instruct patient to avoid pregnancy during paclitaxel therapy. Teach the patient various contraception methods.
- Notify patient that alopecia is reversible but that new hair growth may have a different color or texture. Educate patients not to color hair or have a permanent

when their hair is initially growing back in. The texture is very soft and fine and does not color or take a permanent well.
- Educate patient about fatigue and its causes and any interventions to promote well-being. Encourage patient to plan a minimal exercise program while undergoing therapy. Studies have demonstrated that patients who continue to do some form of minimal exercise tolerate chemotherapy better with fewer symptoms of nausea and fatigue.
- Instruct patient to take no over-the-counter medications or herbal or vitamin supplements without checking with his or her health care provider.
- Educate patient on local resources available and support groups related to their particular diagnosis.

PAMIDRONATE DISODIUM

BRAND NAMES
Aredia

CLASS OF AGENT
Bisphosphonate

CLINICAL PHARMACOLOGY

Mechanism of Action

Pamidronate binds to hydroxyapatite, the chief structural component of bone, preventing the dissolution of calcium and phosphate into the bloodstream. In the neoplastic setting, tumors secrete chemical signals that in turn stimulate osteoclasts and mobilize the release of skeletal calcium. Pamidronate interferes with osteoclast hyperactivity in this setting. **Therapeutic Effect:** Inhibits bone resorption and reduces risk of skeletal-related events.

Absorption and Distribution

In animal studies, 50%-60% was rapidly taken up by bone. Other areas of uptake are the liver, spleen, teeth, and tracheal cartilage. *Half-life:* Early elimination half-life is 28 ± 7 hours. Terminal elimination rate from bone has not yet been determined.

Metabolism and Excretion

Does not inhibit the cytochrome P450 metabolic pathway. Elimination of the drug is exclusively through renal excretion. Dosing pamidronate disodium at 30, 60, and 90 mg over 4 hours and at 90 mg over 24 hours resulted in the recovery of $46 \pm 16\%$ of the drug in the urine over 120 hours.

HOW SUPPLIED/AVAILABLE FORMS
Powder for Injection: 30 mg, 90 mg.
Injection Solution: 3 mg/mL, 6 mg/mL,
9 mg/mL as 10-mL vials

INDICATIONS AND DOSAGES
Treatment of Hypercalcemia of Malignancy
60-90 mg IV over 2-24 hours. Retreatment
can be considered after a minimum of
7 days if the calcium level did not normalize. The retreatment dose is the same as
the initial dose.
Treatment of Osteolytic Lesions
Multiple myeloma: 90 mg IV over 4 hours
every 4 weeks.
Breast cancer: 90 mg IV over 2 hours
every 3-4 weeks.
Treatment of Paget's Disease
30 mg IV over 4 hours daily for
3 consecutive days.
**Dosage Adjustment
in Hepatic Dysfunction**
No adjustments required.
Dosage Adjustment in Renal Dysfunction
No dose adjustments required for mild to
moderate renal dysfunction. Do not administer to patients with severe baseline renal
dysfunction. For patients whose condition
is stabilized with zoledronic acid, renal
deterioration is defined as follows:
Increase of 0.5 mg/dL for patients with
normal baseline serum creatinine.
Increase of 1 mg/dL for patients with an
abnormal baseline serum creatinine.
If renal deterioration is observed, drug
should be held in patients with Paget's
disease, multiple myeloma, and breast cancer. If the creatinine level returns to within
10% of baseline, the patient may be rechallenged with caution and close observation.
If increasing renal dysfunction is observed
in patients being treated for hypercalcemia
of malignancy, a careful evaluation should
ensue and a decision must then be made to
determine whether the potential benefit of
treating outweighs the potential risks.

UNLABELED USES
Hyperparathyroidism, immobilization-related
hypercalcemia, postmenopausal osteoporosis, prophylaxis of glucocorticoid-induced
osteoporosis

PRECAUTIONS
• Renal dysfunction may develop or progress
to full renal failure requiring dialysis. Do
not exceed the maximum recommended
dose of 90 mg. Prolonged infusion for
2-24 hours may reduce risk for renal

toxicity. Assess serum creatinine level
before each infusion.
• Osteonecrosis of the jaw has been reported. Most incidents of osteonecrosis of
the jaw were associated with tooth extraction, but some have also been noted in
patients without this procedure. Many of
these patients also had evidence of local
infection, occasionally progressing to osteomyelitis. Common signs and symptoms
include a "heavy jaw" sensation, pain,
edema, halitosis resulting from superimposed infection, loose teeth, discharge, and
exposed bone, which is sometimes sharp
and spiculated. If osteonecrosis is suspected or diagnosed, patient should be
referred to an oral surgeon. Surgical intervention may actually worsen the situation;
however, minimal bony débridement may
be necessary to remove sharp edges of
bone. Intermittent or continuous antibiotic
therapy may be of benefit along with
0.12% chlorhexidine gluconate oral rinses.
Patients should be encouraged to maintain
excellent oral hygiene routines and to immediately report any suspicious symptoms.
A complete dental examination is strongly
recommended before institution of therapy.
• May decrease serum calcium and phosphorus levels. Magnesium levels may
also be affected. Supplementation may
be required.
• Use with caution when patients are
treated with aspirin-sensitive asthma
as bronchoconstriction has been
reported in patients treated with other
bisphosphonates.
Pregnancy Risk Category: D
Pamidronate may impair fertility and
may cause fetal harm in pregnant women.
Drug excretion into human breast milk is
unknown/not recommended in nursing
women.

CONTRAINDICATIONS
Severe renal insufficiency; incompletely
healed dental extraction sites and osseointegrated dental implants; hypersensitivity
to pamidronate, other bisphosphonates,
mannitol or any other component of the
formulation

DRUG PREPARATION/ADMINISTRATION/
SAFE HANDLING ISSUES
◀ ALERT ▶ Strict adherence to the administration recommendations is necessary to
minimize the risk of renal dysfunction.
• Do not mix with calcium-containing solutions (e.g., lactated Ringer's solution).

- Lyophilized powder: reconstitute with 10 mL of sterile water for injection to each vial resulting in solutions of 30 or 90 mg/10 mL.
- Dilute pamidronate further into sterile 0.45% or 0.9% NaCl or 5% dextrose for injection bags of 250 mL, 500 mL, and 1000 mL.
- Administered over 2-24 hours.
- Drug should be administered as a single IV solution in a line separate from all other drugs.

STORAGE AND STABILITY
- Store intact vials at room temperature.
- Once drug is reconstituted with sterile water for injection, it may be stored for up to 24 hours under refrigeration.

INTERACTIONS
Drug
Loop diuretics (bumetanide, furosemide, ethacrynic acid, torsemide): Use with caution due to enhanced risk of hypocalcemia and hypomagnesemia in the hypercalcemia setting.
Nephrotoxic drugs (aminoglycosides): Increased risk of nephrotoxicity.
Pamidronate: Is not known to inhibit the cytochrome P450 pathway.
Herbal
None known.

LAB EFFECTS/INTERFERENCE
Serum creatinine must be monitored before every dose. Monitor periodically for serum calcium, phosphate, and magnesium levels and CBC.

Y-SITE COMPATIBLES
Hetastarch, palonosetron, pemetrexed, teniposide, thiotepa, voriconazole

INCOMPATIBLES
Do not mix with calcium-containing solutions (e.g., lactated Ringer's solution).

SIDE EFFECTS
Serious Reactions
Renal failure, osteonecrosis of the jaw, severe allergic reactions
Other Side Effects
Frequent (10%-50%):
Anorexia, arthralgias, bone pain, fatigue, infusion site reaction, myalgias, nausea, reduced electrolyte levels (calcium, phosphorus, magnesium, and potassium), transient low-grade fever

Occasional (1%-10%):
Anemia, constipation, diarrhea, headache, hypertension, leukopenia, neutropenia, osteonecrosis of the jaw, renal insufficiency (moderate worsening), somnolence, syncope, tachycardia, thrombocytopenia, vomiting
Rare (Less Than 1%):
Allergic reaction, ocular disorders (uveitis, iritis, scleritis, and episcleritis)

SPECIAL CONSIDERATIONS
Baseline Assessment
- Ensure that a routine dental examination has been completed before institution of therapy. If dental extraction is indicated, adequate time for healing should be allowed before therapy is begun.
- Reinforce need for properly fitting dentures.
- Review all baseline laboratory test results including serum creatinine, BUN, serum calcium, magnesium, phosphate, and serum albumin levels and CBC. Serum creatinine should be assessed before every dose.
- Review all current prescriptions and OTC medications.
- Verify any patient allergies
Intervention and Evaluation
- Complete oral examination periodically.
- If osteonecrosis of the jaw is either suspected or diagnosed, refer patient to an oral surgeon for consultation and drug may need to be interrupted.
- Be aware that intermittent or continuous antibiotic therapy may be necessary to prevent secondary soft-tissue infection or osteomyelitis.
- Know that optimal antibiotics include penicillin VK 500 mg 4 times daily or amoxicillin 500 mg 4 times daily, and if patient is allergic to penicillin, clindamycin 150-300 mg 4 times/day, Vibramycin 100 mg once daily, or erythromycin 400 mg 3 times/day.
- Be aware that oral rinses with 0.12% chlorhexidine gluconate may also be helpful.
- Check serum creatinine before every dose.
- Hold drug for patients who meet the criteria for worsening renal dysfunction (increase of 0.5 mg/dL for patients with normal baseline creatinine levels and increase of 1 mg/dL for patients with abnormal baseline creatinine levels). Reinstitute drug when creatinine level returns to within 10% of baseline.

- Be aware that patient with clinically significant declines of calcium, phosphate, and magnesium levels may need supplementation.
- Treat flu-like symptoms with antiemetics for nausea and bone pain, arthralgias, and myalgias with acetaminophen. If renal insufficiency is not an issue, treatment with NSAIDs may be allowed.

Education

- Explain to patient why he or she is receiving pamidronate (hypercalcemia of malignancy, Paget's disease, multiple myeloma, or breast cancer).
- Review potential side effects.
- Inform patient that flu-like symptoms may occur and that they usually subside within 24-48 hours and typically do not recur after the first or second infusion.
- Brief patient that although a transient low-grade fever may occur, it can be controlled with acetaminophen and usually resolves within 24-48 hours. Reassure patient that fever is due to the flu-like reaction and is not a true infection. If fever persists, educate patient to seek medical attention.
- Educate patient on the need to monitor laboratory work, especially serum creatinine level before every infusion.
- Stress the importance of maintaining adequate hydration.
- If patient is being treated for hypercalcemia of malignancy, teach patient to follow a low calcium diet.
- Reinforce the need for excellent dental hygiene and routine professional dental cleanings.
- Instruct patient to avoid any jaw or dental procedure that would require the healing of bone (i.e., tooth extractions or dental implants)
- Encourage patient to report any new symptoms.
- Instruct patient to take no over-the-counter medications or herbal or vitamin supplements without checking with his or her health care provider.

PEGFILGRASTIM

BRAND NAMES
Neulasta

CLASS OF AGENT
Granulocyte colony-stimulating factor

CLINICAL PHARMACOLOGY
Mechanism of Action
A colony-stimulating factor that stimulates production of granulocytes within bone marrow. **Therapeutic Effect:** Increases ANCs to fight off infection in patients with nonmyeloid malignancies who received chemotherapy. Decreases incidence of infection.

Absorption and Distribution
Readily absorbed after subcutaneous administration. Distribution is limited to plasma compartment. Serum concentrations of the drug remain elevated during chemotherapy-related neutropenia and fall rapidly at the onset of neutrophil recovery.
Half-life: 15-80 hours. Pegfilgrastim is the long-acting formulation of filgrastim.

Metabolism and Excretion
Elimination of pegfilgrastim is almost entirely via a saturable neutrophil receptor-mediated clearance; serum clearance decreases with increasing doses and it is directly related to the number of neutrophils.

HOW SUPPLIED/AVAILABLE FORMS
Solution for Injection: 6 mg in a single dose syringe (10 mg/mL).

INDICATIONS AND DOSAGES
To Reduce Incidence of Infections in Patients Receiving Myelosuppressive Therapy for Nonmyeloid Malignancies
Give as a single 6-mg subcutaneous injection once per chemotherapy cycle. Pegfilgrastim should not be administered in the period between 14 days before and 24 hours after administration of cytotoxic chemotherapy. The 6-mg fixed-dose formulation should not be used in infants, children, and smaller adolescents weighing less than 45 kg.

Dosage Adjustment in Hepatic/Renal Dysfunction
Dosing adjustment is not necessary.

UNLABELLED USES
As component in dose-dense chemotherapy.

PRECAUTIONS
Use pegfilgrastim cautiously in patients who concurrently use medications with myeloid properties and in those with sickle cell disease.

Pregnancy Risk Category: C
Drug excretion into human breast milk is unknown/not recommended in nursing women.

CONTRAINDICATIONS

Hypersensitivity to filgrastim, to *Escherichia coli*–derived products, or to any component of the formulation.

DRUG PREPARATION/ADMINISTRATION/ SAFE HANDLING ISSUES

- Store in refrigerator, but may warm to room temperature up to 48 hrs before use. Discard if left at room temperature for longer than 48 hrs.
- Protect from light.
- Avoid freezing, but if accidentally frozen, may allow to thaw in refrigerator before administration. Discard if freezing takes place a second time.
- Discard if discoloration or precipitate is present.

INTERACTIONS

Drug

Lithium: May potentiate the release of neutrophils.

MONITORING PARAMETERS

CBC including WBC with differential periodically; in addition, routine chemistry to include LDH, alkaline phosphatase, and uric acid levels.

SIDE EFFECTS

Serious Reactions

- Allergic reactions such as anaphylaxis, rash, and urticaria occur rarely.
- Cytopenia resulting from an antibody response to growth factors occurs rarely.
- Splenomegaly occurs rarely with reports of splenic rupture; assess for left upper abdominal or shoulder pain.
- Adult respiratory distress syndrome (ARDS) may occur in patients with sepsis.

Other Side Effects

Frequent (10%-50%):
Abdominal pain, alopecia, anorexia, arthralgia, bone pain, constipation, diarrhea, dizziness, fatigue, generalized weakness, LDH increase, mucositis, nausea, peripheral edema, stomatitis, vomiting

Occasional (1%-10%):
Alkaline phosphatase increased, uric acid increased

Rare (Less Than 1%):
Allergic reactions, ARDS, sickle cell crisis, splenic rupture

SPECIAL CONSIDERATIONS

Baseline Assessment

- Assess CBC with differential, platelet count, electrolyte, BUN, creatinine, uric acid, and LDH levels, and liver functions tests.
- Assess patient for any evidence of splenomegaly.
- Evaluate for any history of allergic reactions to prior growth factor use.
- Obtain baseline weight, and evaluate for evidence of peripheral edema.
- Assess for any evidence of dermatologic conditions, especially a history of Sweet's syndrome.

Intervention and Evaluation

- Assess laboratory parameters before each dose.
- Evaluate patient for weight gain while receiving this agent.
- Monitor patient for allergic reactions, such as erythema, edema, or urticaria.
- Assess patient for evidence of strength of bone pain and need for analgesia.
- Examine patient for peripheral edema, particularly behind the medial malleolus, which is usually the first area to show peripheral edema.
- Assess patient's mucous membranes for evidence of mucositis (such as red mucous membranes, white patches, and extreme mouth soreness) and stomatitis.
- Evaluate patient's muscle strength as weakness and myalgias may occur with this agent.
- Assess patient's pattern of daily bowel activity and stool consistency.
- Evaluate patients with sepsis for signs and symptoms of ARDS, such as rales, rhonchi, nasal flaring, and dyspnea.

Education

- Instruct patient on when to contact his or her health care provider: fever greater than 38° C (greater than 101° F), cough, shortness of breath, edema, right upper quadrant pain, dizziness, or evidence of skin infections such as rash or sores on lower extremities.
- Educate patient on usual side effects of this agent: fever, bone pain, arthralgias, myalgias, rashes.
- Instruct patient on symptoms of allergic reactions such as rash, erythema edema, shortness of breath, or throat swelling.
- Advise patient of the need for frequent laboratory monitoring.

- Educate patient not to take any OTC medications and herbal or vitamin supplements without first checking with his or her health care provider.

PEMETREXED
BRAND NAMES
Alimta

CLASS OF AGENT
Antifolate

CLINICAL PHARMACOLOGY
Mechanism of Action
An antimetabolite that disrupts folate-dependent enzymes essential for cell replication. It is a multitargeted antifolate compound chemically similar to methotrexate. Pemetrexed gains entry into the cell via the reduced folate carrier and is a good substrate for the enzyme folylpolyglutamate synthase, which leads to extensive intracellular polyglutamation; the predominant intracellular form is the pentaglutamate, which is substantially more potent than pemetrexed itself or its monoglutamate. Polyglutamation is a time- and concentration-dependent process that occurs in tumor cells and, to a lesser extent, in normal tissues. Polyglutamated metabolites have an increased intracellular half-life, resulting in prolonged drug action in malignant cells. Pemetrexed and its polyglutamates inhibit at least four enzymes involved in folate metabolism and DNA synthesis: thymidylate synthase, dihydrofolate reductase, glycinamide ribonucleotide formyl transferase, and aminoimidazole carboxamide ribonucleotide formyltransferase.

Absorption and Distribution
Administered by the IV route only. In vitro studies indicate that pemetrexed is approximately 81% bound to plasma proteins. It has a small volume of distribution of 6-9 L/m^2, suggesting that the drug has limited tissue distribution. Pemetrexed total area under the curve (AUC) and maximum plasma concentration increase proportionally with dose. Pemetrexed has a steady-state volume of distribution of 16.1 L. *Half-life:* The elimination half-life of pemetrexed ranges from 2 to 4 hours in patients with normal renal function (CrCl of 90 mL/min).

Metabolism and Excretion
Metabolic pathways have not been identified. Pemetrexed appears to undergo minimal metabolism (hepatic or other) based on urinary excretion data. Pemetrexed is primarily eliminated in the urine, with 70%-90% of the dose recovered unchanged within the first 24 hours following administration. The total systemic clearance of pemetrexed is 91.8 mL/minute. Drug clearance decreases and exposure (AUC) increases as renal function decreases. Total body clearance is dependent upon CrCl and folate deficiency. In folate-deficient patients, a reduction in clearance by approximately 35% can be expected.

HOW SUPPLIED/AVAILABLE FORMS
Powder for Injection: 500 mg.

INDICATIONS AND DOSAGES
Malignant Pleural Mesothelioma
Combination therapy: 500 mg/m^2 IV followed by cisplatin 75 mg/m^2 IV every 3 weeks.
Non-Small Cell Lung Cancer
Single agent: 500 mg/m^2 IV every 3 weeks.
Note: *Cutaneous reactions:* Skin rash has been reported more frequently in patients not pretreated with a corticosteroid. Pretreatment with dexamethasone (or equivalent) reduces the incidence and severity of cutaneous reactions. In clinical trials, dexamethasone 4 mg was given by mouth twice daily the day before, the day of, and the day after pemetrexed administration.
Note: *Vitamin supplementation:* To reduce toxicity, instruct patients treated with pemetrexed to take a low-dose oral folic acid preparation or multivitamin with folic acid on a daily basis. At least five daily doses of folic acid must be taken during the 7-day period preceding the first dose of pemetrexed; dosing should continue during the full course of therapy and for 21 days after the last dose of pemetrexed. Patients must also receive one IM injection of vitamin B$_{12}$ during the week preceding the first dose of pemetrexed and every three cycles thereafter. Subsequent vitamin B$_{12}$ injections may be given on the same day as pemetrexed. In clinical trials, the dose of folic acid studied ranged from 350 to 1000 mcg, and the dose of vitamin B$_{12}$ was 1000 mcg. The most commonly used dose of oral folic acid in clinical trials was 400 mcg.

Dosage Adjustment

Discontinue pemetrexed therapy if a patient experiences any hematologic or nonhematologic grade 3 or 4 toxicity after two dose reductions (except grade 3 transaminase elevations) or immediately if grade 3 or 4 neurotoxicity is observed.

Hematologic Toxicities

Dose adjustments at the start of a subsequent cycle should be based on nadir hematologic counts or maximum nonhematologic toxicity from the preceding cycle of therapy. In studies, laboratory analyses were performed on day 1 before each dose and on days 8 and 15. Treatment may be delayed to allow sufficient time for recovery. Do not have patients begin a new cycle of treatment unless the ANC is 1500 cells/mm³ or more, the platelet count is 100,000 cells/mm³ or more, and CrCl is 45 mL/min or more. Upon recovery, retreat patients using the guidelines in the following table, which are suitable for using pemetrexed as a single agent or in combination with cisplatin:

Dose Reduction for Pemetrexed (Single Agent or in Combination with Cisplatin) Hematologic Toxicities

Nadir ANC <500/mm³ and nadir platelets ≥50,000/mm³	75% of previous dose (both drugs)
Nadir platelets <50,000/mm³ regardless of nadir ANC	50% of previous dose (both drugs)

Nonhematologic Toxicities

If patients develop nonhematologic toxicities (excluding neurotoxicity) of grade 3 or higher (except grade 3 transaminase elevations), withhold pemetrexed until toxicities resolve to less than or equal to the patient's pretherapy value. Resume treatment according to guidelines in the table below:

Dose Reduction for Pemetrexed (Single Agent or in Combination with Cisplatin) Nonhematologic Toxicities*

Neurotoxicity

In the event of neurotoxicity, the recommended dose adjustments for pemetrexed

CTC Grade	Dose of Pemetrexed (mg/m²)	Dose of Cisplatin (mg/m²)
0-1	100% of previous dose	100% of previous dose
2	100% of previous dose	50% of previous dose

and cisplatin are shown in the following table. Discontinue therapy if grade 3 or 4 neurotoxicity is experienced.

Dose Reduction for Pemetrexed (Single Agent or in Combination with Cisplatin) Neurotoxicity 1

Renal Function Impairment

Concomitant Use with NSAIDs

Exercise caution when administering pemetrexed concurrently with NSAIDs to patients whose CrCl is less than 80 mL/minute. Patients with mild to moderate renal insufficiency should avoid taking NSAIDs with short elimination half-lives for a period of 2 days before, the day of, and 2 days after administration of pemetrexed. In the absence of data on potential interactions between pemetrexed and NSAIDs with longer half-lives, all patients taking these NSAIDs should interrupt dosing for at least 5 days before, the day of, and 2 days after pemetrexed administration. If co-administration of an NSAID is necessary, closely monitor patients for toxicity, especially myelosuppression and renal and GI toxicity.

Dosage Adjustment in Hepatic Dysfunction

Pemetrexed is not extensively metabolized by the liver. Dose adjustments based on hepatic impairment experienced during treatment with pemetrexed are provided in the "Dose Reduction for Pemetrexed (Single Agent or in Combination with Cisplatin) Nonhematologic Toxicities" table shown previously.

Dosage Adjustment in Renal Dysfunction

In clinical studies, patients with CrCl of 45 mL/minute or higher required no dose adjustments other than those recommended for all patients. Insufficient numbers of patients with CrCl less than 45 mL/minute have been treated to make dosage recommendations for this group of patients. Therefore, use of pemetrexed for patients whose CrCl is less than 45 mL/minute is not recommended.

PRECAUTIONS

Pregnancy Risk Category: D

Pleural Effusion or Ascites

The effect of third space fluid, such as pleural effusion and ascites, on pemetrexed is unknown. In patients with clinically significant amounts of third space fluid, consider draining the effusion before pemetrexed administration.

	Dose of Pemetrexed (mg/m^2)	Dose of cisplatin (mg/m^2)
Any grade 3† or 4 toxicities except mucositis*	75% of previous dose	75% of previous dose
Any diarrhea requiring hospitalization (irrespective of grade) or grade 3 or 4 diarrhea	75% of previous dose	75% of previous dose
Grade 3 or 4 mucositis	50% of previous dose	100% of previous dose

*National Cancer Institute Common Toxicity Criteria (CTC), excluding neurotoxicity.
†Except grade 3 transaminase elevation.
From Alimta (pemetrexed for injection) prescribing information. Eli Lilly and Company, 2006.

CONTRAINDICATIONS
Hypersensitivity reaction to pemetrexed or ingredients used in the preparation

DRUG PREPARATION/ADMINISTRATION/ SAFE HANDLING ISSUES
◀ ALERT ▶ Pemetrexed is administered by IV infusion over 10 mins. The manufacturer recommends use of protective gloves when handling the drug. If pemetrexed comes in contact with skin or mucosa, affected skin areas should be washed immediately and thoroughly with soap and water and affected mucosa should be thoroughly rinsed with copious amounts of water. Do not use waterless or antibacterial soap as either can enhance the skin reaction. If an eye splash occurs use, copious amounts of water or 0.9% NaCl to irrigate the eyes going from inner to outer canthus. Pemetrexed is not a vesicant. Extravasation should be managed according to local standards of practice; there is no specific antidote for extravasation of pemetrexed. Vials containing 500 mg of pemetrexed should be reconstituted using 20 mL of 0.9% NaCl injection without preservatives, making a solution containing 25 mg/mL. This solution is further diluted in 0.9% NaCl injection without preservatives to a volume of 100 mL before administration. **Note:** Pemetrexed is incompatible with diluents containing calcium (e.g., lactated Ringer's injection or Ringer's injection). Because reconstituted and/or diluted pemetrexed solutions contain no preservatives, any unused portions of these solutions should be discarded. When reconstituted and/or diluted as directed, pemetrexed solutions are stable for 24 hrs at controlled room temperature under ambient lighting.

STORAGE AND STABILITY
Store at 25° C (77° F) with excursions to 15-30° C (59-86° F) permitted. Reconstituted and infusion solutions are stable for up to 24 hrs after initial reconstitution when stored refrigerated (2-8° C [36-46° F]) or at 25° C (77° F) for excursions.
Pemetrexed reconstituted with 0.9% NaCl to a concentration of 25 mg/mL packaged in polypropylene syringes was found to be stable for 2 days at room temperature and 31 days refrigerated.

INTERACTIONS
Drug
Nephrotoxic drugs: Coadministration of nephrotoxic drugs could result in delayed clearance of pemetrexed. Coadministration of substances that also are tubularly secreted (e.g., probenecid) could potentially result in delayed clearance of pemetrexed. *NSAIDs (e.g., ibuprofen):* Daily ibuprofen doses of 400 mg 4 times/day reduce clearance of pemetrexed clearance about 20% (and increase AUC 20%) in patients with normal renal function. Use caution when administering ibuprofen concurrently with pemetrexed to patients with mild to moderate renal insufficiency (CrCl 45-79 mL/minute), and avoid giving NSAIDs with short elimination half-lives 2 days before, the day of, and 2 days after pemetrexed administration. Interrupt dosing in all patients taking NSAIDs with long elimination half-lives for at least 5 days before, the day of, and 2 days after pemetrexed administration. If coadministration of an NSAID is necessary, closely monitor patients for toxicity, especially myelosuppression and renal and GI toxicity.
Herbal
None known.

Y-SITE COMPATIBLES
No information has been published as yet.

INCOMPATIBLES
Use only 0.9% NaCl to reconstitute; flush the line before and after the infusion. Do not add any other medications to the IV line.

SIDE EFFECTS
Serious Reactions
Myelosuppression, manifested as neutropenia, thrombocytopenia, or anemia, may occur.
Other Side Effects
Frequent (10%-50%):
Arthralgias have been reported in 24% of patients treated. In combination with cisplatin for the treatment of malignant melanoma, grade 3 or 4 nausea and vomiting were reported in 12% and 11% of patients, respectively. Rash and/or desquamation is frequently observed (see ALERT above). Fatigue has also been reported and may be prevented with dexamethasone.

Occasional (1%-10%):
(8%-4%) Stomatitis, pharyngitis, diarrhea, anorexia, hypertension, chest pain
(Less Than 3%) Constipation, depression, dysphagia.
Reversible and usually mild renal dysfunction has been observed in up to 25% of patients receiving the every 21-day regimen; a lower frequency is seen with 500 compared with 600 mg/m^2 doses. Renal impairment appears nonprogressive in the face of continued treatment. However, the presence of renal impairment significantly increases the overall toxicity of pemetrexed; dose reduction and close monitoring of serum creatinine levels are indicated in this setting.

Rare (Less Than 1%):
Hypersensitivity reactions have been reported in patients treated with pemetrexed and cisplatin.

SPECIAL CONSIDERATIONS
Baseline Assessment
- Assess patient's CBC with differential, platelet count, electrolyte, BUN, and creatinine levels, and liver function tests.
- Evaluate patient's history of renal and hepatic disease.
- Monitor patient for any evidence of dermatologic conditionsav.
- Assess patient for a history of diabetes as steroids are usually part of the premedications to reduce side effects.

Intervention and Evaluation
- Evaluate patient's blood counts and renal and liver function tests before each dose.
- Assess patient's medication history and introduction of any new agents at each visit.
- Monitor for evidence of dermatologic reactions, arthralgias, and increasing fatigue.
- Evaluate patient for evidence of myelosuppression, evidence of infection, easy bruising, bleeding, or significant fatigue or dyspnea upon exertion.
- Premedicate patient as ordered with corticosteroids.
- Monitor patient for any evidence of hypersensitivity reactions.
- Have emergency/anaphylaxis kit available at bedside along with an oxygen setup and an Ambu bag when administering this agent. The anaphylaxis kit should include the following:
  Diphenhydramine 50 mg
  Hydrocortisone 50 mg
  Epinephrine 1:1000: 1 mL to be administered at 0.3 mL each time; may repeat dose as needed
  Syringes
  Needles
  2 by 2 gauze pad to break epinephrine ampule
  Alcohol wipes

Education
- Instruct patient on when to contact his or her health care provider: fever greater than 38° C (greater than 101° F), chills, shortness of breath, easy bruising or bleeding, the inability to drink at least 1500 mL of fluid in 24 hours, nausea lasting greater than 24 hours, or diarrhea lasting greater than 24 hours.
- Educate patient about the need for premedications and their side effects.
- Educate patient to take folic acid every day and dexamethasone twice daily the day before, the day of, and the day after pemetrexed or as directed by the oncologist.
- Instruct patient to report any evidence of arthralgias, myalgias, or neuropathy.
- Educate patient on symptoms of neuropathy: numbness and tingling in fingers and toes and feelings of pins and needles in extremities.
- Monitor patient for any new medications and herbal or vitamin supplements at each provider visit; instruct patient to avoid initiation of new agents without discussing with the provider.
- Educate patient to avoid all NSAIDs.
- Provide patient with information on local resources and support groups available for his or her specific diagnosis.

PENTOSTATIN

BRAND NAMES
Nipent

CLASS OF AGENT
Antineoplastic agent, antibiotic derivative, antimetabolite

CLINICAL PHARMACOLOGY
Mechanism of Action
An antimetabolite that is isolated from fermentation cultures of *Streptomyces antibioticus*. Acts as an inhibitor of the enzyme adenosine deaminase (ADA), resulting in elevated levels of deoxy-adenosine 5'-triphosphate, which in turn blocks DNA synthesis. May also inhibit RNA synthesis and produce DNA damage. Has its greatest activity in T cells of lymphoid system. **Therapeutic Effect:** Inhibits DNA and RNA synthesis.

Absorption and Distribution
Tissue distribution is within all tissues and with little in the CNS. Distribution half-life: 11 mins. Volume of distribution: 36 L. Protein binding: 4%.
Half-life: 5.7 hours (half-life increased with impaired renal function).

Metabolism and Excretion
Excreted primarily in urine unchanged or as active metabolite (90%).

HOW SUPPLIED/AVAILABLE FORMS
Powder for Injection: 10 mg.

INDICATIONS AND DOSAGES
Hairy Cell Leukemia
4 mg/m^2 IV every 2 weeks until complete response attained (without any major toxicity). Discontinue if no response in 6 months, partial response in 12 months, or 2 doses after a complete response. Prehydrate with 500-1000 mL of fluid and posthydrate with 500 mL of fluid.

Dosage Adjustment in Hepatic Dysfunction
No information.

Dosage Adjustment in Renal Dysfunction
Reduce dose to 2-3 mg/m^2 in patients with CrCl between 50 and 60 mL/minute. Benefits should clearly outweigh any risks of nephrotoxicity in these patients.

UNLABELED USES
Treatment of Hodgkin's lymphoma, myelodysplastic syndrome, T-cell lymphoma

PRECAUTIONS
Use cautiously in patients with preexisting myelosuppression, cardiac disease, or impaired hepatic or renal function. Use cautiously in patients with current or recent infection, chickenpox, or herpes zoster.
Pregnancy Risk Category: D
Drug excretion into human breast milk is unknown/not recommended in nursing women.

CONTRAINDICATIONS
Hypersensitivity to pentostatin

DRUG PREPARATION/ADMINISTRATION/ SAFE HANDLING ISSUES
◀ ALERT ▶ Because pentostatin may be carcinogenic, mutagenic, or teratogenic, wear nitrile or latex, but not vinyl, gloves when handling the drug. If the drug comes in contact with skin, wash the skin thoroughly with soap and water. Do not use waterless hand soap or any antibacterial soap as either can increase the reaction from the agent. If the drug comes in contact with mucous membranes, flush the area with water.
◀ ALERT ▶ Withhold or discontinue administration in patients with severe reactions to pentostatin, CNS toxicity, active underlying infections, increased serum creatinine levels, and ANC less than 200/mm^3 with a baseline count greater than 500/mm^3.
- Reconstitute each 10-mg vial with 5 mL of 0.9% NaCl to provide a concentration of 2 mg/mL.
- Shake thoroughly to ensure dissolution.
- Hydrate patient adequately before and immediately after administration (decreases risk of adverse renal effects).
- Administer prehydration of 500-1000 mL of 5% dextrose in 0.5% NaCl or equivalent and posthydration of 500 mL.
- For IV push, give over 5 mins.
- For IV infusion, further dilute with 25-50 mL of D5W or 0.9% NaCl and give over 20-30 minutes.

STORAGE AND STABILITY
- Refrigerate vial (2-8° C [36-46° F]).
- This medicavation contains no preservatives. After reconstitution or dilution, use within 8 hours when given at room temperature and stored in environmental light.

INTERACTIONS
Drug
Bone marrow depressants: May increase bone marrow depression.

Fludarabine: May increase pulmonary toxicity.
High-dose cyclophosphamide: Concomitant use before bone marrow transplant has been reported to cause fatal cardiac toxicity
Live-virus vaccines: May potentiate virus replication, increase vaccine side effects, and decrease patient's antibody response to vaccine.
Vidarabine: May increase effects and toxicity of vidarabine.
Herbal
None known.

LAB EFFECTS/INTERFERENCE
May increase AST (SGOT), ALT (SGPT), alkaline phosphatase, LDH, uric acid, and creatinine levels.

Y-SITE COMPATIBLES
Fludarabine (may increase pulmonary toxicity), melphalan, ondansetron, paclitaxel, sargramostim

INCOMPATIBLES
No information.

SIDE EFFECTS
Serious Reactions
• Bone marrow depression is manifested as hematologic toxicity. No dosage reduction is recommended at the start of therapy in patients with anemia, neutropenia, or thrombocytopenia. Hold drug if ANC is less than 200 cells/mm^3 (baseline greater than 500 cells/mm^3), and resume when count returns to predose levels.
• Doses higher than recommended (20-50 mg/m^2 in divided doses for more than 5 days) may produce fatal renal, hepatic, pulmonary, or CNS toxicity.
Other Side Effects
Frequent (10%-50%):
Anorexia, arthralgia, diarrhea, chills, cough, fatigue, fever, headache, hematologic toxicity, lethargy, nausea, pain, pharyngitis, rash, sinusitis, skin discoloration, sweating, upper respiratory tract infection, vomiting
Occasional (1%-10%):
Anxiety, blurred vision, chest pain, confusion, conjunctivitis, depression, dizziness, myalgia, peripheral edema
Rare (Less Than 1%):
Coma, dysuria, hematuria, hypersensitivity reactions, thrombophlebitis

SPECIAL CONSIDERATIONS
Baseline Assessment
• Assess baseline CBC with differential, platelets, electrolytes, BUN, and creatinine levels, and liver function tests.
• Evaluate patient's prior emetic history.
• Assess patient's allergy history.
• Monitor patient for any history of depression or altered mental status.
• Obtain a baseline neurologic examination.
• Assess patient for any history of dermatologic problems.
• Obtain baseline weight, and evaluate any peripheral edema.
Intervention and Evaluation
• Assess patient's laboratory data prior to each dosing.
• Premedicate patient with antiemetics before each dose.
• Weigh patient before each dose, and evaluate for any evidence of peripheral edema.
• Evaluate patient for any changes in mental status, confusion, restlessness, agitation, or insomnia.
• Assess patient for any evidence of skin toxicity, rash, pruritus, or conjunctivitis.
• Evaluate patient before each dose for evidence of pulmonary changes, rales, rhonchi, shortness of breath, or dyspnea.
• Monitor for evidence of myelosuppression, fever, chills, bleeding, bruising, or increasing fatigue.
• If severe rash, pulmonary compromise, or altered mental status is present, do NOT administer dose, and check with health care provider before dosing.
Education
• Instruct patient on when to contact his or her health care provider: fever greater than 38° C (greater than 101° F), chills, cough, shortness of breath, easy bruising, bleeding or increasing fatigue, nausea lasting greater than 24 hours, diarrhea lasting greater than 24 hours, or the inability to drink at least 1500 mL of fluids in 24 hours.
• Educate patient and caregivers that altered mental status can occur with this agent and to call the health care provider immediately if any increasing confusion, agitation, or insomnia is noted.
• Educate patient on neutropenic precautions as necessary:
  Practice good handwashing technique.
  Avoid individuals who are ill.
  Wash and cook all foods well.

Avoid crowds.
Avoid fresh fruits and vegetables.
• Educate patient to look for any rashes or skin changes and to report to the health care provider.
• Advise patient that there have been reports of pulmonary toxicity with this agent and to report any changes in respiratory pattern, cough, shortness of breath, or dyspnea upon exertion.
• Instruct patient that visual changes may occur and to report any blurred vision or eye irritation to the health care provider.
• Instruct patient to avoid receiving any vaccinations without first checking with the health care provider.
• Educate patient to drink at least 2 L of fluids per day to maintain good renal function.
• Advise patient and caregiver to monitor for any evidence of edema or weight gain and to report to the health care provider.
• Instruct patient to take no over-the-counter medications or herbal or vitamin supplements without checking with his or her health care provider.
• Provide patient with information on local resources and support groups available for his or her specific diagnosis.

PROCARBAZINE

BRAND NAMES
Matulane, Natulan [Canada]

CLASS OF AGENT
Antineoplastic agent, alkylating agent

CLINICAL PHARMACOLOGY
Mechanism of Action
Procarbazine is a methylhydrazine derivative that inhibits DNA, RNA, and protein synthesis. It may also directly damage DNA. Procarbazine is a prodrug that must be converted to its active 2-azoxyprocarbazine metabolites, which exhibit cytotoxic or mutagenic properties. It is metabolized rapidly either spontaneously or by an enzymatic reaction mediated by the cytochrome P450 system. After conversion, the precise mechanism of action is uncertain but is believed to involve the formation of O-methylguanine DNA adducts. It is proposed that its mechanisms involve inhibition of protein synthesis by inhibiting or damaging the action of DNA, RNA, or transfer RNA.
Cell cycle phase specific for the S phase of cell division. **Therapeutic Effect:** Causes cell death.

Absorption and Distribution
Procarbazine is only administered PO. It is completely absorbed. It distributes into lymph node tissue and bone marrow. It also crosses the blood-brain barrier.
Half-life: After IV administration, its plasma half-life is only 10 minutes. The overall elimination half-life is 1 hour.

Metabolism and Excretion
It is metabolized by red blood cells and by hepatic microsomal enzymes to azoprocarbazine. The main sites of metabolism are the liver and kidney, which convert the parent compound to N-isopropylterephthalamic acid (inactive). About 70% of procarbazine is excreted as metabolites. Only 5% of the drug is excreted unchanged in the urine.

HOW SUPPLIED/AVAILABLE FORMS
Capsules: 50 mg.

INDICATIONS AND DOSAGES
Advanced Hodgkin's Disease
Procarbazine is almost always used in conjunction with the MOPP (mechlorethamine, vincristine [oncovorin], procarbazine, and prednisone) regimen for the treatment of Hodgkin's disease or the C (cyclophosphamide)-MOPP regimen. The dose is 100 mg/m² (rounded to the nearest 50 mg) given daily by mouth for 7-14 days every month.
Pediatric: 50-100 mg/m²/day for 10-14 days of a 28-day cycle. Continue until maximum response occurs, leukocyte count falls below 4000/mm³, or platelet count falls below 100,000/mm³. Maintenance dose: 50 mg/m²/day.

Dosage Adjustment in Hepatic Dysfunction
The dosage of procarbazine should be reduced in patients with liver dysfunction.

Dosage Adjustment in Renal Dysfunction
The dosage of procarbazine should be reduced in patients with renal dysfunction.

UNLABELED USES
Procarbazine is rarely used in treatment of lung carcinoma, malignant melanoma, multiple myeloma, non-Hodgkin's lymphoma, polycythemia vera, or primary brain tumors. As a single agent, it is used in a dose of 2-4 mg/kg PO per day.

PRECAUTIONS
Pregnancy Risk Category: D

CONTRAINDICATIONS
Known hypersensitivity to procarbazine or inadequate marrow reserves

DRUG PREPARATION/ADMINISTRATION/ SAFE HANDLING ISSUES

STORAGE AND STABILITY
Store at room temperature in airtight containers and protected from light.

INTERACTIONS
Drug
Most of the following interactions are related to the monoamine oxidase inhibitor (MAOI) properties of procarbazine and high tyramine-containing foods.
Alcohol: May cause a disulfiram-like reaction.
Anticholinergics, antihistamines: May increase the anticholinergic effects of these drugs.
Bone marrow depressants: May increase myelosuppression.
Buspirone, caffeine-containing medications: May increase B/P.
Carbamazepine, cyclobenzaprinave, MAOIs, maprotiline: May cause hyperpyretic crisis, seizures, or death.
CNS depressants: May increase CNS depression.
Insulin, oral antidiabetic drugs: May increase the effects of these drugs.
Live-virus vaccines: May develop infections after live vaccine injection because of immunosuppression of procarbazine.
Meperidine: May produce coma, seizures, immediate excitation, rigidity, severe hypertension or hypotension, severe respiratory distress, diaphoresis, and vascular collapse.
Sympathomimetics: May increase cardiac stimulant and vasopressor effects.
Tricyclic antidepressants: May increase anticholinergic effects; may cause seizures and hyperpyretic crisis.
Herbal
None known.

LAB EFFECTS/INTERFERENCE
None known.

SIDE EFFECTS
Serious Reactions
• The major toxic effects of procarbazine are myelosuppression manifested as hematologic toxicity (mainly leukopenia, thrombocytopenia, and anemia) and hepatotoxicity manifested as jaundice and ascites.
• Urinary tract infections (UTIs) may occur due to leukopenia.
Other Side Effects
Frequent (10%-50%):
Severe nausea, vomiting, respiratory disorders (cough, effusion), myalgia, arthralgia, drowsiness, nervousness, insomnia, nightmares, diaphoresis, hallucinations, seizures
Occasional (1%-10%):
Hoarseness, tachycardia, nystagmus, retinal hemorrhage, photophobia, photosensitivity, urinary frequency, nocturia, hypotension, diarrhea, stomatitis, paraesthesia, unsteadiness, confusion, decreased reflexes, foot drop
Rare (Less Than 1%):
Hypersensitivity reaction (dermatitis, pruritus, rash, urticaria), hyperpigmentation, alopecia

SPECIAL CONSIDERATIONS
Baseline Assessment
• Assess CBC with differential, platelet count, electrolyte, BUN, and creatinine levels, and liver function tests before initiation of therapy.
• Evaluate patient for prior therapy and tolerance related to emesis.
• Assess patient's history for insomnia, hallucinations, anxiety disorder, and any prior seizures.
• Assess patient's weight before therapy as edema and ascites may occur with this agent.
• Evaluate patient for any history of active liver disease before therapy.
• Monitor patient for history of allergic reactions as hypersensitivity can occur.
• Assess patient for any history of recurrent UTIs or pulmonary disorders.
• Obtain baseline vital signs, monitoring especially for hypotension.
• Refer patient for dietary consultation as needed.
• Inspect skin and oral cavity before initiating therapy.
Intervention and Evaluation
• Evaluate CBC with differential, platelet count, electrolyte, BUN, and creatinine levels, and liver function tests at each visit.
• Weigh patient and monitor vital signs at each visit; include assessment of oxygen saturation as pulmonary changes can occur.
• Assess patient for significant nausea, vomiting, or food intolerance with this agent.

- Evaluate for UTIs or pulmonary symptoms at each visit.
- Assess patient for any neurologic symptoms, anxiety, hallucinations, nightmares, or seizures at each visit.
- Evaluate for symptoms of pancytopenia, anemia, leukopenia, or thrombocytopenia, and initiate colony-stimulating factors as ordered.
- Evaluate patient's nutrition at each visit.
- Premedicate as ordered for nausea, vomiting, and possible hypersensitivity reaction.
- Assess skin and oral cavity at each visit, and initiate a skin and oral care regimen as needed. A usual oral care regimen would include use of a soft toothbrush at least 3 times/day and at bedtime. Instruct patient to rinse oral cavity with cool water and, if wanted, add 1 tsp of baking soda and 1 tsp of salt in 8 ounces of water to swish and spit at least 3 times/day and at bedtime.
- Initiate a skin care regimen to include moisturizers, such as Aquaphor, Eucerin, or Absorbase, for any areas of irritation or desquamation.

Education
- Educate patient on when to contact his or her health care provider: fever greater than 38° C (greater than 101° F), chills, shortness of breath, respiratory distress, altered mental status, increasing anxiety disorder, nausea lasting greater than 24 hours, diarrhea lasting greater than 24 hours, severe right upper quadrant pain, or the inability to take in at least 1500 mL of fluid in 24 hours.
- Instruct patient to take medication as instructed, to avoid skipping doses, and to report any missed doses.
- Advise patient on symptoms of neutropenia: fevers, fatigue, and chills. Instruct patient to make sure good hygiene procedures are followed.
- Educate patient on thrombocytopenic precautions: no straight razors, no rectal suppositories, no aerobic exercises, soft toothbrush, no flossing of teeth, and no dental work without prior authorization from the health care provider.
- Instruct patient on symptoms of anemia: fatigue, shortness of breath, and difficult breathing with exercise.
- Instruct patient on both oral care regimens and skin care protocols.
- Instruct patient to avoid all OTC medications and herbal and vitamin supplements without first checking with the health care provider

- Provide patient with information on local resources and support groups available for his or her specific diagnosis.

RITUXIMAB
BRAND NAMES
Rituxan

CLASS OF AGENT
Chimeric monoclonal antibody

CLINICAL PHARMACOLOGY
Mechanism of Action
Binds to CD20, the antigen found on the surface of pre-B and mature B lymphocytes. CD20 is expressed in greater than 90% of B-cell non-Hodgkin's lymphomas. In vitro data demonstrate B-cell lysis, possibly by complement-dependent cytotoxicity and antibody-dependent cell-mediated cytotoxicity. **Therapeutic Effect:** Depletes B lymphocytes and reduces tumor burden.
Absorption and Distribution
Drug is given IV. Serum levels are proportional to dose. The peak and trough serum levels of rituximab are inversely correlated with number of circulating CD20-positive B cells and amount of disease burden.
Half-life: 3.2 days after first infusion and 8.6 days after fourth infusion.
Metabolism and Excretion
No information.

HOW SUPPLIED/AVAILABLE FORMS
Injection: 10 mg/mL as 100-mg and 500-mg vials.

INDICATIONS AND DOSAGES
Relapse or Refractory Low-Grade or Follicular CD20-Positive Non-Hodgkin's Lymphoma
375 mg/m^2 IV once weekly for 4-8 weeks. May administer a second 4-week course.
First-Line Diffuse Large B-cell CD20-Positive Non-Hodgkin's Lymphoma
375 mg/m^2 IV on day 1 of each chemotherapy cycle.
Rheumatoid Arthritis after Inadequate Response of at Least One Tumor Necrosis Factor Antagonist
Two doses of 1000 mg/dose IV separated by 2 weeks.
As Part of Zevalin Regimen (Ibritumomab Tiuxetan)
250 mg/m^2 IV over 4 hours as part of the Zevalin regimen (ibritumomab tiuxetan).

Dosage Adjustment in Hepatic Dysfunction
No information.

Dosage Adjustment in Renal Dysfunction
No information.

UNLABELED USES
Chronic lymphoid leukemia, graft-versus-host disease, hairy cell leukemia, immune thrombocytopenic purpura, Waldenström's macroglobulinemia

PRECAUTIONS
Fatal infusion reactions have occurred with rituximab administration. They usually appear with the first dose and within 30-120 minutes. Stop or reduce rate infusion, and administer supportive medications as ordered. Once symptoms resolve, most patients can tolerate the infusion resumed at 50% of the previous rate. Discontinue infliximab if symptoms are severe: pulmonary infiltrates, acute respiratory distress syndrome, MI, ventricular fibrillation, and cardiogenic shock.

Tumor lysis syndrome has resulted in acute renal failure, hyperkalemia, hypocalcemia, hyperuricemia, or hyperphosphatemia. Supportive care including dialysis, electrolyte correction and monitoring fluid balance, and renal function may be required. Severe mucocutaneous reactions including paraneoplastic pemphigus, Stevens-Johnson syndrome, lichenoid dermatitis, vesiculobullous dermatitis, and toxic epidermal necrolysis have been reported. Patients should not receive any further rituximab.

Fulminant hepatitis, hepatic failure, and death have been reported in patients with hepatitis B reactivation. Median time to diagnosis was 4 months after starting rituximab therapy.

Pregnancy Risk Category: C
Rituximab should only be used in pregnant women if clearly indicated. Women who are nursing should be advised to discontinue nursing until drug levels are undetectable.

CONTRAINDICATIONS
Known hypersensitivity to murine proteins or any component of the formulation

DRUG PREPARATION/ADMINISTRATION/SAFE HANDLING ISSUES
• Withdraw amount of drug needed and dilute into a 0.9% sodium chloride or 5% D4W bag to make a final concentration of 1-4 mg/mL.
• Do not administer as an IV bolus or push.
• First infusion: administer IV at an initial rate of 50 mg/hour. Increase infusion rate in 50 mg/hour increments every 30 minutes to a maximum of 400 mg/hour. If hypersensitivity or infusion-related reaction develops, temporarily stop or slow the infusion and upon improvement of symptoms, resume at half the previous rate.
• Subsequent infusions can be initiated at a rate of 100 mg/hour and increased in 100 mg/hour increments at 30-minute intervals to a maximum of 400 mg/hour if the patient tolerated the first infusion. Stop or slow infusion as before if the patient develops hypersensitivity or infusion-related reaction.

STORAGE AND STABILITY
• Vials are stored at 2-8° C (36-46° F). Protect from direct sunlight. Do not freeze or shake.
• Diluted infusion bags are stable for 24 hours refrigerated and an additional 24 hours at room temperature. The manufacturer recommends refrigeration, as the solution does not contain preservatives.

INTERACTIONS
Drug
Cisplatin: Increases risk of renal toxicity.
Herbal
None known.

LAB EFFECTS/INTERFERENCE
LDH level may increase.

Y-SITE COMPATIBLES
According to the manufacturer, there is no information, and they recommend that rituximab not be mixed with any other medication. MicroMedex lists acyclovir, amifostine, ampicillin, bleomycin, busulfan, calcium gluconate, carboplatin, carmustine, cefazolin, cimetidine, cyclophosphamide, dactinomycin, daunorubicin, dexamethasone, dexrazoxane, diphenhydramine, docetaxel, filgrastim, fluorouracil, gemcitabine, gentamicin, granisetron, heparin, hydrocortisone succinate, idarubicin, ifosfamide, irinotecan, leucovorin, lorazepam, magnesium, mannitol, mesna, methotrexate,

methylprednisolone, metoclopramide, mitomycin, mitoxantrone, morphine sulfate, paclitaxel, potassium chloride, prochlorperazine, and ranitidine.

INCOMPATIBLES
Do not mix rituximab with any other medications according to the manufacturer. MicroMedex lists aldesleukin, amphotericin B colloidal, ciprofloxacin, daunorubicin, doxorubicin HCl, furosemide, levofloxacin, minocycline, ofloxacin, ondansetron, sodium bicarbonate, topotecan, and vancomycin.

SIDE EFFECTS
Serious Reactions
- Hypersensitivity reactions marked by hypotension, bronchospasm, and angioedema may occur. They usually occurs with the first dose.
- Arrhythmias may occur, particularly in those with a history of preexisting cardiac conditions.
- Tumor lysis syndrome may occur, especially in patients with a heavy tumor burden or high numbers of circulating malignant cells.
- Rare but serious and severe mucocutaneous reactions have been reported. Do not readminister rituximab.

Other Side Effects
Frequent (10%-50%):
Abdominal pain, angioedema, asthenia, back pain, chills, cough, fever, headache, hypotension, infections, leukopenia, nausea, neutropenia, night sweats, rash or pruritus, rhinitis, thrombocytopenia
Occasional (1%-10%):
Anemia, anxiety, bronchospasm, diarrhea, dizziness, dyspnea, flushing, hyperglycemia, hypertension, LDH level increase, myalgia, peripheral edema, rhinitis, sinusitis, throat irritation, urticaria, vomiting
Rare (Less Than 1%):
Fulminant hepatic failure, lichenoid dermatitis, paraneoplastic pemphigus, Stevens-Johnson syndrome, toxic epidermal necrolysis, vesiculobullous dermatitis

SPECIAL CONSIDERATIONS
Baseline Assessment
- Assess CBCs with differential, electrolyte, BUN, and creatinine levels, liver function tests, and hepatitis serologies.
- Assess patient's respiratory function.

- Evaluate disease burden as increased burden can increase risk reactions such as tumor lysis syndrome.
- Evaluate patient for any evidence of prior cardiac or pulmonary disease.
- Assess patient for history of drug allergies, as this is a monoclonal agent, and patients with multiple allergies can be at increased risk of reactions.

Intervention and Evaluation
- Assess laboratory data before each dose of this agent. Although they are less common, rituximab can cause grade 3 and 4 cytopenias: lymphopenia (40%), neutropenia (6%), leukopenia (4%), anemia (3%), and thrombocytopenia (2%). Aplastic anemia (pure red cell aplasia) and hemolytic anemia were reported rarely.
- Administer premedications as ordered, usually acetaminophen and diphenhydramine. Patients with rheumatoid arthritis should receive methylprednisolone 100 mg IV or equivalent before each dose.
- Assess patient for any prior reactions to this medication.
- Have anaphylaxis kit available at bedside along with an oxygen setup and an Ambu bag when administering this agent. The anaphylaxis kit should include the following:
  Hydrocortisone 50 mg
  Diphenhydramine 50 mg
  Epinephrine 1:1000: draw up in syringe, inject only 0.3 mL at a time, and repeat as necessary
  Needles and syringes
- Monitor vital signs as per institutional policy, especially with the first infusion.
- Increase rate at no more than every 30 minutes.
- Monitor patient for evidence of respiratory or cardiac symptoms, chest pain, and shortness of breath.

Education
- Instruct patient on when to contact his or her health care provider: fever greater than 38° C (greater than 101° F), chills, shortness of breath, chest pain, palpitations, myalgias, or arthralgias.
- Educate patient to inform the health care provider if he or she had any difficulty tolerating prior infusions of this agent.
- Advise patient on the necessity of premedications before taking this agent to prevent allergic reactions such as fever and chills.

- Educate patient this is a monoclonal antibody and not a chemotherapeutic agent; therefore, he or she will not experience the usual side effects of nausea, vomiting, diarrhea, or hair loss.
- Instruct patient to avoid taking any OTC medications and herbal or vitamin supplements without first checking with the health care provider.
- Provide patient with information on local resources and support groups available for his or her specific diagnosis.

SARGRAMOSTIM, GRANULOCYTE-MACROPHAGE COLONY-STIMULATING FACTOR

BRAND NAMES
Leukine

CLASS OF AGENT
Human granulocyte-macrophage colony-stimulating factor, hematopoietic growth factor

CLINICAL PHARMACOLOGY
Mechanism of Action
A colony-stimulating factor that regulates production of neutrophils, monocytes, macrophages, and myeloid-derived dendritic cells. May also activate mature neutrophils and macrophages. **Therapeutic Effect:** Decreases incidence of infection.
Absorption and Distribution
Readily absorbed after subcutaneous administration; detected in serum 15 minutes with peak levels at 1-3 hours after injection. *Half-life:* 2-3 hours.
Metabolism and Excretion
No information.

HOW SUPPLIED/AVAILABLE FORMS
Lyophilized Powder for Injection: 250 mcg/mL.
Liquid for Injection: 500 mcg/mL.

INDICATIONS AND DOSAGES
Mobilization of Progenitor Cells
250 mcg/m^2/day IV over 24 hours or subcutaneous every day; begin immediately after progenitor cell infusion. Reduce dose by 50% if WBC count is greater than 50,000 cells/mm^3.
Bone Marrow Transplant
250 mcg/m^2/day IV over 2 hours; begin 2-4 hours after bone marrow infusion.

Continue until ANC greater than or equal to 1500/mm^3 for 3 consecutive days.
Bone Marrow Transplant Failure or Engraftment Delay
250 mcg/m^2/day IV over 2 hours for 14 days; repeat after 7 days if needed.
Recovery of Acute Myelogenous Leukemia Induction Chemotherapy
250 mcg/m^2/day IV over 4 hours; begin 4 days after completing induction chemotherapy. Continue until ANC is greater than or equal to 1500/mm^3 for 3 consecutive days or a maximum of 42 days.
Note: Dose reduce by 50% or interrupt treatment if severe adverse effects occur or if ANC is greater than 20,000 cells/mm^3 or platelet count is greater than 500,000/mm^3. Check CBC with differential twice a week to avoid excessive leukocytosis (WBC greater than 50,000 cells/mm^3 or ANC greater than 20,000 cells/mm^3).
Dosage Adjustment in Hepatic Dysfunction
No adjustments required.
Dosage Adjustment in Renal Dysfunction
No adjustments required.

UNLABELED USES
Treatment of AIDS-related neutropenia; myelodysplastic syndrome; agranulocytosis; aplastic anemia; metastatic renal cell carcinoma, metastatic melanoma

PRECAUTIONS
Use sargramostim cautiously in patients with malignancy with myeloid characteristics (because of the potential for granulocyte colony-stimulating factor to act as a growth factor), preexisting fluid retention, pulmonary infiltrates, CHF, or cardiac conditions. The liquid formulation of sargramostim or lyophilized powder reconstituted with bacteriostatic water contains benzyl alcohol and should not be used in neonates. Do not administer 24 hours before or after chemotherapy.
Pregnancy Risk Category: C
Sargramostim should only be used in pregnant or nursing women if clearly indicated with benefit.

CONTRAINDICATIONS
Patients with greater than 10% leukemic myeloid blasts in bone marrow or peripheral blood; known hypersensitivity to sargramostim, yeast-derived products, or any component of the formulation; concomitant

chemotherapy and radiotherapy (administer sargramostim 24 hours after chemotherapy or radiotherapy).

DRUG PREPARATION/ADMINISTRATION/ SAFE HANDLING ISSUES

◀ ALERT ▶ Begin sargramostim therapy at least 24 hours after last dose of chemotherapy; discontinue at least 24 hours before next dose of chemotherapy.

- May be given by subcutaneous injection or IV infusion (2-24 hours).
- Reconstitute lyophilized powder with 1 mL of sterile water or bacteriostatic water. Direct diluent to side of vial and swirl gently. Do not shake or agitate.
- For IV infusion, use 0.9% sodium chloride injection, USP. Per manufacturer, if the final concentration is less than 10 mcg/mL, albumin (human) at a final concentration of 0.1% should be added to the saline before addition of sargramostim to prevent adsorption to the components of the drug delivery system. To obtain a final concentration of 0.1% albumin, add 1 mg of albumin per 1 mL of 0.9% sodium chloride injection (e.g., use 1 mL of 5% albumin in 50 mL of 0.9% NaCl).
- Do not use an in-line filter for IV infusion.

STORAGE AND STABILITY

- Refrigerate liquid and lyophilized vials.
- Stable only in 0.9% NaCl.
- Liquid sargramostim is stable for 20 days at 2-8° C (36-46° F) once the vial has been punctured.
- Reconstituted lyophilized powder with sterile water contains no preservatives and therefore should be used within 6 hours after reconstitution and or dilution for IV infusion. Discard solution after 6 hours.
- Reconstituted lyophilized powder with bacteriostatic water may be stored for up to 20 days at 2-8° C (36-46° F). Discard solution after 20 days.

INTERACTIONS
Drug

Corticosteroids: May potentiate myeloproliferative effects, use with caution.
Lithium: May potentiate myeloproliferative effects, use with caution.

Herbal
None known.

LAB EFFECTS/INTERFERENCE
May decrease serum proteins and prolong prothrombin time. May cause transient increases in liver enzymes.

Y-SITE COMPATIBLES
Bleomycin, carboplatin, carmustine, cisplatin, cyclophosphamide, cytarabine, dacarbazine, dactinomycin, doxorubicin, etoposide, floxuridine, fluorouracil, granisetron, idarubicin, ifosfamide, mechlorethamine, mesna, methotrexate, mitoxantrone, pentostatin, rituximab, teniposide, trastuzumab, vinblastine, vincristine

INCOMPATIBLES
Do not mix with other medications. Acyclovir, amphotericin B conventional (Fungizone), ampicillin, cefoperazone, chlorpromazine, ganciclovir, haloperidol, hydrocortisone, hydromorphone, hydroxyzine, imipenem-cilastatin, lorazepam, methylprednisolone, mitomycin, morphine, nalbuphine, ondansetron, piperacillin, sodium bicarbonate, tobramycin

SIDE EFFECTS
Serious Reactions
- Arrhythmias and tachycardia occur rarely.
- Edema, capillary leak syndrome, and pleural and/or pericardial effusion have been reported.

Other Side Effects
Frequent (10%-50%): Arthralgia, asthenia, bone pain, chills, diarrhea, fever, fatigue, "first-dose reaction" (dyspnea, hypoxia, flushing, hypotension, syncope, tachycardia, fever, nausea and vomiting, back pain), headache, myalgia
Occasional (1%-10%):
Dyspnea, injection site reactions, peripheral edema, pericardial effusion, rash, weight gain
Rare (Less Than 1%):
Arrhythmia, dizziness, eosinophilia, fainting, hypotension, pain (abdominal, back, chest), tachycardia, thrombosis, transient liver function

SPECIAL CONSIDERATIONS
Baseline Assessment
- Assess CBC with differential, platelet count, electrolyte, BUN, and creatinine

levels and liver function tests before initiating this agent.

- Assess patient for any cardiac history, arrhythmias, tachycardia, or palpitations.
- Evaluate for history of pulmonary or peripheral edema.
- Obtain baseline weight.

Intervention and Evaluation

- Monitor weight at each visit.
- Assess vital sign status, evaluating for any evidence of cardiac changes.
- Obtain CBC with differential, platelet count, liver function tests, and electrolyte, BUN, and creatinine levels as needed.
- Evaluate patient for any evidence of edema or pulmonary changes.
- Assess injection sites for any evidence of reactions or skin rashes.
- Monitor for evidence of bone pain, headache, arthralgias, or myalgias.
- Assess patient for ability to self-inject medication; evaluate compliance with a daily injection.

Education

- Educate patient on the rationale for use of this agent: to increase neutrophil count to protect against infection after chemotherapy or biotherapy or to be used to increase stem cells for collection.
- Instruct patient on when to contact his or her health care provider: fever greater than 38° C (greater than101° F, chills, shortness of breath, chest pain, palpitations, diarrhea lasting greater than 24 hours, nausea lasting greater than 24 hours, or the inability to drink at least 1500 mL of fluid in 24 hours.
- Advise patient to report weight gain of greater than 2 kg in 24 hours.
- Educate patient on self-injection technique as appropriate.
- Instruct patient to monitor injection sites, rotate sites daily, and keep a diary of injection sites.
- Educate patient and significant others that pain may occur as granulocytes are recovering.
- Instruct patient to use acetaminophen for mild pain and to contact the health care provider for severe pain.
- Educate patient to avoid crowds and persons with colds or flu when his or her WBC count may be low.

SORAFENIB

BRAND NAMES

Nexavar

CLASS OF AGENT

Antineoplastic agent, tyrosine kinase inhibitor, vascular endothelial growth factor (VEGF) Inhibitor

CLINICAL PHARMACOLOGY

Mechanism of Action

A multikinase inhibitor that targets serine/threonine and receptor tyrosine kinase. It binds to multiple intracellular (CRAF, BRAF, and mutant BRAF) and cell surface kinases (KIT, Flt-3, VEGF receptor-2, VEGF receptor-3, platelet-derived growth factor receptor-β); VEGF, is thought to be involved with angiogenesis. **Therapeutic Effect:** Inhibits the growth of cancer cells.

Absorption and Distribution

Pharmacokinetic studies have shown that the mean relative bioavailability is 38%-49% compared with that of an oral solution. Bioavailability was reduced by 29% when sorafenib was administered with a high-fat meal. Peak plasma levels are reached approximately 3 hours after PO administration. Steady-state plasma concentrations are achieved within 7 days. Protein binding: 99.5%.

Half-life: 25-48 hours.

Metabolism and Excretion

Metabolized primarily in the liver and undergoes oxidative metabolism, which is facilitated by cytochrome P450 (CYP) 3A4 and glucuronidation mediated by UGT1A9. The main active metabolite, pyridine *N*-oxide, shows in vitro activity similar to that of sorafenib. Elimination is mainly through the feces (77%) and urine (19%). Unchanged drug is found in feces (51% of the dose) but not in the urine.

HOW SUPPLIED/AVAILABLE FORMS

Tablets: 200 mg.

INDICATIONS AND DOSAGES

Advanced Renal Cell Carcinoma

400 mg twice daily on an empty stomach. Continue treatment until there is no clinical benefit or intolerable adverse effects occurs.

Dose Adjustment for Toxicity

Reduce dose in increments of 400 mg. Reduce from 400 mg twice daily to once daily and if dose reduction is

Skin Toxicity Grade	Occurrence	Suggested Dose Modification
Grade 1: Numbness, dysesthesia, paresthesia, tingling, painless swelling, erythema, or discomfort of the hands or feet that does not disrupt normal activities	Any occurrence	Continue treatment and consider topical therapy for symptomatic relief.
Grade 2: Painful erythema and swelling of the hands or feet and/or discomfort affecting normal activities	First occurrence	Continue treatment and consider topical therapy for symptomatic relief. If no improvement within 7 days, see below.
	No improvement within 7 days or second or third occurrence	Interrupt treatment until toxicity resolves to grade 0 to 1. When resuming treatment, decrease dose by one dose level (400 mg daily or 400 mg every other day).
	Fourth occurrence	Discontinue sorafenib.
Grade 3: Moist desquamation, ulceration, blistering, or severe pain of the hands or feet or severe discomfort that causes inability to work or perform activities of daily living	First or second occurrence	Interrupt treatment until toxicity resolves to grade 0 to 1. When resuming treatment, decrease dose by one dose level (400 mg daily or 400 mg every other day).
	Third occurrence	Discontinue sorafenib.

From Sorafenib (Nexavar) Prescribing Information. Bayer Pharmaceuticals Corp., December 2005.

required again, reduce to 400 mg every other day.
Suggested Sorafenib Dose Modifications for Skin Toxicity
Dosage Adjustment in Hepatic Dysfunction
No adjustments required for mild to moderate hepatic dysfunction. There are no data in patients with severe impairment (e.g., Child-Pugh C).
Dosage Adjustment in Renal Dysfunction
No adjustments necessary for mild to moderate renal dysfunction. No information available for patients with CrCl less than 30 mL/minute or patients undergoing dialysis.

UNLABELED USES
No information.

PRECAUTIONS
Hand-foot syndrome, hypertension, serious bleeding events, and cardiac ischemia/infarction have been reported in clinical trials.
Pregnancy Risk Category: D
Use adequate contraceptive methods for at least 2 weeks after discontinuation of sorafenib. Drug excretion into breast milk is unknown/not recommended in nursing women.

CONTRAINDICATIONS
Hypersensitivity to sorafenib or any of its excipients.

DRUG PREPARATION/ADMINISTRATION/ SAFE HANDLING ISSUES
• Take PO on an empty stomach (1 hour before or 2 hours after a meal).

STORAGE AND STABILITY
Store at 25° C (excursions allowed 15-30° C [59-86° F]).

INTERACTIONS
Drug
CYP 3A4 inducers (aminoglutethimide, carbamazepine, dexamethasone, nafcillin, nevirapine, phenobarbital, phenytoin, rifampin, rifabutin, rifapentine): May decrease the levels and effects of sorafenib. Avoid if possible.
CYP 3A4 inhibitors: Unlikely to affect changes. Ketoconazole, a potent inhibitor, did not affect the area under the curve of sorafenib even though in vitro data indicate that sorafenib is metabolized by CYP 3A4.
CYP 2C19, CYP 2D6, CYP 3A4 substrates: Unlikely to effect changes. Even though sorafenib is a competitive inhibitor of these substrates, studies

show that sorafenib did not alter the metabolism of midazolam (CYP3A4 substrate), dextromethorphan (CYP2D6 substrate), and omeprazole (CYP2C19 substrate).

CYP2C9 substrates: Unlikely to effect changes. Even though sorafenib is a competitive inhibitor of CYP2C9, studies with warfarin (CYP2C9 substrate) did not demonstrate marked changes in prothrombin time-international normalized ratio (INR). (See warfarin drug interaction below.)

CYP 2B6 and 2C8: Unknown clinical effect. May increase concentrations of drugs known to be CYP 2B6 and 2C8 substrates, as sorafenib was shown in vitro to be a CYP 2B6 and 2C8 inhibitor.

UGT1A1 and UGT1A9 substrates: In vitro studies demonstrate that sorafenib inhibits glucuronidation of the UGT1A1 and UGT1A9 pathways and may increase UGT1A1 and UGT1A9 substrate concentrations.

Doxorubicin: May increase concentration of doxorubicin. Watch for doxorubicin toxicities.

Irinotecan: May increase concentrations of irinotecan (UGT1A1 substrate). Watch for irinotecan toxicities.

Warfarin: Infrequent bleeding events or elevation in INR has been reported in some patients. Monitor prothrombin time or INR closely.

Herbal
St John's Wort: May increase metabolism and decrease serum sorafenib concentration. Avoid use.

LAB EFFECTS/INTERFERENCE
May decrease phosphate, Hgb, and Hct levels and neutrophil and platelet counts. May increase lipase and amylase levels and transaminases.

SIDE EFFECTS
Serious Reactions
- Cardiac ischemia and or infarction have been reported.
- Hand-foot syndrome is commonly reported and may require drug interruption, dosage reduction, or drug discontinuation.
- Hypertension may occur and is usually mild to moderate. Monitor blood pressure weekly during the first 6 weeks of sorafenib therapy and initiate antihypertensive therapy as clinically indicated.
- Severe hemorrhage has been reported.

Other Side Effects
Frequent (10%-50%):
Alopecia (mild), anorexia, asthenia, constipation, cough, diarrhea, dry skin, dyspnea, erythema, fatigue, hand-foot syndrome, hemorrhage (all sites), hypertension, hypophosphatemia, rash/desquamation, increased lipase and amylase levels, leukopenia, lymphopenia, nausea, pain (abdomen, joint, headache), pruritus, sensory neuropathy, vomiting, weight loss

Occasional (1%-10%):
Acne, anemia, arthralgia, depression, decreased appetite, dyspepsia, dysphagia, erectile dysfunction, exfoliative dermatitis, fever, flushing, influenza-like illness, mucositis, myalgia, neutropenia, rhinorrhea, stomatitis, thrombocytopenia

Rare (Less Than 1%):
Eczema, erythema multiforme, folliculitis, gastritis, GI reflux, gynecomastia, hypersensitivity, hypertensive crisis, infection, INR abnormality, myocardial ischemia, MI, pancreatitis, tinnitus

SPECIAL CONSIDERATIONS
Baseline Assessment
- Assess CBC with differential, platelet count, electrolyte, BUN, creatinine, amylase, and lipase levels, and liver function tests.
- Assess patient for any history of neuropathy.
- Evaluate for any dermatologic conditions, rash, or desquamation.
- Assess cardiac history for chest pain, angina, or MI.
- Evaluate history for any evidence of renal, hepatic, or pancreatic dysfunction.
- Review current medications.
- Assess baseline vital signs for evidence of hypertension.
- Assess patient's ability to comply with an oral medication regimen.

Intervention and Evaluation
- Monitor vital signs at each visit or at least weekly for the first 6 weeks with this agent.
- Instruct patient to take this agent on an empty stomach 1 hour before or 2 hours after eating.
- Monitor compliance with medication; have patient bring medication bottles to the clinic to assess patient's ability to take as directed.
- Assess for evidence of peripheral neuropathy: numbness and tingling in fingers and toes or any other evidence such as

stumbling, difficulty signing name, or picking up coins. Dose reduction is required based on severity.

- Evaluate laboratory data, CBC with differential, platelet count, electrolyte, BUN, creatinine, amylase, and lipase levels, and liver function tests at each visit.
- Monitor for any evidence of cardiac changes, chest pain, tachycardia, palpitations, and increasing episodes of angina or headaches.
- Evaluate for skin changes as hand-foot syndrome (palmar plantar erythrodysthesia) or desquamation of skin may occur with this agent. Initiate skin care program as needed. Dose reductions may be required based on severity.
- Apply moisturizers such as Aquaphor, Eucerin, or Absorbase cream at first sign of erythema of extremities.
- Assess patient's intake and output, and monitor weight.
- Assess patient for any signs or symptoms of diarrhea, and initiate antidiarrheal medication as necessary.
- Monitor need for consultation with a nutritionist or a low-sodium diet if hypertension is noted.
- Evaluate for gastric reflux and anorexia.
- Monitor for fatigue and flu-like symptoms as these can occur with this agent.
- Conduct an abdominal assessment at each visit as amylase and lipase levels can rise with this agent.
- Review all medications patient is taking at each visit, and instruct patient to avoid all OTC medications and herbal and vitamin supplements without first checking with his or her health care provider.

Education

- Instruct patient on when to contact his or her health care provider: fever greater than 38° C (greater than 101° F), chills, chest pain, shortness of breath, severe headaches, nausea lasting greater than 24 hours, the inability to take in at least 1500 mL of fluid in 24 hours, numbness and tingling in fingers and toes that affects activities of daily living, rash, or sores on palms of hands and soles of feet.
- Review medication guidelines at each visit.
- Educate patient to maintain a drug diary and to bring medication and diary to each visit.
- Advise patient to administer medication on an empty stomach 1 hour before or 2 hours after a meal.

- Instruct patient on how to use loperamide for diarrheal symptoms.
- Educate patient on a low-sodium diet, or initiate a consultation with a nutritionist if hypertension is noted.
- Instruct patient to avoid all OTC medications and herbal and vitamin supplements without first checking with the health care provider.
- Educate patient on skin care if any sores or rashes develop: use of moisturizers at least 3 times/day, and use of any petroleum-based moisturizer, such as Vaseline, to hands and feet. Make sure patient knows to pay particular attention to hand and foot hygiene to prevent infection of these areas.
- Advise patient some alopecia may occur with this agent.
- Provide patient with information on local resources and support groups available for his or her specific diagnosis.

SUNITINIB MALATE

BRAND NAMES
Sutent

CLASS OF AGENT
Antineoplastic agent, endothelial growth factor receptor (EGFR)/vascular endothelial growth factor (VEGFR) inhibitor, platelet-derived growth factor receptor (PDGFR) inhibitor, tyrosine kinase inhibitor

CLINICAL PHARMACOLOGY
Mechanism of Action
Inhibits phosphorylation of multiple receptor tyrosine kinases (RTK). Studies have demonstrated the ability of sunitinib to inhibit growth of tumor cells expressing dysregulated target RTKs (PDGFR, VEGFR, Flt-3, colony-stimulation factor-1 receptor, RET, or KIT) in vitro and inhibit PDGFR- and VEGFR-dependent tumor angiogenesis in vivo. These receptors are found on both normal and cancer cells and are involved with tumor proliferation, pathologic angiogenesis, and metastatic progression of cancer. **Therapeutic Effect:** Inhibits the growth and spread of cancer cells.

Absorption and Distribution
Peak plasma concentration is observed 6-12 hours after PO administration. Steady-state concentrations of sunitinib and its primary active metabolite are achieved in 10-14 days. Food has no effect on bioavailability. Protein binding: 95%

and 90% (metabolite). Volume of distribution: 2230 L.

Half-life: 40-60 hours and 80-110 hours (metabolite).

Metabolism and Excretion

Metabolized by cytochrome P450 (CYP) 3A4 to produce the primary active metabolite, which is further metabolized by CYP 3A4. Eliminated primarily via feces (61%) and urine (16%). Oral clearance ranged from 34 to 62 L/hour with an interpatient variability of 40%.

HOW SUPPLIED/AVAILABLE FORMS

Capsules: 12.5 mg, 25 mg, 50 mg.

INDICATIONS AND DOSAGES

GI Stromal Tumor (GIST) after Imatinib Failure and Renal Cell Carcinoma

50 mg PO daily for 4 weeks followed by 2 weeks rest.

Dose Adjustment for Left Ventricular Dysfunction

Interrupt or reduce dose in patients without clinical evidence of CHF, but with ejection fraction less than 50% and greater than 20% below baseline. Discontinue sunitinib if presented with clinical evidence of CHF.

Dose Adjustment for Drug-Drug Interactions

Adjust by 12.5-mg increments based on individual safety and tolerability. Selection of an alternative concomitant medication with no or minimal enzyme effect is recommended. If alternatives are not available, and sunitinib is administered concomitantly with strong CYP 3A4 inhibitors or inducers, then adjust dosage accordingly:

> *CYP 3A4 inhibitors:* Decrease sunitinib dose to minimum 37.5 mg daily.
> *CYP 3A4 inducers:* Increase sunitinib dose to maximum 87.5 mg daily.

Dosage Adjustment in Hepatic Dysfunction

No recommendations available. Studies excluded patients with ALT (SGOT) or AST (SGPT) greater than $2.5 \times$ ULN or, if due to underlying disease, greater than $5 \times$ ULN.

Dosage Adjustment in Renal Dysfunction

No recommendations available. Studies excluded patients with serum creatinine levels greater than $2 \times$ ULN. Pharmacokinetic analyses demonstrated that sunitinib pharmacokinetics were unchanged in patients with CrCl of 42-347 mL/minute.

UNLABELED USES

No information.

PRECAUTIONS

Use with caution in patients with cardiac risk factors as decreases in left ventricular ejection fraction and hypertension have been reported. Monitor for CHF. Serious hemorrhagic events such as GI perforation occur rarely. Adrenal function abnormalities have been reported; monitor for adrenal insufficiency in patients who experience stress such as surgery, trauma, or severe infection.

Pregnancy Risk Category: D

Sunitinib may cause fetal harm when administered during pregnancy. Excretion into human milk is unknown/not recommended in nursing women.

CONTRAINDICATIONS

Hypersensitivity to sunitinib or any of its excipients.

DRUG PREPARATION/ADMINISTRATION/ SAFE HANDLING ISSUES

- Take PO without regard to food.
- Overdose information is not available. Overdose should be treated with general supportive measures. Induction of emesis or use of gastric lavage should be considered in appropriate setting.

STORAGE AND STABILITY

Store at 25° C (77° F) (excursions allowed 15-30° C [59-86° F]).

INTERACTIONS

Drug

CYP 3A4 inducers (aminoglutethimide, carbamazepine, nafcillin, nevirapine, phenobarbital, phenytoin, rifampin, rifabutin, rifapentine): May decrease the levels and effects of sunitinib. Avoid if possible. If alternatives are not available, increase sunitinib dose to maximum 87.5 mg and reduce when CYP 3A4 inducer is discontinued.

CYP 3A4 inhibitors (ciprofloxacin, clarithromycin, diclofenac, doxycycline, erythromycin, imatinib, isoniazid, itraconazole, ketoconazole, nefazodone, nicardipine, propofol, protease inhibitors, quinidine, telithromycin, troleandomycin, verapamil, voriconazole): May increase the levels and effects of sunitinib. Decrease sunitinib dose to minimum 37.5 mg and increase dose when CYP 3A4 inhibitor is discontinued.

Herbal

St John's Wort: May increase metabolism and decrease serum levels of sunitinib concentration unpredictably. Avoid use.

Food
Grapefruit inhibits CYP 3A4 enzymes and can potentially enhance sunitinib effects.

LAB EFFECTS/INTERFERENCE
Elevations in liver function test results and creatinine, lipase, amylase, and uric acid levels. Decrease in left ventricular ejection fraction (LVEF), myelosuppression, and acquired hypothyroidism. Electrolyte abnormalities including hyperkalemia, hypokalemia, hypernatremia, hyponatremia, and hypophosphatemia.

SIDE EFFECTS
Serious Reactions
- In two Medical Research Council of Canada studies and a GIST study, 15% ($n = 25$) and 11% ($n = 22$) of patients, respectively, experienced a decreased LVEF.
- MI, deep vein thrombosis (DVT), pulmonary embolism, and seizures have been reported.

Other Side Effects
Frequent (10%-50%):
General: fatigue, fever
GI: diarrhea, nausea, mucositis, vomiting, constipation, abdominal pain
Cardiac: hypertension, peripheral edema, decreased LVEF
Dermatologic: rash, skin discoloration, hand-foot syndrome
Hematologic: neutropenia, lymphopenia, anemia, thrombocytopenia
Hemorrhage: bleeding (epistaxis most common; rectal, gingival, upper GI, genital, wound bleeding)
Metabolism: anorexia, asthenia
Neurologic: altered taste, dizziness, headache
Musculoskeletal: arthralgia, back pain, myalgia/limb pain
Respiratory: dyspnea, cough
Occasional (1%-10%):
Alopecia, appetite disturbance, blistering of skin, oral pain, periorbital edema, hair color changes, hyperkalemia, hypokalemia, hypernatremia, hyponatremia, hypophosphatemia, increased lacrimation, hyperuricemia, abnormal liver enzymes, increased pancreas enzymes
Rare (Less Than 1%):
Pancreatitis, seizure

SPECIAL CONSIDERATIONS
Baseline Assessment
- Assess CBC with differential, platelet count, electrolyte, BUN, creatinine, uric acid, amylase and lipase levels, liver function tests, and thyroid function tests.
- Assess for history of cardiac disease, DVT, or seizure disorders.
- Evaluate cardiac ejection fraction before initiation of therapy.
- Assess patient for history of hypertension.

Intervention and Evaluation
- Monitor laboratory data at each visit.
- Assess vital signs at each visit, and evaluate for increasing B/P, tachycardia, and arrhythmias as this agent may induce these symptoms.
- Evaluate for neutropenia, thrombocytopenia, and anemia.
- Initiate patient on neutropenic and thrombocytopenic precautions as necessary.
- Assess for GI symptoms, nausea, vomiting, and diarrhea.
- Initiate antiemetic and antidiarrheal medications as needed.
- Monitor for evidence of bleeding and epistaxis or bleeding from oral cavity, rectum, or wounds.
- Assess for evidence of thrombosis, lower extremity weakness, lower extremity pain, or erythema.
- Evaluate for skin reactions such as rash, desquamation, folliculitis, and palmar-plantar erythrodysesthesia, and initiate skin care as needed.
- Assess for mucositis and initiate an oral care regimen as needed. An example is 1 tsp each of salt and baking soda dissolved in 1 glass of water, to swish and spit at least 3 times/day and at bedtime.

Education
- Instruct patient on when to contact his or her health care provider: fever greater than 38° C (greater than 101° F), chills, cough, shortness of breath, nosebleeds lasting greater than 10 mins or bleeding from any area, rectal or urinary problems, swelling of lower extremities, nausea lasting greater than 24 hours, diarrhea lasting greater than 24 hours, or the inability to take in at least 1500 mL of fluid in 24 hours.
- Educate patient on neutropenic precautions as necessary:
  Practice good handwashing technique.
  Avoid individuals who are ill.
  Wash and cook all foods well.
  Avoid crowds.
  Avoid fresh fruits and vegetables.
- Educate patient on thrombocytopenic precautions:
  Use of a soft bristle toothbrush.

No flossing if platelet count is less than 50,000/mm^3.
No IM injections.
No rectal suppositories.
No aerobic exercise.

- Instruct patient to avoid all OTC medications and herbal and vitamin supplements without first checking with the health care provider.
- Advise patient on use of skin care products if is rash noted and to contact the health care provider if rash becomes blistered or weeping.
- Educate patient that partial alopecia may occur, and hair will regrow, although it may be of different color or consistency.
- Provide patient with information on local resources and support groups available for his or her specific diagnosis.

STREPTOZOCIN

BRAND NAMES
Zanosar

CLASS OF AGENT
Antineoplastic agent, alkylating agent

CLINICAL PHARMACOLOGY
Mechanism of Action
An alkylating agent of the nitrosourea type that interferes with DNA replication and RNA synthesis and is cell cycle phase nonspecific. Exact mechanism of action is unknown. It is non-cross-resistant with other nitrosoureas. **Therapeutic Effect:** Disrupts nucleic acid function.
Absorption and Distribution
Drug disappears from the blood quickly and concentrates in liver and kidneys.
Half-life: 35 minutes.
Metabolism and Excretion
Metabolized rapidly through the liver. Primarily excreted in urine as metabolites (60%-70%).

HOW SUPPLIED/AVAILABLE FORMS
Powder for Injection: 1 g (Zanosar).

INDICATIONS AND DOSAGES
Pancreatic Islet Cell Carcinoma
Daily schedule: 0.5-1 g/m^2/day IV for 5 consecutive days. Repeat every 4-6 weeks or until maximum benefit or treatment-limiting toxicity is reached.
Weekly schedule: 1-1.5 g/m^2/dose IV at weekly intervals for the first 2 doses. May

increase dose in subsequent courses based on therapeutic response and toxicity. Maximum single dose: 1.5 g/m^2.

Dosage Adjustment in Hepatic Dysfunction
No specific adjustments are known. Use with caution in patients with severe hepatic toxicity.

Dosage Adjustment in Renal Dysfunction
Because renal toxicity is a dose-limiting adverse effect of streptozocin, caution should be used in patients with preexisting renal insufficiency.

CrCl	Dosage Administer
CrCl 10-50 mL/minute	Administer 75% of dose
CrCl <10 mL/minute	Administer 50% of dose

UNLABELED USES
Carcinoid tumor, colon cancer, hepatic carcinoma, Hodgkin's lymphoma, pancreatic islet cell carcinoma

PRECAUTIONS
Use extremely cautiously in patients with preexisting renal disease. Be aware that renal toxicity is dose related and cumulative. It may be severe or fatal. Do not use with other potentially nephrotoxic agents. Be aware that streptozocin may be carcinogenic.
Pregnancy Risk Category: D
Streptozocin use should be avoided during pregnancy, especially in the first trimester. Be aware that streptozocin use may cause fetal harm, and it is unknown whether the drug is distributed in breast milk. Breast-feeding is not recommended in this patient population.

CONTRAINDICATIONS
Hypersensitivity to streptozocin or any component of the formulation

DRUG PREPARATION/ADMINISTRATION/ SAFE HANDLING ISSUES
◀ ALERT ▶ Streptozocin dosage is individualized on the basis of patient's clinical response and tolerance of the drug's adverse effects. When used in combination therapy, consult specific protocols for optimum dosage and sequence of drug administration.
◀ ALERT ▶ Because streptozocin may be carcinogenic, mutagenic, or teratogenic, wear nitrile or latex gloves when handling the drug. If the drug comes in contact

with skin, wash the skin thoroughly with soap and water. Do not use antibacterial or waterless soap to wash area as either can enhance the skin reaction. If the drug comes in contact with mucous membranes, flush the area with copious amounts of water or normal saline.

- Streptozocin is a vesicant. Treat extravasations according to institutional protocol.
- Reconstitute 1-g vial with 9.5 mL of 0.9% NaCl or D5W. The resulting concentration is 100 mg of streptozocin and 22 mg of citric acid per mL.
- Dilute further with a 0.9% NaCl or D5W bag if desired.
- Administer as short infusion (30-60 minutes) or as a 6-hour infusion; may be given by rapid IV push.

STORAGE AND STABILITY

- Store unopened vials in refrigerator (2-8° C [36-46° F]) and protect from light.
- Reconstituted solutions should be used within 12 hours if kept at room temperature.
- Because this drug contains no preservatives, the vial should not be used for more than one dose.

INTERACTIONS
Drug
Doxorubicin: Streptozocin has increased half-life of doxorubicin, resulting in increased myelosuppression.
Bone marrow depressants: May increase the risk of bone marrow depression.
Live-virus vaccines: May potentiate viral replication, increase vaccine side effects, and decrease patient's antibody response to the vaccine.
Nephrotoxic medication (amphotericin B, aminoglycosides, cisplatin): May increase risk of renal dysfunction.
Phenytoin: May decrease streptozocin efficacy.
Herbal
None known.

LAB EFFECTS/INTERFERENCE
May increase Hct, BUN, plasma creatinine concentrations, urinary protein concentration, ALT (SGPT), alkaline phosphatase, and AST (SGOT), bilirubin, and LDH. May decrease albumin, blood glucose, and phosphate levels.

Y-SITE COMPATIBLES
Amifostine, etoposide, filgrastim, gemcitabine, granisetron, melphalan, ondansetron (Zofran), paclitaxel, palonosetron, rituximab, vinorelbine

INCOMPATIBLES
Acyclovir, allopurinol, aztreonam, cefepime, levofloxacin, pantoprazole, piperacillin, tazobactam, trastuzumab

SIDE EFFECTS
Serious Reactions
- Major adverse reactions are bone marrow depression resulting in hematologic toxicity as evidenced by severe leukopenia, anemia, and severe thrombocytopenia. Nadir is 7-14 days with recovery in 21 days.
- Nephrotoxicity is dose-related and cumulative and may be severe or fatal. Monitor CrCl before each cycle.
- Severe acute and delayed nausea and vomiting are highly likely. Premedicate patient with a 5-hydroxytryptamine$_3$ receptor antagonist (e.g., ondansetron, granisetron, or palonosetron) and dexamethasone. Other antiemetics such as aprepitant, lorazepam, prochlorperazine, or metoclopramide, may be added to the antiemetic regimen as needed.
- If using aprepitant with dexamethasone, reduce steroid dosage by 50% due to decreased steroid metabolism.
- Abnormalities in glucose tolerance have occurred and are usually mild to moderate and easily treatable. However, insulin shock secondary to hypoglycemia has been reported.
Other Side Effects
Frequent (10%-50%):
Nausea, vomiting (greater than 90%), renal toxicity (65%)
Occasional (1%-10%):
Diarrhea, hypoglycemia, pain or redness at site of injection
Rare (Less Than 1%):
Hepatotoxicity, leukopenia or infection, thrombocytopenia

SPECIAL CONSIDERATIONS
Baseline Assessment
- Assess CBC with differential and platelet count before each dose, and monitor weekly while patient is receiving therapy.
- Assess renal function tests and BUN and creatinine levels before and after each course of therapy; continue to monitor weekly.

- Assess 24-hour urine CrCl before initial course of therapy.
- Assess liver function tests before each course of therapy, and monitor weekly while patient is receiving therapy.
- Assess baseline glucose level.

Intervention and Evaluation
- Perform renal function tests before and after each course of therapy.
- Obtain serial urinalysis (quantify proteinuria with a 24-hour collection if abnormal), plasma creatinine, serum electrolyte, and BUN levels, and CrCl before and weekly during and 4 weeks after drug administration.
- Monitor CBC with differential and platelet count and liver function tests weekly.
- Premedicate patient as ordered with antiemetic therapy at least 30 minutes before dose administration.
- Monitor patient for signs and symptoms of neutropenia, thrombocytopenia, and anemia.
- Monitor patient for signs and symptoms of impaired renal function, weight gain, edema, and any changes in respiratory pattern.
- Monitor patient's prior peripheral IV sites for any signs or symptoms of erythema, pain, or burning.
- Evaluate patient for potential central line placement if patient develops significant skin reactions at prior IV sites.
- Monitor patient for protracted nausea, vomiting, and diarrhea after dosing.
- Instruct patient to contact his or her health care provider if he or she is unable to tolerate 1500 mL of fluid in 24 hours or for nausea continuing greater than 24 hours after dosing.
- Monitor patient for signs and symptoms of infection, fever, and chills; make sure patient has a thermometer at home and can read it.
- Make sure patient has a 24-hour number to contact the health care provider.
- Monitor for any skin toxicity.
- Monitor patient for any signs or symptoms of hypoglycemia, feeling faint, lightheaded, or dizzy, or nausea.

Education
- Instruct patient on signs and symptoms of infection, renal impairment, and changes in color of urine or stool, which would be indicative of hepatic changes.
- Instruct patient on signs and symptoms of hypoglycemia.

- Instruct patient on when to contact his or her health care provider: fever greater than 38° C (greater than 101° F), diarrhea lasting greater than 24 hours, or the inability to take in at least 1500 mL of in 24 hours.
- Instruct patient on delivery of growth factors as appropriate.
- Instruct patient on the possibility of skin changes.
- Caution women of childbearing age to avoid pregnancy. Educate patient regarding contraception options.
- Stress to patient that he or she should not receive live vaccinations without the physician's approval as streptozocin lowers the body's resistance and that he or she should avoid contact with anyone who recently received a live-virus vaccine.
- Instruct patient to take no over-the-counter medications or herbal or vitamin supplements without checking with his or her health care provider.
- Educate patient on local resources available and support groups related to their particular diagnosis.

TAMOXIFEN

BRAND NAMES
Nolvadex, Soltamox

CLASS OF AGENT
Antineoplastic agent, selective estrogen receptor modulator

CLINICAL PHARMACOLOGY
Mechanism of Action
A nonsteroidal antiestrogen that competes with estradiol for estrogen receptor binding sites in tumors and target tissues. Tamoxifen acts as an antagonist in breast and brain tissues, an agonist in bone, liver, and the cardiovascular system, and as a mixed agonist/antagonist in the uterus. **Therapeutic Effect:** Inhibits DNA synthesis and estrogen response.

Absorption and Distribution
Well absorbed from the GI tract. Protein binding: 99%.
Half-life: 7 days.

Metabolism and Excretion
Metabolized in the liver via cytochrome P450 (CYP) 3A4 and CYP2D6. Primarily eliminated in feces by the biliary system (26%-51%); urine excretion 9%-13%.

HOW SUPPLIED/AVAILABLE FORMS
Tablets: 10 mg, 20 mg.
Oral Liquid Solution: 10 mg/5 mL.

INDICATIONS AND DOSAGES
- Adjunctive treatment after resection and breast irradiation
- Treatment of metastatic breast cancer
- Ductal carcinoma in situ (DCIS): invasive cancer risk reduction
- Prevention of breast cancer in high-risk women

20-40 mg PO daily. Give doses greater than 20 mg/day in divided doses.

UNLABELED USES
Gynecomastia; induction of ovulation; McCune-Albright syndrome of precocious puberty; ovulation induction: 5-40 mg PO twice daily for 4 days

PRECAUTIONS
Use tamoxifen cautiously in patients with leukopenia and thrombocytopenia and in patients with a history of thromboembolic events.

Pregnancy Risk Category: D
Tamoxifen should be avoided during pregnancy, especially during the first trimester, because it may cause fetal harm. It is unknown whether tamoxifen is distributed in breast milk; however, breast-feeding should be avoided. Tamoxifen has been known to inhibit lactation. Avoid pregnancy for 2 months after discontinuation of tamoxifen.

CONTRAINDICATIONS
History of known hypersensitivity to tamoxifen or any of its components; history of significant thromboembolic disease; concomitant use with coumarin-type anticoagulants in women receiving tamoxifen for risk reduction or women with DCIS

DRUG PREPARATION/ADMINISTRATION/ SAFE HANDLING ISSUES
- Give tamoxifen PO without regard to food.
- Give doses greater than 20 mg/day in divided doses.

STORAGE AND STABILITY
Store at room temperature: 15-25° C (59-77° F).

INTERACTIONS
Drug
Tamoxifen is a substrate for CYP 3A, 2C9, and 2D6.
Aminoglutethimide: Decreases tamoxifen plasma concentrations.
CYP 3A4 and CYP 2C8/9 inducers (carbamazepine, glucocorticoids, nevirapine, phenobarbital, phenytoin, rifamycin):
May decrease tamoxifen serum levels.
CYP 3A4 inhibitors (ciprofloxacin, clarithromycin, diclofenac, doxycycline, erythromycin, imatinib, isoniazid, ketoconazole, nefazodone, nicardipine, protease inhibitors, quinidine, verapamil):
May increase tamoxifen serum levels.
CYP 2C8/9 inhibitors (delavirdine, fluconazole, gemfibrozil, ketoconazole, nicardipine, NSAIDs, pioglitazone, sulfonamides): May increase tamoxifen serum levels.
CYP 2D6 inhibitors (cimetidine, codeine, fluoxetine, haloperidol, paroxetine): May increase tamoxifen serum levels.
Estrogens: May decrease the effects of tamoxifen.
Letrozole: Decreases letrozole serum levels by 37%.
Warfarin (coumarin-type anticoagulants): Significant increased risk for bleeding
Herbal
St John's Wort: May decrease tamoxifen serum levels.

LAB EFFECTS/INTERFERENCE
Decrease in platelet count and leukopenia have infrequently been reported.

SIDE EFFECTS
Serious Reactions
Uterine malignancies, stroke, and pulmonary emboli associated with tamoxifen have been known to cause fatalities.
Other Side Effects
Frequent (10%-50%):
Men and women: Arthralgia, asthenia, fatigue, hot flashes, myalgia, nausea, sweating, vasodilation
Occasional (1%-10%):
Women: Changes in menstruation, endometrial hyperplasia or polyps, genital itching, vaginal discharge
Men: Decreased libido, impotence
Men and women: Bone pain, cataracts, confusion, constipation, diarrhea, dizziness, fractures, headache, hypercholesterolemia, hypertension, insomnia, nausea, osteoporosis, peripheral edema, rash, somnolence, thromboembolic events, visual disturbances, vomiting, weakness, weight gain
Rare (Less Than 1%):
Endometrial cancer, hypercalcemia, retinopathy, uterine sarcoma

SPECIAL CONSIDERATIONS
Baseline Assessment
- Check the results of patient's estrogen receptor assay test, if ordered, before beginning tamoxifen therapy.

- Monitor patient's CBC with differential, with platelet count, and serum calcium levels before and periodically during tamoxifen therapy.

Intervention and Evaluation
- Monitor patient adherence with daily dosing.
- Assess all medications patient is currently taking, including OTC medications and herbal and vitamin supplements for possible hormonal supplementation.
- Be alert for reports of increased bone pain and provide adequate pain relief as ordered.
- Monitor patient's intake and output and weight.
- Examine patient for peripheral edema.
- Assess patient for signs and symptoms of hypercalcemia, including constipation, deep bone or flank pain, excessive thirst, hypotonicity of muscles, increased urine output, nausea and vomiting, and renal calculi. Tamoxifen flare response usually occurs in patients with extensive bony metastases and is characterized by hypercalcemia, bone pain, and/or localized disease swelling and redness. Monitor serum calcium 3-7 days after tamoxifen initiation. May need to treat hypercalcemia.
- If patient has a vascular access device in place, monitor on a monthly basis to assess for possibility of thrombus.
- Instruct patient to report any changes in menstrual bleeding or vaginal discharge.
- Advise patient not to use any OTC medications for the signs and symptoms of menopause without checking with her health care provider.

Education
- Instruct all patients to notify their health care provider for leg cramps, weakness, or weight gain and female patients for vaginal bleeding, itching, or discharge.
- Inform patient that he or she may initially experience an increase in bone and/or tumor pain, which has been known to correlate with positive response to this agent and usually subsides over time.
- Educate patient on the importance of compliance with this medication and to not stop this agent unless the health care provider is notified.
- Educate patient on appropriate pain control.
- Instruct patient to report any nausea and vomiting which does not resolve in 24 hours.

- Instruct patient to use contraceptive methods other than birth control pills.
- Instruct patient to not use any herbal remedies or OTC preparations without first checking with the health care provider.
- Instruct female patients to get annual gynecologic examinations.
- Instruct patient to get periodic eye examinations, especially if he or she experiences symptoms of cataracts.

TEMOZOLOMIDE

BRAND NAMES
Temodal (Australia), Temodar

CLASS OF AGENT
Alkylating agent

CLINICAL PHARMACOLOGY
Mechanism of Action
Temozolomide is an imidazotetrazine derivative that was developed as an oral form of the active metabolite of dacarbazine. It is a prodrug and is converted to a highly active cytotoxic metabolite, 5-(3-methyltriazen-1-yl)-imidazole-4-carboxamide (MTIC), which alkylates the O-6 and N-7 positions of guanine. Its cytotoxic effect is associated with methylation of DNA. **Therapeutic Effect:** Inhibits DNA replication, causing cell death.

Absorption and Distribution
Rapidly and completely absorbed after PO administration. Peak plasma concentration occurs in 1 hour. However, a high-fat meal decreases and delays absorption of temozolomide. Protein binding to albumin is about 15%. Temozolomide crosses the blood-brain barrier and distributes into the cerebrospinal fluid. It has a large volume of distribution ranging from 0.45 to 0.6 L/kg. The mean value is 28 L in adults and 10-14 L in children.
Half-life: After PO, IV, or intra-arterial administration, the mean halflife ranged from 1.2 to 2.4 hours and was similar in both adults and children.

Metabolism and Excretion
Temozolomide is degraded in vivo to MTIC, which is an active metabolite of dacarbazine. Unlike dacarbazine, formation of MTIC from temozolomide does not required metabolic activation by the liver. Temozolomide is eliminated primarily in urine (38%). Less than 1% is eliminated in the feces.

TEMOZOLOMIDE INTERRUPTIONS OR DISCONTINUATIONS DURING CONCOMITANT PHASE

Toxicity	Interrupt Temozolomide	Discontinue Temozolomide
ANC	≥ 0.5 and $<1.5 \times 10^9$/L	$<0.5 \times 10^9$/L
Platelets	≥ 10 and $<100 \times 10^9$/L	$<10 \times 10^9$/L
CTC nonhematologic toxicity (except for alopecia, nausea, or vomiting)	Grade 2	Grade 3 or 4

From Temodar (temozolomide) Product Information, Schering Corp., 2005.

TEMOZOLOMIDE DOSE LEVELS FOR MAINTENANCE

Dose Level	Dose (mg/m²/day)	Remarks
−1	100	Reduction for prior toxicity
0	150	Dose during cycle 1
1	200	Dose during cycles 2-6 in absence of toxicity

From Temodar (temozolomide) Product Information, Schering Corp., 2005.

TEMOZOLOMIDE DOSE REDUCTIONS OR DISCONTINUATIONS DURING MAINTENANCE PHASE

Toxicity	Reduce by 1 Dose Level	Discontinue Temozolomide
ANC	$<1 \times 10^9$/L	If dose reduction to <100 mg/m² required
Platelets	$<50 \times 10^9$/L	If dose reduction to <100 mg/m² required
CTC nonhematologic toxicity (except for alopecia, nausea, or vomiting)	Grade 3	Grade 4 or if same grade 3 nonhematologic toxicity (except for alopecia, nausea, or vomiting) recurs after dose reduction

From Temodar (temozolomide) Product Information, Schering Corp., 2005.

TEMOZOLOMIDE DOSE ADJUSTMENTS DURING SUBSEQUENT CYCLES BASED ON LOWEST RECORDED LABORATORY VALUES

ANC <1000/mL or platelets $<50,000$/mL	Postpone therapy until ANC >1500/mL and platelet count $>100,000$mL; reduce dose by 50 mg/m²/day for subsequent cycle
ANC 1000-1500/mL or platelet count 50,000-100,000/mL	Postpone therapy until ANC >1500/mL and platelet count $>100,000$/mL; maintain initial dose
ANC >1500/mL or platelet count $>100,000$/mL	Increase dose to or maintain dose at 200 mg/m²/day for 5 days for subsequent cycle

From Temodar (temozolomide) Product Information, Schering Corp., 2005.

HOW SUPPLIED/AVAILABLE FORMS
Capsules: 5 mg, 20 mg, 100 mg, 250 mg.

INDICATIONS AND DOSAGES
High-Grade Glioma
Concomitant Phase
75 mg/m²/day for 42 days concomitant with focal radiotherapy. Continue at full dose for the entire 42 concomitant period up to 49 total days, except to hold or discontinue temozolomide for toxicity (do not reduce dose).
Interruptions: Treatment with concomitant temozolomide could be continued when all of the following conditions were met: absolute neutrophil count = 1.5×10^9/L; platelet count = 100×10^9/L; National Cancer Institute Common Toxicity Criteria (CTC)

non-hematologic toxicity is grade 1 (except for alopecia, nausea, or vomiting).
Maintenance Phase Cycle 1
Begins 4 wks after concomitant phase: 150 mg/m²/day for 5 days followed by 23 days without treatment.
Maintenance Phase Cycles 2-6
At the start of cycle 2, the dose is escalated to 200 mg/m²/day, if the CTC nonhematologic toxicity for cycle 1 is grade 2 (except for alopecia, nausea, and vomiting), ANC is 1.5×10^9/L, and platelet count is 100×10^9/L. The dose remains at 200 mg/m²/day for the first 5 days of each subsequent cycle except if toxicity occurs. If the dose was not escalated at cycle 2, escalation should not be done in subsequent cycles.

Maintenance Phase Dose Reductions
During treatment a CBC should be obtained on day 22 (21 days after the first dose of temozolomide) or within 48 hours of that day and weekly until the ANC is greater 1.5×10^9/L (1500/microliter) and the platelet count exceeds 100×10^9/L (100,000/microliter). The next cycle of temozolomide should not be started until the ANC and platelet count exceed these levels. Dose reductions during the next cycle should be based on the lowest blood counts and worst nonhematologic toxicity during the previous cycle.

Anaplastic Astrocytoma
Initially, 150 mg/m2/day for 5 consecutive days of a 28-day treatment cycle. Subsequent doses are based on platelet count and ANC during the previous cycle. For ANC greater than 1500/microliter and platelet count greater than 100,000/microliter, maintenance 200 mg/m^2/day for 5 days every 4 weeks. Continue until disease progression. Minimum: 100 mg/m^2/day for 5 days every 4 weeks.

Dosage Adjustment in Hepatic Dysfunction
No guideline for dose adjustment in patients with hepatic dysfunction has been published.

Dosage Adjustment in Renal Dysfunction
Although no guideline has been published, it is recommended that dose reduction be considered in patients with severe renal dysfunction.

UNLABELED USES
Other brain tumors: use doses similar to that for astrocytoma; malignant melanoma: use doses similar to that for astrocytoma

PRECAUTIONS
Pregnancy Risk Category: D

CONTRAINDICATIONS
Hypersensitivity to temozolomide, dacarbazine

DRUG PREPARATION/ADMINISTRATION/ SAFE HANDLING ISSUES
Oral capsules should be handled carefully. It is recommended that patients do not handle the capsule but rather use a dispensing cup for administration.

STORAGE AND STABILITY
Store temozolomide capsules at controlled room temperature of 25° C (77° F); brief excursions permitted to 15-30° C (59-86° F).

INTERACTIONS
Drug
Live-virus vaccines: May potentiate viral replication, increase vaccine side effects, and decrease patient's antibody response to the vaccine.
Valproic acid: Decreases the clearance of temozolomide by 5% (clinical importance is unknown).
Herbal
None known.

LAB EFFECTS/INTERFERENCE
May decrease blood Hgb levels and neutrophil, platelet, and WBC counts.

SIDE EFFECTS
Serious Reactions
Elderly patients and women are at increased risk for developing severe myelosuppression, characterized by neutropenia and thrombocytopenia and usually occurring within the first few cycles. Neutrophil and platelet counts reach their nadirs approximately 26-28 days after administration and recover within 14 days of the nadir.

Other Side Effects
Frequent (10%-50%):
Nausea, vomiting, headache, fatigue, constipation, diarrhea, asthenia, fever, dizziness, peripheral edema, incoordination, insomnia
Occasional (1%-10%):
Paresthesia, drowsiness, anorexia, urinary incontinence, anxiety, pharyngitis, cough
Rare (Less Than 1%):
No information.

SPECIAL CONSIDERATIONS
Baseline Assessment
• Assess CBC with differential, platelet count, electrolytes, BUN, and creatinine levels, and liver function tests.
• Evaluate prior experience with chemotherapy agents and amount of emesis experienced.
• Assess baseline weight and any evidence of peripheral edema.
• Evaluate patient's ability to comply with dose administration as this is an oral agent.
Intervention and Evaluation
• Assess CBC with differential, platelet count, electrolyte, BUN, and creatinine levels, and liver function tests on a routine basis. For the treatment phase with concomitant radiation therapy, a CBC should

be obtained weekly. For the 28-day treatment cycles, a CBC should be obtained on day 22 (21 days after the first dose). Blood counts should be performed weekly until recovery if the ANC falls below 1.5×10^9/L and the platelet count falls below 100×10^9/L.

- Patients receiving concomitant radiation (high-grade glioma regimen) should also be receiving *Pneumocystis carinii* pneumonia antibiotic prophylaxis.
- Monitor weight and evaluate for peripheral edema at each visit
- Assess patients for evidence of neutropenia, thrombocytopenia, and anemia.
- Evaluate patient for any evidence of toxicity, nausea, vomiting, constipation, increasing fatigue, weakness, edema, or evidence of incontinence.
- Assess patients for adherence issues related to dosing administration; have patient bring medication bottles to each visit to determine doses taken.
- Reeducate patient as needed about when and how to take this agent.
- Assess patient for any evidence of altered mental status, confusion, weakness, coordination problems, or anxiety.
- Evaluate patient for any evidence of paresthesias, numbness, or tingling while taking this agent.

Education

- Instruct patient on when to contact his or her health care provider: fever greater than 38° C (greater than 101° F), shaking, chills, cough, shortness of breath, dyspnea upon exertion, easy bruising, bleeding, diarrhea lasting greater than 24 hours, nausea or vomiting lasting greater than 24 hours, or the inability to take at least 1500 mL of fluid in 24 hours.
- Instruct patient to take on drug on an empty stomach to reduce nausea and vomiting.
- Educate patient that constipation may result from this agent, and instruct patient to take stool softeners and senna at night if bowel movements are not occurring in their usual pattern.
- Advise patient that he or she may experience weakness, coordination difficulties, numbness and tingling in hands and feet, and some mental status changes and to contact the health care provider if these occur.
- Instruct patient on appropriate dosing of this agent, and make sure patient

takes as directed and contact the health care provider if unable to take the medication because of side effects.

- Educate patient to monitor his or her weight and to contact the health care provider if any evidence of edema or urinary incontinence is noted.
- Instruct patient to take no over-the-counter medications or herbal or vitamin supplements without checking with his or her health care provider.
- Provide patient with information on local resources and support groups available for his or her specific diagnosis.

TENIPOSIDE

BRAND NAMES
Vumon

CLASS OF AGENT
Antineoplastic agent, podophyllotoxin

CLINICAL PHARMACOLOGY
Mechanism of Action
An epipodophyllotoxin that induces single- and double-strand breaks in DNA, inhibiting or altering DNA synthesis. Teniposide impairs mitochondrial electron transport in the respiratory chain at the NADH dehydrogenase level. It causes irreversible metaphase arrest as well as premitosis lesion, blocking cell cycle traverse possibly through impairment of cellular respiration and energy production. It acts in the late S and early G_2 phases of the cell cycle. **Therapeutic Effect:** Prevents cells from entering mitosis.

Absorption and Distribution
The drug is given by IV administration. The volume of distribution is 3.1 L/m². The steady-state volume of distribution ranges from 8 to 44 L/m² in adults and 3 to 11 L/m² in children. It is extensively bound to protein (>99%). Less than 1% appears in the cerebrospinal fluid.
Half-life: Parent compound: 5 hours.

Metabolism and Excretion
Primarily metabolized by the liver, but only 10% of the drug is excreted in the feces. Between 10% and 21% of the drug is excreted by the kidneys.

HOW SUPPLIED/AVAILABLE FORMS
Injection Solution: 50 mg/5 mL ampules.

INDICATIONS AND DOSAGES
Induction Therapy in Patients with Refractory Childhood Acute Lymphoblastic Leukemia (in Combination with Other Antineoplastic Agents)
Pediatrics: Dosage is individualized on the basis of patient's clinical response and tolerance of the drug's adverse effects. When used in combination therapy, consult specific protocols for optimum dosage or sequence of drug administration.

Dosage Adjustment in Hepatic Dysfunction
Because most of a dose of teniposide is metabolized in the liver, the manufacturer states that a dose adjustment may be necessary in patients with significant hepatic impairment. However, no specific recommendations are given.

Dosage Adjustment in Renal Dysfunction
Although specific guidelines have not been published, dose reduction may be necessary in patients with severe renal dysfunction.

PRECAUTIONS
Pregnancy Risk Category: D

CONTRAINDICATIONS
ANC less than 500/mm³; hypersensitivity to Cremophor EL (polyoxyethylated castor oil), etoposide, or teniposide; platelet count less than 50,000/mm³

DRUG PREPARATION/ADMINISTRATION/ SAFE HANDLING ISSUES
◂ ALERT ▸
- Dilute teniposide with either 5% dextrose or 0.9% NaCl to a final concentration of 0.1, 0.2, 0.4, or 1 mg/mL. Teniposide concentrations of 0.1, 0.2, or 0.4 mg/mL are stable at room temperature for up to 24 hours after preparation. Final diluted concentrations of 1 mg/mL should be given within 4 hours of preparation to reduce the chance of precipitation.
- Do not refrigerate diluted solutions.
- Do not agitate solutions more than is recommended when preparing, as precipitation may occur even at the recommended final concentrations.
- Do not flush administration sets with heparin as precipitation may result. Administration sets should be thoroughly flushed with either 5% dextrose or 0.9% NaCl.

STORAGE AND STABILITY
- Store teniposide under refrigeration at 2-8° C (36-46° F) and protect from light. Freezing will not adversely affect teniposide.
- Final diluted concentrations of 1 mg/mL should be given within 4 hours of preparation to reduce the chance of precipitation.

INTERACTIONS
Drug
Bone marrow depressants: May increase myelosuppression.
Live-virus vaccines: May potentiate viral replication, increase vaccine side effects, and decrease patient's antibody response to the vaccine.
Fosphenytoin, phenobarbital, phenytoin: Because of cytochrome P450 (CYP) 3A4 induction, these drugs will increase teniposide drug clearance and may decrease its effects.
Glucosamine: This agent has induced resistance to the topoisomerase II inhibitor teniposide in vitro in EMT6 cancer cells and induced resistance to the topoisomerase II inhibitors etoposide and doxorubicin in vitro in human colon and ovarian cancer cells. The clinical effect of glucosamine taken orally is unknown; it is possible that glucosamine may confer resistance to teniposide in humans. Avoid glucosamine in patients being treated with teniposide.
Methotrexate: May increase intracellular accumulation of this drug.
Sodium salicylate, sulfamethizole, tolbutamide: In a study in which 34 different drugs were tested, therapeutically relevant concentrations of tolbutamide, sodium salicylate, and sulfamethizole displaced protein-bound teniposide in fresh human serum to a small but significant extent. Because of the extremely high binding of teniposide to plasma proteins, these small decreases in binding could cause substantial increases in free drug levels in plasma that could result in potentiation of drug toxicity. Therefore, caution should be used in administering teniposide to patients receiving these other agents.
Vincristine: May increase the severity of peripheral neuropathy.
Herbal
None known.

LAB EFFECTS/INTERFERENCE
None significant.

Y-SITE COMPATIBLES

Amifostine, aztreonam, bleomycin, carboplatin, carmustine, cisplatin, cladribine, cyclophosphamide, cytarabine, dacarbazine, dactinomycin, daunorubicin, dexrazoxane, doxorubicin, etoposide, etoposide phosphate, floxuridine, fludarabine, fluorouracil, gemcitabine, granisetron hydrochloride, heparin, ifosfamide, irinotecan, leucovorin, mechlorethamine, melphalan, mesna, mitomycin, mitoxantrone, ondansetron, oxaliplatin, paclitaxel, palonosetron, pamidronate, rituximab, sargramostim, thiotepa, topotecan, trastuzumab, vinblastine, vincristine, vinorelbine

INCOMPATIBLES

Amphotericin B liposomal (AmBisome), dantrolene, idarubicin, phenytoin

SIDE EFFECTS
Serious Reactions
- Myelosuppression manifested as hematologic toxicity (principally leukopenia, neutropenia, and thrombocytopenia) may be severe and may increase the risk of infection or bleeding.
- Hypersensitivity reaction may include anaphylaxis (marked by chills, fever, tachycardia, bronchospasm, dyspnea, and facial flushing).

Other Side Effects
Frequent (10%-50%):
Mucositis, nausea, vomiting, diarrhea, anemia
Occasional (1%-10%):
Alopecia, rash, hepatic dysfunction, fever, renal dysfunction, peripheral neurotoxicity
Rare (Less Than 1%):
No information

SPECIAL CONSIDERATIONS
Baseline Assessment
- Monitor CBC with differential, platelet count, electrolyte, BUN, and creatinine levels, and liver function tests before dosing.
- Assess patient's allergy history as this agent may be associated with hypersensitivity reactions.
- Evaluate patient for any evidence of skin reactions.

Intervention and Evaluation
- Administer premedications as required for emetic control along with hypersensitivity reactions as ordered.
- Monitor for side effects of nausea, vomiting, diarrhea, and skin reactions before each dose.
- Assess laboratory data including renal function before each dose.
- Evaluate for any signs of peripheral neuropathy.
- Monitor for signs or symptoms of mucositis, and initiate an oral care regimen as needed.
- Have anaphylaxis kit available at bedside along with an oxygen setup and an Ambu bag before administration of this agent. The anaphylaxis kit should include the following:
  Diphenhydramine 50 mg
  Hydrocortisone 50 mg
  Epinephrine 1:1000: draw up in syringe and inject only 0.3 mL at a time for each injection; repeat as necessary
  Needles and syringes

Education
- Instruct patient on when to contact his or her health care provider: fever greater than 38° C (greater than 101° F), shaking, chills, nausea or vomiting lasting greater than 24 hours, diarrhea lasting greater than 24 hours, or the inability to take in at least 1500 mL of fluid in 24 hours.
- Educate patient on an oral care regimen as needed. An example is 1 tsp each of salt and baking soda dissolved in 1 glass of water to swish and spit at least after each meal and at bedtime.
- Advise patient of the possibility of peripheral neuropathy and the symptoms associated with it: numbness and tingling in fingers and toes, pain, or temperature alterations.
- Educate patient that alopecia may occur and will last after the last dose for at least 3-4 months. When hair recovers, it may have a different color and consistency.
- Instruct patient that a skin rash may develop from this agent and to report any significant rashes to the health care provider.
- Advise patient to use contraception to prevent pregnancy while receiving this agent.
- Instruct patient on neutropenic precautions:
  Practice good handwashing techniques.
  Avoid crowds.
  Avoid salad bars in restaurants.
  Wash and cook all foods well to prevent transmission of infection.

- Instruct patient to take no over-the-counter medications or herbal or vitamin supplements without checking with his or her health care provider.
- Provide patient with information on local resources and support groups available for his or her specific diagnosis.

THALIDOMIDE

BRAND NAMES
Thalomid

CLASS OF AGENT
Angiogenesis inhibitor, immunosuppressant agent, tumor necrosis factor (TNF) blocking agent

CLINICAL PHARMACOLOGY
Mechanism of Action
An immunomodulator whose exact mechanism is unknown. Possesses antiangiogenic and immunosuppressive activity. Several proposed mechanisms include inhibition in production of TNF-α, resulting in down-modulation of cell surface adhesion molecules involved in leukocyte migration, reduction of angiogenic-promoting factors, and enhancement of the immune system by stimulating T cells. **Therapeutic Effect:** Kills malignant myeloma cells.

Absorption and Distribution
Slowly absorbed with a mean time to peak plasma concentration from 3-6 hours postdose. Protein binding: 55% for R isomer and 65% for S isomer.
Half-life: 6-8 hours.

Metabolism and Excretion
Undergoes nonenzymatic hydrolysis in plasma to multiple metabolites. Eliminated in urine as metabolites (less than 1%) 12-24 hours after dosing.

HOW SUPPLIED/AVAILABLE FORMS
Capsules: 50 mg, 100 mg, 200 mg. Available only through prescribers and pharmacies registered with the System for Thalidomide Education and Prescribing Safety (S.T.E.P.S.). Informed consent, compliance with mandatory patient registry, and surveys for each prescription are required for both male and female patients. (Contact: Celgene Customer Care Center toll-free at 1-888-4-CELGENE.)

INDICATIONS AND DOSAGES
◀ ALERT ▶ Treatment should not be initiated if ANC is less than 750/mm^3.
Erythema Nodosum Leprosum
Initiate at 100-300 mg PO daily as a single bedtime dose, at least 1 hour after the evening meal. For patients who previously required higher doses, initiate at up to 400 mg PO daily. Continue until an active reaction subsides, then reduce dose every 2-4 weeks in 50-mg increments.
Maintenance therapy should be kept at the lowest effective dose. Tapering off medication should be attempted every 3-6 months in 50-mg increments every 2-4 weeks.
Multiple Myeloma (Unlabeled)
100-800 mg PO daily with dexamethasone or as part of DTPACE (continuous infusion cisplatin, doxorubicin, cyclophosphamide, and etoposide) regimen. Refer to individual protocol.
Dosage Adjustment in Hepatic/Renal Dysfunction
No information available. The pharmacokinetics in patients with hepatic and renal impairment has not been determined.

UNLABELED USES
Treatment of Crohn's disease, recurrent aphthous ulcers in patients with HIV infection, multiple myeloma, wasting syndrome associated with HIV infection or cancer, graft-versus-host disease

PRECAUTIONS
Peripheral neuropathy may resolve slowly or be permanent and generally occurs after months of usage but may occur long after drug is discontinued. Use with caution in patients with preexisting neuropathy. Neutropenia has been reported and can be significant. Treatment should not be initiated if ANC is less than 750/mm^3. Monitor regularly and consider drug interruption or discontinuation if neutropenia persists.

CONTRAINDICATIONS
Pregnant women or women capable of becoming pregnant (unless there are no treatment alternatives and patient takes precaution to avoid pregnancy); patients who cannot adhere to the S.T.E.P.S program; hypersensitivity to thalidomide or any of its excipient ingredients
Pregnancy Risk Category: X
Thalidomide may cause severe birth defects or death to an unborn baby. Even a single

dose taken by a pregnant woman can cause birth defects. Excretion into human breast milk is unknown/not recommended in nursing women.

DRUG PREPARATION/ADMINISTRATION/ SAFE HANDLING ISSUES

◀ **ALERT** ▶ Swallow capsules as single bedtime dose, at least 1 hour after the evening meal.
* Do not break, chew, or open capsules.
* Overdosage of 14.4 g did not result in fatality.

STORAGE AND STABILITY
Store at room temperature.

INTERACTIONS
Drug
Alcohol, other CNS depressants: May increase sedative effects.
Medications associated with peripheral neuropathy (isoniazid, lithium, metronidazole, phenytoin): May increase peripheral neuropathy.
Medications that decrease effectiveness of hormonal contraceptives (carbamazepine, protease inhibitors, rifampin): May decrease the effectiveness of the contraceptive; patient must use two other methods of contraception.
Herbal
None known.

LAB EFFECTS/INTERFERENCE
Decreases neutrophil, platelet, hemoglobin, and Hct

SIDE EFFECTS
Serious Reactions
* Neutropenia and peripheral neuropathy may occur and require drug interruption or reduction.
* Thromboembolism events have been reported.
* HIV RNA levels increased in HIV-positive patients. The clinical significance of this is unknown. Both studies were conducted before the availability of highly active antiretroviral therapy.
Other Side Effects
Frequent (10%-50%): Dizziness, rash, somnolence
Occasional (1%-10%):
Alopecia, asthenia, back pain, chills, constipation, dry mouth, dry skin, facial edema, headache, hypothyroidism, increased appetite, malaise, mood changes, nausea, nail

disorder, peripheral neuropathy, pruritus, rash, weight gain
Rare (Less Than 1%):
Abdominal pain, impotence

SPECIAL CONSIDERATIONS
Baseline Assessment
* Perform a pregnancy test 24 hours before initiation of thalidomide.
* Assess CBC with differential, platelet count, electrolyte, BUN, and creatinine levels, liver function tests, and thyroid function before initiating therapy.
* Assess patient for any history of peripheral neuropathy or history of deep vein thrombosis.
* Monitor for history of hypertension and any evidence of bradycardia.
* Evaluate patient for history of depression and mood swings.
* Obtain baseline weight.

Intervention and Evaluation
* Monitor blood counts at each visit, paying particular attention to CBC with differential.
* Weigh patient at each visit.
* Monitor patient for any evidence of deep vein thrombosis, swelling, or erythema in the lower extremities or in arm if patient has a vascular access device.
* Monitor for pregnancy via the S.T.E.P.S. program as per guidelines, counsel patient, and reinforce information as necessary. Pregnancy tests should be performed weekly during the first month and monthly thereafter in women with regular menstrual cycles. If menstrual cycles are irregular, the pregnancy testing should occur every 2 weeks. Effective contraception must be used for at least 1 month before beginning therapy, during therapy, and for 1 month after discontinuation of thalidomide therapy unless the woman has been postmenopausal for 24 months or has had a hysterectomy. Male patients must use latex condoms when having sexual intercourse with women of childbearing potential, even if he has undergone successful vasectomy.
* Monitor vital signs at each visit to assess hypertension status.
* Evaluate for signs and symptoms of peripheral neuropathy: numbness and tingling in fingers and toes, and pain and burning in lower extremities.
* Initiate neutropenic precautions as needed based upon differential.

- Assess patient for signs and symptoms of anemia: shortness of breath, increasing fatigue, and dyspnea upon exertion.
- Evaluate patient for any evidence of rash, pruritus or desquamation on skin recommend that patient use creams to keep skin moisturized as needed.

Education

- Instruct patient on when to contact his or her health care provider: fever greater than 38° C (greater than 101° F), chills, shortness of breath, increasing fatigue, nausea lasting greater than 24 hours, diarrhea lasting greater than 24 hours, swelling in lower extremities, pain or erythema of area or swelling in arm on side of vascular access device, significant constipation, or the inability to take in at least 1500 mL of fluid in 24 hours.
- Educate patient on signs and symptoms of peripheral neuropathy: numbness and tingling of fingers and toes.
- Reinforce as appropriate the need for contraception at each visit and the risk of significant birth defects.
- Advise patient on neutropenic precautions: Practice good handwashing techniques. Avoid fresh fruits or vegetables, and cook all food well. Avoid persons with colds or flu like symptoms. Do no work with fresh flowers or plants. Avoid cleaning up after pets, and avoid litter boxes.
- Educate patient on symptoms of fatigue and anemia.
- Instruct patient to avoid all OTC medications and herbal and vitamin supplements without first checking with the health care provider.
- Provide patient with information on local resources and support groups available for his or her specific diagnosis.

THIOGUANINE

BRAND NAMES
Tabloid

CLASS OF AGENT
Antineoplastic agent, antimetabolite

CLINICAL PHARMACOLOGY
Mechanism of Action
A purine analog that is converted into 6-thioguanylic acid. There are several possible mechanisms of action including feedback inhibition of de novo purine synthesis, inhibition of purine nucleotide interconversions, and incorporation into DNA and RNA as fraudulent bases. Cell cycle specific for the S phase of the cell cycle. **Therapeutic effect:** Inhibits synthesis and utilization of purine nucleotides.

Absorption and Distribution
Incomplete and variable absorption; bioavailability 30% (range 14%-46%). Food may affect absorption. Peak serum concentration achieved in 8 hours postdose. Poor penetration into the CNS.
Half-life: 11 hours.

Metabolism and Excretion
Metabolized in the liver to 2-amino-6-methylthiopurine and other metabolites of variable activity. Unlike mercaptopurine, detoxification of thioguanine is not dependent on xanthine oxidase and, therefore, is not affected by xanthine oxidase inhibitors such as allopurinol. Primarily excreted in urine, mostly as the methylated metabolite. Unlikely to be removed by hemodialysis.

HOW SUPPLIED/AVAILABLE FORMS
Tablets: 40 mg.

INDICATIONS AND DOSAGES
Please refer to individual disease protocol as doses and schedules vary.
Acute Nonlymphocytic Leukemia
2-3 mg/kg/day PO calculated to the nearest 20 mg or 75-200 mg/m^2/day PO in 1-2 divided doses for 5-7 days or until remission.
Dosage Adjustment in Hepatic/Renal Dysfunction
No recommendations available. Consider dose reduction.

UNLABELED USES
Chronic myelogenous leukemia, inflammatory bowel disease, psoriasis

PRECAUTIONS
Use with caution in patients with renal or liver dysfunction. Patients who have a thiopurine S-methyltransferase (TPMT) deficiency or demonstrate low/intermediate TPMT activity will require dose reductions and have a higher risk for myelosuppression. If patient shows clinical or laboratory evidence of severe toxicity, TPMT genotyping or phenotyping should be considered.

Pregnancy Risk Category: D
Thioguanine may cause fetal harm when
administered during pregnancy. Excretion
into human milk is unknown/not recommended in nursing women.

CONTRAINDICATIONS
Hypersensitivity to thioguanine or any of
its excipients; patients whose disease has
demonstrated prior resistance to mercaptopurine or thioguanine

**DRUG PREPARATION/ADMINISTRATION/
SAFE HANDLING ISSUES**
- ◀ ALERT ▶ Thioguanine is considered a
  hazardous agent. Wash hands before and
  after contact with the bottle or tablets.
- Do not crush or chew on tablet. If tablet
  is accidentally crushed, immediately wipe
  it up with a damp cloth and discard in a
  closed container such as a plastic bag.
- Be aware that thioguanine dosage is individualized on the basis of patient's clinical response and tolerance of the drug's
  adverse effects.
- Administer preferably on an empty stomach (1 hour before and 2 hours after a
  meal). Absorption may vary with food.
- Overdose signs and symptoms may be
  immediate, such as nausea, vomiting,
  malaise, hypertension, and diaphoresis,
  or delayed, such as bone marrow suppression and renal failure. Induce emesis if
  clinically indicated.

STORAGE AND STABILITY
Store at 15-25° C (59-77° F).

INTERACTIONS
Drug
*Aminosalicylate derivatives (olsalazine,
mesalazine, sulfasalazine):* Inhibits TPMT
enzymes and may reduce thioguanine
metabolism.
Bone marrow depressants: May increase
risk of bone marrow depression.
Busulfan: Increased risk of hepatotoxicity.
Live-virus vaccines: May potentiate viral
replication, increase vaccine side effects,
and decrease patient's antibody response to
the vaccine.
Herbal
None known.

LAB EFFECTS/INTERFERENCE
May elevate serum alkaline phosphatase,
bilirubin, AST (SGOT), ALT (SGPT), and
uric acid levels.

SIDE EFFECTS
Serious Reactions
- Long-term use may cause liver toxicity.
- Leukopenia, infection, and thrombocyto-
  penia may occur.
- Hyperuricemia and uric acid nephropathy
  have been reported.
Other Side Effects
Frequent (10%-50%):
Anemia, leukopenia, thrombocytopenia
Occasional (1%-10%):
Anorexia, diarrhea, drug fever, esophageal
varices, GI necrosis and perforation, hepa-
tomegaly, hyperpigmentation, hyperurice-
mia, intrahepatic cholestasis, jaundice, nau-
sea, stomach pain, stomatitis, vomiting
Rare (Less Than 1%):
Mucositis, rash, unsteady gait

SPECIAL CONSIDERATIONS
Baseline Assessment
- Assess CBC with differential, platelet
  count, electrolyte, BUN, creatinine, and
  uric acid levels, and liver function tests.
- Assess patient for any prior dermatologic
  problems.
- Evaluate patient for any prior liver
  problems.
Intervention and Evaluation
- Monitor CBC with differential, platelet
  count, electrolyte, BUN, creatinine, and
  uric acid levels and liver function tests on
  a regular basis while patient is receiving
  this agent.
- Assess patient for medication compliance
  issues with oral daily dosing.
- Administer preferably on an empty stomach (1 hour before or 2 hours after a
  meal). Absorption varies with food.
- Evaluate patient for neutropenia,
  thrombocytopenia, and anemia.
- Assess skin for any evidence of hyperpigmentation, dermatitis, and areas of
  desquamation.
- Evaluate patient for any evidence of
  hepatic dysfunction, right upper quadrant
  pain, abdominal pain and fullness, clay-
  colored stools, or altered urine color.
- Hyperuricemia may occur as a consequence of rapid cell lysis. Minimize
  effects with increased hydration or initiation of allopurinol.
- Monitor patient for signs or symptoms of
  gout-like disorders or kidney stones.
- Initiate an oral care regimen as needed for
  mucositis, and inspect the oral cavity at
  each visit or each shift in the inpatient
  setting.

Education

- Advise patient to be sure to take the medication as prescribed and notify his or her health care provider if unable to take medication doses.
- Advise patient to take medication preferably on an empty stomach (1 hour before or 2 hours after a meal).
- Instruct patient on when to contact his or her health care provider: fever greater than 38° C (greater than 101° F), shaking, chills, easy bruising, bleeding, fatigue, nausea lasting greater than 24 hours, diarrhea lasting greater than 24 hours, or the inability to take at least 1500 mL in 24 hours.

Educate patient on the possibility of oral ulcers and instruct patient on an oral care regimen. An example is 1 tsp each of salt and baking soda dissolved in 1 glass of water, to swish and spit at least 3 times/day and at bedtime.

- Instruct patient on neutropenic precautions:
  - Practice good handwashing techniques.
  - Avoid crowds and persons with known infections.
  - Cook all food well.
- Advise patient on altered liver function symptoms, right upper quadrant pain, or abdominal fullness, pruritus, clay-colored stools, and cola-colored urine.
- Educate patient to practice good skin care, and use moisturizers as needed to keep skin intact.
- Instruct patient to drink 2 L of fluids daily to prevent renal toxicity.
- Teach patient to wash hands before and after contact with the bottle or tablet. People not taking thioguanine should not be exposed to it.
- Advise patient to avoid all OTC preparations and herbal and vitamin supplements without first checking with the health care provider.
- Provide patient with information on local resources and support groups available for his or her specific diagnosis.

THIOTEPA

BRAND NAMES
Thioplex

CLASS OF AGENT

Antineoplastic agent, alkylating agent chemically related to nitrogen mustard

CLINICAL PHARMACOLOGY
Mechanism of Action

An alkylating agent that inhibits DNA and RNA protein synthesis by cross-linking with DNA and RNA strands. Secondly, thiotepa releases ethyleneimine radicals, which disrupts bonds of DNA. It is cell cycle phase nonspecific. **Therapeutic Effect:** Interferes with DNA and RNA function.

Absorption and Distribution

Oral absorption from the GI tract is variable because the drug is unstable in acidic pH. It should not be given PO.

After intravesical administration, systemic absorption from the bladder mucosa ranges from 10% to almost 100% of the instilled dose and is enhanced by extensive tumor infiltration or acute mucosal inflammation, after endoscopic surgical procedures or radiation therapy, and in the presence of vesicoureteral reflux.

After intraperitoneal administration of 30 to 80 mg/m^2 doses of thiotepa, peak intraperitoneal concentrations, which occurred immediately after administration, were about 4-22 mcg/mL; systemic absorption ranges between 80% and 100% of the administered dose.

After IV administration, thiotepa and its active metabolite N,N',N''-triethylene-phosphoramide (TEPA) distribute widely into several tissues including brain, heart, kidney, lung, and skeletal muscle. It is not known whether thiotepa or TEPA distribute into breast milk, but it is likely.

Volume of distribution: 0.25-1.6 L/kg.
Half-life: 2-3 hours (parent) and 13-21 hours (metabolite).

Metabolism and Excretion

Metabolized extensively by cytochrome P450 (CYP) enzymes in the liver to TEPA. TEPA is the major metabolite and possesses cytotoxic activity. Clearance from the body may be impaired by hepatic dysfunction. Urinary excretion is 63%. Less than 2% of administered dose is excreted as thiotepa and TEPA in urine. Thiotepa is dialyzable. After high doses as are used in stem cell transplant, the drug is excreted substantially in sweat.

HOW SUPPLIED/AVAILABLE FORMS

Powder for Injection: 15 mg, 30 mg.

INDICATIONS AND DOSAGES
Adenocarcinoma of Breast and Ovary, Lymphosarcoma, Hodgkin's Disease

IV administration: 0.3-0.4 mg/kg every 1-4 weeks. Maintenance dose adjusted weekly based on blood counts.

Control of Intracavitary Effusions from Neoplastic Disease
Intracavitary injection: 0.6-0.8 mg/kg every 1-4 weeks.

Papillary Carcinoma of Urinary Bladder
Intravesical instillation: 60 mg in 30-60 mL instilled weekly for 4 weeks.

Leptomeningeal Metastasis (Unlabeled)
Intrathecal administration: 10-15 or 5-11.5 mg/m^2

Dosage Adjustment in Hepatic/Renal Dysfunction
No recommendations available. Use with extreme caution and adjust dose.

UNLABELED USES
Treatment of lung carcinoma, leptomeningeal metastasis

PRECAUTIONS
Use with caution in patients with preexisting hepatic, renal, or bone marrow diseases. Systemic drug absorption may occur with intravesical administration and cause bone-marrow suppression.

Pregnancy Risk Category: D
Thiotepa may cause fetal harm when administered to a pregnant woman. Drug excretion into human breast milk is unknown/not recommended in nursing women.

CONTRAINDICATIONS
Severe myelosuppression (leukocyte count less than 3000/mm^3 or platelet count less than 150,000/mm^3), hypersensitivity to thiotepa or to its formulation

DRUG PREPARATION/ADMINISTRATION/ SAFE HANDLING ISSUES
◀ ALERT ▶ Because thiotepa may be carcinogenic, mutagenic, or teratogenic, wear nitrile or latex, but not vinyl, gloves when handling the drug. If the drug comes in contact with skin, wash the skin thoroughly with soap and water. Do not use waterless hand soap or any antibacterial soap as either can increase the reaction from the agent. If the drug comes in contact with mucous membranes, flush the area with water. Personnel handling bedding or clothing of patients who have received high-dose thiotepa should exercise caution.

• Reconstitute a 15-mg vial with 1.5 mL of sterile water for a concentration of 10 mg/mL. For a 30-mg vial, reconstitute with 3 mL of sterile water.
• Withdraw calculated dose and further dilute in 0.9% NaCl or D5W before administration.
• Before administration, filter with a 0.22-micron filter to eliminate haze; reconstituted solutions should be clear.
• For IV administration, administer as a bolus or rapidly (10-60 minutes).
• For intrathecal administration, dilute drug in 1-5 mL of nonpreservative 0.9% NaCl.
• For intracavitary administration, administer drug through the same tubing as used to remove the fluid from the cavity.
• For intravesical administration, instill thiotepa 60 mg in 30-60 mL of NaCl into the bladder by catheter. Solution should be retained for 2 hours. Dehydrate patient for 2 hours before instillation. Reposition patient every 15 minutes for maximum area contact.

STORAGE AND STABILITY
• Store vials under refrigeration at 2-8° C (36-46° F). Protect from light.
• Vials reconstituted with sterile water should be stored in the refrigerator and used within 8 hours. Reconstituted solutions further diluted with NaCl should be used immediately per manufacturer.

INTERACTIONS
Drug
Bone marrow depressants: May increase myelosuppression.
Live-virus vaccines: May potentiate virus replication, increase vaccine side effects, and decrease patient's antibody response to the vaccine.
Succinylcholine: May prolong apnea by inhibiting pseudocholinesterase activity.
Herbal
None known.

LAB EFFECTS/INTERFERENCE
May cause decreases in WBC, neutrophil, and platelet counts and Hgb.

Y-SITE COMPATIBLES
Allopurinol (Aloprim), bumetanide (Bumex), calcium gluconate, carboplatin (Paraplatin), cyclophosphamide (Cytoxan), dexamethasone (Decadron), diphenhydramine (Benadryl), doxorubicin (Adriamycin), etoposide (VePesid), fluorouracil, gemcitabine (Gemzar), granisetron (Kytril), heparin, hydromorphone (Dilaudid), leucovorin, lorazepam (Ativan), magnesium sulfate, morphine, ondansetron (Zofran), paclitaxel (Taxol), potassium chloride, vincristine (Oncovin), vinorelbine (Navelbine)

INCOMPATIBLES
Cisplatin (Platinol-AQ), filgrastim (Neupogen)

SIDE EFFECTS
Serious Reactions
- Hematologic toxicity, manifested as leukopenia, anemia, thrombocytopenia, and pancytopenia, may result from bone marrow depression. It may also occur with systemic drug absorption through intravesical administration.
- Although the WBC count falls to its lowest point 10-14 days after initial therapy, the initial effects on bone marrow may not evident for 30 days.

Other Side Effects
Frequent (10%-50%):
Fatigue, myelosuppression
Occasional (1%-10%):
Abdominal pain, alopecia, anorexia, cystitis, dizziness, dysuria, headache, hematuria (after intravesical dose), nausea, pain at injection site, stomatitis, urinary retention, vomiting, weakness
Rare (Less Than 1%):
Amenorrhea, blurred vision, hypersensitivity reactions, interference with spermatogenesis, rash

SPECIAL CONSIDERATIONS
Baseline Assessment
- Assess CBC with differential, platelet count, electrolyte, BUN, and creatinine levels, and liver function tests.
- Evaluate patient's history for evidence of significant emesis with prior chemotherapy.
- Assess patient's history for prior allergic reactions as these can occur with this agent.
- Evaluate patient for central venous access as needed.

Intervention and Evaluation
- Assess all laboratory data before initiating premedications for this agent.
- Premedicate with antiemetics as ordered.
- Monitor patient for potential allergic reactions, hives, bronchospasm, and dermatitis.
- Assess infusion rate and any notation of pain at injection site as this agent is an irritant; monitor the need for a central venous access device at each administration.
- Assess patient for neutropenia with each dose of this agent.
- Initiate neutropenic and thrombocytopenic precautions as needed per institutional guidelines.

- Evaluate patient for signs and symptoms of mucositis.
- Initiate an oral care regimen as necessary. An example is 1 tsp each of salt and baking soda in 8 ounces of water to swish and spit at least 3 times/day and at bedtime.
- Assess patient for any evidence of cystitis or symptoms of urinary tract infection.

Education
- Educate patient on when and for how long to take antiemetic therapy.
- Instruct patient on when to contact his or her health care provider: fever greater than 38° C (greater than 101° F), chills, rigors, nausea lasting greater than 24 hours, diarrhea lasting greater than 24 hours, severe abdominal cramping, or the inability to take in at least 1500 mL of fluid in 24 hours.
- Advise patient to report any signs or symptoms of allergic-type reactions with this agent: hives, rash, shortness of breath, or difficulty breathing.
- Instruct patient on signs and symptoms of myelosuppression, neutropenia, thrombocytopenia, and anemia.
- Instruct patient on neutropenic precautions:
  Practice good handwashing techniques.
  Avoid crowds and any persons who are ill.
  Wash and cook all food well.
  Avoid all raw fruits and vegetables.
- Educate patient on thrombocytopenic precautions:
  Do not take temperatures rectally or administer enemas.
  Do not give IM injections.
  Do not perform heavy lifting or strenuous exercises.
  Do not floss teeth, and use a soft toothbrush.
- Educate patient on signs and symptoms of mucositis and a mouth care regimen to use if mucositis occurs.
- Educate patient on the need for contraception while receiving this agent as this agent can induce birth defects. Sterility may be reversible; amenorrhea usually reverses in 6-8 mos depending on the age of patient. Discuss sperm or egg banking options if this is appropriate.
- Instruct patient to avoid all OTC medications and herbal and vitamin supplements without first checking with the health care provider.

- Educate patient that alopecia may occur rarely with this agent.
- Provide patient with information on local resources and support groups available for his or her specific diagnosis.

TOPOTECAN

BRAND NAMES
Hycamtin

CLASS OF AGENT
Antineoplastic agent, topoisomerase I inhibitor

CLINICAL PHARMACOLOGY
Mechanism of Action
A DNA topoisomerase inhibitor that interacts with topoisomerase I, an enzyme that allows DNA replication by producing reversible single-strand breaks in DNA to relieve torsional strain. Topotecan prevents religation of the DNA strand, resulting in damage to double-strand DNA during DNA synthesis. **Therapeutic Effect:** Kills cancer cells.

Absorption and Distribution
Extensively distributed into tissues. Protein binding: 35%.
Half-life: 2-3 hours (increased in impaired renal function).

Metabolism and Excretion
Topotecan undergoes a reversible pH-dependent hydrolysis to its active form after IV administration. Liver metabolism to the *N*-demethylated metabolite is a minor metabolic pathway. Excreted in urine (30%).

HOW SUPPLIED/AVAILABLE FORMS
Powder for Injection: 4 mg (single-dose vial).

INDICATIONS AND DOSAGES
Refer to individual protocols for dosage regimens. Alternative schedules of 3-day and weekly continuous infusion are currently under evaluation.

Ovarian Carcinoma, Small Cell Lung Cancer
1.5 mg/m^2/day IV over 30 minutes for 5 consecutive days, beginning on day 1 of a 21-day course. Minimum of four courses recommended.

Cervical Cancer
0.75 mg/m^2/day IV over 30 minutes for 3 consecutive days, followed by cisplatin 50 mg/m^2/day IV on day 1 repeated every 21 days.

Dosage Adjustment in Myelosuppression
If severe neutropenia (neutrophil count less than 1500/mm^2) occurs or platelet count falls below 25,000 cells/mm^3 during treatment, reduce dose for subsequent courses by 0.25 mg/m^2 or administer filgrastim (granulocyte colony-stimulating factor) no sooner than 24 hours after the last dose of topotecan. Allow for neutrophil recovery greater than 1000 cells/mm^3, platelet count greater than 100,000 cells/mm^3, and Hgb of 9.0 g/dL before subsequent course treatments.

Dosage Adjustment in Hepatic Dysfunction
No adjustments necessary (total bilirubin less than 1.5 to less than 10 mg/dL).

Dosage Adjustment in Renal Dysfunction
Mild renal impairment (CrCl of 40-60 mL/minute): no adjustments necessary.
Moderate renal impairment (CrCl of 20-39 mL/minute): adjust dose to 0.75 mg/m^2.
Severe renal impairment: No recommendations available.

UNLABELED USES
Treatment of solid tumors including osteosarcoma, neuroblastoma, gliomas, pediatric leukemia, myelodysplastic syndrome, rhabdomyosarcoma

PRECAUTIONS
Use with caution in patients with renal impairment or mild myelosuppression.

Pregnancy Risk Category: D
Because of the risk of fetal harm, pregnant women should not take topotecan. Breast-feeding is not recommended for patients taking this drug.

CONTRAINDICATIONS
Baseline neutrophil count less than 1500 cells/mm^3, breast-feeding, pregnancy, severe myelosuppression

DRUG PREPARATION/ADMINISTRATION/ SAFE HANDLING ISSUES
◄ ALERT ▶ Do not initiate topotecan if patient's baseline ANC is less than 1500 cells/mm^3 and platelet count is less than 100,000/mm^3.
- Reconstitute powder with 4 mL of sterile water for injection to make a concentration of 1 mg/mL.
- Further dilute with 50-100 mL of 0.9% NaCl or D5W.

- Administer the drug by IV infusion over 30 minutes.
- Extravasation is associated with only mild local reactions, such as ecchymosis and erythema.

STORAGE AND STABILITY
- Store vials at room temperature in original cartons.
- Reconstituted vials diluted for infusion are stable at room temperature in ambient lighting for up to 24 hours; however, because it contains no preservatives, the manufacturer recommends doses to be administered immediately after reconstitution and dilution.

INTERACTIONS
Drug
In vitro studies indicate that there are no effects the cytochrome P450 enzyme family.
Bone marrow depressants: May increase the risk of myelosuppression.
Cisplatin: May increase the severity of myelosuppression; may be sequence related.
Live-virus vaccines: May potentiate viral replication, increase vaccine side effects, and decrease patient's antibody response to the vaccine.
Herbal
None known.

LAB EFFECTS/INTERFERENCE
May increase serum bilirubin, AST (SGOT), and ALT (SGPT) levels. May decrease RBC, leukocyte, neutrophil, and platelet counts.

Y-SITE COMPATIBLES
Carboplatin (Paraplatin), cisplatin (Platinol AQ), cyclophosphamide (Cytoxan), dactinomycin, doxorubicin (Adriamycin), etoposide (VePesid), gemcitabine (Gemzar), granisetron (Kytril), ifosfamide, methylprednisolone, ondansetron (Zofran), oxaliplatin, paclitaxel (Taxol), palonosetron, prochlorperazine, teniposide, thiotepa, vincristine (Oncovin)

COMPATIBLES
Dexamethasone (Decadron), 5-fluorouracil, mitomycin (Mutamycin), pantoprazole, pemetrexed, ticarcillin and clavulanate, rituximab, trastuzumab

SIDE EFFECTS
Serious Reactions
- Severe neutropenia (neutrophil count less than 500 cells/mm^3) occurs in 60% of patients, usually during the first course of therapy. The neutrophil nadir usually occurs at a median of 12 days after starting therapy.
- Thrombocytopenia (platelet count less than 25,000/mm^3) occurs in 27% of patients, and severe anemia (RBC count less than 8 g/dL) occurs in 37% of patients. The platelet and RBC nadirs usually occur at a median of 15 days after the first course of therapy is started.

Other Side Effects
Frequent (10%-50%):
Anemia, anorexia, asthenia, blood transfusions, diarrhea, total alopecia, dyspnea, fatigue, nausea, neutropenia, thrombocytopenia, vomiting
Occasional (1%-10%):
Abdominal pain, chest pain, constipation, coughing, headache, paresthesia, rash, stomatitis, sepsis
Rare (Less Than 1%):
Anaphylactoid reaction, arthralgia, increased hepatic enzymes, malaise, myalgia, severe dermatitis, severe pruritus, severe bleeding

SPECIAL CONSIDERATIONS
Baseline Assessment
- Assess patient's CBC with differential and platelet count before each topotecan dose.
- Know that myelosuppression may precipitate life-threatening anemia, hemorrhage, and infection.
- Premedicate patient with antiemetics, as ordered, on the day of treatment, starting at least 30 minutes before topotecan administration. Topotecan has a low emetic potential.
- In elderly patients, age-related renal impairment may require dosage adjustment.
- The safety and efficacy of topotecan have not been established in children.

Intervention and Evaluation
- Monitor patient's CBC with differential and platelet count frequently during topotecan treatment for evidence of myelosuppression and thrombocytopenia.
- Assess patient for dyspnea, headache, anemia, bleeding, and signs of infection.
- Monitor patient's serum electrolyte levels, hydration status, and intake and output because diarrhea and vomiting are common side effects of topotecan.
- Assess patient's ability to take in at least 1500 mL of fluid in 24 hours.
- Initiate neutropenic precautions as needed per institutional protocol.

- Initiate thrombocytopenic precautions when platelet count is less than 50,000/mm^3.
- Assess patient's nutritional status, and if needed, obtain a consultation with a nutritionist.
- Help patient manage the drug's side effects, for example, by providing small, frequent meals and antiemetics to help prevent or treat nausea and vomiting.

Education

- Instruct patient on when to call his or her health care provider and make sure patient has a 24-hour number for the provider.
- Instruct patient on signs and symptoms of infection and thrombocytopenia: fever greater than 38° C (greater than 101° F), chills, epistaxis, or bleeding from any site.
- Instruct patient to contact provider if unable to take in at least 1500 mL of fluid in 24 hours, diarrhea greater than three stools over baseline, and nausea and vomiting lasting greater than 24 hours with antiemetics provided.
- Instruct patient in neutropenic precautions as needed:
    Practice good handwashing techniques.
    Cook all foods.
    Avoid fresh fruits and vegetables.
    Avoid fresh flowers.
    Avoid all persons with infection, and avoid crowds.
- Instruct patient on thrombocytopenic precautions:
    Use soft toothbrush.
    Avoid flossing.
    Avoid straight razors; use electric razor only.
    Instruct women to avoid shaving legs.
    Avoid heavy lifting and strenuous activities.
- Instruct patient that alopecia will occur with 2-3 weeks of drug initiation and resolution takes 2-4 months after completion of therapy; new hair growth may have a different color or texture.
- Explain that diarrhea may develop late in therapy. Teach patient to watch for signs and symptoms of dehydration and electrolyte depletion.
- If ordered, provide instructions for using antiemetic and antidiarrheal medications.
- Urge patient to avoid receiving vaccinations and coming in contact with anyone who has recently received a live-virus vaccine.

- Advise patient to avoid all OTC preparations and herbal and vitamin supplements without first checking with the health care provider.
- Educate patient on local resources available and support groups related to their particular diagnosis.

TOREMIFENE CITRATE

BRAND NAMES
Fareston

CLASS OF AGENT
Selective estrogen receptor modulator (SERM)

CLINICAL PHARMACOLOGY
Mechanism of Action
A nonsteroidal, triphenylethylene derivative that competes with estrogen for estrogen receptors on tumors and target tissues. As with other SERMs, toremifene can act estrogenic or antiestrogenic, depending on the context in which it is examined. In humans it acts predominantly antiestrogenic and binds to estrogen receptors effectively blocking it from estrogen. **Therapeutic Effect:** Blocks growth-stimulating effects of estrogen in hormone-responsive tumors and target tissues.
Absorption and Distribution
Well absorbed after oral administration with peak plasma concentrations within 3 hours. Steady-state concentrations achieved within 4-6 weeks. Volume of distribution: 580 L. Protein binding: 99%, mainly albumin.
Half-life: 5 days.
Metabolism and Excretion
Metabolized in the liver by cytochrome P450 (CYP) 3A4 to *N*-demethyltoremifene (weak antiestrogen). Eliminated as metabolites in feces (major); undergoes enterohepatic circulation. Urine excretion (10%).

HOW SUPPLIED/AVAILABLE FORMS
Tablets: 60 mg.

INDICATIONS AND DOSAGES
Metastatic Breast Cancer in Postmenopausal Women with Estrogen Receptor-Positive or Unknown Tumors
60 mg PO daily until disease progression is observed.
Dosage Adjustment in Hepatic Dysfunction
No recommendations available.

**Dosage Adjustment
in Renal Dysfunction**
No dosage adjustments necessary.

UNLABELED USES
Treatment of desmoid tumors, endometrial carcinoma

PRECAUTIONS
Patients with history of thromboembolic diseases and preexisting endometrial hyperplasia
Pregnancy Risk Category: D
Toremifene may cause fetal harm when administered during pregnancy. Drug excretion into human milk is unknown/not recommended in nursing women.

CONTRAINDICATIONS
Hypersensitivity to toremifene or any of its excipients.

DRUG PREPARATION/ADMINISTRATION/ SAFE HANDLING ISSUES
- Take once daily without regard to food.
- Overdosage of 680-mg repeated doses resulted in vertigo, headache, and dizziness. Symptoms resolved within 2 days after discontinuation of drug. Monitor vital signs and provide supportive care.

STORAGE AND STABILITY
Store at room temperature. Protect from light and heat.

INTERACTIONS
Drug
CYP 3A4 inducers (carbamazepine, phenobarbital, phenytoin, ranitidine, rifampin): May decrease toremifene blood concentration and effectiveness.
CYP 3A4 inhibitors (ciprofloxacin, clarithromycin, diclofenac, doxycycline, erythromycin, isoniazid, itraconazole, ketoconazole, nefazodone, nicardipine, propofol, protease inhibitors, quinidine, verapamil): Increases toremifene blood concentration. Monitor for adverse effects.
Warfarin (coumarin-derivative anticoagulants): Increases the risk of bleeding. Monitor international normalized ratio or prothrombin time regularly.
Herbal
St John's Wort: May increase metabolism and decrease serum toremifene concentration. Avoid use.

LAB EFFECTS/INTERFERENCE
May increase serum alkaline phosphatase, bilirubin, calcium, and AST (SGOT) levels.

SIDE EFFECTS
Serious Reactions
- Symptoms of tumor flare, such as musculoskeletal pain and erythema with increased size of tumor lesions, that later regress may occur during the first few weeks after drug initiation in patients with extensive metastatic disease to bones. Monitor for hypercalcemia and give supportive care as indicated.
- Ocular toxicity (cataracts, glaucoma, and decreased visual acuity), cardiac events (MI, arrhythmia, angina pectoris, and cardiac failure) and hypercalcemia occur rarely.
- Endometrial hyperplasia has been reported rarely.

Other Side Effects
Frequent (10%-50%):
Diaphoresis, hot flashes, nausea, vaginal discharge
Occasional (1%-10%):
Cataracts, dizziness, dry eyes, edema, elevated liver enzyme levels, hypercalcemia, vaginal bleeding, vomiting
Rare (Less Than 1%):
Abnormal vision, anorexia, arthritis, corneal keratopathy, depression, diplopia, endometrial hyperplasia, fatigue, glaucoma, ischemic attack, lethargy, leukopenia, pulmonary embolism, thrombocytopenia, thrombophlebitis, vaginal bleeding

SPECIAL CONSIDERATIONS
Baseline Assessment
- Assess baseline CBC with differential, platelet count, electrolyte, BUN, creatinine, calcium, and phosphorus levels, and liver function tests.
- Assess patient for any evidence of hypercalcemia.
- Evaluate patient for any history of glaucoma and cataracts.
- Obtain baseline weight, and assess for any evidence of edema.
- Assess patient for any history of deep vein thrombosis.
- Evaluate patient for any history of endometrial cancer.
Intervention and Evaluation
- Evaluate new laboratory data at each visit.

- Assess patient for signs and symptoms of hot flashes, diaphoresis, and decreased visual acuity.
- Evaluate patient for any evidence of nausea, vomiting, or vaginal discharge or bleeding.
- Monitor patient for weight changes and evidence of peripheral edema.
- Assess patient for usual fluid intake.
- Assess patient for any evidence of deep vein thrombosis or tumor flare.
- Monitor patient for any evidence of depression and intervene as needed.

Education
- Instruct patient on when to contact his or her health care provider: nausea lasting greater than 24 hours, the inability to take at least 1500 mL of fluid in 24 hours, vaginal bleeding, or decreased visual acuity.
- Assess patient for adherence in taking this medication, and instruct patient to contact the health care provider if he or she has any difficulties in taking this agent on a regular basis.
- Advise patient that this agent causes a slight risk of endometrial cancer, so any evidence of vaginal bleeding or discharge needs to be reported to the health care provider.
- Educate patient to see an optician or ophthalmologist on a regular a basis to evaluate for any evidence of cataracts or glaucoma.
- Advise patient that dry eyes and dizziness may occur.
- Educate patient that a tumor flare manifesting as increased pain may occur and to report this to the health care provider.
- Instruct patient on signs and symptoms of deep vein thrombosis, erythema, pain, and edema of the lower extremities.
- Advise patient on symptoms of hypercalcemia, nausea, vomiting, constipation, abdominal pain, weakness, lethargy, frequent urination and nocturia and to contact the health care provider if any of these symptoms occur.
- Instruct patient to take no over-the-counter medications or herbal or vitamin supplements without checking with his or her health care provider.
- Provide patient with information on local resources and support groups available for his or her specific diagnosis.

TOSITUMOMAB AND IODINE I 131 TOSITUMOMAB

BRAND NAMES
Bexxar

CLASS OF AGENT
Antineoplastic agent, monoclonal antibody, radiopharmaceutical

CLINICAL PHARMACOLOGY
Mechanism of Action
An antineoplastic radioimmunotherapeutic monoclonal antibody-based regimen composed of the murine IgG monoclonal antibody, tositumomab, and the radiolabeled monoclonal antibody, iodine I 131 tositumomab. The antibody portion binds specifically to the CD20 antigen, which is found on pre-B and B lymphocytes and on more than 90% of B-cell non-Hodgkin lymphomas, resulting in formation of a complex. Possible mechanisms of action include induction of apoptosis, complement-dependent cytotoxicity, and antibody-dependent cellular cytotoxicity mediated by the antibody. May also induce cell death with ionizing radiation from the radioisotope. **Therapeutic Effect:** Depletes circulating CD20-positive cells. At 7 weeks, the median number of circulating CD20 cells was zero. Lymphocyte recovery began approximately 12 weeks post-treatment.

Absorption and Distribution
Widely absorbed and distributed in tissues. *Half-life:* The I 131 half-life is 8 days. The effective half-life of I 131 tositumomab is 65 days. Patients with a high tumor burden, splenomegaly, or bone marrow involvement have a faster clearance, shorter half-life, and larger volume of distribution.

Metabolism and Excretion
Elimination of iodine 131 occurs by decay and excretion in urine.

HOW SUPPLIED/AVAILABLE FORMS
Dosimetric step: tositumomab 225 mg/16.1 mL (two vials), tositumomab 35 mg/2.5 mL (one vial), and iodine 131 tositumomab 0.1 mg/mL (one vial). *Therapeutic step:* tositumomab 225 mg/16.1 mL (two vials), tositumomab 35 mg/2.5 mL (one vial), and iodine 131 tositumomab 1.1 mg/mL (one or two vials).

Dosing Schedule

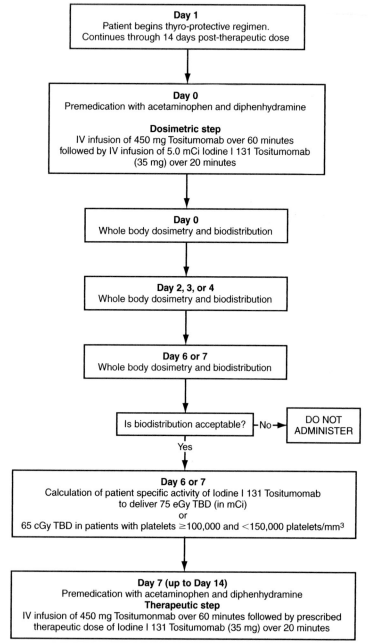

Day 1
Patient begins thyro-protective regimen.
Continues through 14 days post-therapeutic dose

Day 0
Premedication with acetaminophen and diphenhydramine

Dosimetric step
IV infusion of 450 mg Tositumomab over 60 minutes
followed by IV infusion of 5.0 mCi Iodine I 131 Tositumomab
(35 mg) over 20 minutes

Day 0
Whole body dosimetry and biodistribution

Day 2, 3, or 4
Whole body dosimetry and biodistribution

Day 6 or 7
Whole body dosimetry and biodistribution

Is biodistribution acceptable? —No→ DO NOT ADMINISTER

Yes

Day 6 or 7
Calculation of patient specific activity of Iodine I 131 Tositumomab
to deliver 75 eGy TBD (in mCi)
or
65 cGy TBD in patients with platelets ≥100,000 and <150,000 platelets/mm³

Day 7 (up to Day 14)
Premedication with acetaminophen and diphenhydramine
Therapeutic step
IV infusion of 450 mg Tositumonmab over 60 minutes followed by prescribed
therapeutic dose of Iodine I 131 Tositumomab (35 mg) over 20 minutes

From Tositumomab and iodine I 131 Tositumomab (Bexxar) prescribing information. GlaxoSmithKline, October 2005.

INDICATIONS AND DOSAGES
Non-Hodgkin's Lymphoma (Including Rituximab-Refractory Non-Hodgkin's Lymphoma)
Dosimetric step: Day 0: tositumomab 450 mg/50 mL NaCl over 60 minutes. Then, tositumomab 35 mg and iodine I 131 tositumomab containing 5.0 mCi of iodine-131.
Therapeutic step: Day 6 or 7: tositumomab 450 mg/50 mL NaCl over 60 minutes. Then, tositumomab 35 mg and the calculated dose of iodine I 131 tositumomab to deliver 75 cGy total body irradiation for patients with platelets greater than or equal to 150,000/mm^3 or 65 cGy total body irradiation for patients with platelets 100,000-150,000/mm^3.
Note: Patients are required to have ANC greater than 1500 cells/mm^3 and platelet count greater than or equal to 100,000/mm^3.
Note: Patients should not receive the dosimetric dose if they have not received at least 3 doses of saturated solution of potassium iodide (SSKI,) 3 doses of Lugol's solution, or one 130-mg potassium iodide tablet 24 hours before the dosimetric dose. Premedicate with thyroid protective agents including SSKI 4 drops orally 3 times/day, Lugol's solution 20 drops orally 3 times/day, or potassium iodide tablets 130 mg orally daily. Thyroid agents should be initiated at least 24 hours before administration of the iodine I 131 tositumomab dosimetric dose and continued until 2 weeks after administration of the iodine I 131 tositumomab therapeutic dose.
Note: Premedicate with acetaminophen 650 mg PO and diphenhydramine 50 mg PO 30 minutes before both dosimetric and therapeutic steps.
Dosage Adjustment in Hepatic Dysfunction
No information.
Dosage Adjustment in Renal Dysfunction
No information. However, drug clearance is delayed.

UNLABELED USES
No information.

PRECAUTIONS
Prolonged and severe cytopenias manifested as neutropenia and thrombocytopenias may occur and lead to infections and hemorrhage. CBCs with differential and platelet counts should be obtained before initiation of the tositumomab therapeutic regimen and monitored weekly for at least 10-12 weeks after completion of therapy or until severe cytopenias have completely resolved; more frequent monitoring is recommended in patients with evidence of moderate or severe cytopenias.
For hypothyroidism, thyroid-blocking agents should be initiated at least 24 hours before receiving the dosimetric dose and continued until 14 days after the therapeutic dose. Patients who cannot take thyroid-blocking agents should not be treated with this regimen.

CONTRAINDICATIONS
Hypersensitivity to any components of tositumomab and iodine I 131 tositumomab or murine proteins; pregnancy; ANC less than 1500 cells/mm^3 and platelet count less than 100,000/mm^3; greater than 25% of intratrabecular marrow space involved by lymphoma
Pregnancy Risk Category: X
Components of this regimen may cause fetal harm when administered during pregnancy. According to the manufacturer, transplacental passage of radioiodine may cause severe and possibly irreversible hypothyroidism in neonates. Contraception should be used with male and female patients during treatment and for 12 months post-treatment. Radioiodine is excreted in breast milk. Formula feedings should be implemented. Women should be advised to discontinue nursing.

DRUG PREPARATION/ADMINISTRATION/ SAFE HANDLING ISSUES
◄ ALERT ► Tositumomab and iodine I 131 tositumomab are radiopharmaceuticals and should be used only by physicians and other professionals qualified by training and experienced in the safe use and handling of radionuclides. This agent must be handled using strict radioactivity guidelines. Proper aseptic technique and precautions should be used. Waterproof gloves should be used in the preparation and during the determination of radiochemical purity of iodine I 131 tositumomab. Appropriate shielding should be used during radiolabeling, and use of a syringe shield is recommended during administration to patient. Radiation safety precautions must be used to administer this agent. Patient must be placed in appropriate isolation after receipt of this agent.

◀ **ALERT** ▶ Patients are required to have ANC >1500 cells/mm^3 and platelet count greater than or equal to 100,000/mm^3.

◀ **ALERT** ▶ Patients should not receive the dosimetric dose if they have not received at least 3 doses of SSKI, 3 doses of Lugol's solution, or one 130-mg potassium iodide tablet 24 hours before the dosimetric dose.

• Premedicate with acetaminophen 650 mg PO and diphenhydramine 50 mg PO 30 minutes before both dosimetric and therapeutic steps.

• For preparation of the dosimetric step and therapeutic step, refer to the manufacturer's prescribing information.

• Calculation of the dose for the therapeutic step can be done manually or automatically using the GlaxoSmithKline software program. (Contact: Bexxar Service Center at 877-423-9927 [877-4-bexxar]).

STORAGE AND STABILITY

• Store vials of tositumomab in refrigerator 2-8° C (36-46° F). Protect from light. Do not shake.

• Diluted solutions of tositumomab are stable for up to 24 hours when stored refrigerated and for upto 8 hours at room temperature. Does not contain any preservatives.

• Iodine I 131 tositumomab should be stored frozen in the original lead pots (−20° C or below) until it is removed for thawing before administration to patient.

• Thawed dosimetric and therapeutic doses of iodine I 131 tositumomab are stable for up to 8 hours refrigerated or at room temperature.

• Solutions of iodine I 131 tositumomab diluted for infusion contain no preservatives and should be stored refrigerated before administration.

INTERACTIONS
Drug
Anticoagulants (heparin, low molecular weight heparins, thrombolytics, warfarin): May increase potential for prolonged and severe thrombocytopenia and increase risk of bleeding.

Antiplatelet drugs (aspirin, clopidogrel, glycoprotein Iib/IIIa antagonists, NSAIDs, ticlopidine): May increase potential for prolonged and severe thrombocytopenia and increase risk of bleeding.

Bone marrow depressants: May increase bone marrow depression.

Live-virus vaccines: May potentiate virus replications, increase vaccine side effects, and decrease patient's antibody response to vaccine.

Herbal
Herbals with antiplatelet activity.

LAB EFFECTS/INTERFERENCE

May decrease blood Hct and Hgb levels, platelet and WBC counts, and thyroid-stimulating hormone level.

Y-SITE COMPATIBLES

No information.

INCOMPATIBLES

Do not mix with any other medications.

SIDE EFFECTS
Serious Reactions

• Infusion toxicity characterized by bronchospasm, angioedema, fever, rigors, diaphoresis, hypotension, dyspnea, and others may occur during or within 48 hours of the infusion. Slowing and/or interrupting the infusion-managed infusional toxicities.

• Grade 3 or 4 thrombocytopenia (53%) or grade 3 or 4 neutropenia (63%) may occur. The time to nadir was 4-7 weeks, and the duration of cytopenias was 30 days. CBCs should be obtained weekly for 10-12 weeks.

• Infections may occur in 45% of patients.

• Hemorrhage may occur in 12% of patients.

• Secondary malignancies such as myelodysplastic syndrome, acute leukemia have been reported in patients in clinical studies and expanded access programs (4%).

Other Side Effects
Frequent (10%-50%):
Abdominal pain, anorexia, asthenia, chills, cough, diarrhea, dyspnea, fever, general pain, headache, hematologic toxicity infection, myalgia, nausea, pharyngitis, rash, vomiting
Occasional (1%-10%):
Arthralgia, back pain, chest pain, constipation, dizziness, dyspepsia, hypotension, hypothyroidism, neck pain, peripheral edema, pneumonia, pruritus, rhinitis, somnolence, sweating, vasodilatation, weight loss
Rare (Less Than 1%):
Grade 3 or 4 arthralgia, back pain, chills, constipation, cough, dyspepsia, hypotension, infection, myalgia, neck pain, pain, rash, sweating, vomiting, weigh loss

SPECIAL CONSIDERATIONS
Baseline Assessment
- Assess CBC with differential, platelet count, electrolyte, BUN, and creatinine levels, liver function tests, and thyroid function tests before dosing.
- Rule out pregnancy.
- Review radiation safety instructions before administering this agent.
- Be aware that a bone marrow biopsy report is required to determine that no more than 25% disease is noted in bone marrow; bone marrow failure has been reported in patients with higher than 25% disease involvement in bone marrow.

Intervention and Evaluation
- Assess CBC with differential, platelet count, and electrolyte levels weekly for 12 weeks, and if severe cytopenias persistent, until they have resolved.
- Administer premedications as ordered before receipt of this agent.
- Ensure that patient receives the required amount of thyroid-protective agent before the dosimetric step. Continue this agent throughout therapy and for up to 2 weeks post-treatment.
- Monitor for 48 hours after dosing for any evidence of hypersensitivity reactions, fevers, chills, rigors, hypotension, dyspnea, or nausea.
- Assess thyroid function on an annual basis.
- Assess patient for any evidence of sepsis.
- Assess for any evidence of GI toxicity. Nausea, vomiting, and abdominal pain were often reported within days of infusion. Diarrhea generally occurs days to weeks after infusion.
- Implement radiation safety precautions per institutional protocol.
- Monitor patient's blood counts at each return visit as this agent can induce severe and prolonged myelosuppression. Assess patient for any evidence of neutropenia, thrombocytopenia, or anemia as nadir is prolonged. Assess need for hematologic support (granulocyte colony-stimulating factor, erythropoietin, platelet transfusion, and red blood cell transfusions).
- Evaluate patient for any evidence of tinnitus, pruritus, or arthralgias or asthenia.

Education
- Educate patient that this is a murine monoclonal antibody, and severe hypersensitivity reactions can occur.
- Advise patient that premedications will be given before dosing this agent.
- Instruct patient on when to contact his or her health care provider: infection, fever greater than 38° C (greater than 101° F), shaking, chills, shortness of breath or dyspnea upon exertion, easy bruising, bleeding, nausea lasting greater than 24 hours, diarrhea lasting greater than 24 hours, or the inability to take in at least 1500 mL of fluid in 24 hours.
- Educate patient on the need for lifelong thyroid replacement therapy and the importance of taking medication appropriately.
- Educate patient on radiation safety precautions after discharge: allow no young children or women of childbearing age to be closer than 3 feet for the first week, allow no sharing of utensils, flush toilet at least twice each time it is used, and limit visitors to the household during the first week.
- Educate patient on contraception usage for both male and female patients during treatment and for up to 12 months after treatment.
- Advise patient that symptoms of fatigue, weakness, or myalgias may occur.
- Provide patient with information on local resources and support groups available for his or her specific diagnosis.

TRASTUZUMAB

BRAND NAMES
Herceptin

CLASS OF AGENT
Monoclonal antibody

CLINICAL PHARMACOLOGY
Mechanism of Action
Binds to the human epidermal growth factor receptor 2 (HER-2 or erbB2) protein, which is overexpressed in 25%-30% of primary breast cancers, thereby inhibiting proliferation of tumor cells. HER-2 overexpression can be determined by using immunohistochemistry (IHC), and gene amplification can be determined using fluorescence in situ hybridization; patients were eligible in clinical trials if they had 2+ or 3+ overexpression by IHC. **Therapeutic Effect:** Inhibits the growth of tumor cells and mediates antibody-dependent cellular cytotoxicity.

Absorption and Distribution
Volume of distribution: 44 mL/kg. It is not known whether trastuzumab crosses the blood-brain barrier or the placenta. Partial

distribution into the cerebrospinal fluid (CSF) or breast milk in humans is not known, but transfer into the placenta and CSF has been observed in monkeys *Half-life:* 5.8 days (range: 1-32 days). Mean half-life increased and clearance decreased with increasing dose levels.

Metabolism and Excretion
According to the British Columbia Cancer Agency, trastuzumab undergoes degradation through irreversible receptor binding. The metabolism of trastuzumab is not completely known. It appears that elimination of the drug involves binding to IgG and clearance of IgG-drug complex through the reticuloendothelial system.

HOW SUPPLIED/AVAILABLE FORMS
Injection, Powder for Reconstitution: 440 mg multidose vial.

INDICATIONS AND DOSAGES
Breast Cancer
Loading dose of 4 mg/kg IV as a 90-minute infusion, then 2 mg/kg IV weekly as a 30-minute infusion.
(unlabeled) 4 mg/kg IV as 90-minute infusion every 2 weeks.
(unlabeled) 8 mg/kg loading dose followed by 6 mg/kg IV as a 90-minute infusion every 3 weeks.
Dosage Adjustment in Hepatic/Renal Dysfunction
No information.

UNLABELED USES
Solid tumors with HER-2 overexpression (e.g., ovarian carcinoma)

PRECAUTIONS
Cardiotoxicity in the form of CHF, MI, stroke, and heart failure is the most common serious adverse effect with trastuzumab. Risk factors include age, preexisting cardiac dysfunction/disease, and prior treatment with doxorubicin and cyclophosphamide. Left ventricular ejection fraction (LVEF) should be obtained before treatment and during treatment. A dose delay or discontinuation should be considered per protocol, depending on the severity of cardiotoxicity. Discontinue treatment if LVEF is less than 40% or if there is a marked decrease in function.
Pregnancy Risk Category: B
Nursing women should be advised to discontinue nursing during therapy and for 6 months afterward per the manufacturer.

CONTRAINDICATIONS
Preexisting cardiac disease; known hypersensitivity to trastuzumab, benzyl alcohol, murine components, or any component of the formulation

DRUG PREPARATION/ADMINISTRATION/SAFE HANDLING ISSUES
◄ **ALERT** ► Practice aseptic technique when handling this product. Use nitrile or latex gloves.
• Each vial of trastuzumab should be reconstituted with 20 mL of bacteriostatic water for injection, USP, or 1.1% benzyl alcohol preserve.
• The multidose solution concentration is 21 mg/mL.
• Do not shake solution.
• Withdraw the calculated dose amount of volume and inject into a 250-mL 0.9% NaCl bag.
• Administer the loading dose over 90 minutes (4 mg/kg). If no problems arise, then administer subsequent doses over 30 minutes (2 mg/kg).

STORAGE AND STABILITY
• Store vials refrigerated at 2-9° C (36-46° F). A reconstituted vial of trastuzumab with bacteriostatic water for injection is stable for 28 days after reconstitution when refrigerated.
• If unpreserved sterile water for injection is used (e.g., for patients with benzyl alcohol allergies), then the solution should be used immediately and any unused proportion should be discarded.
• A diluted bag that contains trastuzumab may be store refrigerated for up to 24 hours.

INTERACTIONS
Drug
Anthracyclines (doxorubicin, epirubicin): May increase the risk of cardiac dysfunction.
Cyclophosphamide: May increase the risk of cardiac dysfunction.
Myelosuppressive agents: May increase risk of neutropenia.
Herbal
None known.

LAB EFFECTS/INTERFERENCE
None known.

Y-SITE COMPATIBLES
None known.

INCOMPATIBLES
Do not mix trastuzumab with any other medications or with D5W.

SIDE EFFECTS
Serious Reactions
- Cardiomyopathy, ventricular dysfunction, and CHF occur rarely. Left ventricular function should be assessed before and during treatment. A dose delay or discontinuation should be considered, depending on the severity of cardiotoxicity. Discontinue treatment if LVEF is less than 40% or if there is a marked decrease in function.
- Infusion reactions including anaphylaxis reactions and pulmonary events may occur and have been reported in the black box warning.

Other Side Effects
Frequent (10%-50%):
Abdominal pain, anorexia, asthenia, back pain, chills, cough, diarrhea, dyspnea, fever, headache, infection, nausea, pain, vomiting
Occasional (1%-10%):
Allergic reaction, anemia, arthralgia, bone pain, CHF, depression, dizziness, edema, flu-like symptoms, herpes simplex reactivation, insomnia, leukopenia, paresthesia, pharyngitis, rash, rhinitis, sinusitis, tachycardia, urinary tract infection
Rare (Less Than 1%):
Anaphylactoid reaction, apnea, ataxia, confusion, convulsions, electrolyte abnormality, hematuria, hemorrhage, hepatic failure, hypotension, hypothyroidism, intestinal obstruction, kidney failure, myopathy, neuropathy, pneumothorax, radiation injury, shock, syncope

SPECIAL CONSIDERATIONS
Baseline Assessment
- Assess CBC with differential, electrolyte, BUN, and creatinine levels, and liver function tests.
- Obtain baseline echocardiogram or multiple gated acquisition scan before dosing; ejection fraction (EF) needs to be at least 50% for safe dosing.
- Evaluate cardiac history for any evidence of heart failure or other cardiac diseases.
- Evaluate patient's allergy history to assess for the need to premedicate before giving this monoclonal antibody.
- Obtain baseline weight, and assess for any evidence of pretibial or pedal edema.

- Assess for any evidence of peripheral neuropathy from prior chemotherapies or comorbid diseases.

Intervention and Evaluation
- Premedicate patient to prevent hypersensitivity reactions as ordered.
- Check for EF data before dosing.
- Monitor patient's CBC with differential, along with electrolyte, BUN, and creatinine levels, and liver function tests on a scheduled basis per institutional guidelines.
- Assess patient for any evidence of increasing cough, dyspnea, nausea, or vomiting since last dose.
- Evaluate patient for any increasing pain since starting this agent.
- Assess patient for any evidence of herpes simplex on lips or in the oral cavity or genital area as this agent may reactivate herpes simplex.
- Assess patient for increasing peripheral neuropathy if it is being given with paclitaxel or if patient has a history of diabetic neuropathy.
- Monitor cardiac assessment, B/P, tachycardia, tachypnea, and increasing heart sounds for evidence of CHF, edema of lower extremities, and pretibial or pitting edema.
- Monitor weights on a regular basis.

Education
- Instruct patient this is a monoclonal antibody, and because of a small murine component, some patients may have a hypersensitivity reaction and will be given premedications as necessary.
- Educate patient that timing of the agent will decrease as they tolerate the agent. The first dose is usually given over 90 minutes, and subsequent doses will be given over 30 minutes if the agent is tolerated.
- Instruct patient on when to contact his or her health care provider: fever greater than 38° C (greater than 101° F), shaking, chills, cough, shortness of breath, weight gain or edema of lower extremities, or any evidence of easy bruising, bleeding, or increasing fatigue.
- Educate patient on symptoms to report: headaches, abdominal pain, back pain, bone pain, or any new pain.
- Instruct patient that this agent can alter cardiac function so if new symptoms of shortness of breath, dyspnea upon exertion, or increasing cough or palpitations occur to contact the health care provider.

- Advise patient that cardiac testing will be planned on a regular basis per guidelines to monitor for any cardiac changes.
- Educate patient and caregiver that this agent can induce peripheral neuropathy or increase existing neuropathy.
- Advise patient to inform the health care provider if he or she is taking any new OTC medications or herbal products as they may interfere with or enhance toxicity of this agent.
- Provide patient with information on local resources and support groups available for his or her specific diagnosis.

TRETINOIN, ALL-*TRANS*-RETINOIC ACID (ATRA)

BRAND NAMES
Vesanoid

CLASS OF AGENT
Vitamin A derivative, retinoic acid derivative, antineoplastic agent

CLINICAL PHARMACOLOGY
Mechanism of Action
Exact mechanism is unknown. To induce remission in patients with acute promyelocytic leukemia (APL), French-American-British (FAB) classification M3 (including the M3 variant), tretinoin works by producing an initial maturation of the primitive promyelocytes derived from the leukemic clone, followed by a repopulation of the bone marrow and peripheral blood by normal, polyclonal hematopoietic cells. **Therapeutic Effect:** Decreased proliferation of APL cells.
Absorption and Distribution
ATRA is well absorbed with or without food. Time to peak concentration is between 1 and 2 hours. A single 45 mg/m^2 (approximately 80 mg) PO dose to patients with APL resulted in a mean ± SD peak tretinoin concentration of 347 ± 266 ng/mL. ATRA is greater than 95% bound in plasma, predominately to albumin.
Half-life: 0.5-2 hours.
Metabolism and Excretion
ATRA metabolites have been identified in plasma and urine. Cytochrome P450 (CYP) enzymes have been implicated in the oxidative metabolism of ATRA. It is believed that ATRA induces its own metabolism, with the plasma level decreasing to one

third of the initial level after 1 week of continuous therapy; however, increasing the dose to "correct" for this change is not necessary. In patients with APL, daily administration of a 45 mg/m^2 dose resulted in an approximately 10-fold increase in the urinary excretion of 4-oxo-*trans*-retinoic acid glucuronide after 2-6 weeks of continuous dosing compared with baseline values. Approximately two thirds of a dose administered is recovered in the urine, with the remaining recovered in the feces.

HOW SUPPLIED/AVAILABLE FORMS
Capsules: 10 mg
Topical (Noncancer Indication): liquid, gel cream.

INDICATIONS AND DOSAGES
Acute promyelooytic leukemia (APL)
Remission induction: 45 mg/m^2/day in 2-3 divided doses with food for up to 30 days after complete remission (maximum duration of treatment: 90 days).
Remission maintenance: 45-200 mg/m^2/day in 2-3 divided doses for up to 12 months.
Note: Optimal consolidation or maintenance regimens have not been determined. All patients should therefore receive a standard consolidation or maintenance chemotherapy regimen for APL after induction therapy with tretinoin unless otherwise contraindicated.
Dosage Adjustment in Hepatic/Renal Dysfunction
No information available.

UNLABELED USES
No information available.

PRECAUTIONS
Patients with APL are at high risk and can have severe adverse reactions to tretinoin. Administer under the supervision of a physician who is experienced in the management of patients with acute leukemia and in a facility with laboratory and supportive services sufficient to monitor drug tolerance and to protect and maintain the condition of a patient compromised by drug toxicity, including respiratory compromise.
About 25% of patients with APL who have been treated with tretinoin have experienced a syndrome called the retinoic acid (RA)-APL syndrome, which is characterized by fever, dyspnea, weight gain, radiographic pulmonary infiltrates, and pleural

or pericardial effusions. This syndrome has occasionally been accompanied by impaired myocardial contractility and episodic hypotension. It has been observed with or without concomitant leukocytosis. Endotracheal intubation and mechanical ventilation have been required in some patients because of progressive hypoxemia, and several patients have died of multiorgan failure. The syndrome usually occurs during the first month of treatment, with some cases reported after the first dose. Management of the syndrome has not been defined, but high-dose steroids given at the first suspicion of the RA-APL syndrome appear to reduce morbidity and mortality. At the first signs suggestive of the syndrome, immediately initiate high-dose steroid therapy (dexamethasone 10 mg IV) every 12 hours for 3 days or until resolution of symptoms, regardless of the leukocyte count. The majority of patients do not require termination of tretinoin therapy during treatment of the RA-APL syndrome. During treatment, approximately 40% of patients will develop rapidly evolving leukocytosis, which is associated with a higher risk of life-threatening complications. If signs and symptoms of the RA-APL syndrome are present together with leukocytosis, initiate high-dose steroid treatment immediately. Consider adding full-dose chemotherapy (including an anthracycline, if not contraindicated) to the tretinoin therapy on day 1 or 2 for patients presenting with a WBC count of more than 5×10^9/L or immediately for patients presenting with a WBC count of less than 5×10^9/L or if the WBC count reaches 6×10^9/L by day 5, 10×10^9/L by day 10, or 15×10^9/L by day 28.

Initiation of therapy with tretinoin may be based on the morphologic diagnosis of APL. Confirm the diagnosis of APL by detection of the t(15;17) genetic marker by cytogenetic studies. If these are negative, PML (promyelocytic leukemic)/RAR (retinoic acid receptor) fusion should be sought using molecular diagnostic techniques. The response rate of other acute myelogenous leukemia subtypes to tretinoin has not been demonstrated. Retinoids have been associated with pseudotumor cerebri (benign intracranial hypertension), especially in children. Concurrent use of other drugs associated with this effect (e.g., tetracyclines) may increase risk. Early signs and symptoms include papilledema,

headache, nausea, vomiting, and visual disturbances.

Pregnancy Risk Category:
Tretinoin should not be used in women of childbearing potential unless the woman is capable of complying with effective contraceptive measures. Therapy is normally begun on the 2nd or 3rd day of the next normal menstrual period; two reliable methods of effective contraception must be used during therapy and for 1 month after discontinuation of therapy, unless abstinence is the chosen method. Within 1 week before the institution of tretinoin therapy, blood or urine should be collected for a serum or urine pregnancy test with a sensitivity of at least 50 million international units/L. When possible, delay tretinoin therapy until a negative result from this test is obtained. When a delay is not possible, make sure that patient is using two reliable forms of contraception. Repeat pregnancy testing and contraception counseling monthly throughout the period of treatment.

CONTRAINDICATIONS
Sensitivity to parabens, vitamin A, other retinoids, or any component of the formulation; pregnancy

DRUG PREPARATION/ADMINISTRATION/ SAFE HANDLING ISSUES
• Take capsules with food.

STORAGE AND STABILITY
Store capsules at room temperature: 15-30° C (59-86° F). Protect from light.

INTERACTIONS
Drug
Substrate (minor) of cytochrome P450 (CYP) 2A6, 2B6, and 2C8/9; inhibits CYP 2C8/9 (weak); induces CYP 2E1 (weak)
Antifibrinolytic agents (aminocaproic acid, aprotinin, tranexamic acid): Concurrent use may increase risk of thrombosis.
Ketoconazole: Increases the mean plasma area under the curve of tretinoin.
Tetracyclines: Concurrent use may increase risk of pseudotumor cerebri.
Herbal
No information available.

LAB EFFECTS/INTERFERENCE
Up to 60% of patients experience hypercholesterolemia or hypertriglyceridemia, which are reversible upon completion of treatment. Elevated liver function test

results occur in 50%-60% of patients during treatment. Carefully monitor liver function test results during treatment and consider a temporary withdrawal of tretinoin if test results reach more than 5 × UNL.

SIDE EFFECTS
Serious Reactions
- The RA-APL syndrome occurs in about 25% of patients with APL.

Other Side Effects
Frequent (10%-50%):
Virtually all patients experience some drug-related toxicity, in particular, headache, fever, weakness, and fatigue. These adverse effects are seldom permanent or irreversible nor do they usually require therapy interruption.
- Cardiovascular: Peripheral edema, chest discomfort, edema, arrhythmias, flushing, hypotension, hypertension
- CNS: Headache, fever, malaise dizziness, anxiety, insomnia, depression, confusion
- Dermatologic: Skin/mucous membrane dryness, pruritus, rash, alopecia
- Endocrine and metabolic: Hypercholesterolemia and/or hypertriglyceridemia
- GI: Nausea/vomiting, liver function test results increased, GI hemorrhage, abdominal pain, mucositis, diarrhea, constipation, dyspepsia, abdominal distension, weight gain, weight loss, xerostomia, anorexia
- Hematologic: Hemorrhage, leukocytosis, disseminated intravascular coagulation
- Miscellaneous: Infections, shivering, RA-PML syndrome, increased diaphoresis
- Neuromuscular and skeletal: Bone pain, myalgia, paresthesia
- Ocular: Visual disturbances
- Otic: Earache/ear fullness
- Renal: Renal insufficiency
- Respiratory: Upper respiratory tract disorders, dyspnea, respiratory insufficiency, pleural effusion, pneumonia, rales, expiratory wheezing, dry nose

Occasional (1%-10%):
- Cardiovascular: Cerebral hemorrhage, pallor, cardiac failure, cardiac arrest, MI, enlarged heart, heart murmur, ischemia, stroke, myocarditis, pericarditis, pulmonary hypertension, secondary cardiomyopathy
- Central nervous system: Intracranial hypertension, agitation, hallucination, agnosia, aphasia, cerebellar edema, cerebral hemorrhage, seizures, coma, CNS depression, dysarthria, encephalopathy, hypotaxia, light reflex absent, dementia, somnolence, slow speech
- Dermatologic: Cellulitis, photosensitivity
- Endocrine and metabolic: Acidosis
- GI: Hepatosplenomegaly, hepatitis, ulcer
- Hepatic: Ascites, hepatitis
- Miscellaneous: Face edema
- Neuromuscular and skeletal: Tremor, leg weakness, hyporeflexia, dysarthria, facial paralysis, hemiplegia, flank pain, asterixis, abnormal gait, bone inflammation
- Ocular: Dry eyes, visual acuity change, visual field deficit
- Otic: Hearing loss
- Renal: Acute renal failure, renal tubular necrosis
- Respiratory: Lower respiratory tract disorders, pulmonary infiltration, bronchial asthma, pulmonary/larynx edema

Rare (Less Than 1%):
Arterial thrombosis, basophilia, cataracts, conjunctivitis, corneal opacities, erythema nodosum, increased erythrocyte sedimentation rate, gum bleeding, decreased hematocrit, decreased hemoglobin, hypercalcemia, hyperhistaminemia, hyperuricemia, inflammatory bowel syndrome, irreversible hearing loss, mood changes, myositis, optic neuritis, pancreatitis, pseudomotor cerebri, renal infarct, Sweet's syndrome, vasculitis, venous thrombosis

SPECIAL CONSIDERATIONS
Baseline Assessment
- Inform women of childbearing potential of risk to fetus if pregnancy occurs. Instruct in need for use of two reliable forms of contraception concurrently during therapy and for 1 month after discontinuation of therapy, even in infertile, premenopausal women. A pregnancy test should be obtained within 1 week before institution of therapy. Be aware that it is unknown whether tretinoin is distributed in breast milk; do not administer to nursing mothers. Tretinoin may have a teratogenic and embryotoxic effect.
- Obtain initial liver function tests, and cholesterol, lipid, and triglyceride levels.

Intervention and Evaluation
- Assess therapeutic response to tretinoin therapy.
- Monitor liver function tests, CBC with differential and platelet count, prothrombin test, partial prothrombin test,

international normalized ratio, and cholesterol and triglyceride levels.
- Monitor signs/symptoms of pseudotumor cerebri in children.

Education
- Instruct patient using the topical formulation to avoid exposure to sunlight or sunbeds and to use sunscreens and protective clothing. Affected areas should also be protected from wind and cold. If skin is already sunburned, do not use until fully resolved. Keep tretinoin away from eyes, mouth, angles of nose, and mucous membranes. Do not use medicated, drying, or abrasive soaps; wash face no more than 2-3 times/day with bland soap. Avoid use of preparations containing alcohol, menthol, spice, or lime such as shaving lotions, astringents, and perfume. Mild redness and peeling is expected; decrease frequency or discontinue medication if excessive reaction occurs. Nonmedicated cosmetics may be used; however, cosmetics must be removed before tretinoin application. Improvement is noted during the first 24 weeks of therapy. Therapeutic results are noted in 2-3 weeks with optimal results in 6 weeks.
- Advise patient taking oral tretinoin to take with food. Do not open or chew capsules.
- Obtain frequent blood tests while patient is taking medication.
- Maintain adequate hydration. Report persistent vomiting or diarrhea.
- Instruct patient to report any nausea or vomiting with agent.

TRIPTORELIN PAMOATE

BRAND NAMES
Trelstar Depot, Trelstar LA

CLASS OF AGENT
Antineoplastic agent, luteinizing hormone-releasing hormone (LHRH) agonist, gonadotropin-releasing hormone (GnRH) agonist

CLINICAL PHARMACOLOGY
Mechanism of Action
A potent LHRH (also known as GnRH) agonist analog that inhibits luteinizing hormone secretion through a negative feedback mechanism from the anterior pituitary gland. Circulating levels of luteinizing hormone, follicle-stimulating hormone, testosterone, and estradiol rise initially and then subside

with continued therapy. Onset of suppression occurs 2-4 weeks after initiation of therapy and is reversible after discontinuation.
Therapeutic Effect: In males, produces pharmacologic castration and decreases the growth of abnormal prostate tissue.
Absorption and Distribution
Not absorbed orally. Volume of distribution: 30-33 L. No protein binding.
Half-life: 2.81 hours; moderate to severe renal impairment: 6.56-7.65 hours; liver disease: 7.58 hours.
Metabolism and Excretion
Metabolism is unknown but is unlikely to involve cytochrome P450. Excretion via liver and kidneys.

HOW SUPPLIED/AVAILABLE FORMS
Powder for Injection (Trelstar Depot): 3.75 mg.
Powder for Injection (Trelstar LA): 11.25 mg.

INDICATIONS AND DOSAGES
Palliative Treatment for Advanced Prostate Cancer
3.75 mg IM once every 28 days; 11.25 mg IM every 84 days in buttock.
Dosage Adjustment in Hepatic/Renal Dysfunction
No recommendations available.

UNLABELED USES
Endometriosis, in vitro fertilization, ovarian cancer

PRECAUTIONS

CONTRAINDICATIONS
Hypersensitivity to triptorelin or any component of its formulation, LHRH, or LHRH agonists; pregnancy
Pregnancy Risk Category: X
Triptorelin may cause fetal harm when administered during pregnancy. Drug excretion into human breast milk is unknown/not recommended in nursing women.

DRUG PREPARATION/ADMINISTRATION/ SAFE HANDLING ISSUES
- Reconstitute vial with 2 mL of sterile water. Shake well. Reconstituted suspension should appear milky.
- Administer 3.75 mg every 28 days or 11.25 mg every 84 days IM (long-acting).
- Refer to manufacturer package insert for instructions on use of Clip'n'Ject.

STORAGE AND STABILITY
Store at room temperature.

INTERACTIONS
Drug
Hyperprolactinemic drugs: Reduce the number of pituitary GnRH receptors.
Herbal
None known.

LAB EFFECTS/INTERFERENCE
May alter serum pituitary-gonadal function test results. May cause transient increase in serum testosterone levels, usually during first week of treatment.

COMPATIBLES
Reconstitute only with sterile water.

SIDE EFFECTS
Serious Reactions
* Worsening symptoms or onset of new symptoms may occur in the first week after initiation of LHRH agonists and are due to a transient increase in hormones. Patients receiving LHRH agonists have had uretal obstruction and spinal cord compression as part of these symptoms.
* Anaphylactic shock, angioedema, and spinal cord compression (with weakness or paralysis of the lower extremities) have been reported.
Other Side Effects
Frequent (10%-50%):
Hot flashes, skeletal pain
Occasional (1%-10%):
Anemia, dizziness, fatigue, headache, hypertension, impotence, insomnia, pain (back, leg, arms, injection site), pruritus, vomiting
Rare (Less Than 1%):
Asthenia, conjunctivitis, diarrhea, dyspnea, eye pain, gynecomastia, leg cramps, peripheral edema, pharyngitis, rash, urine retention, urinary tract infections (UTIs)

SPECIAL CONSIDERATIONS
Baseline Assessment
* Assess CBC with differential, platelet count, electrolyte, BUN, and creatinine levels, and liver function tests.
* Assess for any risk of spinal cord compression and uretal obstruction before initiating therapy.
* Obtain baseline evaluation for history of or current hypertension.
* Assess for pain score before initiating therapy.

* Evaluate for any history of visual problems, infections, dry eyes, or conjunctivitis.
* Assess skin integrity for routing injections from this agent.
* Evaluate patient for history of UTIs and their frequency.
Intervention and Evaluation
* Monitor laboratory data at each visit, paying particular attention to the CBC and liver function tests.
* Assess pain score at each visit.
* Assess patient for headaches, weakness, paralysis, or eye problems such as dry eyes, conjunctival drainage, or infections.
* Monitor patient's vital signs, noting any increase in B/P, evidence of peripheral edema or weight gain, or evidence of UTI symptoms: frequency, urgency, or burning upon urination.
* Evaluate all prior injections sites for evidence of erythema, edema, and pain.
* Assess patient for symptoms of hot flashes, irritability, insomnia, and depression.
* Monitor patient for evidence of gynecomastia, libido changes, and impotence. Make appropriate psychosocial referrals as needed.
Education
* Instruct patient on when to contact his or her health care provider: fever greater than 38° C (greater than 101° F), chills, frequency, urgency or burning upon urination, headaches, drainage from eyes, increase in skeletal pain, or weakness in lower extremities.
* Advise patient of usual side effects of hot flashes, night sweats, irritability, insomnia, and depression.
* Inform patient of possible body image changes such as painful or swollen breasts and changes in sexual function such as decreased libido and impotence.
* Counsel patient to report evidence of edema and weight gain.
* Instruct female patients of the importance of use of nonhormonal contraceptive agents while receiving therapy. Advise patients that 1 or more successive missed dose of triptorelin may result in breakthrough bleeding or ovulation with the potential for pregnancy.
* Instruct patient to take no over-the-counter medications or herbal or vitamin supplements without checking with his or her health care provider.

- Provide patient with information on local resources and support groups available for his or her specific diagnosis.

VALRUBICIN
BRAND NAMES
Valstar

CLASS OF AGENT
Antineoplastic agent, anthracycline

CLINICAL PHARMACOLOGY
Mechanism of Action
An anthracycline antibiotic that inhibits incorporation of nucleosides into nucleic acids after penetrating cells. **Therapeutic Effect:** Causes chromosomal damage, arresting cells in the G2 phase of cell division, and interferes with DNA synthesis.
Absorption and Distribution
Well absorbed into bladder wall. During the 2-hour dose retention period, only nanogram quantities are absorbed into the plasma. If the bladder wall is compromised, there might be significant absorption.
Half-life: Not applicable.
Metabolism and Excretion
During dose retention, the metabolism of valrubicin to its metabolites N-trifluoroacetyladriamycin and N-trifluoroacetyladriamycinol is negligible. After retention, voiding the instillate excretes the drug.

HOW SUPPLIED/AVAILABLE FORMS
Solution for Intravesical Instillation:
200 mg/5 mL vials. Product discontinued. (Future product availability may be through Valera Pharmaceuticals, Inc., Cranbury, NJ, 888-282-5372.)

INDICATIONS AND DOSAGES
Bacillus Calmette-Guérin–Refractory Carcinoma in Situ (CIS) of the Urinary Bladder in Patients for Whom Immediate Cystectomy Would Be Associated with Unacceptable Morbidity or Mortality
Intravesical instillation in urinary bladder 800 mg once weekly for 6 weeks.
Dosage Adjustment in Hepatic/Renal Dysfunction
No information available.

UNLABELED USES
No information available.

PRECAUTIONS
Delay of cystectomy after valrubicin therapy may lead to metastatic bladder cancer. If a complete response of CIS to treatment is not seen after 3 months or if CIS recurs, cystectomy must be reconsidered. Use with caution in patients with severe irritable bladder symptoms; bladder spasm and spontaneous discharge of drug may occur.
Pregnancy Risk Category: C
May cause fetal harm when administered during pregnancy. Such exposure could occur if there is perforation of the urinary bladder. Men and women should use contraception while receiving valrubicin therapy. Drug excretion into human breast milk is unknown/not recommended in nursing women.

CONTRAINDICATIONS
Use in perforated bladder will lead to significant systemic absorption and potential severe systemic adverse effects including hematologic toxicity; severe irritated bladder; small bladder capacity (inability to tolerate 75 mL), urinary tract infection (UTI); known hypersensitivity to valrubicin or anthracyclines or Cremophor EL.

DRUG PREPARATION/ADMINISTRATION/SAFE HANDLING ISSUES
◄ ALERT ► Because valrubicin may be carcinogenic, mutagenic, or teratogenic, wear nitrile or latex, but not vinyl, gloves when handling the drug. If the drug comes in contact with skin, wash the skin thoroughly with soap and water. Do not use waterless hand soap or any antibacterial soap as either can increase the reaction from the agent. If the drug comes in contact with mucous membranes, flush the area with water.
- Administration should be delayed at least 2 weeks after transurethral resection and/or fulguration.
- For each instillation, four 5-mL vials (200 mg valrubicin/5-mL vial) should be brought to room temperature, but not heated.
- Valrubicin 20 mL should be withdrawn from the 4 vials and diluted with 55 mL of 0.9% NaCl, providing 75 mL of diluted solution.
- Solutions should be prepared and stored in glass, polypropylene, or polyolefin containers and tubing. Do not use polyvinyl chloride bags to prevent leaching.

- A urethral catheter is inserted into patient's bladder, the bladder is drained, and 75 mL of diluted solution is instilled slowly via gravity flow over a period of several minutes.
- The catheter is withdrawn after solution is instilled.
- Patient should retain the drug for 2 hours before voiding. Some patients are unable tolerate the drug for 2 full hours.
- Patients should be instructed to maintain adequate hydration following treatment.

STORAGE AND STABILITY
- Store vials under refrigeration at 2-8° C (36-46° F).
- Diluted valrubicin in 0.9% NaCl solution is stable for 12 hrs at temperatures up to 25° C.
- At temperatures below 4° C, Cremophor EL may begin to form a waxy precipitate. The vial should be warmed in the hand until the solution is clear.

INTERACTIONS
Drug
No information as the drug is not significantly absorbed systemically.
Herbal
No information available.

LAB EFFECTS/INTERFERENCE
No information available.

Y-SITE COMPATIBLES
Do not mix with other medications.

INCOMPATIBLES
Do not mix with other medications.

SIDE EFFECTS
Serious Reactions
- Severe leukopenia and neutropenia may develop 2 weeks after drug instillation if systemic exposure to valrubicin occurs. Administration of drug should be delayed until bladder integrity is restored in patients with a perforated bladder or those in whom the integrity of the bladder mucosa has been compromised.
Other Side Effects
Frequent (10%-50%):
Local intravesical reactions (usually resolve in 1-7 days: local bladder symptoms, urinary frequency or urgency, dysuria, hematuria, bladder pain, cystitis, bladder spasms), abdominal pain, nausea, UTI

Occasional (1%-10%):
Local intravesical reactions (nocturia, local burning, urethral pain, pelvic pain, gross hematuria), diarrhea, vomiting, urine retention, microscopic hematuria, asthenia, headache, malaise, back pain, chest pain, dizziness, rash, anemia, fever, vasodilation
Rare (Less Than 1%):
Flatus, peripheral edema, hyperglycemia, pneumonia, myalgia

SPECIAL CONSIDERATIONS
Baseline Assessment
- Assess CBC with differential, platelet count, electrolyte, BUN, and creatinine levels, and liver function tests.
- Ensure the integrity of the bladder to prevent inadvertent systemic absorption.
- Evaluate patient for any evidence of prior cardiac dysfunction, chest pain, heaviness, or cardiac disease, angina, or MI.
- Assess patient for any prior reaction to anthracyclines and Cremophor as this agent contains both of these.
- Evaluate patient for any evidence of UTI before dosing with this agent.
- Assess patient for evidence of diabetes as 1% of patients may develop hyperglycemia.
Intervention and Evaluation
- Assess laboratory data before each dosing.
- Evaluate patient for any evidence of bladder irritation, frequency, urgency, or burning upon urination.
- Premedicate patient as ordered for nausea; this occurs rarely, but if noted after the first dose, premedicate before subsequent doses.
- Assess cardiac function before each dosing; cardiac effects such as chest pain, tightness, or heaviness occur rarely.
- Before bladder instillation evaluate patient for any evidence of new urinary tract symptoms and do not administer this agent if bladder is injured or inflamed.
- Assess patient for any evidence of diarrhea and frequency of stools.
Education
- Instruct patient on when to contact his or her health care provider: fever greater than 38° C (greater than 101° F), chills, shortness of breath, chest pain, chest tightness, frequency, urgency, or burning upon urination, nausea lasting for greater than 24 hours, diarrhea lasting for greater than 24 hours, or the inability to take in at least 1500 mL of fluid in 24 hours.

- Instruct patient that urine will be red or pink tinged for 24 hours after dosing.
- Instruct patient to empty bladder before each dose and avoid drinking fluids for several hours before dosing.
- Instruct patient to collect or handle urine as chemotherapy waste for 6 hours after each dose. If patient has children or pets, instruct patient to keep the toilet lid closed and to flush twice.
- Educate diabetic patients that this agent may induce hyperglycemia and to monitor glucose more closely after bladder instillation.
- Instruct patient on usual urinary tract symptoms: frequency, urgency, burning, bladder spasms, cystitis, urinary retention, and pain in the pelvis and urethra. Instruct patient to contact the health care provider if these symptoms worsen.
- Educate patient on pain symptoms that may result from this agent: headaches, dizziness, back pain, weakness, and myalgias. Instruct patient to contact the health care provider if these symptoms worsen.
- Instruct patient to avoid all OTC medications and herbal and vitamin supplements without first checking with the health care provider.
- Provide patient with information on local resources and support groups available for his or her specific diagnosis.

VINBLASTINE SULFATE

BRAND NAMES
Oncovin (Australia), Velban, Velbe (Australia)

CLASS OF AGENT
Vinca alkaloid

CLINICAL PHARMACOLOGY
Mechanism of Action
Binds to microtubular protein of mitotic spindle, causing alterations in microtubule assembly and metaphase arrest. Also affects microtubules involved in chemotaxis and directional migration, membrane trafficking, and transmission of receptor signals. It is considered a cell cycle-specific drug. **Therapeutic Effect:** Inhibits cell division.
Absorption and Distribution
In its parent state is not absorbed by the oral route. Although it is taken up rapidly into cells, it does not cross the blood-brain

barrier. Plasma protein binding ranges from 43% to 99%. It binds extensively to blood elements, especially platelets. Volume of distribution: 27.3 L/kg.
Half-life: Plasma disappearance is triexponential with a rapid distribution half-life of less than 5 minutes. The second phase plasma half-life ranges from 53 to 99 minutes, and the terminal half-life is 24.8 hours.
Metabolism and Excretion
Metabolized in the liver to at least one active metabolite, deacetylvinblastine. Cytochrome P450 (CYP) 3A4 is primarily responsible for biotransformation of vinblastine. Primarily eliminated as metabolites in bile and then feces.

HOW SUPPLIED/AVAILABLE FORMS
Injection: 1 mg/mL as 10 mL and 25 mL vials.
Powder for Injection: 10-mg vials.

INDICATIONS AND DOSAGES
Remission Induction in Advanced Testicular Carcinoma or Germ Cell Tumors, Advanced Mycosis Fungoides, Breast Carcinoma, Choriocarcinoma, Disseminated Hodgkin's Disease, Non-Hodgkin's Lymphoma, Kaposi's Sarcoma, or Letterer-Siwe Disease (Histiocytosis X).
Initially, 3.7 mg/m^2 IV as a single dose. Increase dose by about 1.8 mg/m^2 at weekly intervals until desired therapeutic response is attained, WBC count falls below 3000/mm^3, or maximum weekly dose of 18.5 mg/m^2 is reached. Administer one increment less than dose required to produce WBC count of 3000/mm^3. Each subsequent dose is given when WBC count returns to 4000/mm^3 and at least 7 days have elapsed since previous dose.
Pediatrics: Initially, 2.5 mg/m^2 IV as a single dose. Increase dose by about 1.25 mg/m^2 at weekly intervals until desired therapeutic response is attained, WBC count falls below 3000/mm^3, or maximum weekly dose of 7.5-12.5 mg/m^2 is reached. Administer one increment less than dose required to produce WBC count of 3000/mm^3. Each subsequent dose is given when WBC count returns to 4000/mm^3 and at least 7 days have elapsed since previous dose.
Dosage Adjustment in Hepatic Dysfunction
Bilirubin level of 1.5-3 mg/dL or AST (SGOT) of 60-180 units/L necessitates a 50% dose reduction. Bilirubin level of

3-5 mg/dL is 25% of usual dose. Hold therapy for bilirubin greater than 5 mg/dL or AST greater than 180 units/L.
Dosage Adjustment in Renal Dysfunction
No dosage adjustment necessary.

UNLABELED USES
Bladder, transitional cell, cervical, esophageal, non–small cell lung and renal cell cancers; melanoma; bladder, head and neck, kidney, or lung carcinoma; chronic myelocytic leukemia; germ cell ovarian tumors; neuroblastoma

PRECAUTIONS
Pregnancy Risk Category: D

CONTRAINDICATIONS
Bacterial infection, severe leukopenia, significant granulocytopenia (unless it stems from disease being treated), hypersensitivity, intrathecal route

DRUG PREPARATION/ADMINISTRATION/ SAFE HANDLING ISSUES
◀ ALERT ▶ Fatal if given intrathecally. Special outer bag labeling as with vinblastine: "Accidental administration by the intrathecal route can be fatal." There have been several accidental deaths as a result of inadvertent intrathecal administration of vinca alkaloids. Syringes should include a safety outerwrap that states: "DO NOT REMOVE COVERING UNTIL MOMENT OF INJECTION. FATAL IF GIVEN INTRATHECALLY. FOR INTRAVENOUS USE ONLY." Syringes themselves should include an auxiliary sticker that states: "FATAL IF GIVEN INTRATHECALLY. FOR INTRAVENOUS USE ONLY." As a patient safety strategy, some institutions require that vinblastine only be sent to the ward or clinic in a small minibag. This practice may decrease the incidence of sentinel events in health systems.
• Lyophilized powder vial should be reconstituted with 10 mL of bacteriostatic sodium chloride injection to make a final concentration of 1 mg/mL. Nonpreservative sodium chloride may be used, if unused portions are discarded immediately.
• As per manufacturer recommendations, inject vinblastine into either the tubing of a running IV infusion or directly into a vein over 1 minute. To prevent cellulitis or phlebitis, secure the needle within the vein so that no solution extravasates. To further minimize extravasation, rinse syringe and needle with venous blood before withdrawal of needle. Do not dilute the dose in large volumes of diluent (i.e., 100-250 mL) or give IV for prolonged periods (e.g., 30 mins), because this often results in vein irritation and increases the chance of extravasation.
• Because of the enhanced possibility of thrombosis, do not inject solution into an extremity in which circulation is impaired or potentially impaired by conditions such as compressing or invading neoplasm, phlebitis, or varicosity.

STORAGE AND STABILITY
After reconstitution with bacteriostatic sodium chloride injection and removal of a portion from the vial, refrigerate the remainder for 28 days without loss of potency. Refrigerate unopened vials at 2-8° C (36-46° F).

INTERACTIONS
Drug
Antigout medications: May decrease the effects of these drugs.
Bone marrow depressants: May increase myelosuppression.
CYP 3A4 inhibitors: All the substrates and inhibitors of CYP3A4 such as the azole antifungals (itraconazole and ketoconazole), erythromycin, cyclosporine, isoniazid, and nifedipine have a very high propensity to interfere with vinblastine metabolism. Because vinblastine is metabolized by CYP3A4, similar to vincristine, cytotoxicity may be enhanced and result in greater toxicity. Vinblastine should be used with caution in combination with these drugs and its dosage may have to be reduced to provide patient safety. The combination of erythromycin and vinblastine has been reported to enhance bone marrow toxicity.
CYP 3A4 inducers (carbamazepine, dexamethasone, phenobarbital, phenytoin, etc.): In the presence of CYP 3A4 inducers, the metabolism of vinblastine is increased, which may result in decreased plasma concentrations and efficacy.
Live-virus vaccines: May potentiate viral replication, increase vaccine side effects, and decrease patient's antibody response to the vaccine.
Mitomycin: There have been several case reports of pulmonary toxicity in patients with

breast cancer and lung cancer treated with the combination of vinblastine and mitomycin. Symptoms include acute respiratory distress, shortness of breath, dyspnea, or wheezing—a picture of obstructive pulmonary disease that differs from mitomycin pulmonary toxicity, which is a slower onset syndrome associated with microangiopathy. The incidence of pulmonary toxicity associated with the vinblastine-mitomycin combination has ranged from 3% to 39%. Symptoms occur with a rapid onset, usually 1-5 hours, after vinblastine administration. The acute symptoms can be managed with IV corticosteroid therapy. The mechanism for this interaction is unknown, and it is uncertain whether there is a pharmacokinetic basis. It appears to be an enhanced pharmacodynamic effect on the pulmonary parenchyma or a hypersensitivity-like reaction.

Phenytoin: Patients receiving phenytoin may demonstrate decreased serum concentrations due to inhibition of CYP 3A4 metabolism by vinblastine. Phenytoin levels should be monitored more closely in patients receiving vinblastine.

Herbal

St John's Wort: May increase drug metabolism and reduce the effectiveness of vinblastine.

Food

Grapefruit inhibits CYP 3A4 enzymes and can potentially enhance the effects of vinblastine.

LAB EFFECTS/INTERFERENCE

May increase serum uric acid levels.

Y-SITE COMPATIBLES

Allopurinol (Aloprim), amifostine, bleomycin, carboplatin, cisplatin (Platinol AQ), cyclophosphamide (Cytoxan), dactinomycin, doxorubicin (Adriamycin), doxorubicin liposomal, etoposide (VePesid), etoposide phosphate, filgrastim, fludarabine, 5-fluorouracil, gemcitabine (Gemzar), granisetron (Kytril), heparin, ifosfamide, leucovorin, melphalan, methotrexate, mitomycin, ondansetron (Zofran), paclitaxel (Taxol), palonosetron, pemetrexed, rituximab, sargramostim, teniposide, thiotepa, trastuzumab, vincristine, vinorelbine (Navelbine)

INCOMPATIBLES

Amphotericin B liposomal (AmBisome), cefepime (Maxipime), furosemide (Lasix), lansoprazole, pantoprazole

SIDE EFFECTS
Serious Reactions

- Hematologic toxicity is manifested as leukopenia and, less commonly, as anemia. The WBC count reaches its nadir 4-0 days after initial therapy and recovers within 7-14 days (21 days with high vinblastine doses).
- Thrombocytopenia is usually mild and transient, with recovery occurring in few days.
- Hepatic insufficiency may increase the risk of toxic drug effects.
- Acute shortness of breath or bronchospasm may occur, particularly when vinblastine is administered concurrently with mitomycin.
- Vinblastine is fatal if given intrathecally.

Other Side Effects
Frequent (10%-50%):

Nausea, vomiting, alopecia, myelosuppression

Occasional (1%-10%):

Constipation or diarrhea, rectal bleeding, headache, paraesthesia (occur 4-6 hours after administration and persist for 2-10 hours); malaise; asthenia; dizziness; pain at tumor site; jaw or face pain; depression; dry mouth

Rare (Less Than 1%):

Dermatitis, stomatitis, phototoxicity, hyperuricemia

SPECIAL CONSIDERATIONS
Baseline Assessment

- Assess CBC with differential, platelet count, electrolyte, BUN, and creatinine levels, and liver function tests.
- Assess patient for prior hepatic or neurologic toxicity.
- Evaluate patient for any pulmonary compromise.
- Assess peripheral access for necessity of central line placement as this agent is a vesicant.
- Avoid any situation in which vinblastine could accidentally be administered intrathecally.

Intervention and Evaluation

- Monitor laboratory parameters before each dose, paying particular attention to CBC with differential and platelet count.
- Make sure liver function tests are normal before dosing as patient's side effects can increase if the liver is not functioning normally.
- Infuse this agent slowly as rapid infusion can result in severe jaw pain.

- Have an extravasation kit at bedside if delivering this agent peripherally, and follow institutional guidelines if leakage is noted.
- Monitor patient for increasing symptoms of peripheral neuropathy before each dosing.
- Evaluate patient for constipation, and initiate bowel regimen as necessary.
- Monitor for evidence of changes in mental status, dizziness, malaise, or depression.

Education
- Instruct patient to take fluids to prevent constipation.
- Instruct patient on when to contact his or her health care provider: fever greater than 38° C (greater than 101° F), chills, cough, shortness of breath, dyspnea upon exertion, nausea lasting for greater than 24 hours, diarrhea lasting for greater than 24 hours, or the inability to take in at least 1500 mL of fluids in 24 hours.
- Instruct patient to report any symptoms of pain, burning, or tingling while receiving this agent.
- Instruct patient that this agent is a vesicant. Educate patient on risk of leakage into subcutaneous tissue that may result in tissue damage.
- Instruct patient on bowel regimen as needed.
- Instruct patient that alopecia usually occurs within 2-3 weeks after dosing and when hair recovers it may have a different color and texture.
- Encourage patient to wear sunglasses when going outside as some patients develop photosensitivity.
- Instruct patient to avoid taking any OTC medications or herbal or vitamin supplements without first checking with the health care provider.
- Provide patient with information on local resources and support groups available for his or her specific diagnosis.

VINCRISTINE SULFATE
BRAND NAMES
Oncovin, Vincasar PFS

CLASS OF AGENT
Vinca alkaloid

CLINICAL PHARMACOLOGY
Mechanism of Action
Binds to microtubular protein of mitotic spindle, causing alterations in microtubule assembly and metaphase arrest. It also affects microtubules involved in chemotaxis and directional migration, membrane trafficking, and transmission of receptor signals. **Therapeutic Effect:** Inhibits cell division.

Absorption and Distribution
After IV administration, it is distributed rapidly into body tissues. It does not cross the blood-brain barrier. Within 15-30 minutes after IV administration, greater than 90% of the drug is distributed from blood into tissue where it remains tightly, but not irreversibly, bound. Penetration across the blood-brain barrier is poor. Protein binding: 75%.
Half-life: Studies in cancer patients show a triphasic serum decay pattern after rapid IV injection. Initial, middle, and terminal half-lives are 5 minutes, 2.3 hours, and 85 hours, respectively; the range of the terminal half-life is 19 to 155 hours.

Metabolism and Excretion
Extracted in the liver and then secreted into bile, where it is excreted by the biliary system into the feces. About half of the dose is recovered as metabolites. About 10% of the drug is excreted in the urine. The liver is the major excretory organ; approximately 80% of a dose appears in feces and 10%-20% in urine. Hepatic dysfunction may alter elimination kinetics and augment toxicity.

HOW SUPPLIED/AVAILABLE FORMS
Injection: 1 mg/mL in 1-mL, 2-mL, 5-mL vials.

INDICATIONS AND DOSAGES
Acute Leukemia, Advanced Non-Hodgkin's Lymphoma, Disseminated Hodgkin's Disease, Neuroblastoma, Rhabdomyosarcoma, Wilms' Tumor
0.4-1.4 mg/m² IV once a week. Some protocols cap dose at 2 mg.
Pediatrics: 1-2 mg/m² once a week. Some protocols cap dose at 2 mg.
Children weighing less than 10 kg or with a body surface area less than 1 m² should be given a dose of 0.05 mg/kg.
Dosage Adjustment in Hepatic Dysfunction
Bilirubin level of 1.5-3 mg/dL or AST (SGOT) of 60-180 units/L necessitates a 50% dose reduction. Bilirubin level of 3-5 mg/dL necessitates 25% of usual dose. Hold therapy for bilirubin level greater than 5 mg/dL or AST greater than 180 units/L.

Dosage Adjustment in Renal Dysfunction
No dosage adjustment necessary.

UNLABELED USES
Treatment of breast, cervical, colorectal, lung, and ovarian carcinomas; chronic lymphocytic and chronic myelocytic leukemias; germ cell ovarian tumors; idiopathic thrombocytopenic purpura; malignant melanoma; multiple myeloma; mycosis fungoides

PRECAUTIONS
Use cautiously in patients with hepatic impairment, neurotoxicity, or preexisting neuromuscular disease.
Pregnancy Risk Category: D

CONTRAINDICATIONS
Patients receiving radiation therapy through ports that include the liver, patients with the demyelinating form of Charcot-Marie-Tooth syndrome, hypersensitivity, intrathecal route

DRUG PREPARATION/ADMINISTRATION/ SAFE HANDLING ISSUES
◂ ALERT ▸ Fatal if given intrathecally. Special outer bag labeling as with vinblasline: "Accidental administration by the intrathecal route can be fatal." There have been several accidental deaths as a result of inadvertent intrathecal administration of vinca alkaloids. Syringes should include a safety outerwrap that states: "DO NOT REMOVE COVERING UNTIL MOMENT OF INJECTION. FATAL IF GIVEN INTRATHECALLY. FOR INTRAVENOUS USE ONLY." Syringes themselves should include an auxiliary sticker that states: "FATAL IF GIVEN INTRATHECALLY. FOR INTRAVENOUS USE ONLY." As a patient safety strategy, some institutions require that vincristine only be sent to the ward or clinic in a small minibag. This practice may decrease the incidence of sentinel events in health systems.
◂ ALERT ▸ Dosage is individualized on the basis of patient's clinical response and tolerance of the drug's adverse effects. When administering this drug in combination therapy, consult specific protocols for optimum dosage and sequence of drug administration.
◂ ALERT ▸ Because vincristine may be carcinogenic, mutagenic, or teratogenic, handle the drug with extreme care during preparation and administration.

◂ ALERT ▸ Give by IV injection only. Use extreme caution in calculating the dosage and administering the drug because overdose may result in serious or fatal outcomes.
- Refrigerate unopened vials.
- The solution normally appears clear and colorless. Discard the solution if it becomes discolored or contains a precipitate.
- May be given undiluted.
- Inject the dose into the tubing of a running IV infusion or directly into a vein over more than 1 min.
- Do not inject into an extremity with impaired or potentially impaired circulation caused by an invading neoplasm, phlebitis, or varicosity.
- Be aware that extravasation produces burning, edema, and stinging at the injection site. If this occurs, stop the injection immediately, notify the physician, inject hyaluronidase locally, if ordered, and apply heat to the affected area to disperse vincristine and minimize cellulitis and discomfort.

STORAGE AND STABILITY
Stored under refrigeration. Preserved, undiluted vials are stable at room temperature for 6 mos.

INTERACTIONS
Drug
Asparaginase: When given before vincristine, asparaginase will enhance neurotoxicity by decreasing hepatic clearance of vincristine. Give vincristine 12-24 hours before asparaginase.
Neurotoxic medications: Vincristine may increase the risk of neurotoxicity, ESPECIALLY with cisplatin.
Cytochrome P450 (CYP) 3A4 inhibitors: All the substrates and inhibitors of CYP3A4 such as the azole antifungals (itraconazole and ketoconazole), erythromycin, cyclosporine, isoniazid, and nifedipine have very high propensity to interfere with vincristine metabolism. Because vincristine is metabolized by CYP3A4, cytotoxicity may be enhanced and result in greater toxicity. Vincristine should be used with caution in combination with these drugs and its dosage may have to be reduced to provide patient safety.
CYP 3A4 inducers (carbamazepine, dexamethasone, phenobarbital, phenytoin, etc.): In the presence of CYP 3A4 inducers, the metabolism of vincristine is

increased, which may result in decreased plasma concentrations and efficacy.

Live-virus vaccines: May potentiate viral replication, increase vaccine side effects, and decrease patient's antibody response to the vaccine.

Mitomycin: May enhance pulmonary toxicity.

Herbal
St John's Wort: May increase drug metabolism and reduce effectiveness of vincristine.

Food
Grapefruit inhibits CYP 3A4 enzymes and can potentially enhance the effects of vincristine.

LAB EFFECTS/INTERFERENCE
May increase serum uric acid levels.

Y-SITE COMPATIBLES
Allopurinol (Aloprim), amifostine, bleomycin sulfate, carboplatin, carmustine, cisplatin (Platinol AQ), cladribine, cyclophosphamide (Cytoxan), cytarabine (Ara-C, Cytosar), dactinomycin, daunorubicin, dexrazoxane, docetaxel, dolasetron, doxorubicin (Adriamycin), doxorubicin liposomal, etoposide (VePesid), etoposide phosphate, filgrastim, fludarabine, 5-fluorouracil, gemcitabine (Gemzar), granisetron, heparin sodium, granisetron (Kytril), ifosfamide, leucovorin calcium, melphalan, mesna, metoclopramide, methotrexate, mitomycin, mitoxantrone, ondansetron (Zofran), palonosetron, paclitaxel (Taxol), rituximab, sargramostim, teniposide, thiotepa, trastuzumab, topotecan, vinblastine, vinorelbine (Navelbine)

INCOMPATIBLES
Amphotericin B conventional (Fungizone), Cefepime HCl (Maxipime), diazepam, furosemide (Lasix), idarubicin HCl (Idamycin), lansoprazole, nafcillin, pantoprazole, phenytoin, sodium bicarbonate

SIDE EFFECTS
Serious Reactions
- Acute shortness of breath and bronchospasm may occur, especially when vincristine is administered concurrently with mitomycin.
- Prolonged or high-dose therapy may produce foot or wrist drop, difficulty walking, slapping gait, ataxia, and muscle wasting.
- Vincristine is a vesicant.

- Vincristine is fatal if given intrathecally.
- Acute uric acid nephropathy may occur.

Other Side Effects
Frequent (10%-50%):
Peripheral neuropathy (occurs in nearly every patient; first clinical sign is depression of Achilles tendon reflex and is the dose-limiting effect), alopecia, constipation or obstipation (upper colon impaction with empty rectum), abdominal cramps, headache, jaw pain, hoarseness, diplopia, ptosis or drooping of eyelid, urinary tract disturbances

Occasional (1%-10%):
Nausea, vomiting, diarrhea, abdominal distention, stomatitis, fever

Rare (Less Than 1%):
Mild leukopenia, mild anemia, thrombocytopenia

SPECIAL CONSIDERATIONS
Baseline Assessment
- Monitor patient's CBC with differential and platelet count, electrolyte, BUN, creatinine, and serum uric acid levels, and liver function test results.
- Assess patient for any history of peripheral neuropathy.
- Assess patient's normal bowel habits for any history of constipation or difficulty passing stools.
- Assess for any cranial nerve palsies, paying particular attention to third and seventh cranial nerves.
- Assess patient for acceptable peripheral access as this agent is a vesicant.
- Have an extravasation kit at bedside before drug delivery.
- Make sure needle is inserted via a one-pass technique if using a peripheral vein.
- Avoid any situation in which vincristine could accidentally be administered intrathecally.

Intervention and Evaluation
- Monitor all laboratory data, paying particular attention to liver function abnormalities. The dose of this agent must be reduced with an elevated bilirubin level.
- Assess for any evidence of extravasation and initiate institutional protocol if necessary.
- Evaluate patient's peripheral access for the possibility of requiring central line placement.
- Assess patient for symptoms of peripheral neuropathy such as any numbness or

tingling in fingers or toes and loss of deep tendon reflexes (Achilles tendon).

- Assess for and evaluate bowel sounds, stool consistency, and pattern of daily bowel activity. Initiate a bowel regimen for assistance in passing stools. Do not administer drug until patient has had a bowel movement on day of drug administration.
- Monitor patient for any evidence of diplopia or ptosis.
- Monitor patient's fluid status, advocating for intake of at least 2 L of fluid per day.

Education

- Instruct patient on when to contact his or her health care provider: fever greater than 38° C (greater than 101° F), chills, shortness of breath, dyspnea wwavupon exertion, nausea lasting for greater than 24 hours, severe constipation, or the inability to take in at least 1500 mL of fluid in 24 hours.
- Warn patient to immediately notify the person administering drug if pain or burning occurs at the injection site during drug delivery.
- Instruct patient to report any signs or symptoms of jaw pain or hoarseness while receiving agent.
- Instruct patient to report any constipation while receiving this agent, and initiate bowel regimen to include laxatives and a stool softener as necessary
- Encourage intake of at least 2 L of fluid daily for the next several days to assist with passing stools.
- Encourage patient to be stay physically active to stimulate the colon.
- Instruct patient to report any numbness or tingling in fingers and toes, along with any changes in ability to walk or to get up from a sitting position.
- Make sure patient has a thermometer at home and knows how to read it.
- Inform patient that hair loss is reversible but that new hair growth may have a different color and texture.
- Urge patient not to receive live-virus vaccinations and to avoid contact with crowds and those with known infections.
- Instruct patient to avoid OTC medications and herbal and vitamin supplements without first checking with the health care provider.
- Provide patient with information on local resources and support groups available for his or her specific diagnosis.

VINORELBINE TARTRATE

BRAND NAMES
Navelbine

CLASS OF AGENT
Vinca alkaloid

CLINICAL PHARMACOLOGY
Mechanism of Action
Semisynthetic vinca alkaloid with antitumor activity that interferes with microtubule assembly. The vinca alkaloids are structurally similar compounds composed of two multiringed units, vindoline and catharanthine. Unlike other vinca alkaloids, the catharanthine unit is the site of structural modification for vinorelbine. The antitumor activity of vinorelbine is thought to be due primarily to inhibition of mitosis at metaphase through its interaction with tubulin. Like other vinca alkaloids, vinorelbine may also interfere with the following: (1) amino acid, cyclic AMP, and glutathione metabolism; (2) calmodulin-dependent $Ca2+$-transport ATPase activity; (3) cellular respiration; and (4) nucleic acid and lipid biosynthesis. Whereas vincristine produces depolymerization of axonal microtubules at 5 mcM, vinblastine and vinorelbine do not have this effect until concentrations of 30 and 40 mcM, respectively. These data suggest relative selectivity of vinorelbine for mitotic microtubules. It may thus be less neurotoxic than vincristine. **Therapeutic Effect:** Prevents cell division.

Absorption and Distribution
Oral vinorelbine is rapidly absorbed (1.5-3 hours) with an elimination half-life of 40 hours. Absorption of oral vinorelbine is not delayed in elderly patients and bioavailability (38%) is similar to that in younger patients (40%). After oral administration, blood concentrations of vinorelbine in elderly patients are within the range of values observed in younger patients. Compared with the intravenous drug, oral vinorelbine demonstrated linear pharmacokinetics as well an absolute bioavailability of 40%. Food has no influence on the pharmacokinetic profile of oral vinorelbine even if nausea and vomiting are less frequent and less severe in the fed patients than in the fasting patients. Despite all this information on oral vinorelbine, there currently is not an oral form

that is commercially available in the United States.

Plasma protein binding in cancer patients ranges from 79.6% to 91.2%. Binding is not altered in the presence of cisplatin, fluorouracil, or doxorubicin. The drug is widely distributed after IV administration.

Half-life: 28-43 hours.

Metabolism and Excretion

All of the metabolites of oral vinorelbine have been identified and, among these, only deacetylvinorelbine presented activity demonstrating that for both PO and IV routes of administration, the drug has the same metabolism pattern.

Oral vinorelbine is eliminated primarily as the unconjugated form in the bile. In this process, the cytochrome P450 (CYP) 3A4 isoform of cytochrome P450 is mostly involved. Reliable dose correspondences are 80 mg/m^2 (oral) to 30 mg/m^2 (intravenous) and 60 mg/m^2 (oral) to 25 mg/m^2 (intravenous). Therefore, intravenous and oral forms show similar interindividual variability, the same metabolism pattern, reproducible intrapatient blood exposure, and the same pharmacokinetic-pharmacodynamic relationship. Vinorelbine is metabolized in the liver and eliminated primarily in the feces by the biliary system.

HOW SUPPLIED/AVAILABLE FORMS

Injection: 10 mg/mL (1-mL, 5-mL vials).

INDICATIONS AND DOSAGES

Unresectable, Advanced Non–Small Cell Lung Cancer (as Monotherapy or in Combination with Cisplatin)

30 mg/m^2 IV administered weekly over 6-10 minutes (as monotherapy).

25 mg/m^2 IV every week or 30 mg/m^2 IV on days 1 and 29, then every 6 weeks (in combination with cisplatin).

Dosage Adjustment Guidelines

Dosage adjustments should be based on granulocyte count obtained on the day of treatment, as follows:

Dosage Adjustment in Hepatic Dysfunction

Vinorelbine should be adjusted for the following bilirubin levels:

Granulocyte Count on Day of Treatment (cells/mm^3)	Dose (mg/m^2)
≥1500 or higher	30
1000-1499	15
<1000	Do not administer

Data from Vinorelbinec product information, Bedford Labs, 2005.

Dosage Adjustment in Renal Dysfunction

No dosage adjustment necessary.

Total Bilirubin (mg/dL)	Dose (mg/m^2)
≤2	30
2.1-3	15
>3	7.5

Data from Vinorelbinec product information, Bedford Labs, 2005.

UNLABELED USES

Breast cancer, cisplatin-resistant ovarian carcinoma, Hodgkin's disease

PRECAUTIONS

Pregnancy Risk Category: D

CONTRAINDICATIONS

Granulocyte counts of less than 1000 cells/mm3, known hypersensitivity reactions, intrathecal route

DRUG PREPARATION/ADMINISTRATION/ SAFE HANDLING ISSUES

◀ ALERT ▶ Vinorelbine must be administered carefully as it is a vesicant.

- The usual initial dose is 30 mg/m^2 administered weekly. The recommended method of administration is an IV injection over 6-10 minutes either in a syringe or bag. Administer the diluted vinorelbine into the side port of a free-flowing IV line closest to the IV bag followed by flushing with 75-125 mL of one of the solutions.
- Syringe: Dilute the calculated dose of vinorelbine to a concentration between 1.5 and 3 mg/mL. The following solutions may be used for dilution: 5% dextrose Injection or 0.9% NaCl injection.
- IV bag: Dilute the calculated dose of vinorelbine to a concentration between 0.5 and 2 mg/mL. The following solutions may be used for dilution: 5% dextrose injection; 0.45% or 0.9% NaCl injection; 5% dextrose and 0.45% NaCl injection; Ringer's injection; or lactated Ringer's injection.

STORAGE AND STABILITY

When stored under refrigeration at 2-8° C (36-46° F) and protected from light in the carton, unopened vials are stable until the date indicated on the package.

When stored at temperatures up to 25° C (77° F), unopened vials are stable for up to 72 hours. Protect from light. Do not freeze. Do not administer if particulate matter is seen.

Diluted vinorelbine may be used for up to 24 hours under normal room light when stored in polypropylene syringes or polyvinyl chloride bags at 5-30° C (41-86° F).

INTERACTIONS
Drug

Bone marrow depressants: May increase the risk of myelosuppression.

Cisplatin: Significantly increases the risk of granulocytopenia.

CYP 3A4 inhibitors: All the substrates and inhibitors of CYP 3A4 such as the azole antifungals (itraconazole and ketoconazole), erythromycin, cyclosporine, isoniazid, and nifedipine have very high propensity to interfere with vinorelbine metabolism. Because vinorelbine is also metabolized by CYP 3A4, similar to vincristine, cytotoxicity may be enhanced and result in greater toxicity. Vinorelbine should be used with caution in combination with these drugs, and its dosage may have to be reduced to provide patient safety.

CYP 3A4 inducers (carbamazepine, dexamethasone, phenobarbital, phenytoin, etc.): In the presence of CYP 3A4 inducers, the metabolism of vinorelbine is increased, which may result in decreased plasma concentrations and efficacy.

Live-virus vaccines: May potentiate viral replication, increase vaccine side effects, and decrease patient's antibody response to the vaccine.

Mitomycin: There have been several case reports of pulmonary toxicity in breast cancer and lung cancer patients treated with the combination of vinorelbine and mitomycin. Symptoms include acute respiratory distress, shortness of breath, dyspnea, or wheezing—a picture of obstructive pulmonary disease that differs from mitomycin pulmonary toxicity, which is a slower onset syndrome associated with microangiopathy. The incidence of pulmonary toxicity associated with the vinorelbine-mitomycin combination has ranged from 3% to 39%. Symptoms occur with a rapid onset, usually 1-5 hours after vinorelbine administration. The acute symptoms can be managed with IV corticosteroid therapy. The mechanism for this interaction is unknown, and it is uncertain whether there is a pharmacokinetic basis for the interaction between mitomycin and

vinorelbine. It appears to be an enhanced pharmacodynamic effect on the pulmonary parenchyma or a hypersensitivity-like reaction.

Paclitaxel and docetaxel: When vinorelbine precedes paclitaxel, bone marrow toxicity is significantly greater than with the reverse sequence of drug administration. Thus, paclitaxel and docetaxel should be administered before vinorelbine.

Phenytoin: Patients receiving phenytoin may demonstrate decreased serum concentrations due to induction of CYP 3A4 metabolism by vinorelbine. Phenytoin levels should be monitored more closely in patients receiving vinorelbine.

Herbal

St John's Wort: May increase drug metabolism and reduce the effectiveness of vinorelbine.

Food

Grapefruit inhibits CYP 3A4 enzymes and can potentially enhance the effects of vinorelbine.

LAB EFFECTS/INTERFERENCE

May increase total serum bilirubin and AST (SGOT) levels, liver function test results. Decreases granulocyte, leukocyte, thrombocyte, RBC counts.

Y-SITE COMPATIBLES

Amifostine, bleomycin, calcium gluconate, carboplatin (Paraplatin), carmustine, cisplatin (Platinol AQ), cyclophosphamide (Cytoxan), cytarabine (Ara-C, Cytosar), dacarbazine (DTIC-Dome), dactinomycin, daunorubicin (Cerubidine), dexamethasone (Decadron), dexrazoxane, diphenhydramine (Benadryl), docetaxel, doxorubicin (Adriamycin), etoposide (VePesid), etoposide phosphate, filgrastim, floxuridine, fludarabine, fluorouracil, gemcitabine (Gemzar), granisetron (Kytril), hydromorphone (Dilaudid), idarubicin (Idamycin), ifosfamide, irinotecan, leucovorin, mechlorethamine, melphalan, mesna, methotrexate, morphine, ondansetron (Zofran), oxaliplatin, paclitaxel, palonosetron, pemetrexed, rituximab, streptozocin, teniposide (Vumon), trastuzumab, vinblastine (Velban), vincristine (Oncovin)

INCOMPATIBLES

Acyclovir (Zovirax), allopurinol (Aloprim), aminophylline, amphotericin B (Fungizone), amphotericin B complex

(Abelcet, AmBisome, Amphotec), ampicillin (Omnipen), cefazolin (Ancef), cefepime, cefoperazone (Cefobid), cefotetan (Cefotan), cefoxitin, ceftriaxone (Rocephin), cefuroxime (Zinacef), chloramphenicol, dantrolene, diazepam, 5-fluorouracil, foscarnet, furosemide (Lasix), ganciclovir (Cytovene), heparin, ketorolac, lansoprazole, methylprednisolone (Solu-Medrol), mitomycin, nafcillin, nitroprusside, pantoprazole, phenobarbital, phenytoin, piperacillin, sodium bicarbonate, sulfamethoxazole-trimethoprim, thiopental

SIDE EFFECTS
Serious Reactions
- Bone marrow depression is manifested mainly as granulocytopenia, which may be severe. Other hematologic toxicities, including neutropenia, thrombocytopenia, leukopenia, and anemia increase the risk of infection and bleeding.
- Acute shortness of breath and severe bronchospasm occur infrequently, particularly in patients with preexisting pulmonary dysfunction and in those receiving mitomycin concurrently.

Other Side Effects
Frequent (10%-50%):
Asthenia (35%); mild or moderate nausea (34%); constipation (29%); erythema, pain, or vein discoloration at injection site (28%); fatigue (27%); peripheral neuropathy manifested as paraesthesia and hyperesthesia (25%); diarrhea (17%); alopecia (12%)
Occasional (1%-10%):
Phlebitis (10%), dyspnea (7%), loss of deep tendon reflexes (5%)
Rare (Less Than 1%):
Chest pain, jaw pain, myalgia, arthralgia, rash

SPECIAL CONSIDERATIONS
Baseline Assessment
- Assess baseline CBC with differential, electrolyte, BUN, and creatinine levels, and liver function tests.
- Assess patient for any prior history of peripheral neuropathy or pulmonary compromise.
- Evaluate patient's peripheral access as this agent can induce necrosis of skin if leakage occurs into subcutaneous tissue.
- Assess patient's history of nausea with any prior chemotherapy as this agent can induce emesis.

- Avoid any situation in which vinorelbine could accidentally be administered intrathecally.

Intervention and Evaluation
- Monitor patient's CBC with differential and platelet count, do not administer if ANC is less than 1000/mm^3.
- Assess patient for any evidence of drug leakage during administration.
- Evaluate need for vascular access device in patients with poor peripheral access at each dosing.
- Monitor patient for jaw pain during drug administration.
- Premedicate patient with antiemetics before administration.
- Assess of vital signs and conduct pulmonary examination before dosing as this agent can induce bronchospasm.
- Evaluate patient for evidence of neutropenia, thrombocytopenia, and anemia before each dose.
- Assess patient for any evidence of constipation or diarrhea before each dose.
- Monitor patient for increasing fatigue.
- Assess patient for evidence of increasing peripheral neuropathy, paresthesias, dysesthesias, and hypoesthesias.
- Provide counselling and support to patient on potential impending alopecia.

Education
- Instruct patient on when to contact his or her health care provider: infection, fever greater than 38° C (greater than 101° F), chills, cough, shortness of breath, dyspnea upon exertion, easy bruising or bleeding, nausea lasting for greater than 24 hours, diarrhea lasting for greater than 24 hours, or the inability to take in at least 1500 mL in 24 hours.
- Advise patient on symptoms of peripheral neuropathy: numbness and tingling in fingers and toes, and weakness. Instruct patient notify the health care provider if they occur.
- Educate patient on how to take antiemetics for nausea.
- Instruct patient on a bowel regimen if constipation is an issue, making sure patient has a stool softener and a stimulant laxative such as senna.
- Encourage patient to drink at least 2 L of fluid per day.
- Instruct patient that alopecia may occur and provide opportunities for counseling regarding this issue. Inform patient that

new hair growth may have a different color and texture.
- Advise patient to avoid all OTC medications and herbals and vitamin supplements without first checking with the health care provider.
- Provide patient with information on local resources and support groups available for his or her specific diagnosis.

ZOLEDRONIC ACID
BRAND NAMES
Zometa

CLASS OF AGENT
Bisphosphonate

CLINICAL PHARMACOLOGY
Mechanism of Action
Inhibits the activity of osteoclasts and induces apoptosis of osteoclastic cells. In a neoplastic setting, tumors secrete certain chemical signals that in turn stimulate osteoclasts and mobilize the release of skeletal calcium. Zoledronic acid has been shown to impede this process by limiting the tumor cells' capacity to invade and adhere to the bone. **Therapeutic Effect:** Inhibit bone resorption and reduce risk of skeletal-related events.
Absorption and Distribution
The majority of drug is quickly taken up by bone; 22% is bound to plasma proteins independent of concentration.
Half-life: Early elimination half-life is 1.75 hours. Terminal elimination is prolonged with very low levels of drug detectable in plasma up to 28 days postinfusion. Terminal elimination half-life is 146 hours.
Metabolism and Excretion
Studies have demonstrated a lack of drug metabolism when administered IV. Zoledronic acid does not inhibit the cytochrome P450 metabolic pathway. Elimination is primarily through renal excretion; $39 \pm 16\%$ is recovered in the urine 24 hours postinfusion. Excretion through feces was less than 3%. The remainder of drug is presumably directly bound to bone. The bound drug is slowly released back into the plasma where it is then excreted through the kidneys. Clearance of drug is dependent on creatinine clearance and independent of dose.

HOW SUPPLIED/AVAILABLE FORMS
Injection Solution: 4 mg/5 mL.

INDICATIONS AND DOSAGES
Hypercalcemia of Malignancy, Osteolytic Lesions Associated with Solid Tumors and Multiple Myeloma
4 mg IV over at least 15 minutes. For hypercalcemia, repeat dosing should occur no more frequently than every 7 days if calcium level has not adequately returned and remained in the normal range. For osteolytic lesions associated with solid tumors and multiple myeloma, dosing is repeated every 3-4 weeks indefinitely.
Dosage Adjustment in Hepatic Dysfunction
No dosage adjustment necessary.
Dosage Adjustment in Renal Dysfunction
There is a real risk of clinically significant deterioration of renal function, which in some cases may progress to renal failure even after a single dose of zoledronic acid. Patients with serum creatinine greater than 3.0 mg/dL were excluded in studies in patients with bone metastasis. In patients with hypercalcemia of malignancy and renal insufficiency, treatment should only be considered after carefully evaluating the risks and benefits. Mild to moderate renal impairment requires reduced dosing based on CrCl. The Cockcroft-Gault formula determines the glomerular filtration rate or CrCl.
CrCl (mL/min) = $(140 \times$ age$) \times$ weight (kg) $\times 0.85$ (for females)/$72 \times$ serum creatinine
The following table designates dosage adjustments for patients with renal insufficiency and the corresponding drug volume.

Baseline Creatinine Clearance (mL/min)	Dose (mg)	Volume (mL)
>60	4.0	5.0
50-60	3.5	4.4
40-49	3.3	4.1
30-39	3.0	3.8

Do not administer to patients with severe baseline renal dysfunction. For patients stabilized with administration of zoledronic acid, renal deterioration is defined as follows:
Increase of 0.5 mg/dL for patients with a normal baseline serum creatinine level.
Increase of 1.0 mg/dL for patients with an abnormal baseline serum creatinine level.
If renal deterioration is observed, drug should be held in patients with multiple myeloma or osteolytic lesions from solid

tumors. If the creatinine level returns to within 10% of baseline, patient may be re-challenged with caution and close observation. If increasing renal dysfunction is observed in patients being treated for hypercalcemia of malignancy, a careful evaluation should ensue and a decision must then be made to determine whether the potential benefit of treating outweighs the potential risks.

UNLABELED USES

Osteoporosis, Paget's disease, prophylaxis of bone loss in men with nonmetastatic prostate cancer on androgen deprivation therapy

PRECAUTIONS

• Renal dysfunction may develop or progress to full renal failure requiring dialysis. Do not exceed maximum dose of 4 mg infused over 15 minutes. Infusion times less than 15 minutes increase the risk for renal dysfunction. Assess serum creatinine before each infusion.
• Osteonecrosis of the jaw has been reported. Most incidents of osteonecrosis of the jaw were associated with tooth extraction but have also been noted in patients without this procedure. Many of these patients also had evidence of local infection, occasionally progressing to osteomyelitis. Common signs and symptoms include a "heavy jaw" sensation, pain, edema, halitosis resulting from superimposed infection, loose teeth, discharge, and exposed bone, which is sometimes sharp and spiculated. If osteonecrosis is suspected or diagnosed, a referral to an oral surgeon should be made. Surgical intervention may actually worsen the situation; however, minimal bony débridement may be necessary to remove sharp edges of bone. Intermittent or continuous antibiotic therapy may be of benefit along with 0.12% chlorhexidine gluconate oral rinses. Patients should be encouraged to maintain excellent oral hygiene routines and to immediately report any suspicious symptoms. A complete dental examination is strongly recommended before institution of therapy.
• May decrease serum calcium and phosphorus levels. Magnesium levels may also be affected. Supplementation may be required.

• Use with caution when treating patients with aspirin-sensitive asthma as bronchoconstriction has been reported in patients treated with other bisphosphonates.

Pregnancy Risk Category: D
May impair fertility and may cause fetal harm in pregnant women. Drug excretion into human breast milk is unknown/not recommended in nursing women.

CONTRAINDICATIONS

Severe renal insufficiency (defined as creatinine clearance less than 39 mL/min); incompletely healed dental extraction sites and osseointegrated dental implants; hypersensitivity to zoledronic acid, other bisphosphonates, mannitol, or any other component of the formulation

DRUG PREPARATION/ADMINISTRATION/SAFE HANDLING ISSUES

◀ ALERT ▶ Strict adherence to the administration recommendations is necessary to minimize the risk of renal dysfunction.
• Do not mix with calcium-containing solutions (e.g., lactated Ringer's solution).
• 5 mL of concentrated zoledronic acid should be immediately diluted in 100 mL of sterile 0.9% NaCl or 5% dextrose injection. See table under "Dosage Adjustment in Renal Dysfunction" for appropriate volumes for patients with renal insufficiency.
• Drug should be administered as a single IV solution in a line separate from all other drugs.
• Dose must be infused over no less than 15 minutes.
• Patients receiving zoledronic acid for bone metastases should also receive an oral calcium supplement (500 mg) and an oral multiple vitamin containing vitamin D (400 international units) daily.

STORAGE AND STABILITY

• Store intact vial at room temperature.
• Once drug is reconstituted with sterile water for injection, it may be stored for up to 24 hours under refrigeration.

INTERACTIONS

Drug
Zoledronic acid is not known to inhibit the cytochrome P450 pathway.
Loop diuretics (bumetanide, ethacrynic acid, furosemide, torsemide): Use with

caution because of the enhanced risk of hypocalcemia and hypomagnesemia in the hypercalcemia setting.

Nephrotoxic drugs (aminoglycosides): Increased risk of nephrotoxicity

Thalidomide: In the setting of multiple myeloma, combined treatment may potentiate the risk of renal dysfunction.

Herbal
None known.

LAB EFFECTS/INTERFERENCE

Serum creatinine must be monitored before every dose. Monitor periodically for serum calcium, phosphate, and magnesium levels, CBC.

Y-SITE COMPATIBLES

Administer as a single IV solution in a line separate from all other drugs.

COMPATIBLES

Do not mix with calcium-containing solutions (e.g., lactated Ringer's solution).

SIDE EFFECTS
Serious Reactions
Renal failure, osteonecrosis of the jaw, and severe allergic reactions have occurred.
Frequent (10%-50%):
Agitation, anemia, anorexia, anxiety, constipation, dehydration, depression, diarrhea, electrolyte imbalance (calcium, phosphorus, magnesium, and potassium), fever, flu-like syndrome (chills, fatigue, nausea, vomiting, arthralgias, myalgias, and bone pain), headache, hypotension, insomnia, neutropenia, renal insufficiency (reduced or worsening), thrombocytopenia
Occasional (1%-10%):
Chest pain, mucositis, osteonecrosis of the jaw
Rare (Less Than 1%):
Acute renal failure, allergic reaction, conjunctivitis

SPECIAL CONSIDERATIONS
Baseline Assessment
- Ensure that routine dental examination has been completed before institution of therapy. If dental extraction is indicated, adequate time for healing should be allowed before therapy is begun.
- Reinforce the need for properly fitting dentures.
- Review all baseline laboratory tests including serum creatinine, BUN, serum

calcium, magnesium, and phosphate, and serum albumin levels and CBC. Assess serum creatinine levels before every dose.
- Review patient's current prescriptions and use of OTC products.
- Verify any patient allergies.

Intervention and Evaluation
- Advise patient to have periodic oral examinations.
- Refer patient to oral surgeon for consultation if osteonecrosis of the jaw is either suspected or diagnosed; drug may need to be interrupted.
- Be aware that intermittent or continuous antibiotic therapy may be necessary to prevent secondary soft-tissue infection or osteomyelitis. Optimal antibiotics include penicillin VK 500 mg 4 times/day and amoxicillin 500 mg 4 times/day. If patient is allergic to penicillin, clindamycin 150-300 mg 4 times/day, doxycycline (Vibramycin) 100 mg daily, or erythromycin 400 mg 3 times/day can be used.
- Oral rinses with 0.12% chlorhexidine gluconate may also be helpful.
- Assess serum creatinine level before every dose.
- Hold drug in patients who meet the criteria for worsening renal dysfunction (increase of 0.5 mg/dL for patients with normal baseline creatinine levels and increase of 1 mg/dL for patients with abnormal baseline creatinine levels). Reinstitute drug when creatinine returns to within 10% of baseline.
- Be aware that patients with clinically significant declines of calcium, phosphate, and magnesium levels may need supplementation.
- Treat flu-like symptoms with antiemetics for nausea and acetaminophen for the bone pain, arthralgias, and myalgias. Treat with NSAIDs may be allowed if renal insufficiency is not an issue.

Education
- Explain to patient why he or she is receiving zoledronic acid (hypercalcemia of malignancy, multiple myeloma, or osteolytic lesions associated with solid tumors).
- Review potential side effects.
- Inform patient that if flu-like symptoms occur, they usually subside within 24-48 hours and typically do not recur after the first or second infusion.
- Brief patient that although a high fever (101.4° F) may occur, it can be controlled

with acetaminophen and usually resolves within 24-48 hours. Reassure patient that fever is due to the flu-like reaction and not a true infection. Instruct patient to contact the health care provider if fever persists.

* Educate patient on the need to monitor laboratory analyses, in particular the serum creatinine level, before every infusion.
* Stress the importance for maintaining adequate hydration.
* Instruct patient to consume a low-calcium diet if he or she being treated for hypercalcemia of malignancy.
* Reinforce the need for excellent dental hygiene and routine professional dental cleanings.
* Instruct patient to avoid any jaw or dental procedure that would require the healing of bone (i.e., tooth extractions, dental implants, and others)
* Encourage patient to report any new symptoms.

BIBLIOGRAPHY

Alberts DS, Jiang C, Liu PY, et al. Long-term follow-up of a phase II trial of oral altretamine for consolidation of clinical complete remission in women with stage III epithelial ovarian cancer in the Southwest Oncology Group. *Int J Gynecol Cancer* 2004;14: 224-228.

Allen, 1994a

Andre P, Cisternino S, Chiadmi F, et al. Stability of bortezomib 1-mg/mL solution in plastic syringe and glass vial. *Ann Pharmacother* 2005;39:1462-1466.

Avastin (bevacizumab) prescribing information. Genetech, South San Francisco, CA. 2006.

BiCNU intravenous solution (carmustine) prescribing information. 2003

Cerubidine (daunorubicin) prescribing information. 1999.

Chan JK, Loizzi V, Manetta A, et al. Oral altretamine used as salvage therapy in recurrent ovarian cancer. *Gynecol Oncol* 2004;92:368-371.

Chou WC, Dang CV. Acute promyelocytic leukaemia: recent advances in therapy and molecular basis of response to arsenic therapies. *Curr Opin Hematol* 2005;12:1-6.

Cytoxan (cyclophosphamide) prescribing information. 2000.

Doxil (doxorubicin) prescribing information. 1999.

DTIC-Dome (dacarbazine) prescribing information. 1998.

Eloxatin (oxaliplatin) prescribing information. 2004.

Ethyol (amifostine) prescribing information. 2002.

Feldweg AM, Lee CW, Matulonis UA, Castells M. Rapid desensitisation for hypersensitivity reactions to paclitaxel and docetaxel: a new standard protocol used in 77 successful treatments. *Gynecol Oncol* 2005;96:824-829.

Gabizon et al, 1994a

Gliadel (polifeprosan 20 with carmustine) prescribing information. 1999.

Jagannath S, Barlogie B, Berenson J, et al. A phase 2 study of two doses of bortezomib in relapsed or refractory myeloma. *Br J Haematol* 2004; 127:165-172.

Jeyabalan N, Hirte HW, Moans F. Treatment of advanced ovarian carcinoma with carboplatin and paclitaxel in patients with renal failure. *Int J Gynecol Cancer* 2000;10:463-468.

Kornblith A, Herndon JE 2nd, Silverman LR, et al. Impact of azacitidine on the quality of life of patients with myelodysplastic syndrome treated in a randomized phase III trial: a Cancer and Leukemia Group B study. *J Clin Oncol* 2002;20:2441-2452.

Lee CW, Matulonis UA, Castells M. Carboplatin hypersensitivity: a 6-h 12-step protocol effective in 35 desensitizations in patients with gynecological malignancies and mast cell/IgE-mediated reactions. *Gynecol Oncol* 2004;95:370-376.

Ludwig H, Khayat D, Giaccone G, et al. Proteasome inhibition and its clinical prospects in the treatment of hematologic and solid malignancies. *Cancer* 2005;104:1794-1807.

Maier SK, Hammond JM. Role of lenalidomide in the treatment of multiple myeloma and myelodysplastic syndrome. *Ann Pharmacother.* 2006;40:286-289.

Marcucci G, Silverman L, Eller M, et al. Bioavailability of azacitidine subcutaneous versus intravenous in patients with the myelodysplastic syndromes. *J Clin Pharmacol* 2005;45:597-602.

Markman M, Kennedy A, Webster K, et al. Paclitaxel-associated hypersensitivity reactions: experience of the gynecologic oncology program of the Cleveland Clinic Cancer Center. *J Clin Oncol* 2000;18:102-105.

Messaad D, Sablayrolles P, Pujol JL, Demoly P. Successful docetaxel tolerance induction. *Allergy* 2003;58:1320-1321.

Mutamycin (mitomycin) prescribing information. 1997

Richardson P, Barlogie B, Berenson J, Singhal S, Jagannath S, Irwin D, et al. A phase 2 study of bortezomib in relapsed, refractory myeloma. *N Engl J Med* 2003;348:2609-2617.

Richardson P, Sonnevald P, Schuster MW, et al. Bortezomib or high-dose dexamethasone for relapsed multiple myeloma. *N Engl J Med* 2005;352:2487-2498.

Riggs, 1984

Robinson JB, Singh D, Bodurka-Bevers DC, et al. Hypersensitivity reactions and the utility of oral and intravenous desensitization in patients with gynecologic malignancies. *Gynecol Oncol* 2001;82:550-558.

Rose PG, Fusco N, Smrekar M, et al. Successful administration of carboplatin in patients with clinically documented carboplatin hypersensitivity. *Gynecol Oncol* 2003;89:429-433.

Shen ZX, Chen GO, Ni JH, et al. Use of arsenic trioxide (As^2O_3) in the treatment of acute promyelocytic leukemia (APL): II. Clinical efficacy and pharmacokinetics in relapsed patients. *Blood* 1997;89:3354-3360.

Silverman L, Demakos EP, Peterson BL, et al. Randomized controlled trial of azacitidine in patients with the myelodysplastic syndrome: a Study of the Cancer and Leukemia Group B. *J Clin Oncol* 2002;20:2429-2440.

Sullivan M, Hahn K, Kolesar J. Azacitidine: a novel agent for myelodysplastic syndromes. *Am J Health-Syst Pharm* 2005;62:1567-1573.

Targretin capsules (bexarotene) prescribing information. St. Petersburg, FL: R. P. Scherer, 2001.

Uttamsingh V, Lu C, Miwa G, et al. Relative contributions of the five major human cytochromes P450, 1A2, 2C9, 2C19, 2D6 and 3A4, to the hepatic metabolism of the proteosome inhibitor bortezomib. Drug Metab Dispos 2005;33:1723-1728.

Velcade (bortezomib) package insert. Cambridge, MA: Millennium Pharmaceuticals; 2005.

Vidaza (azacitidine) package insert. Boulder, CO: Pharmion Corporation; 2004.

Watanabe M, Aoki Y, Tomita M, et al. Paclitaxel and carboplatin combination chemotherapy in a hemodialysis patient with advanced ovarian cancer. *Gynecol Oncol* 2002;84:335-338.

Weber D. Thalidomide and its derivatives: new promise for multiple myeloma. *Cancer Control* 2003;10:375-383.

Xue et al, 1986

INTRODUCTION

Pediatric cancers are relatively rare occurrences in the United States, having an incidence of 1 in 7000 children, aged 0–14 years.[1,2] They account for only about 2% of all cancers in Western industrialized nations.[3] Table 2–1 lists the most common cancers in children and adolescents. Behind accidents, cancer is the second most common cause of death in children younger than 15 years of age.[4]

Early detection and prompt treatment are the pivotal components to ensuring a good outcome for a child with cancer. To achieve this goal, a high index of suspicion is needed by the pediatric practitioner, and early referral to a pediatric oncologist is essential. Early diagnosis is a difficult task due to theI insidious nature of the disease. Approximately 15% of patients complain of unusual signs and symptoms that mimic those of other more common disorders.[5] In addition, very young children are often unable to make their complaints known.

As with any disease process, it is critical to obtain a detailed and thorough history, focusing on the chief complaint. Many symptoms that parents may associate with cancer are those that occur in adults with cancer, such as a sore that does not heal, a lump or thickening in the breast, indigestion, or difficulty swallowing. Although these signs and symptoms are useful as warning signs to the adult population, they are of little help in children. Thus, it is important to have knowledge of the child's past medical history and family history. Many genetic conditions can predispose a child to an increased risk of malignancy (Tables 2–2 and 2–3). A history of a previous cancer also puts a child at an increased risk of a secondary malignancy due either to the treatment received or to a genetic predisposition. Once a malignancy is suspected, the child should be referred to a pediatric oncologist for complete staging and initial treatment.

Fortunately, many pediatric cancers that previously have had low survival rates now have 5-year event-free survival rates greater than 70%. This chapter focuses on the most common pediatric cancers and the treatment used for each; specifically these include acute leukemias, lymphomas, and common solid tumors.[4]

ACUTE LEUKEMIAS

The acute leukemias are the most common pediatric malignancies. They result from a proliferation of hematopoietic precursors. The hallmark of these diseases is the leukemic "blast cell," a visibly immature and abnormal cell in the peripheral blood that often replaces the bone marrow and thus interferes with normal hematopoiesis. These blast cells proliferate in the marrow and inhibit the normal cellular elements, resulting in anemia, neutropenia, and thrombocytopenia.[5]

The acute leukemias are categorized according to their cell of origin[6] (Table 2–4). Acute lymphoblastic leukemia (ALL) arises from the precursor lymphoid cells. Acute myelogenous leukemia (AML) arises from the precursor myeloid cell. Treatment of the acute leukemias, especially ALL, and the number of survivors have increased dramatically in the last 30+ years. In addition, "risk-based" treatment strategies have been developed in an attempt to match the aggressiveness of therapy to the presumed risk of relapse and death.[7]

Table 2–1 **Most Common Childhood Malignancies in Children Younger Than Age 15 and Adolescents Aged 15–19**

CHILDREN YOUNGER THAN AGE 15		ADOLESCENTS AGED 15–19	
Malignancy	Incidence (%)	Malignancy	Incidence (%)
Acute leukemia	28.2	Lymphoma	25.1
CNS tumors	22.1	Germ cell/gonadal	12.4
Lymphoma	9.3	Acute leukemia	9.9
Neuroblastoma	7.9	CNS tumors	9.8
Wilms' tumor	6	Malignant melanoma	7.6

CNS, Central nervous system.
National Cancer Institute surveillance and epidemiology data, 2005.

Table 2–2 **Common Hereditary Disorders Associated with Childhood Cancers**

Chromosomal Abnormality	Cancer
Down syndrome	Leukemia, testicular, retinoblastoma
Turner syndrome	Neurogenic, gonadal, endometrial
Klinefelter syndrome	Leukemia, germ cell
Other sex aneuploidy	Retinoblastoma
XY gonadal dysgenesis	Gonadoblastoma, dysgerminoma
Trisomy 13	Teratoma, leukemia, neurogenic
Trisomy 18	Neurogenic, Wilms' tumor
XYY, XYY mosaic	Osteoblastoma and medulloblastoma

Table 2–3 **Other Genetic Disorders**

Disorder	Cancer
Xeroderma pigmentosa	Basal, squamous cell, melanoma
Bloom syndrome	Leukemia, lymphoma, gastrointestinal
Fanconi syndrome	Leukemia, hepatoma, squamous cell
Ataxia-telangiectasia	Lymphoma, leukemia, Hodgkin's disease, brain, gastric, ovarian, other epithelial tumors
Neurofibromatosis type I	Gliomas, malignant peripheral nerve sheath tumors
Tuberous sclerosis	Rhabdomyosarcoma, brain tumors
Von Hippel Lindau disease	Renal cell, pheochromocytomas

Table 2–4 **Types of Acute Leukemias**

Cell of Origin	Frequency (%)	Disease-Free Survival at 5 Yr (%)
Lymphoid		
B-precursor	72	80
B-precursor + myeloid	10	15
T-cell	16	50
B-cell	2	60
Myeloid	50	25
Promyeloid	7	30
Myelomonocytoid	16	25
Monocytoid	16	35
Erythroid	2	
Megakaryocytoid	6	50
Chronic myeloid	3	30

INCIDENCE AND EPIDEMIOLOGY

In the pediatric population, leukemia accounts for one third of all childhood malignancies. Acute leukemia is the most common malignancy in children younger than 15 years of age, with 3000–4000 new cases diagnosed annually in the United States.[3] The incidence in the United States is approximately 2.8 cases per 100,000 children.[3]

For children, the 5-year event-free survival rate for ALL is nearly 80%. This degree of success can be attributed to use of risk-directed treatment strategies and to enrollment of patients in clinical trials. AML is, by definition, a high-risk disease with a 5-year survival of only 50%.[6]

Acute Lymphocytic Leukemia

ALL accounts for 75%–80% of childhood leukemia and has a peak incidence in the 2- to 5-year age range. ALL is diagnosed in approximately 3000 children annually. The mean age of onset is 4 years (range of 2–5 years).[2,8] The incidence of ALL among children aged 2–3 years is approximately fourfold that for infants and almost 10-fold that for children who are 19 years old. At diagnosis, 85% of patients are between the ages of 2 and 10 years.[9] ALL occurs more commonly in boys than in girls.[10] In the United States, the incidence of ALL is more common in Caucasian children than for African Americans, American Indians, and Hispanic ethnicities.[5]

In ALL, the majority of cells will have an antigen on the cell surface, called the *common ALL antigen.*[12] Most will be of immature B-cell origin and less commonly of T-cell or mature B-cell origin. Before the advent of chemotherapy, this disease was fatal within 3–4 months, with virtually no survivors at 1 year after diagnosis.

Acute Myelogenous Leukemia

Approximately 500 new cases of AML are diagnosed in children annually, and although AML accounts for less than 20% of all leukemias, it represents 33% of deaths from leukemia in children and teenagers. There is a bimodal peak of AML, first at 2 years of age, after which there is a steady decline in cases to age 9; it then peaks again at around age 16.[6,13]

ETIOLOGY OF THE ACUTE LEUKEMIAS

The cause of the acute leukemias is still unknown; multiple influences related to genetics, socioeconomics, age of infection with viral illness, environment, hematopoietic development, and chance may all play a role. In most instances, however, there is no reasonable or obvious explanation for the development of leukemia.

The influence of genetics in leukemia is supported by several observations. For example, among identical twins, the occurrence of ALL is associated with as much as a 25% chance of the disease developing in the other twin within 1 year.[12] Individuals with chromosome abnormalities have an increased risk of leukemia. Patients with Down syndrome have a 20-fold increased risk of developing leukemia compared with the rest of the population.[6]

Nongenetic risk factors for ALL are few. An increased risk of ALL is associated with a higher socioeconomic status. This relationship is presumed to be related to hygiene and exposure to infectious agents. It is postulated that less social contact in early infancy, and thus a late exposure to some common infectious agents may have some impact.[12] Prenatal or postnatal exposure to radiation has been associated with the development of pediatric leukemias. There is evidence to suggest that most cases of ALL in children have a prenatal origin. Each child's disease is unique and can be characterized by specific immunoglobulin and T-cell receptor rearrangements. Evidence of these rearrangements can be found at birth.[14,15]

Box 2–1   Conditions Associated with Increased Risk of Acute Myelogenous Leukemia

Congenital
Diamond-Blackfan anemia
Neurofibromatosis
Down syndrome
Wiskott-Aldrich syndrome
Kostmann syndrome
Li-Fraumeni syndrome

Chromosomal instability
Fanconi's anemia

Acquired risk factors
Ionizing radiation
Cytotoxic chemotherapeutic agents
Benzenes

Risk factors for the development of AML include environmental factors such as exposure to toxins and organic chemicals, ethnicity, and genetics. Congenital conditions and chromosomal instability syndromes associated with an increased risk of AML as shown Box 2–1. However, the vast majority of children have no identifiable risk factors.[5]

Of increasing concern in the pediatric population is the increased prevalence of AML as a secondary malignancy, resulting from chemotherapy and radiation treatment for previous cancers. Topoisomerase inhibitors, such as etoposide, and alkylating agents, such as ifosfamide and cyclophosphamide, in particular, have been linked to an increased risk of myelodysplastic syndrome and AML.[16]

PATHOGENESIS OF ACUTE LEUKEMIAS

All blood cells are produced from a common hematopoietic precursor or *stem cell.* According to *Stedman's Medical Dictionary,* the definition of leukemia is "a progressive proliferation of abnormal leukocytes found in hemopoietic tissues, other organs, and usually in the blood in increased numbers." In contrast with normal white cells, leukemic cells arise from dysregulated clonal expansion of immature lymphoid or myeloid precursors that are blocked at a particular stage of differentiation and result in blast cells. As these cells expand, they acquire one and more chromosomal abnormalities.[16] Although the number of blast cells may vary from person to person, a critical mass of cells can eventually invade the peripheral circulation and infiltrate normal tissues.[17] As blast cells accumulate, they suppress the production of other normal cells. The clinical signs of this suppression of normal cellular elements are anemia, neutropenia, and thrombocytopenia.[6]

CLASSIFICATION

For all patients with newly diagnosed leukemia, an aspirate of the liquid marrow and a bone marrow core biopsy are obtained.[17] Morphologic and cytochemical analysis of these samples distinguishes three subtypes of ALL (L1, L2, and L3) and eight subtypes of AML (M0–M7) as classified by the recent French-American-British (FAB) scheme (Table 2–5).[5] This system is based purely on morphology and cytochemistry with consideration of nuclear appearance and degree of differentiation. However, this scheme is rapidly losing favor as newer schemes based on features that can be identified only by immunologic cell surface markers and molecular cytogenetic evaluation are being used.[6]

Table 2–5 French-American-British Subtypes of Acute Myeloid Leukemia

FAB Classification	Common Name	Clinical Features	Cytogenetic Associations	Distribution in Childhood (Age)	
				<2 Yr	<2 Yr
M0	Acute myeloid leukemia, minimally differentiated	Leukocytosis	inv (3q26), t(3;3)		1%
M1	Acute myeloblastic leukemia without maturation	Leucocytosis		17%	23%
M2	Acute myeloblastic leukemia with maturation	Myeloblastoma or chloroma	t(8;21) t(6;9); rare		26%
M3	Acute promyelocytic leukemia	Disseminated intravascular coagulation	t(15;17); rarely, t(11;17) or (5;17)		4%
M4	Acute myelomonoblastic leukemia	Hyperleukocytosis, CNS involvement, skin and gum infiltration	11 q23, inv 3, t(3;3), t(6;9), t(1;22)	30%	24%
M4Eo	Acute myelomonoblastic leukemia with abnormal eosinophils	Hyperleukocytosis, CNS involvement, skin and gum infiltration	inv 16, t(16;16)	rare	rare
M5	Acute monoblastic leukemia	Hyperleukocytosis, CNS involvement, skin and gum infiltration	11 q23, t(9;11), t(8;16), t(1;22)	46%	15%
M6	Erythroleukemia	Fatigue, joing pain, pallor, thrombocytopenia	favorable t(8;21), inv 16/t(16;16), and +14; unfavourable with −5/5q, − 7/7q-, inv3, 11q, 17p, del20q, +13, t(9;22),	rare	2%
M7	Acute megakaryoblastic leukemia		t(1;22) Down syndrome frequent (< 2 years of age)	7%	5%

FAB = French–American–British classification; CNS = central nervous system.
Modified from Current Pediatrics: Chapter 28. Major Pediatric Neoplastic Diseases. From Albano E, Bassal M, Porter C, et al. Neoplastic diseases. In Hay W, Levin M, Sondheimer J, Deterding R, eds. *Current Pediatrics: Diagnosis and Treatment*, 17th ed.

Specifically, the World Health Organization has developed a classification of AML that is based on the above characteristics and clinical features. These factors taken together more accurately characterize the distinct biologic and clinical behavior of the disease. Although this classification is used for both adult and pediatric populations, it appears to have more applicability to adults.[18] Of patients with AML, 80% will have cytogenetic clonal abnormalities that are often predictive of outcome.[12]

In addition, immunophenotyping by flow cytometry has become an increasingly important factor in the diagnosis of leukemia. This approach takes advantage of the development of monoclonal antibodies targeted to cell surface antigens that are differentially expressed during hematopoietic differentiation.[12] The antigens are referred to as *antibody cluster determinants,* or *CD,* which define cells at various stages of development, and these markers can easily separate ALL from AML and T-cell ALL from pre-B-cell ALL.[19] The detailed information offered by flow cytometric analysis plus the recognition of several prognostic cytogenetic features combines to more narrowly predict prognosis and develop risk-directed therapies for both ALL and AML.[17]

ALL can be derived from either B cells or T cells. Approximately 70%–80% of childhood ALLs are of B-cell precursor lineages (CD10[+], CD19[+], and CD20[+]). Leukemic lymphoblasts with the L3 morphology usually have markers for mature B-cell ALL (CD10[+], CD19[+], CD20[+], CD22[+], CD25[+], and surface immunoglobulin). T-cell ALLs (15%–17% of all ALLs) will be positive for CD2, CD3, CD4, CD5, CD7, and CD8 and are associated with a poorer prognosis.

Cytogenetic studies from ALL lymphoblasts are used to classify ALL and are also used for assignment to a particular treatment risk group. Standard karyotype analysis frequently is complemented by molecular analysis of known predictive chromosomal abnormalities using fluorescence in situ hybridization. Both numerical and structural abnormalities of the chromosomes in ALL are associated with prognosis and influence selection of treatment:

- t(9;22) BCR/ABL translocation (Philadelphia chromosome) is present in 3%–4% of patients with ALL and often occurs in older children.
- t(1;19) E2A/PBX1 translocation in B-precursor ALL is present in about 5% of patients with ALL and is associated with an increased white blood cell (WBC) count.
- t(4;11) MLL/AF4 rearrangement is present in 5% of pediatric patients with ALL and 60% of infants with ALL.
- t(8;14) MYC/IGH translocation in mature B-cell ALL with FAB L3 morphology is present in 1% of patients with ALL.
- t(1;14) TAL1/TCR translocation is present in approximately 3% of patients with ALL and is associated with male sex, T-cell disease, and increased WBC count[15]

CLINICAL PRESENTATION

The onset of symptoms for the acute leukemias can be acute or insidious. Most symptoms result from expansion of the leukemic clone in the bone marrow and involvement of the peripheral blood and extramedullary sites such as lymph nodes, liver, spleen, and the central nervous system (CNS). Most children present with a short history of nonspecific symptoms such as fatigue, weakness, and fever.[6]

Intermittent fevers are common, due to either cytokine influence or leukopenia. Between 21% and 33% of patients experience bone pain, especially in the pelvis, vertebral bodies, and legs. This is usually due to leukemic involvement of the periosteum but may also be caused by aseptic osteonecrosis because of bone marrow involvement. The patient may limp or refuse to bear weight on a limb. Musculoskeletal pain may be mistaken for rheumatologic pain.[17,18]

Approximately 50% of children with ALL will present with lymphadenopathy, an indication of extramedullary leukemic spread. A good rule of thumb is that if a lymph node is bigger than 10 mm in its greatest dimension, it is considered to be enlarged. Epitrochlear nodes are considered enlarged if they are greater than 5 mm and inguinal nodes are enlarged if they are greater than 15 mm. These nodes will be nontender, firm, and rubbery and may have coalesced together and feel matted. Painless enlargement of the testes can also be a presenting sign of ALL.

Anemia, the most common presenting symptom, manifests as pallor, tiredness, and general fatigue. Patients with thrombocytopenia often present clinically with petechiae and ecchymosis. Neutropenic patients may be febrile and have signs and symptoms of infection.

The patient may have a completely normal physical examination or may have signs of bone marrow infiltration, including pallor, petechiae or purpura, hepatomegaly, or splenomegaly (present in more than 60% of patients). Lymphadenopathy, either localized or disseminated (cervical, axillary, and inguinal), is common. The testes may be unilaterally or bilaterally enlarged due to leukemic infiltration. Superior vena cava syndrome may be caused by mediastinal adenopathy compressing the superior vena cava. A prominent venous pattern may develop over the upper chest from collateral vein enlargement. The neck may feel full from venous engorgement, and there may be facial plethora as well as periorbital edema. If a mediastinal mass is present, tachypnea, orthopnea, and respiratory distress can result.[17,18]

Leukemic infiltration of cranial nerves can cause cranial nerve palsies with mild nuchal rigidity. The optic fundi may show exudates of leukemic infiltration and hemorrhage from thrombocytopenia. Anemia can cause a flow murmur, tachycardia, and, rarely, congestive heart failure. Bone and joint pain may be found on examination, particularly in the pelvis, lower spine, and femur.[17,18]

The distinction between ALL and AML generally requires at minimum a bone marrow biopsy and aspirate. In ALL, the bone marrow at diagnosis is usually hypercellular with normal hematopoiesis being replaced by leukemic blasts. For AML, the presence of greater than 20% blasts in the bone marrow is diagnostic.[13] In both AML and ALL, a lumbar puncture is performed to determine whether CNS leukemia is present.

PROGNOSTIC FACTORS
Acute Lymphocytic Leukemia
In children with ALL, clinical trials have identified several risk factors that correlate with outcome. Prognostic features identified include age, WBC count, cytogenetic abnormalities, ploidy, leukemic cell immunophenotype, and degree of initial response to therapy during induction. When these factors are combined, they predict groups of patients with varying degrees of risk for treatment failure.[17]

Infants as a whole do poorer than older children, but infants younger than 3 months have even a higher incidence of treatment failure. Again, this is thought to be due to the unique biology of the tumor. A large percentage of infants with ALL have a specific rearrangement of a gene at chromosome band 11q23, called the *MLL* gene. Infants who do not have this rearrangement have a better outcome.[20]

In children with B-precursor ALL, a higher WBC count at diagnosis portends an increased risk for treatment failure. The transition point appears to be a WBC count of 50,000/mm^3. The elevation of the WBC count is a surrogate marker for other high-risk prognostic factors, such as unfavorable chromosomal translocations t(4;11) and t(9;22).[21] The presence or absence of leukemic cells in the CNS obtained by lumbar puncture has prognostic significance as well. If performance of the lumbar puncture is traumatic, then the presence of blasts in the cerebrospinal fluid (CSF) specimen may be falsely positive, as some cells may have occurred in the blood because of trauma to the lumbar space. The presence of blasts in the CSF is associated with a high risk for relapse.[22]

Girls with ALL often have a better outcome than boys. One possible reason for the difference is the chance of relapse in the testes of boys. Furthermore, boys appear to have an increased risk for bone marrow and CNS relapse for unclear reasons.[23,24]

Survival rates differ with ethnicity. African American and Hispanic children have lower survival rates compared with Caucasian and Asian children. The explanation for this difference is not known.[25,26]

Finally, the rapidity of response to induction treatment has prognostic significance, reflecting the sensitivity of leukemic blasts to chemotherapy. Patients recognized as rapid early responders or slow early responders (based on the percentage of blasts present in bone marrow aspirates within 7–14 days after induction begins) have significantly different outcomes. Rapid responders have a higher cure rate than slow responders.

Acute Myelogenous Leukemia

The major prognostic factors in newly diagnosed AML are age, subtype (FAB M2), and chromosome status. Among children, male sex, platelet count less than $20,000/mm^3$, hepatomegaly, greater than 15% bone marrow blasts at day 14 of induction, and FAB subtype M5 are all associated with lower remission rates. The absence of these features and a normal chromosome 16 were associated with more favorable outcomes.[27]

TREATMENT GOALS

The primary objective in treating patients with acute leukemia is to achieve a complete remission. Remission is defined as the absence of all clinical evidence of disease with restoration of normal hematopoiesis. For both ALL and AML, remission induction is achieved with the use of highly myelosuppressive chemotherapy.

Treatment of Acute Lymphoblastic Leukemia

The treatment of acute leukemia, especially ALL, has improved over the past several years with the number of survivors increasing dramatically. Survival rates have increased as a result, with 5-year disease-free survival rates approaching 80%, largely due to the fact that 75%–80% of all children with newly diagnosed ALL are enrolled in a clinical trial designed by the Children's Oncology Group and approved by the National Cancer Institute. The treatment for ALL consists of three main elements: remission induction, intensification (consolidation), and continuation/maintenance phases of treatment. Therapy to eradicate subclinical CNS leukemia is also an integral part of therapy for ALL (Box 2–2).[7]

Specific prognostic features help determine the intensity of the treatment. Current treatment protocols for ALL in children emphasize risk-based therapy to reduce toxicity in patients with a low risk of relapse while ensuring appropriate, more aggressive therapy for those with a high risk of relapse. Criteria for risk stratification include WBC count, age at time of diagnosis, cytogenetics, immunophenotype, and response to induction therapy.[28–30]

Remission Induction. The primary objective of treatment is to eliminate all morphologic evidence of disease and restore normal hematopoiesis.[21] Induction consists of a standard three-drug regimen: a glucocorticoid (prednisone or dexamethasone), vincristine, and asparaginase or pegylated asparaginase. For patients with high-risk ALL, daunorubicin is added to the standard three-drug regimen.[17] Dexamethasone is now replacing prednisone in some standard-risk protocols because of its longer half-life and better CNS penetration. Even though dexamethasone possesses more favorable pharmacologic characteristics than prednisone, its use may be associated with more life-threatening infections and septic deaths than prednisone.[31]

Intensification (Consolidation). After completion of induction and restoration of morphologically normal hematopoiesis, patients begin intensification (consolidation) therapy. The goal of this phase is to administer dose-intensive chemotherapy to further reduce the burden of residual leukemic cells. In children, the intensity of the consolidation treatment is now determined not only by the child's initial risk classification but also by the rate of leukemic cytoreduction during induction. As a part of this intensification regimen, the Berlin-Frankfurt-Munster study group introduced a treatment element called *delayed intensification* (or reinduction) therapy. This therapy consists of a repetition of the initial remission induction therapy administered approximately

---

Box 2–2 Representative Chemotherapy for Pediatric Acute Lymphocytic Leukemia[5]

Induction (1 month)
Intrathecal cytarabine on day 0
Prednisone 40 mg/m^2 per day or dexamethasone 6 mg/m^2 per day orally for 28 days
Vincristine 1.5 mg/m^2 per dose (maximum 2 mg) IV weekly for 4 doses
Pegylated asparaginase 2500 units/m^2 IM for 1 dose of asparaginase 6000 units/m^2 per dose IM
Monday, Wednesday, and Friday for 6 doses
Intrathecal methotrexate weekly for 2–4 doses

Consolidation (1 month)
Mercaptopurine 50–75 mg/m^2 per dose PO at bedtime for 28 days
Vincristine 1.5 mg/m^2 per dose (maximum 2 mg) IV on day 0
Intrathecal methotrexate weekly for 1–3 doses

Delayed intensification (2 months)
Dexamethasone 10 mg/m^2 per day PO on days 0–6 and 14–20
Vincristine 1.5 mg/m^2 per dose (maximum 2 mg) IV weekly for 3 doses
Pegylated asparaginase 2500 units/m^2 per dose IM for 1 dose
Doxorubicin 25 mg/m^2 per dose IV on days 0, 7, and 14
Cyclophosphamide 1000mg/m^2 per dose IV on day 28
Thioguanine 60 mg/m^2 per dose orally at bedtime on days 28–41
Cytarabine 75 mg/m^2 per dose subcutaneous or IV on days 28–31 and 35–38
Intrathecal methotrexate on days 0 and 28

Maintenance (12-week cycles) lasting approximately 100 weeks
Methotrexate 20 mg/m^2 per dose orally at bedtime or IM weekly with dose escalation as tolerated
Mercaptopurine 75 mg/m^2 per dose PO at bedtime on days 0–83
Vincristine 1.5 mg/m^2 per dose (maximum 2 mg) IV on days 0, 28, and 56
Dexamethasone 6 mg/m^2 per day PO on days 0–4, 28–32, and 56–60
Intrathecal methotrexate on day 0

---

3 months after remission. Most institutions have now adopted this regimen, as it appears to improve long-term outcome.[32]

Continuation/Maintenance. The purpose of maintenance therapy is to further eliminate leukemic cells and produce a continuing complete remission. The two most important agents in maintenance chemotherapy are oral methotrexate and mercaptopurine. Improved survival has been associated with increasing mercaptopurine dosage to the limit of individual tolerance, based on absolute neutrophil count.[32] The addition of intermittent "pulses" of vincristine and a steroid (dexamethasone or prednisone) to the antimetabolite backbone improves outcome and is a part of most modern continuation regimens.[7,25,28–30,33]

Central Nervous System Prophylaxis

Effective treatment of CNS leukemia has made a remarkable impact on the overall survival for childhood ALL. The justification for CNS prophylaxis is based on two clinical findings. First, the CNS is a frequent sanctuary for leukemia, and undetectable leukemic cells are present in the CNS in many patients at the time of diagnosis. Second, many chemotherapeutic agents do not easily cross the blood-brain barrier.[5]

CNS prophylaxis typically includes intrathecal chemotherapy (methotrexate, cytarabine, and corticosteroids), systemic chemotherapy with dexamethasone and high-dose methotrexate, and/or the addition of craniospinal irradiation in selected high-risk patients. Even though craniospinal irradiation is the most effective modality, its use is associated with learning disabilities, neuroendocrine abnormalities, growth retardation, secondary brain tumors, and other complications. Thus, intrathecal drug therapy has largely replaced cranial irradiation for all except those patients with a very high risk of CNS relapse.[34]

Bone marrow transplantation (hematopoietic stem cell transplantation [HSCT]) is rarely used as the initial treatment for ALL. Patients whose blasts contain certain chromosomal abnormalities, such as t(9;22) or hypodiploidy (less than 44 chromosomes), and infants with t(4;11) may have a better cure rate with early HSCT from a matched sibling donor or a matched unrelated donor than with intensive chemotherapy alone. HSCT cures about 50% of patients who have relapses, provided that a second remission is achieved with chemotherapy before the transplant. Children who have a relapse more than 1 year after completion of chemotherapy (late relapse) may be cured with intensive chemotherapy without HSCT.[35-37]

A number of new biologic agents, including tyrosine kinase inhibitors and immunotoxins, are in various stages of research and development.[38]

Treatment of Acute Myelogenous Leukemia

As with ALL, the primary aim in treating patients with AML is to induce remission and thereafter prevent relapse. Treatment of AML is conventionally divided into two phases: remission induction and postremission therapy. Despite multiple strategies to increase the intensity of therapy over the past many years, the overall survival rate has reached a plateau of 50%–60%, suggesting that further intensification of conventional chemotherapy will not greatly improve survival rates.[34]

Remission Induction. The goal of induction chemotherapy in AML is essentially identical to that of ALL, that is, "empty" the bone marrow of all abnormal hematopoietic precursors to allow repopulation with normal cells. The combination of an anthracycline (daunorubicin, doxorubicin, or idarubicin) and the antimetabolite cytarabine forms the backbone of AML induction therapy. The most common induction regimen ("7+3") combines daunorubicin for 3 days with cytarabine on days 1–7.[5] Despite studies in which alternative anthracyclines were used, high-dose cytarabine was substituted for conventional-dose cytarabine, or etoposide and/or thioguanine was added, the 7+3 regimen remains the standard induction regimen (Box 2–3).

Postremission Therapy. Once an initial remission is achieved, further intensive therapy is imperative to prevent relapse. Induction therapy is inadequate, and many leukemia cells survive the initial treatment. At this point, there are three options available for patients: high-dose chemotherapy, allogeneic bone marrow transplantation from an HLA-matched related or unrelated donor, and autologous bone marrow transplantation.[34]

HODGKIN AND NON-HODGKIN LYMPHOMA

Lymphomas are a mixed group of diseases that arise from malignant transformation of immune cells that reside in lymphoid tissues.[39] This transformation distinguishes them from leukemias, which arise in bone marrow cells. Lymphomas are

---

Box 2–3 Representative Chemotherapy for Acute Myelogenous Leukemia[5,6]

Remission induction
Cytarabine 25 mg/m² IV every 6 hours for a total of 20 doses on days 1–5
Daunorubicin 30 mg/m² IV on day 1
Etoposide 150 mg/m² IV on days 1–4
Dexamethasone 2 mg/m² PO every 8 hours on days 1–4
6-Thioguanine 50 mg/m² every 12 hours on days 1–5

Postremission chemotherapy
Cytarabine 3000 mg/m² IV every 12 hours for 4 doses
Alternating with Cytarabine 100 mg/m² IV daily by continuous infusion for 5 days

the third most common cancer in children and adolescents in the United States, accounting for approximately 13% of newly diagnosed malignancies in this age group. Based on their differing histology and clinical and outcome features, lymphomas are classified generally as either Hodgkin or non-Hodgkin lymphomas (Table 2–6). Non-Hodgkin lymphomas (NHLs) account for approximately 60% of these diagnoses, and Hodgkin disease (HD) represents the remaining 40%.[40]

HODGKIN'S LYMPHOMA
Pathogenesis
Hodgkin lymphoma is a clonal malignant lymphoid disease of transformed lymphocytes. It is characterized by a variable number of characteristic multinucleated large lymphocytes called Reed-Sternberg cells. These cells are pathognomonic for the diagnosis and are usually detected in excisional lymph node biopsy specimen. A lymph node involved with HD contains only a small percentage (1%–2%) of Reed-Sternberg cells, along with normal reactive cells, inflammatory cells, and fibrosis.[39] Thus, an adequate surgical specimen and tedious pathologic review are necessary.

HD is subdivided into four histologic groups that are determined in part by the inflammatory milieu of the biopsy specimen. The groups are as follows:

1. Nodular sclerosing Hodgkin lymphoma. This histologic subtype represents approximately 80% of HD in older children and 45% in younger children. In this subtype, large collagenous bands divide the lymph node into nodules, and there is often a Reed-Sternberg cell variant called the lacunar cell identified in the biopsy specimen.[41]
2. Mixed cellularity Hodgkin lymphoma is more common in younger children than in adolescents (~35% versus 10%–20%). Pathologic evaluation of this biopsy specimen will show Reed-Sternberg cells in a background of an abundant number of reactive cells.[41]
3. Lymphocyte-rich classical Hodgkin lymphoma. This subtype can have a nodular appearance, but immunophenotype analysis distinguishes between the two groups. Patients with completely resected stage I lymphocyte-rich classical Hodgkin lymphomas still require chemotherapy with or without radiation therapy, compared with patients with stage I nodular lymphocyte-predominant Hodgkin lymphomas, who may be followed without postsurgical therapy.[41,42]
4. Nodular lymphocyte-predominant Hodgkin lymphoma. This subtype is characterized by large cells with multilobed nuclei often referred to as *popcorn cells.* It is most common in boys younger than 10 years of age. Children with this subtype are often asymptomatic, presenting with localized, nonbulky disease.[42,43]

Nodular sclerosing and mixed cellularity Hodgkin lymphomas are the most common subtypes in children.[44]

Incidence
There is a 4:1 male predominance in the first decade; this predominance slowly decreases as the pediatric population ages until adolescence when the male-to-female ratio approaches that of the adult population. In undeveloped countries, the peak incidence is seen in younger children. In the United States the risk of developing HD is increased in families with higher socioeconomic status and education and lower in large families.

Etiology
The etiology of Hodgkin lymphoma is uncertain. Several studies have suggested that exposure to an infectious agent might increase the risk for the childhood form of Hodgkin lymphoma. Patients infected with the Epstein-Barr virus (EBV) appear

Table 2–6 Histologic Classification of Lymphomas in Children and Adolescents

Major Histopathologic Categories	Category (Working Formulation)	Immunophenotype	Clinical Presentation	Chromosome Translocation	Genes Affected
Lymphoblastic lymphoma, precursor T/leukemia	Lymphoblastic convoluted and nonconvoluted	T cell Pre-B cell	Mediastinal, bone marrow Skin, bone	MTS1/p16ink4a deletion TAL1 t(1;14)(p34; q11), t(11;14)(p13;q11)	TAL1, TCRAO, RHOMB1, HOX11
Burkitt's and Burkitt's-like lymphomas	ML small noncleaved cell	Mature B cell	Intra-abdominal (sporadic) jaw (endemic) head and neck (nonjaw) (sporadic)	t(8;14)(q24 q32), t(2;8) (p11;q24), t(8;22)(q24; q11)	C-MYC, IGH, IGK, IGL
Diffuse large B-cell lymphoma	ML large cell	Mature B cell; maybe CD30+	Nodal; abdomen, bone, primary CNS, mediastinal	Not well characterized in children	
Anaplastic large cell lymphoma, systemic	ML immunoblastic or ML large	CD30+ (Ki-1+) T cell or null cell	Variable, but systemic symptoms often prominent	t(2;5)(p23;q35)	ALK, NMP
Anaplastic large cell lymphoma, cutaneous		CD30+ (Ki-1+ usually) T cell	Skin only; single or multiple lesions	Lacks t(2;5)	

ML, Malignant lymphoma.

to have an increased risk of developing Hodgkin lymphoma. Of note, the onset of Hodgkin lymphoma may occur several months to years after the initial exposure. The large proportion of patients with Hodgkin lymphoma who have high EBV antibody titers suggests that enhanced activation of EBV may precede the development of Hodgkin lymphoma.[45]

Clinical Presentation

Hodgkin lymphoma most commonly presents as painless lymphadenopathy, usually in the cervical area and/or mediastinum. Up to 40% of patients with Hodgkin lymphoma may have constitutional symptoms (also called *B symptoms*) including fever greater than 38° C, weight loss, and drenching night sweats.[39] These symptoms are considered unfavorable prognostic findings and are associated with more advanced disease.[44] *Bulky disease,* defined as a mass that is 10 cm in size or *large mediastinal adenopathy,* is also unfavorable. Involvement of extranodal tissues (lung, liver, and bone marrow) by direct extension from regional nodal disease is considered *E* (extranodal) disease.

An excisional biopsy of a suspicious lymph node should be performed for the initial diagnosis of Hodgkin lymphoma. Staging of HD determines treatment and prognosis. The most common staging system is the Ann Arbor classification system that describes the extent of disease as stages from I to IV and includes the presence or absence of constitutional symptoms.[46,47] It is used for both HD and NHL, although its prognostic value for NHLs is less than with in HD.[46,47] Stage I is involvement of a single lymph node, whereas stage IV involves more than one anatomic site on both sides of the diaphragm. Information about prognostic factors such as mediastinal mass, location of other bulky nodal disease, E disease, and the extent of subdiaphragmatic disease are also included in this staging system.[48]

Nearly half of all patients with HD will have asymptomatic mediastinal disease, either adenopathy or an anterior mediastinal mass. If left unattended, symptoms due to compression of vital structures in the thorax may occur. A chest radiograph should be obtained when lymphoma is being considered. Splenomegaly or hepatomegaly may also be present and has been associated with advanced disease.[49]

Evaluation of disease should also include a physical examination of all lymph node regions, a chest radiograph, a computed tomographic scan of the chest/abdomen/pelvis and nuclear imaging (gallium scans or positive emission tomography), bone scans, and bone marrow biopsy to determine the extent of disease.[44]

Prognosis

Prognostic factors for HD are less well delineated than those for other malignancies, but codependent factors, such as disease stage, bulk of tumor, and biologic aggressiveness appear to be important and will influence treatment strategies. Histology, male sex, and B symptoms were poor prognostic indicators in one study. In another study male sex, stage IIB, IIIB, or IV disease, WBC count 11,500/mm^3 or higher, and hemoglobin lower than 11.0 g/dL were significant for poorer prognosis. Yet, in a third study, the combination of B symptoms and bulky disease was linked with an inferior outcome.[50–52]

Some general observations about prognosis can be made. Current treatment regimens give children with stage I and II HD at least a 90% disease-free survival 5 years after diagnosis. Because two thirds of all relapses occur within 2 years after diagnosis, and because relapse rarely occurs beyond 4 years, 5-year disease-free survival generally equates with cure. In more advanced disease (stages III and IV), 5-year event-free survival rates range from more than 60% to 90%. With more patients being long-term survivors, the risk of secondary malignancies, including both leukemias and sold tumors, is becoming more apparent. The type of tumor depends on the treatments used, but the risk is clearly greatest among those who are younger at diagnosis. Therefore, elucidating the optimal treatment strategy that minimizes such risk should be the goal of future studies.

Treatment of relapsed HD is usually successful and involves radiation therapy in combination with chemotherapy. Autologous or allogeneic HSCT may be an alternative and may improve survival rates.[50-52]

Treatment

In an attempt to minimize late effects, the treatment scheme for Hodgkin lymphoma is divided in to three categories: early favorable, early unfavorable (intermediate), and advanced stage.[48] The standard of care for the majority of children and adolescents with Hodgkin lymphoma is risk-adapted, combined-modality therapy using low-dose, involved-field radiation in combination with multiagent chemotherapy.[45] The basic thesis of this approach is the use of chemotherapy to minimize exposure to radiation, which causes more long-term complications in children.

For patients with early-stage favorable disease, a short duration of chemotherapy of two to four cycles with agents such as Adriamycin (doxorubicin), bleomycin, vinblastine, and dacarbazine (ABVD) plus involved-field radiation is the current approach.[48] Another less commonly used regimen includes mechlorethamine (nitrogen mustard), Oncovin (vincristine), procarbazine, and prednisone (MOPP).

For patients with unfavorable disease, derivative combinations of MOPP and ABVD have been used. Because of the myelosuppressive effects of mechlorethamine, COPP (replacing mechlorethamine with cyclophosphamide) has more recently replaced MOPP. Etoposide has also been added to improve treatment response and reduce the cumulative doses of alkylating and anthracycline chemotherapy.[45] However, the increasing risks of secondary leukemias in patients with Hodgkin lymphoma have tempered the use of this agent except for the patients with the highest stage disease.

Overall survival for pediatric Hodgkin lymphoma is currently about 90%. Of note, the risk of death from failure of treatment is similar to that from other causes, particularly late effects of therapy (refer to section on late effects).[44] Using combined chemotherapy with lower dose, limited-field radiation provides disease control without significant adverse effects. The main challenge in the future will be to develop strategies that decrease late morbidity and mortality but retain the same efficacy of current therapy (Table 2–7 and Box 2–4).[48]

NON-HODGKIN LYMPHOMA

Childhood NHLs are a group of diseases originating in the cells and organs of the immune system as in Hodgkin lymphoma.[53] The three different histologic subtypes of NHL are Burkitt's lymphoma (BL), lymphoblastic lymphoma (LL), and large-cell lymphoma.[45,54] The difference between lymphoblastic lymphoma and acute lymphoblastic leukemia relates to marrow disease (i.e., there is greater than 25% marrow involvement in leukemia).

Incidence

NHLs are a diverse group of cancers accounting for 5%–10% of malignancies in children younger than age 15 (about 500 new cases per year in the United States). The incidence of NHL increases with age. Children aged 15 or younger account for only 3% of all cases of NHL; it is uncommon before the age of 3 years. The median age at presentation is 10 years. There is a male predominance of about 3:1.

Table 2-7 Treatment of Pediatric Hodgkin's Disease

ABVD	Doxorubicin (Adriamycin), bleomycin, vinblastine, dacarbazine
ABVE (DBVE)	Doxorubicin (Adriamycin), bleomycin, vincristine, etoposide
VAMP	Vincristine, doxorubicin (Adriamycin), methotrexate, prednisone
OPPA +/− COPP (females)	Vincristine (Oncovin), prednisone, procarbazine, doxorubicin (Adriamycin), cyclophosphamide, vincristine (Oncovin), prednisone, procarbazine
OEPA +/− COPP (males)	Vincristine (Oncovin), etoposide, prednisone, doxorubicin (Adriamycin), cyclophosphamide, vincristine (Oncovin), prednisone, procarbazine
COPP/ABV	Cyclophosphamide, vincristine (Oncovin), prednisone, procarbazine, doxorubicin (Adriamycin), bleomycin, vinblastine
BEACOPP (advanced stage)	Bleomycin, etoposide, doxorubicin (Adriamycin), cyclophosphamide, vincristine (Oncovin), prednisone, procarbazine
COPP	Cyclophosphamide, vincristine (Oncovin), prednisone, procarbazine
CHOP	Cyclophosphamide, doxorubicin (Adriamycin), vincristine (Oncovin), prednisone
ABVE-PC (DBVE-PC)	Doxorubicin (Adriamycin), bleomycin, vincristine, etoposide, prednisone, cyclophosphamide

---

Box 2-4 Representative Regimen for Hodgkin Lymphoma[45]

Stages II, III, and IV

ABVD
Adriamycin (doxorubicin) 25 mg/m² IV on days 1 and 15
Bleomycin 10 units/m² IV on days 1 and 15
Vinblastine 6 mg/m² IV on days 1 and 15
Dacarbazine 375 mg/m² IV on days 1 and 15

MOPP
Mechlorethamine 6 mg/m² IV on days 1 and 8
Oncovin (vincristine) 1.4 mg/m² IV on days 1 and 8
Procarbazine 100 mg/m² orally on days 1–15
Prednisone 40 mg/m² on days 1–15

COPP
Cyclophosphamide substituted for mechlorethamine
Cyclophosphamide 600 mg/m² IV on days 1 and 8

It is twice as common in Caucasians as in African Americans. In equatorial Africa, NHL accounts for almost 50% of pediatric malignancies.[55]

Staging
In the adult population, the Ann Arbor staging system is used most frequently; however, staging of childhood NHL usually follows the St. Jude Children's Research Hospital scheme. Stage I disease involves a single lymph node. Stage II involves two or more lymph nodes on the same side of the diaphragm. Stage III involves lymph nodes on both sides of the diaphragm. Stage IV is characterized by diffuse involvement of one or more extranodal sites, including the bone marrow or liver, and CNS disease.[56] The main prognostic factor for patients with NHL is tumor burden at presentation.[57]

Etiology
In most cases of NHL, the etiology is not apparent, and the disease may be "spontaneous." Known predisposing conditions include immunodeficiency, autoimmune disorders, AIDS, and post-transplant lymphoproliferative disorders.[53] Infectious agents, such as EBV, may also play a role in the development of NHL, but the association is less apparent than in Hodgkin lymphoma.

Children with congenital or acquired immune deficiencies (Wiskott-Aldrich syndrome, severe combined immunodeficiency syndrome, X-linked lymphoproliferative syndrome, HIV infection, and immunosuppressive therapy after solid organ or marrow transplantation) have an increased risk of developing NHL. It has been estimated that their risk is 100–10,000 times that of age-matched control subjects.[55]

The majority of children who develop NHL are immunologically intact. Some animal data suggest a viral contribution to the pathogenesis of NHL, and there is evidence of viral involvement in human NHL as well. In equatorial Africa, 95% of BLs contain DNA from the EBV, but in North America, less than 20% of BLs contain the EBV genome. The role of other viruses, such as human herpes viruses 6 and 8, disturbances in host immunologic defenses, chronic immunostimulation, and specific chromosomal rearrangements are under investigation as potential triggers in the development of NHL.[55]

Clinical Presentation

There is wide overlap between the clinical presentation of Hodgkin lymphoma and NHL; both involve the same nodal structures, liver, and spleen as well as the mediastinum. For NHL, there are some characteristic presentations that include BL and T-cell NHL.

BL typically presents with a rapidly enlarging abdominal tumor, pain, and changes in bowel habits. Patients with BL, in particular, have a risk for tumor lysis syndrome on initiation of chemotherapy, because of the high sensitivity of tumor to conventional chemotherapy.[56]

Patients with T-lymphoblastic NHL often present with a mediastinal mass commonly associated with a pleural effusion. These patients generally seek medical attention because of severe respiratory distress resulting from airway compression.[40]

Other NHLs present predominantly with peripheral adenopathy and a variety of other organ involvement, which may be distinct from B-cell and T-cell NHL or may, in fact, resemble either of these. Final diagnosis in this multifaceted group of diseases is determined by histology and immunophenotyping.

Prognosis

The major predictors of outcome in pediatric NHL are the treatment protocols used, tumor burden as evidenced by the stage of disease at presentation, and the serum lactate dehydrogenase (LDH) concentration. Of patients with limited stage disease, 85%–95% can expect long-term, disease-free survival. Patients with disease on both sides of the diaphragm, with CNS disease, or with bone marrow involvement in addition to a primary site have a 70%–80% 5-year disease-free survival rate, depending on the treatment protocol used. Relapses occur early in NHL; patients with LL rarely have recurrences after 30 months from diagnosis. Dramatic improvement in survival has been observed in advanced stage BL and Burkitt-like lymphoma (BLL). The addition of cyclophosphamide to the treatment protocols for BL and BLL has resulted in a 75% event-free survival. It is very uncommon for patients with BL or BLL to experience a recurrence beyond 1 year. Patients who do have a relapse may have a chance for cure with the use of autologous or allogeneic HSCT.[58]

Treatment

The main treatment for childhood NHL is combination chemotherapy. Surgery and radiation therapy have minor roles in the treatment scheme, because of the often widespread and systemic nature of the disease.[58]

Most of the regimens designed for the treatment of LL were originally adapted from therapies for the management of ALL.[58] However, these regimens have been modified to become high-intensity short-duration regimens, which lead to improved outcomes. Patients with LL require a longer treatment duration compared with patients with B-cell or large-cell lymphoma. The two most effective protocols are the Berlin-Frankfurt-Munster protocol and a modified version of the LSA_2L_2 protocol (initially used at Memorial Sloan-Kettering Cancer Center in New York), in which high-dose methotrexate is included. These protocols usually combine cyclophosphamide, vincristine, prednisone, doxorubicin, and methotrexate. For patients with more extensive disease, higher-dose methotrexate ($5–8$ g/m^2) and high-dose cytarabine are used. CNS prophylaxis is an essential component in the therapy for lymphomas. Chemotherapy is given over an extended period (12–32 months) during all three phases of treatment including induction, consolidation, and maintenance.[58]

The primary treatment of BL consists of short duration (6 months), intensive alkylating agent therapy (cyclophosphamide) in addition to other agents that are active in lymphomas (intermediate- or high-dose methotrexate, vincristine, anthracyclines, etoposide, and cytarabine).[56] L-Asparaginase has also been incorporated into several successful regimens.[58]

The most common regimen used in large-cell lymphoma is cyclophosphamide, doxorubicin, vincristine, and prednisone (CHOP). The therapy may differ with respect to tumor cell immunophenotype.[58]

Despite dramatic improvements in the treatment of childhood NHL, approximately 20%–30% of patients do not achieve either a complete remission and relapse.[59] Refinement of risk-adapted therapies that minimize long-term adverse effects remains a challenge.

A novel approach for the treatment of NHL incorporates monoclonal antibodies that target specific cell surface lymphoma antigens. Rituximab, an anti-CD20$^+$ monoclonal antibody, along with conventional chemotherapy is being used against CD20$^+$ B-cell NHL This agent has already proven to be effective in the adult population (Box 2–5).[58]

COMMON SOLID TUMORS

CENTRAL NERVOUS SYSTEM TUMORS[60]

CNS tumors are the most common solid tumor in childhood, representing greater than 20% of all pediatric tumors in children younger than 14 years of age and accounting for 26% of all deaths. In the last 15 years, the incidence of pediatric CNS

Box 2–5 Representative Regimen for Non-Hodgkin's Lymphoma[58]

B-Cell Lymphoma (COPAD)
Cyclophosphamide 375 mg/m^2 IV daily on days 1–3
Vincristine (Oncovin) 2 mg/m^2 IV × 1 dose
Prednisone 60 mg/m^2/day divided twice daily PO for 5 days
Adriamycin (Doxorubicin) 60 mg/m^2 IV × 1 dose on day 1

Large-Cell Lymphoma (CHOP)
Cyclophosphamide 750 mg/m^2 IV × 1 dose
Hydroxydaunorubicin (doxorubicin) 50 mg/m^2 IV × 1 dose
Vincristine 1.4 mg/m^2 (maximum 2 mg) IV × 1 dose
Prednisone 100 mg by mouth on days 1–5
Duration varies according to stage

Table 2–8 Childhood Brain Tumors

Tumor	Aged 0–14 (%)	Aged 15–19 (%)
Gliomas (glioblastomas, astrocytoma)	57	46
PNET/medulloblastoma	18.7	7.3
Pituitary	0.7	10.4
Germ cell tumor	3.5	6.8
All others	27.9	33.5

tumors appears to have increased. This is probably due to improvements in detection and radiographic imaging.

Of pediatric CNS tumors, 20% are located in the spinal cord and 80% are in the brain. Of those located in the brain, 50% arise in the posterior fossa and 50% in the supratentorial compartment (Table 2–8). Tumors that are common in adults, such as meningiomas, pituitary tumors, and metastatic tumors, are rare in children. The most common brain tumors in children are gliomas.

Many improvements in survival in childhood cancer have been attributed to clinical trials that are designed to compare new therapy with standard therapy.[61–63] Advances in imaging, surgery, and adjunctive therapies have also led to longer survival for children with brain tumors. Unfortunately, these treatments have long-term sequelae that can ultimately affect neurologic function and quality of life.[61]

Classification

CNS tumors are classified primarily by both their histology and location. As with leukemias, immunohistochemical analysis and cytogenetic and molecular genetic findings are increasingly being used for more precise diagnosis and classification. The distribution and tumor types in children differ greatly from those in adults.[61]

Approximately 60% of CNS tumors in children are infratentorial with most being located in the cerebellum or the adjacent fourth ventricle. Examples of these tumors include cerebellar, astrocytoma, and medulloblastoma. Supratentorial tumors, located in the cerebral hemispheres, comprise approximately 30% to 40% of childhood brain tumors and include low- and high-grade gliomas.

Most childhood brain tumors can be divided into two categories according to the cell of origin: glial tumors, such as astrocytomas, and ependymomas (nonglial tumors), such as medulloblastomas and other primitive neuroectodermal tumors (PNETs). Some tumors may contain both glial and neural elements (e.g., ganglioma), and there is also a group of brain tumors that do not fit either classification (i.e., craniopharyngiomas, germ cell tumors, choroid plexus tumors, and meningiomas). Furthermore, low-grade and high-grade versions of tumors are found in most categories.[61–63]

Clinical Presentation

The signs and symptoms of CNS tumors in children depend more on their age, level of development, and location than on tumor type or histology. Obstruction of CSF flow and resultant increased intracranial pressure (ICP) are among the earliest clinical manifestations of CNS tumors. Thus, the classic triad of signs and symptoms of increased ICP (morning headaches, vomiting without nausea, and papilledema) is present in less than 30% of children at diagnosis. Other indicators of increased ICP, such as increasing head circumference, cranial nerve palsies, dysarthria, ataxia, hemiplegia, hyperreflexia, macroencephaly and the cracked pot sign, have all been reported in children with CNS tumors. The onset and progression of these symptoms are generally slow and advance as the obstruction and pressure increases. Other signs and symptoms include altered gait, visual disturbances, and poor balance.[62,63] Seizures will eventually develop in more than 50% of patients with CNS tumors. Personality changes, blurred vision, diplopia, weakness, decreased coordination, and precocious puberty may also be seen. Poor performance in school and personality changes are common in older children, whereas irritability, failure to thrive, and delayed development are common in very young children. Development of head tilt (torticollis) may be due to a posterior fossa tumor.[61–63]

Clinical findings at presentation vary, depending on the child's age and the tumor's location. Children younger than 2 years of age are more likely to develop infratentorial tumors, usually presenting with nonspecific symptoms such as vomiting, unsteadiness, lethargy, and irritability. There may be few objective signs of the disease. Macrocephaly, ataxia, hyperreflexia, and cranial nerve palsies are some signs that may be present. Papilledema, which is generally a reliable sign of increased ICP, may not be seen in young children because the head can expand. Instead, measuring head circumference and observing gait are essential in evaluating a child for a possible brain tumor. Eye findings and apparent visual disturbances such as difficulty tracking objects can occur in association with optic pathway tumors such as optic glioma.[61–63]

Astrocytoma is the most common brain tumor of childhood; nearly all are low-grade and are found in the posterior fossa. In the majority of children, they are cured by complete resection alone. Medulloblastoma and related PNETs are the most common high-grade brain tumors in children. These usually occur in the first decade of life, with a peak incidence between ages 5 and 10 years, with a male-to-female ratio of 1.3:2.1. Brainstem tumors are the third most common tumors and usually high grade. For brainstem tumors that diffusely infiltrate the brainstem and mainly involve the pons, the chance of long-term survival is less than 15%. The outcome with brainstem tumors that occur above or below the pons and grow in an eccentric or cystic manner is somewhat better. Exophytic tumors in this location may be surgically excised.[61–63]

Older children more commonly have supratentorial tumors, which are associated with headache, visual symptoms, seizures, and focal neurologic deficits. Unfortunately, initial presenting features are often nonspecific. Again poor performance in school and personality changes are common. Upon questioning, these children may describe vague visual disturbances. Although headaches are also common, they usually do not occur during morning hours and may be confused with migraine.[61,62]

Older children with infratentorial tumors characteristically present with signs and symptoms of hydrocephalus, including worsening morning headache, vomiting, gait unsteadiness, double vision, and papilledema. Slowly enlarging tumors, such as cerebellar astrocytomas can have symptoms that worsen over several months. Morning vomiting may be the only symptom of posterior fossa ependymomas, which often originate in the floor of the fourth ventricle near the vomiting center. Children with brainstem tumors may present with facial and extraocular muscle palsies, ataxia, and hemiparesis; hydrocephalus occurs in approximately 25% of these patients at diagnosis.[61,62]

Prognosis

Despite improvements in surgery, chemotherapy, and radiation therapy, the outlook for cure remains poor for children with high-grade glial tumors. The extent of surgical resection appears to correlate positively with prognosis, with a 3-year progression-free survival rate of 17% for patients undergoing biopsy only, 29%–32% for patients undergoing partial or subtotal resections, and 54% for those having 90% of their tumor resected.

An early Children's Cancer Group study showed a 45% progression-free survival rate for children who received radiation therapy and chemotherapy. A follow-up Children's Cancer Group study in which all patients had chemotherapy and radiation therapy showed a 5-year progression-free survival rate of 36%. Effective salvage therapy has also been achieved with high-dose chemotherapy for those who have a relapse.

Biologic factors that may affect survival are being increasingly identified. The prognosis for diffuse pontine gliomas remains very poor, with no benefit obtained from the addition of high-dose chemotherapy to radiation treatment.[61–63]

Treatment

The three treatment modalities for pediatric CNS tumors are surgery, chemotherapy, and radiation therapy. The goal of treatment is to eradicate the most tumor with the least amount of morbidity. Long-term neuropsychologic morbidity is an especially important issue as it relates to deficits caused by the tumor itself and/or the sequelae of treatment.

Surgery is the mainstay of therapy for most CNS tumors in children; it reduces the tumor burden and provides tissue for histologic diagnosis. Effective surgery is always a balance between maximal tumor resection and the preservation of vital structures and function.[61]

New techniques have improved the precision of surgery and may decrease complications and improve outcome. These advances include the use of the operating microscope, the ultrasonic tissue aspirator, and the CO_2 laser (although this is less commonly used in pediatric brain tumor surgery); the accuracy of computerized stereotactic resection and the availability of intraoperative monitoring techniques such as evoked potentials and electrocorticography have increased the feasibility and safety of surgical resection of many pediatric brain tumors. Second-look surgery after chemotherapy is increasingly being used when tumors are incompletely resected at the time of the initial surgery.[61–63]

Before surgery, dexamethasone is started (0.5–1 mg/kg initially, then 0.25–0.5 mg/kg/day in four divided doses). Anticonvulsants are also started if the child has had a seizure of if the surgical approach is likely to induce seizures.[61,62]

A variety of conventional chemotherapy regimens may be used after surgery for further reduction in tumor size (Box 2–6). For children with unresectable low-grade astrocytomas, vincristine and carboplatin are used. Children with more aggressive tumors may receive both high-dose chemotherapy and radiation. High-dose chemotherapy with concurrent autologous bone marrow or peripheral blood stem cell reconstitution is being used in selected patients, but this approach is still considered experimental.[61]

Radiation therapy for brain tumors has evolved considerably over the past decade. More precise techniques diminish radiation exposure to uninvolved adjacent tissue, thus reducing toxicity. For tumors with a high probability of neuraxis dissemination, as is the case with medulloblastoma, craniospinal radiation (CSI) is still

---

Box 2–6 Representative Chemotherapy Regimen for Central Nervous System Tumors[61]

Vincristine 1.5 mg/m^2 (maximum 2 mg) IV push
Carboplatin 560 mg/m^2 IV × 1 day only
May repeat above cycles every 3–4 weeks

the standard therapy in children older than 3 years of age. In other tumors, CSI has been abandoned because neuraxis dissemination at the first relapse is rare. The major limitations of radiation include altered growth and neurocognitive deficits.[7,62]

NEUROBLASTOMA

NEUROBLASTOMA, the most common extracranial solid tumor in childhood, accounts for 8%–10% of all cancers in children.[64] It originates from neural crest cells in the sympathetic nervous system, which extends from the base of the neck to the tailbone. Pathologic diagnosis is not always easy, and neuroblastoma must be differentiated from other "small, round, blue cell" malignancies of childhood, such as Ewing's sarcoma, rhabdomyosarcoma, peripheral PNET, and lymphoma. Of the diagnoses of neuroblastoma, 50% are before the age of 2 years and 90% are before the age of 5 years.[1,64]

Neuroblastoma is an interesting, biologically diverse disease. Spontaneous remissions in infants with stage 4S disease and spontaneous or induced differentiation to a benign neoplasm have been reported. Unfortunately, neuroblastoma can also be an extremely malignant neoplasm. The overall survival rate in advanced disease has changed little in 20 years despite significant advances in our understanding of this tumor at the molecular level.[64] These tumors most often arise in or near the adrenal glands in the abdomen or pelvis. Of these tumors, 70% are metastatic at diagnosis.[5]

Incidence

In the United States, the annual incidence is about 8 new cases per 1 million per year. This translates to about 600 newly diagnosed neuroblastomas annually. The median age of diagnosis is 2 years of age, and approximately 40% of neuroblastoma are diagnosed in children younger than 1 year of age. Few neuroblastomas are diagnosed after 5 years of age.

Clinical Presentation

The presenting signs and symptoms of neuroblastoma in children reflect both the location of the primary tumor and the extent of disease. Patients with localized disease are often relatively asymptomatic, whereas children with metastatic disease appear ill with systemic symptoms such as weight loss, bone pain, and fever. Although most children have a primary abdominal tumor, neuroblastoma can arise from wherever there is sympathetic tissue. Common manifestations include a hard painless mass in the neck, a localized intrathoracic mass found incidentally on a chest radiograph, or a palpable abdominal mass. The most common sites of metastasis are lymph nodes, bone marrow, orbit, liver, bones, skin, and skull. Liver metastasis can be massive, particularly in the newborn. Subcutaneous nodules may be present. On examination they are bluish in color, and when compressed there will be an erythematous flush followed by blanching that is thought to be due to secondary catecholamine release.[64]

Unusual paraneoplastic manifestations are occasionally seen in patients with neuroblastoma. These include chronic watery diarrhea associated with tumor secretion of vasoactive intestinal peptides and opsoclonus-myoclonus (dancing eyes-dancing feet syndrome). It has been suggested that the neurologic syndromes are due to cross-reacting antibodies. These manifestations may persist after therapy.[64]

Approximately 60% of children with neuroblastoma will be anemic due to either chronic disease or marrow infiltration. Thrombocytopenia may also be present. Thrombocytosis is more common than thrombocytopenia; either may have marrow involvement. Urinary catecholamine (vanillylmandelic acid or homovanillic acid) levels are elevated in as many as 90% of patients at diagnosis and should be measured before surgery. Elevated ferritin and LDH levels at diagnosis appear to be of prognostic value when combined with age, stage, and tumor histology.[64,65]

Prognostic Factors

As with most malignancies, the stage of disease at presentation is the most important prognostic factor in neuroblastoma. Several staging systems exist, but all staging is based on the International Neuroblastoma Staging System (INSS). The patient's age and certain biologic features are also used to classify patients into one of three groups: low-risk, intermediate-risk, or high-risk.[66] Infants younger than 1 year of age have markedly better disease-free survival rates than older children with comparable stages of disease and thus are classified separately.

Molecular parameters are essential to supplement clinical staging and aid in treatment planning. Amplification of the *MYCN* proto-oncogene or its gene product can be detected in approximately 20% of patients with neuroblastoma. Either is a reliable marker of aggressive clinical behavior with rapid disease progression. Tumor cell DNA content is also predictive of outcome; diploidy is associated with poor outcome. Common cytogenetic abnormalities associated with high-risk features and adverse outcome include deletion of the short arm of chromosome 1 and gains of 17q genetic material.[64,65]

Treatment

Surgery plays an important role in the management of neuroblastoma for diagnosis, staging, and treatment. The goal is total resection of visible tumor, although tumors are often too large or have invaded vital organs in ways that make complete resection difficult or impossible. In these situations, limited surgery followed by aggressive chemotherapy may allow a delayed, safer surgical resection. In patients with widely metastatic disease, the role of surgery is more to provide diagnostic tissue than tumor debulking; metastatic disease is not resectable.

Low-risk patients with neuroblastoma require minimal treatment. For patients with completely resectable tumors, no further therapy is warranted after surgery. Overall survival for these patients is approximately 90% at 5 years.[64]

Chemotherapy is an important treatment modality for most children with neuroblastoma. Patients with stage III and IV disease and even patients with stage II disease benefit, even though they may have had an apparent gross total resection of tumor (Box 2–7).

These low- and intermediate-risk patients with favorable biologic characteristics are treated with a short course of chemotherapy. In contrast, intermediate-risk patients with unfavorable biologic characteristics and patients with higher-stage tumors receive more prolonged and aggressive chemotherapy.

Box 2–7 Representative Chemotherapy Regimens for Neuroblastoma[62]

Doses may vary according to institution or protocol

Alternating cycles of:
1. Vincristine 1.5 mg/m^2 IV on day 1
   Adriamycin 37.5 mg/m^2 IV on days 1 and 2
   Cyclophosphamide 2100 mg/m^2/day on days 1 and 2
2. Cisplatin 40 mg/m^2 IV daily for 5 days
   Etoposide 100 mg/m^2 IV daily for 5 days

The goal of therapy in high-risk patients is to deliver intensive doses of combination chemotherapy with short intervals between cycles.[67] Current chemotherapeutic regimens include a combination of cyclophosphamide and doxorubicin or cisplatin and etoposide. Some institutions are using stem cell rescue in an effort to further dose intensify the consolidation therapy. Unfortunately, despite intensive interventions, more than 50% of children with high-risk disease still have relapses. In an effort to treat chemotherapy-resistant tumor cells, the differentiation agent 13-*cis*-retinoic acid has been given to high-risk patients after completion of consolidation chemotherapy.[67]

OSTEOSARCOMA

Osteosarcomas are primary malignant tumors of bone that are characterized by the production of osteoid or immature bone by the malignant cells. Osteosarcoma is the most common bone tumor and, among solid tumors, is the fifth most common tumor in children and adolescents. Approximately 400 cases (children and young adults) are diagnosed each year in the United States.[68,69]

Survival of children with malignant bone sarcomas has improved dramatically over the past 30 years, largely as a result of chemotherapeutic advances. Before the era of neoadjuvant chemotherapy, 80% to 90% of patients with osteosarcoma died of their disease, because they developed metastatic disease despite achievement of local control of the tumor. This phenomenon led to the belief that the majority of patients with osteosarcoma had subclinical metastatic disease that was present at the time of diagnosis, without evidence of overt metastases. This was eventually proven to be the case.[68,69]

Incidence and Etiology

Osteosarcoma accounts for only 2.6% of all pediatric malignancies, and the incidence is slightly higher in boys.[70] Most osteosarcomas occur during the first two decades of life, a period characterized by rapid skeletal growth.

The etiology of osteosarcoma is unknown, although rapid bone growth was one of the first associated factors identified. Osteosarcoma, with its peak incidence during the pubertal growth spurt, occurs at the time of maximal expansion of bone. The most common sites of origin are the metaphyses of long bones.[68] These data have led to speculation that bone tumors arise from an aberration of the normal process of bone growth and remodeling at a time when rapidly proliferating cells are particularly susceptible to oncogenic agents, mitotic errors, or other events leading to neoplastic transformation.[1,71]

Various environmental agents have been implicated in causing osteosarcoma, but only ionizing radiation has a well-documented effect. Genetics may also play a role in the development of osteosarcoma. Patients with hereditary retinoblastoma and the Li-Fraumeni familial cancer syndrome have a predisposition to development of osteosarcoma.[70,71]

In children with a solid tumor who receive radiation therapy as part of their treatment regimen, the most frequently diagnosed secondary malignancy is osteosarcoma.[72] Early estimates suggested that approximately 3% of osteosarcomas could be attributed to prior irradiation. However, it is hypothesized that as survival rates improve and patients live long enough after their primary radiotherapy, a higher incidence is likely to be revealed. The interval between the initial radiotherapy irradiation and the appearance of a secondary osteosarcoma ranges from 4 to more than 40 years, with the average being 12–16 years.[72]

Prior exposure to chemotherapy, especially to alkylating agents, is also associated with secondary osteosarcomas and may even potentiate the effect of previous radiation. The risk of a secondary bone cancer is predominantly related to alkylating agents and appears to be dose dependent. At least one report suggested that treatment with anthracyclines may shorten the interval to development of a secondary bone tumor.[72]

Clinical Presentation

The most common sites of osteosarcoma in children are the femur, tibia, and humerus. Pain is perhaps the most frequent presenting symptom. Patients often relate the pain to a recent traumatic event. Systemic symptoms such as fever, weight loss, and malaise are generally absent. The most important finding on physical examination is a soft tissue mass, which is frequently large and tender to palpation. Osteosarcomas have a predilection for the metaphyseal region of the long bones. Swelling around the bone and even a pathologic fracture are not uncommon.[71,73]

At the time of presentation, 10%–20% of patients will have demonstrable overt micrometastatic disease. Distant metastases most commonly involve the lungs, but can also involve the bone.

Prognostic Factors

The most important adverse prognostic factor in osteosarcoma is the presence of metastatic disease. Approximately 15%–20% of patients with newly diagnosed osteosarcoma have metastases detectable on the initial imaging studies. The most common site of metastases is the lung. Tumor location is also associated with prognosis. Children with primary tumors of the tibia and distal femur appear to have a more favorable outcome than those with axial primary tumors. The percentage of tumor necrosis after preoperative chemotherapy is the most consistent and important factor associated with outcome in patients with localized osteosarcoma. Patients who have less than 90% of tumor necrosis after the initial induction period are considered poor responders and have a worse prognosis.[70]

Treatment

Chemotherapy. Over the last 30 years, the recognition of the importance of adjuvant chemotherapy has allowed 70% of patients with osteosarcoma to be cured of their disease. Chemotherapy is an essential part of treatment for osteosarcoma. Chemotherapy is responsible for higher survival rates, and it has also been shown to decrease the number of pulmonary nodules (Box 2–8).[68]

Standard regimens now include both neoadjuvant (preoperative) and adjuvant (postoperative) chemotherapy. The role of neoadjuvant chemotherapy is to induce maximal tumor necrosis and to help facilitate surgical resection. Drugs that have

---

Box 2–8 Representative Chemotherapy Regimens for Osteosarcoma[66–68,70]

Doses may vary according to institution or protocol

Alternating cycles of:
1. Cisplatin 120 mg/m^2/day IV on day 1
   Doxorubicin 75 mg/m^2/day continuous infusion over 72 hours (25 mg/m^2/day)
2. Methotrexate 12 g/m^2 IV over 4 hours with leucovorin rescue
3. Ifosfamide 1.8 g/m^2/day IV daily for 5 days
   Doxorubicin 37.5 mg/m^2 IV daily on days 1 and 2

been successful against osteosarcoma include doxorubicin, cisplatin, ifosfamide (with mesna), and high-dose methotrexate with leucovorin rescue.

For the 20% of patients who present with metastatic disease, the prognosis and outcome are very poor. Treatment consists of very aggressive chemotherapy with resection of both the primary tumor and metastatic lesions. The success of this treatment obviously depends on the size and number of the nodules. Patients with multiple small lesions are not good candidates. Recent reports suggest overexpression of HER2/erbB-2 in some patients with osteosarcoma. Interestingly, HER2/erb-2 is the same marker for an oncogene that is also common in some patients with breast cancer. Thus, the use of anti-HER2 monoclonal antibodies may be an effective strategy for this group of high-risk patients.[12]

Surgery and Radiation Therapy. Definitive cure requires en bloc surgical resection of the tumor with a margin of uninvolved tissue. The goal of surgery in osteosarcoma is to remove all of the affected bone. *Limb sparing* refers to successful resection of the tumor and reconstruction of a viable, functional extremity. This is an attempt to leave enough of the original bone to preserve a moderately functional limb.[68] Before the development of limb-sparing procedures, amputation of the extremity was the standard surgical procedure used to treat and cure patients with osteosarcoma. Amputation is now generally reserved for patients with primary tumors considered unresectable or with widely metastatic disease.

Amputation and limb salvage are equally effective in achieving local control of osteosarcoma. Of course, a limb-sparing procedure is always preferable to an amputation, but complications can occur, including major involvement of the neurovascular bundle by tumor; immature skeletal age, especially for lower extremity tumors; infection in the region of the tumor; inappropriate biopsy site; and extensive muscle involvement that would result in a poor functional outcome. In these instances, an amputation is preferable.

Postsurgical chemotherapy is generally continued until the patient has received approximately 1 year of treatment. Relapses are unusual beyond 3 years, but late relapses can occur.[66,68,70]

The histologic response to neoadjuvant chemotherapy is an excellent predictor of outcome. Patients having 90% tumor necrosis have a 70%–90% long-term, disease-free survival rate. Other favorable prognostic factors include distal skeletal lesions, longer duration of symptoms, age older than 20 years, female sex, and near-diploid tumor DNA index.[66,68,70]

Radiation therapy is of little help in treating osteosarcomas, as they tend to be highly radioresistant lesions. For this reason, radiation therapy has no role in the primary management of osteosarcomas.[66,68,70]

RHABDOMYOSARCOMA

Rhabdomyosarcoma (RMS) is the most common soft-tissue sarcoma of childhood, accounting for approximately 3% of pediatric malignancies. Common sites of disease include the head and neck region, genitourinary tract, and extremities.[74] RMS is thought to originate from immature cells that would normally differentiate or mature into striated skeletal muscle; however, these tumors can arise in locations where skeletal muscle is not typically found.

Incidence and Etiology

Approximately 350 rhabdomyosarcomas are diagnosed annually in the United States. There are two major histologic subtypes of RMS: embryonal and alveolar. Embryonal RMS is the most common subtype in childhood, whereas the alveolar subtype is more often seen in adolescents.[74–76]

RMS is a disease of young children with two thirds of cases being diagnosed in children younger than 6 years of age, and the most frequent incidence being in children younger than 10 years of age. The disease is more common in boys than in girls.[74–76] There is a smaller incidence peak in early to mid adolescence. The incidence in African-American girls is half that in Caucasian girls, whereas the incidence in boys is similar for both groups. Incidence appears to be lower in Asians compared with predominantly Caucasian populations.[74–76]

Although RMS can arise anywhere in the body, distinct patterns link primary sites, histology, and age at diagnosis. For example, head and neck RMS is more common in younger children. When RMS arises in the orbit, they are almost always of the embryonal type. Nearly 80% of genitourinary tract RMSs are of the embryonal type. A unique form of embryonal RMS that arises from the wall of the bladder or vagina, referred to as the *botryoid variant (sarcoma botryoides)*, is seen almost exclusively in infants. However, this variant can also arise within the nasopharynx in older children. Extremity tumors present more commonly in adolescents and are frequently of the alveolar type.

Various studies have suggested an association between RMS and uterine exposure. Some studies reported a higher incidence of RMS in those exposed to radiation in utero, in children from families with a low socioeconomic status, and in those who received antibiotics soon after birth or whose parents used recreational drugs during pregnancy. However, these findings have not been confirmed by other studies.[74–76]

Most cases of RMS appear to be sporadic, but the disease has been associated with familial syndromes such as neurofibromatosis, the Li-Fraumeni syndrome, the Beckwith-Wiedemann syndrome, and the Costello syndrome.[75]

Data suggest that children who develop RMS at age 3 years or younger may have a hereditary predisposition to cancer and should be screened for a specific germline mutation, p53. Furthermore, if a p53 germline mutation is identified, the question then becomes whether the treatment protocol should be modified to reduce exposure to ionizing radiation and/or chemotherapeutic agents, as the p53 mutations are associated with an increased risk for secondary malignancies, which can then be exacerbated by the radiotherapy and certain chemotherapeutic agents. However, there are no standard guidelines, and the approach to such patients has been variable.[75]

Clinical Presentation

The most common primary sites for RMS are the head and neck region (35% to 40%), the genitourinary tract (25%), and the extremities (20%). The impact of the primary site on prognosis is shown in Table 2–9. Head and neck tumors are divided into three major groups: orbital, parameningeal, and nonparameningeal. Orbital RMS commonly presents as proptosis. The parameningeal sites include

Table 2–9 Prognosis of Nonmetastatic Rhabdomyosarcoma

Site of Primary Tumor	n	5-Year Overall Survival (% ± SE)
Genitourinary, nonbladder or prostate	92	94 ± 3
Orbit	48	85 ± 5
Genitourinary (bladder/prostate)	62	80 ± 5
Head and neck, nonparameningeal	48	64 ± 7
Head and neck, parameningeal	135	64 ± 4
Other	67	63 ± 6

Data from Stevens MC, Rey A, Bouvet N, et al. Treatment of nonmetastatic rhabdomyosarcoma in childhood and adolescence: third study of the International Society of Paediatric Oncology—SIOP Malignant Mesenchymal Tumor 89. *J Clin Oncol* 2005;23:2618–2628.

the nasal cavity, paranasal sinuses, middle ear, and infratemporal fossa. Tumors at these sites may present with nasal, sinus, or aural obstruction, often with purulent or bloody discharge. The nonparameningeal sites include the scalp, face, buccal mucosa, oropharynx, and neck. Patients with these tumors typically present with a visible and palpable mass.[66]

Fewer than 25% of patients will have identifiable distant metastatic disease at diagnosis. Most will have only a single site of metastatic involvement, usually a pulmonary site. However, in view of the poor outcomes seen with surgery alone in patients with apparently localized disease, the majority of patients are presumed to have clinically occult micrometastases at diagnosis. Other sites of distant metastatic involvement include bone marrow and bone; visceral involvement and brain metastases are rare.[74-76]

Patients with genitourinary RMS may present with hematuria and urinary flow obstruction. Prostatic primary tumors typically present as large pelvic masses causing symptoms such as urinary frequency or constipation from extrinsic compression of the bladder or intestinal tract. Vaginal tumors, which are generally accompanied by mucosanguineous drainage and a protruding polypoid mass, tend to develop in very young girls. Cervical and uterine tumors are more common in older girls. Paratesticular tumors can produce scrotal or inguinal enlargement in prepubertal or postpubertal boys along with a palpable pelvic mass.[74-76]

RMSs involving an extremity occur most often in adolescents and typically present with a painful mass or swelling. Such tumors frequently spread to the regional lymph nodes.[74-76]

Less common sites of primary disease include the trunk, chest wall, perineal-perianal region, and biliary tract. Primary RMSs of the liver, brain, trachea, heart, breast, and ovary have been reported, but are not common.[74-76]

Prognostic Factors

The staging system for RMS is different from that for other solid tumors. Prognostic determination is made by using the clinical group system developed by the International Rhabdomyosarcoma Study Group and the extent of tumor. The International Rhabdomyosarcoma Study Group recognizes four categories of disease on the basis of the amount of tumor remaining after initial surgery and the degree of local or distant metastases. Patients with localized disease (clinical group I) have a favorable outcome, whereas those with metastatic disease (clinical group IV) have an unfavorable outcome.[74-76] The prognosis for a child or adolescent with RMS is related to age at diagnosis, resectability, presence of metastases, number of metastatic sites, histopathology, and unique biologic characteristics of RMS tumor cells (Table 2-10).

The site of the primary tumor is also predictive of outcome. Children with orbital tumors or with genitourinary tumors that do not arise in the bladder or prostate gland have the best outcome. Patients with parameningeal or extremity tumors have the worst prognosis.

Table 2–10 Rhabdomyosarcoma: Risk Factors for Disease Prognosis

Stage of Disease	5-Year Survival (%)
Localized	70
Residual tumor after surgery	70
No residual tumor after surgery	9
Alveolar histology	Associated with worse outcomes and metastatic disease

Treatment

The development of intensive clinical trials has resulted in significant improvements in outcome. For patients with nonmetastatic disease, a 60%–70% disease-free survival can be expected.[74] As for other solid tumors, the therapeutic approach to RMS includes surgery, radiation therapy, and chemotherapy. All patients are considered to have micrometastatic disease, regardless of the degree of resection. Thus, chemotherapy is given universally.

Once RMS has been diagnosed, the patient should be referred to a pediatric oncology surgeon. Surgery is the most rapid way to achieve disease control. A complete excision of the primary tumor should be considered for localized disease as long as functional and/or cosmetic results are acceptable. If complete resection is not feasible or if disease involves the orbit, vagina, bladder, or biliary tract, the patient will have a diagnostic biopsy and neoadjuvant chemotherapy in an attempt to shrink the tumor to an operable size followed by induction chemotherapy, and then definitive local therapy. In some patients, debulking surgery may be considered, although its utility is unclear.[74–76]

Radiation therapy is indicated for almost all patients except those with embryonal tumors that have been completely resected. In this group, chemotherapy appears to be sufficient.[74–76] Radiation therapy plays a vital role in the management of RMS, particularly in patients with tumors that cannot be completely removed by surgery.

In general, two to three cycles of chemotherapy are administered before radiation therapy. Parameningeal tumors with intracranial extension are the exceptions to this therapy. In this situation, radiation therapy is begun immediately (see below). Delaying radiation therapy beyond 18 weeks decreases the likelihood of achieving local control and should be avoided.[74–76]

Local therapy alone for RMS results in survival rates of less than 20%, presumably due to the presence of micrometastatic disease in the majority of patients. The incorporation of systemic chemotherapy into treatment protocols has increased survival rates in patients with localized disease to approximately 60%–90%.[74–76]

The combination of vincristine, dactinomycin, and cyclophosphamide (VAC) has been considered the gold standard of treatment for RMS. Any other investigational regimen for RMS must be able to produce similar, if not better, results. It should be noted that in sequential International Rhabdomyosarcoma Study Group trials, the addition of many individually active agents such as doxorubicin, cisplatin, etoposide, ifosfamide, and melphalan did not improve outcomes compared with VAC. More recently the camptothecins (topotecan and irinotecan) have been shown to be active against RMS in phase I and II studies, and these agents are being studied in combination with VAC for patients with poor-risk disease (Box 2–9).[74–76] For adjuvant therapy, cyclophosphamide has been eliminated without any compromise in outcome in the subgroup of patients who are classified as low-risk in the prognostic stratification system (Table 2–11).[74–76]

Box 2–9 Representative Regimens for Rhabdomyosarcoma[74]

Alternating cycles of:
1. Vincristine 1.5 mg/m^2 IV × 1 dose on day 1
   Actinomycin D 0.045 mg/kg (maximum 2.5 mg) × 1 dose on day 1 (not given during radiation)
   Cyclophosphamide 2200 mg/m^2 IV on day 1
2. Ifosfamide 1800 mg/m^2 IV daily × 5 days
   Etoposide 100 mg/m^2 IV daily × 5 days
3. Vincristine 1.5 mg/m^2 IV × 1 dose on day 1
   Cyclophosphamide 2200 mg/m^2 IV × 1 dose on day 1

Table 2-11 Rhabdomyosarcoma Prognostic Stratification

Prognosis (EFS)	Stage	Group	Site	Size	Age	Histology	Mets	Nodes	Treatment (IRS-V)
Excellent (>85%)	1	I	Favorable	a or b	<21	EMB	M0	N0	VA
	1	II	Favorable	a or b	<21	EMB	M0	N0	VA + XRT
	1	III	Orbit only	a or b	<21	EMB	M0	N0	VA + XRT
	2	I	Unfavorable	a	<21	EMB	M0	N0 or NX	VA
Very good (70–85%)	1	II	Favorable	a or b	<21	EMB	M0	N1	VAC + XRT
	1	III	Orbit only	a or b	<21	EMB	M0	N1	VAC + XRT
	2	III	Favorable, excluding orbit	a or b	<21	EMB	M0	N0 or N1 or NX	VAC + XRT
	2	II	Unfavorable	a	<21	EMB	M0	N0 or NX	VAC + XRT
	3	I or II	Unfavorable	a	<21	EMB	M0	N1	VAC + (XRT, Gp II)
	3	I or II	Unfavorable	b	<21	EMB	M0	N0 or N1 or NX	VAC + (XRT, Gp II)
Good (50–70%)	2	III	Unfavorable	a	<21	EMB	M0	N0 or NX	VAC ± Topo + XRT
	2	III	Unfavorable	a	<21	EMB	M0	N1	VAC ± Topo + XRT
	3	III	Unfavorable	b	<21	EMB	M0	N0 or N1 or NX	VAC ± Topo + XRT
	1, 2, 3	I, II, III	Favorable or unfavorable	a or b	<21	ALV/UDS	M0	N0 or N1 or NX	VAC ± Topo + XRT
Poor (<30%)	4	I, II, III, or IV	Favorable or unfavorable	a or b	<10	EMB	M1	N0 or N1 or NX	VAC ± Topo + XRT
	4	IV	Favorable or unfavorable	a or b	≥10	EMB	M1	N0 or N1 or NX	CPT-11, VAC + XRT
	4	IV	Favorable or unfavorable	a or b	21	ALV/UDS	M1	N0 or N1 or NX	CPT-11, VAC + XRT

Favorable: Orbit/eyelid, head and neck (excluding parameningeal) genitourinary (not bladder or prostate), and biliary tract; unfavorable: bladder, prostate, extremity, parameningeal, trunk, retroperitoneal, pelvis, other; a: tumor size ≤5 cm in diameter; b: tumor size >5 cm in diameter; EMB, embryonal, botryoid, or spindle cell rhabdomyosarcomas or ectomesenchymomas with embryonal RMS; N0, regional nodes, clinically not involved; N1 not N2: regional nodes clinically involved; NX, node status unknown; VAC, vincristine, actinomycin D, cyclophosphamide; XRT, radiotherapy; Topo: topotecan; Gp: group; CPT-1: irinotecan.

Reproduced with permission from Raney RB, Anderson JR, Barr FG, et al. Rhabdomyosarcoma and undifferentiated sarcoma in the first two decades of life: a selective review of Intergroup Rhabdomyosarcoma Study Group experience and rationale for Intergroup Rhabdomyosarcoma Study V. J Pediatr Hematol Oncol 2001;23:215. Copyright © 2001 Lippincott Williams & Wilkins.

EWING SARCOMA

Ewing sarcoma is a "family of tumors" characterized by small, round cell growths that arise either in bone or soft tissues. These tumors are often referred to as *Ewing sarcoma* or *peripheral primitive neuroectodermal tumors*. The Ewing family of tumors are characterized by a common cytogenetically abnormality: the t(11;22) or t(21;22) translocation.[77] In the last 30 years, advances have been made in the treatment of Ewing sarcoma because of enrollment in clinical trials. Approximately 75% of patients with low-risk nonmetastatic disease can expect a 5-year disease-free survival. Unfortunately, the 5-year disease-free survival of patients with metastatic disease is only 25%.

Incidence and Etiology

The Ewing sarcoma family of tumors is the second most common type of bone cancer after osteosarcoma. In the United States, these tumors account for 3.5% of pediatric tumors between the ages of 10 and 14 years and 2.3% between ages 15 and 19. Approximately 300 new cases of Ewing sarcoma are diagnosed each year in children and adolescents younger than age 20 years. The peak incidence in boys is between the ages of 10 and 14 years, whereas in girls it is between the ages of 5 and 9 years.[77] Approximately one third of tumors are diagnosed in children younger than 10 years of age, another one third diagnosed as young adults up to age 20 and the final third in patients over 20 years of age. Ewing sarcoma is more common in Caucasians and very rare in African Americans and Asians. The reason for this ethnic distribution is unknown, although it is recognized that interethnic differences exist for certain alleles of the Ewing sarcoma gene, which is consistently disrupted in these tumors. Although a slight male predominance is seen, there is little evidence of any familial or genetic predisposition. However, in one series an excess of congenital mesenchymal defects in affected patients was reported, and another suggested an increase in neuroectodermal tumors and stomach cancer in families of patients with Ewing sarcoma.[78–80]

Although specific environmental exposures (e.g., ionizing radiation) have not been identified as risk factors, an association has shown between farming and the development of Ewing sarcoma.[81]

Bone is the principal site of involvement in 60% of patients. The most common sites are the flat bones of the chest wall, pelvis, and extremities, but any bone can be affected.[66]

Clinical Presentation

Ewing sarcoma usually presents during the second decade of life (median age is 13 years) with localized pain, swelling, and a visible palpable mass. Often, physical trauma may lead to physical examination and the ultimate diagnosis. Pain may be mild at first, but often intensifies rapidly, is aggravated by physical activity, and is worse at nighttime. The mass, if present, is generally firmly attached to bone and moderately to markedly tender to palpation. Swelling of the affected limb with erythema around the site of the mass is common.[75,78–80] If the lesion is juxta-articular, the patient may experience loss of joint motion. Rib lesions are associated with direct pleural extension and large extraosseous masses.[75,78–80] Involvement of the spine or sacrum can cause nerve root irritation or compression and can result in back pain, radiculopathy, or symptoms of spinal cord compression (e.g., bowel and/or bladder control issues).[75,78–80]

Of patients with Ewing sarcoma, 10%–20% will have constitutional signs or symptoms at the time of presentation, including fever, fatigue, weight loss, or anemia.

Fever is related to cytokine production by tumor cells and, along with other system symptoms, is associated with advanced disease.[75,78–80]

More than 80% of patients will present with clinically localized disease. However, overt metastases may become evident within weeks to months in the absence of effective treatment.[75,78–80]

Pathologic fractures, typically of the femur, may be present in as many as 15% of patients before diagnosis. Approximately 25% of patients have metastatic disease upon presentation. The most common sites of metastases are the lungs, bones, and bone marrow.[78] Long-term follow-up is imperative as late recurrences are well documented.[75,78–80]

Prognosis

Several clinical and biologic characteristics can assist in defining prognosis and directing the intensity of therapy. These include the presence or absence of metastases, location and size of the primary tumor, age at diagnosis, the response to therapy, and the presence of certain chromosomal translocations.[2,75,78,79]

Of the above-listed characteristics, the key prognostic factor is the presence or absence of metastases. The 20%–25% of patients who have disseminated disease (usually to the lungs) at diagnosis have the worst prognosis, although those with limited lung metastases may have a small, but reasonable, opportunity for cure. In this specific group, approximately 20% will survive years, compared with only 10% of those with bone or bone marrow involvement.[75,78–80]

Patients presenting with localized disease; axial primary tumors (i.e., tumors of the pelvis, rib, spine, scapula, skull, clavicle, and sternum) have a worse treatment outcome than those with extremity lesions (5-year relapse-free survival of 40% versus 61%). Patients with small primary tumors do better than those with larger tumors. Fever, anemia, and elevated serum LDH levels present at diagnosis all correlate with greater volume disease and poorer prognosis.[75,78–80]

In the last 30 years, advances have been made in the treatment of Ewing sarcoma, again because of enrollment in clinical trials. However, local and distant metastases are a common problem; about half of children have a recurrence within 2 years, and about 60% of the recurrences are at distant sites. The 5-year disease-free survival for patients with low-risk nonmetastatic disease is approximately 75%. Unfortunately, patients with metastatic disease or large pelvic primary tumors have a 5-year disease-free survival of 25%.[75,78–80]

Treatment

Combination chemotherapy is the backbone of multimodality treatment for Ewing sarcoma. Current treatment strategies involve the use of neoadjuvant and adjuvant chemotherapy. Surgery is the treatment of choice for local control. Radiation therapy is generally reserved for unresectable disease and for patients with positive or close margins of tumor after surgery.[66,75,78,79] However, only 20% of children are long-term survivors with either surgery or radiation alone.[66]

Chemotherapy is an important part of the treatment, regardless of the degree of resection. Most chemotherapy regimens include combinations of the following agents: doxorubicin, dactinomycin, cyclophosphamide, vincristine, etoposide, and ifosfamide (Box 2–10). As with other tumors, high-dose chemotherapy followed by autologous stem cell rescue is being explored as a treatment option for advanced disease.[78]

The optimal regimen for PNET tumors is not clearly established, but most pediatric oncologists recommend that because of their biologic similarities with Ewing's sarcoma they should be treated in a similar fashion.[66,75,78]

Box 2–10 Representative Regimens for Ewing's Sarcoma[66,77]

Alternating cycles of:
1. Vincristine 1.5 mg/m^2 IV (maximum 2 mg) on day 1
   Doxorubicin 75 mg/m^2 IV continuous infusion over 48 hours
   Cyclophosphamide 1200 mg/m^2 IV on day 1
2. Ifosfamide 1800 mg/m^2 IV daily on days 1–5
   Etoposide 100 mg/m^2 IV daily on days 1–5

WILMS' TUMOR

Wilms' tumor is the most common renal neoplasm of childhood. Advancements in surgery, chemotherapy, and radiation have increased the overall survival for Wilms' tumor to more than 85%.[82] The excellent outcome for these patients has led investigators to consider reductions in the intensity of treatment with the goal of preserving outcome while decreasing toxicity. Other related renal tumors include clear cell sarcoma, rhabdoid tumor of the kidney, and renal cell carcinoma. These tumors have distinctly different outcomes than that for the more common Wilms' tumor.

Incidence and Etiology

Wilms' tumor represents approximately 6% of all childhood malignancies with approximately 650 new cases diagnosed each year in the United States. After neuroblastoma, this is the second most common abdominal tumor in children. The incidence of Wilms' tumor is higher in African-American than in Caucasian or Asian populations. Girls have a slightly higher risk of developing this tumor. The median age at diagnosis is related both to sex, with tumors being diagnosed earlier in boys than in girls, and tumor laterality, with bilateral tumors presenting at a younger age than unilateral tumors. Wilms' tumor occurs most commonly between ages 2 and 5 years, with a mean age at diagnosis of about 3 years. Approximately 5%–10% of patients with Wilms' tumors have bilateral disease.[75,82,83]

Wilms' tumors in most children have no underlying cause. Environmental associations have been implicated, but the findings supporting this view are conflicting. In a few children, Wilms' tumor occurs in the setting of associated malformations including aniridia, hemihypertrophy, genitourinary malformations (e.g., cryptorchidism, hypospadias, gonadal dysgenesis, pseudohermaphroditism, and horseshoe kidney). Wilms' tumor is a well-known part of several identifiable syndromes including Denys-Drash syndrome, Beckwith-Wiedemann syndrome, and Wilms' tumor, aniridia, ambiguous genitalia, and mental retardation (WAGR) syndrome.[75,82,83]

Clinical Presentation

Wilms' tumor typically presents as an asymptomatic abdominal mass found incidentally. The mass is usually smooth, firm, and well demarcated and rarely crosses the midline, although it can extend inferiorly into the pelvis. Abdominal pain, fever, anemia, hematuria, and hypertension are frequent signs and symptoms seen in approximately 20%–30% of patients. Constitutional symptoms (weight loss, bone pain, and cachexia) are uncommon in Wilms' tumor. Wilms' tumor can spread both locally and hematogenously, and the most common sites of metastases are the lungs and liver.[83] Up to 10% of children will have metastatic disease at presentation. Of these, 15% and 80% will have liver and pulmonary involvement, respectively. Bone and brain metastases are uncommon and tend to be associated with more aggressive renal tumors.[75,82,83]

Treatment

Treatment of Wilms' tumor involves multimodality therapy: surgery, chemotherapy, and radiation therapy in metastatic disease. An exploratory laparoscopy is generally indicated and allows inspection and palpation of the contralateral kidney. At this time the liver and lymph nodes are also inspected with suspicious areas being either excised or analyzed by biopsy. Almost all patients with unilateral disease initially undergo a partial or full nephrectomy. An attempt is made to resect the tumor en bloc, and extreme care is exercised to avoid spillage of tumor cells as this would adversely affect staging and have an impact on the therapeutic strategy.[75,83]

Because staging dictates therapy, it is imperative that pediatric surgeons perform the initial surgery. For patients with bilateral disease, resection of the most impaired organ or parts of both may be considered with a secondary surgical procedure planned after chemotherapy.[75,82,83] Furthermore, tumor histology has implications for therapy and prognosis. A favorable histology tumor is one that resembles the classic triphasic Wilms' tumor and its variants. Of Wilms' tumors, 5% are diffusely anaplastic, are associated with a poor prognosis, and are thus determined to be an unfavorable histology.[75,82,83]

In 1969, the National Wilms Tumor Study began a series of clinical trials designed to cure 90% of children with Wilms' tumor. The dose intensity and extent of chemotherapy were matched to the patients' tumor stage and presumed risk of relapse and death. The National Wilms Tumor Study showed in one trial that survival rates could be improved by intensifying therapy during the initial treatment phase while shortening overall duration of treatment. Vincristine and dactinomycin are the most commonly used agents. Patients with more extensive disease also receive doxorubicin (Box 2–11).[82]

Using a stratified approach the 4-year overall survival rates are as follows: stage I favorable histology, 96%; stages II to IV favorable histology, 82%–92%; stages I to III unfavorable histology, 56%–70%; and stage IV unfavorable histology, 17%. Patients with recurrent disease have about a 50% salvage rate with surgery, radiation therapy, and chemotherapy. HSCT is being investigated as a way to improve survival after relapse.[2,75,84]

RETINOBLASTOMA

Epidemiology

Retinoblastoma, a neuroblastic tumor, is the most common intraocular neoplasm in children. Retinoblastoma represents 3% of all pediatric malignancies. The incidence of retinoblastoma is approximately 1 in 20,000 births. Boys and girls are affected equally with no racial preference. Retinoblastoma is a disease of the very young and is often present at birth. The median age at diagnosis for patients with bilateral disease is 12 months and for those with unilateral disease is 24 months. Onset after 6 years of age is extremely rare, but retinoblastoma has been reported in adults.[66,85]

Box 2–11 Representative Regimen for Wilms' Tumor (Favorable Histology)[66]

Alternating cycles of:
1. Vincristine 1.5 mg/m^2 IV × 1 dose
   Actinomycin D 1.35 mg/m^2 IV × 1 dose
2. Vincristine 1.5 mg/m^2 IV × 1 dose + actinomycin D 1.35 mg/m^2 IV × 1 dose + doxorubicin 30 mg/m^2 × 1 dose

The overall survival rate for retinoblastoma has improved dramatically. This can be attributed to better detection methods and to the development of alternative treatment strategies.[86]

Genetics

Retinoblastoma can occur in two different clinical forms. The first is bilateral or multifocal hereditary (40% of cases), characterized by the presence of germline mutations of the *RB1* gene. The second type is unilateral and nonhereditary (60% of cases).[66]

A "two-hit" hypothesis has been suggested to explain the observations that familial tumors are typically bilateral and that patients with random tumors usually present with unilateral disease. The hypothesis proposes that two mutational events in a developing retinal cell lead to the occurrence of retinoblastoma and further suggests that the two events could be mutations of both alleles of the *RB1* gene.[85] The retinoblastoma gene is a tumor suppressor gene, located in chromosome 13q14, that codes for the RB protein.[85]

Genetic Counseling

Retinoblastoma is an interesting disease, because the hereditary form has autosomal-dominant inheritance with almost complete penetrance.[7] There is a 45% chance that any given child of the patient will inherit the disease. There is also a possibility that one of the patient's siblings could develop retinoblastoma. The risk of retinoblastoma varies, depending on the relationship to the family member and the form of mutation.[85] All children with a family history of retinoblastoma should be screened soon after birth by a ophthalmologist to allow for early identification of the disease.[85,86] Current guidelines recommend examination at birth and every 4 months for up to 4 years of age.[86] Prospective parents who have a positive family history of retinoblastoma should be referred for genetic counseling.[85] Even patients with the nonhereditary form of retinoblastoma should receive counseling, because they also have the germline mutation.

Clinical Presentation

Most retinoblastomas are diagnosed while the tumor remains intraocular. Leukocoria, a lack of the normal red reflex of the eye, is present in 60% of patients. The second most frequent sign is strabismus, which usually suggests macular involvement.[66,86] Other manifestations include decreased vision, red eye, discoloration of the iris, inflammation, and tearing.[85]

Most frequently, a parent or relative of the affected child will note an irregularity of the eye that prompts evaluation by a pediatrician.[86] Occasionally, retinoblastoma is first observed after a flash photograph that shows leukocoria.[66]

Evaluation

Current strategies for the diagnosis of intraocular retinoblastoma involve a pediatrician looking for leukocoria with an ophthalmoscope. Retinoblastoma has a creamy pink appearance. However, the presence of retinal detachment or vitreous hemorrhage can make the inspection difficult. Pupillary dilatation and anesthesia are essential in evaluating the entire retina.[66,86] Usually, the diagnosis of retinoblastoma is made without histologic confirmation. Imaging studies that are useful in the detection of retinoblastoma include ultrasonography, computed tomography, and magnetic resonance imaging. Magnetic resonance imaging may be more helpful in detecting tumor extension into the optic nerve.[86]

Staging

The Reese-Ellsworth classification has been recognized as the standard for intraocular disease. This system was initially intended for prediction of outcome after radiation, not enucleation. In this classification, the eyes are divided into five groups based on size, location, number of lesions, and the presence of vitreous seeding.[66] Even though the Reese-Ellsworth system is not necessarily predictive for outcomes using current treatment strategies, it is still the classification used most frequently to evaluate therapeutic outcomes.[86]

Treatment

The treatment of retinoblastoma has changed in the past decade.[85] The goal in managing retinoblastoma should be first to save the child's life and then to preserve vision.[66,86] Therefore, therapy should be individualized on the basis of the overall situation, including concern for metastatic disease, risks for secondary malignancies, location of the tumor, and visual prognosis.[86] The current treatment options for retinoblastoma include enucleation, laser therapy, cryotherapy, radioactive plaques, external beam radiation, and chemotherapy.[66,86]

Surgery. Enucleation is the careful removal of the intact eye and proximal optic nerve without spillage of tumor into the orbit. Before recent advances in chemotherapy and other conservative treatment methods, such as laser treatment and focal therapy, enucleation had been the treatment of choice. Enucleation is still indicated for advanced retinoblastoma in which there is tumor invasion and little chance of preserving vision.[66,86]

Focal Therapy. Examples of focal therapy include photocoagulation with an argon laser, cryotherapy, and transpupillary thermotherapy. These methods are used for small tumors (less than 3–6 mm), usually in patients with bilateral disease and in combination with chemoreduction. The use of focal therapy is especially important in combination with chemotherapy, because the two modalities appear to have a synergistic effect.[66]

Radiation Therapy. Retinoblastoma is a radiosensitive tumor.[66,86] External beam radiotherapy delivers whole-eye irradiation to treat more advanced disease, especially if there is vitreous seeding.[86] The use of radiation alone can cure 75%–85% of patients. The addition of cryotherapy or photocoagulation increases the cure rate to 90%. The risk of recurrence of retinoblastoma after external beam radiation remains a problem; recurrences are seen within the first 1–4 years after treatment.[86]

Radioactive plaque therapy is a form of brachytherapy in which a radioactive plaque is placed on the sclera over the base of the retinoblastoma.[86] It is beneficial in the treatment of localized tumors, because the procedure time is short and exposure is limited to the area of interest with little involvement of extraocular structures.[66]

Chemotherapy. Chemotherapy is usually reserved for those patients with extraocular disease, for the subgroup of patients with intraocular disease with high-risk histologic characteristics, and for patients with bilateral disease in combination with focal therapy. Current regimens include platinum compounds, etoposide, cyclophosphamide, doxorubicin, vincristine, and ifosfamide (Box 2–12).[66]

Late Effects

Because their orbital development is still in progress, children treated for retinoblastoma are at risk of functionally cosmetically important bony orbital abnormalities. These become more evident during early adolescence when orbital growth is complete, and facial deformities can result. Both enucleation and radiation therapy affect orbital growth.[66]

Box 2–12 Example Regimens

Unilateral Retinoblastoma[88]
Carboplatin 560 mg/m^2 IV every 3 weeks for 4 cycles
Vincristine 1.5 mg/m^2 IV weekly for the first 2 weeks of each cycle

Bilateral Retinoblastoma[89]
Vincristine 1.5 mg/m^2 (maximum 2 mg) or 0.05 mg/kg/dose (<10 kg)
Etoposide 100 mg/m^2 IV daily × 3 days or 3.3 mg/kg/day (<10 kg)
Carboplatin 560 mg/m^2 IV × 1 dose
Repeat above every 3 weeks for 6 cycles

Patients with the hereditary form of retinoblastoma seem to have an increased chance of developing secondary tumors. The most frequent types are osteosarcoma, soft tissue sarcoma, and cutaneous melanoma.[85] These malignancies typically start in the second decade of life. The cumulative risk is 1% per year. The risk is increased with external beam radiation treatment to the eye, and the incidence of cancer is greatest when radiotherapy is given to patients younger than 12 months of age.[85,87]

HEPATOBLASTOMA

Hepatoblastoma is the most common liver tumor in children, and the majority of tumors are diagnosed before the age of 5 years. Survival for hepatoblastoma has greatly improved in the past 30 years. In the 1970s, the survival rate was only 30%, whereas now it is approximately 60%–70%. This improvement may be related to the use of effective adjuvant chemotherapy and to the use of liver transplantation for patients with unresectable tumors.[84]

Incidence and Etiology

Primary tumors of the liver are rare in children and account for only 1.3% of malignancies in children younger than 15 years. Hepatoblastoma comprises 60% of the pediatric liver tumors and is largely confined to the very young. The median age of diagnosis of hepatoblastoma is 18 months.[75,84,90]

Two important genetic syndromes are associated with hepatoblastoma in children: familial adenomatous polyposis and Beckwith-Wiedemann syndrome.[84] In families with familial adenomatous polyposis, there is a 200–800 times greater incidence of hepatoblastoma than in the general population. Other than genetic syndromes, there has been an association between hepatoblastoma and maternal exposure to metals, paints, and oil products. Approximately 10% of children with hepatoblastoma have a history of prematurity and prolonged hospitalization. The reason for this relationship is unclear, but it has been postulated that environmental exposures, together with immature or genetically altered metabolic pathways, predispose patients to hepatoblastoma.[75,84,90] This disease occurs more frequently in Caucasians than in African Americans (4 to 5:1) and is slightly more prevalent in boys than in girls (1.4 to 2:1).[75,84,90]

Clinical Presentation

The majority of patients with hepatoblastoma present with an asymptomatic abdominal mass found on a routine physical examination. Anorexia, weight loss, vomiting, and abdominal pain may occur as the disease progresses.

There are several histologic subtypes of this malignancy (Table 2–12) with some having a better outcome than others. Evidence shows that pure fetal histology is associated with a better prognosis, whereas anaplasia is associated with a

Table 2–12 **Hepatoblastoma Histologic Subtypes**

Subtype	Frequency (%)
Epithelial type	56
Fetal	31
Embryonal	19
Macrotrabecular	3
Small cell undifferentiated	3
Mixed mesothelial/mesenchymal	44

poorer prognosis. At diagnosis, the average size of the tumor is 10–12 cm. It is usually well circumscribed, with the right lobe of the liver is generally being more affected than the left.

The concentration of human chorionic gonadotropin, which is produced by hepatoblasts, is often elevated and can lead to signs of precocious puberty, pubic hair, and a deepening voice.[61] The α-fetoprotein level is almost always highly elevated and is a marker for disease. Patients with normal or low levels of α-fetoprotein and those with extremely high levels have a poorer prognosis compared to those patients with intermediate levels.[76,90]

Of interest, the platelet count is often elevated and frequently in the range of 1 million. Metastases are usually confined to the lungs and are seen in only 10% of patients at diagnosis.

Treatment

Treatment for hepatoblastoma is primarily based on stage. Surgery is indicated to determine the extent of hepatic involvement and the presence or absence of metastatic disease. Stage I disease is a tumor that can be completely resected. Stage II is a tumor that has microscopic residual disease at the margins of the resected specimen. Stage III is a tumor that is partially resected or unresected but confined to the liver. Stage IV is the presence of distant metastases. Between 40% and 60% of hepatoblastomas are considered inoperable at diagnosis. These unresectable lesions, however, can potentially be made to be resectable with preoperative chemotherapy.[84] Standard chemotherapy includes ifosfamide, doxorubicin, cisplatin, 5-fluorouracil, and vincristine (Box 2–13). In the current era, aggressive chemotherapy and orthotopic liver transplant are the standards of care for patients with nonmetastatic but locally advanced disease.[75,84,90]

SECONDARY MALIGNANCIES IN PEDIATRICS

With the increasing number of cancer survivors among pediatric patients, the risk of treatment-related sequelae is also increasing. In pediatric cancer patients who have survived longer than 5 years from their initial diagnosis, the most common cause of death remains relapse of their original cancer. However, the second most common cause is treatment-related problems with development of a secondary

---

Box 2–13 Recommended Regimen for Hepatoblastoma[66]

1. Cisplatin 90 mg/m² IV over 6 hours on day 1
   Doxorubicin 20 mg/m²/day IV continuous infusion over 96 hours
2. Vincristine 1.5 mg/m² IV on day 1
   Cisplatin 90 mg/m² IV over 6 hours on day 1
   5-Fluouroucil 600 mg/m² IV on day 2

malignancy.[91] The two most common second malignancies are acute leukemia (including myelodysplastic syndrome) and solid tumors.[59]

RADIATION

Prior radiation is associated with a wide variety of secondary cancers that almost always appear within the radiation field. The risk of radiation-associated tumor is highest when the exposure occurs at a young age and increases with the total dose delivered. Examples of radiation-associated tumors include breast and lung cancer, thyroid cancer, brain tumors, and osteosarcoma.[91] There is often a long latency period from the time of radiation to the occurrence of the second cancer, typically 10–20 years, although earlier onset has been reported. The outcome of treatment for radiation-induced second cancers depends on the type and resectability of the neoplasms.[59] Nonmetastatic tumors are more amenable to surgery, and systemic diseases such as leukemia and myelodysplastic syndrome are not diseases treated by surgery.

Female patients treated with mantle radiation for HD before the age of 21 years have a significantly higher risk of developing radiation-related breast cancer compared with those treated in their adult years. The risk of breast cancer begins to increase about 8 years after radiation. Breast cancer in the majority of these women is diagnosed at a relatively young age. Because the outcome is closely linked to stage at diagnosis, early diagnosis should confer a survival advantage.[91–93]

An increased risk for development of thyroid cancer is well known after radiation that includes the neck for multiple primary cancers, including HD, acute lymphoblastic leukemia, and brain tumors and after total body irradiation (TBI) for HSCT.[91–93]

Radiation therapy increases the risk of bone tumors in a dose-dependent fashion. Therapy with alkylating agents is also linked to bone cancer, with the risk increasing with total drug exposure.[91]

Another example of the interaction of treatment- and nontreatment-related risk factors is lung cancer. Lung cancer has been reported after chest radiation therapy, even though this occurrence is relatively infrequent. However, the risk is known to increase among smokers. As for other tumors, the latency may be long and will increase as the length of follow-up lengthens.

CHEMOTHERAPY

Another example of the multiple interactions between risk factors is the development of secondary myelodysplasia and acute myeloid leukemia. Both of these diseases have been associated with exposure to alkylating agents (e.g., cyclophosphamide and ifosfamide) and topoisomerase II inhibitors, particularly etoposide and teniposide.[94] A dose-dependent relationship is noted with alkylating agents, which typically cause leukemias after latencies of 5–10 years. Alkylating agent–induced secondary leukemias are often associated with chromosome abnormalities of 5 or 7.[59] Among the alkylating agents, the leukemogenic potential is least with cyclophosphamide.

The risk of epipodophyllotoxin-associated leukemia is related more to schedule (i.e., the dose intensity) and less to the total dose.[91–93] The topoisomerase-associated leukemias often have a shorter latency (2–4 years), without the otherwise typical preceding myelodysplastic phase but often with characteristic cytogenetic abnormalities involving chromosome 11q23.[59]

GENETIC FACTORS

Genetic predisposition also plays a role in the development of primary and second neoplasms. For example, an increased risk of secondary sarcomas is well documented in patients with the genetic form of retinoblastoma, and, although related to the dose of radiation, the site of disease may be outside the treatment field. Another example of the role of genetics is the Li-Fraumeni syndrome: multiple first-degree relatives with onset of breast, brain, and bone sarcomas diagnosed before the age of 45 years. Members of families with the Li-Fraumeni syndrome are known to have a significant increased risk for subsequent cancers related to chemotherapy and radiation. It appears that germline mutations in tumor suppressor genes, such as those occurring in the Li-Fraumeni syndrome, might interact with therapeutic exposures, resulting in an increased risk of secondary malignancies.[91]

SCREENING AND MONITORING

Second malignancies are a significant threat to the health of survivors treated for cancer during childhood; thus, vigilant screening after completion of treatment is important. Monitoring should include, at a minimum, yearly complete blood count with differential and platelet count for 10 years after therapy. Screening recommendations for other secondary cancers should consist of annual physical examination of the skin and soft tissues in the radiation field and radiographic or other cancer-screening evaluations.[91]

LATE EFFECTS

In the past 30 years, there have been dramatic improvements in survival after childhood cancer. The overall 5-year survival rate for all pediatric cancer is now 80% versus only about 20%–25% in the early 1970s. As impressive as this survival rate may be, there is an associated increase in the late sequelae of treatment that is related to the increased intensity of treatment as well as to the opportunity to observe such problems among the increasing number of survivors. Currently, it is estimated that 1 in every 900 adults younger than age 45 is a pediatric cancer survivor. It is also estimated that up to 60% of pediatric cancer survivors have a disability that can be attributable to the treatment they received.[93] Because of these treatment-related complications, long-term follow-up of survivors is essential. Complications can develop in virtually any organ, including the brain (neurocognitive), heart and lung, endocrine tissue, kidneys, gastrointestinal tract, and musculoskeletal system and can also cause problems in growth and development.[91,93]

Neurocognitive Complications

Neurocognitive complications after treatment for childhood cancer occur generally as a result of whole-brain or craniospinal radiation. Chemotherapy treatment with high-dose methotrexate and/or cytarabine or intrathecal methotrexate is also being increasingly implicated as a cause as the use of radiation declines. Children having a history of brain tumors, acute lymphoblastic leukemia, or NHL are most likely to be affected. Risk factors include radiation dose and schedule, location and area of the radiation field, young age at the time of diagnosis, additional treatment with systemic or intrathecal chemotherapy, and female sex. The most severe deficits are noted in children with brain tumors, especially those children who received radiation therapy when they were younger than 5 years of age. Such deficits usually manifest within 1–2 years after radiation therapy. The most common are difficulties with receptive and expressive language, attention span, and visual and perceptual motor skills. Intellectual as well as academic achievement deficits are also common.[91]

Personality and Behavior

Survivors who received radiation for their childhood brain tumor may be less socially competent and may demonstrate other behavioral problems. Adolescent survivors may have an increased sense of physical fragility and vulnerability that manifests as hypochondriasis or phobic behaviors. Finally, these survivors are more likely to report symptoms of depression and somatic distress in adulthood. They may require ongoing counseling or other psychologic interventions years after therapy has been completed.[91,93]

Cardiac Complications

Beyond the effects of radiation, children who receive anthracyclines (e.g., doxorubicin and daunomycin) have a significant risk of acute and chronic cardiotoxicity. Cardiotoxicity associated with these agents is dose dependent and is uncommon with low cumulative doses of less than 300 mg/m^2. At least 5% of patients who have received a cumulative doxorubicin dose of more that 550 mg/m^2 will experience cardiac dysfunction. When the cumulative dose exceeds 600 mg/m^2, the incidence of severe cardiomyopathy rises above 30%.[91,95]

The mechanism of cardiotoxicity is believed to be free radical formation and oxidative stress on the myocardium from drug and metabolites, resulting in cardiomyopathy, pericarditis, and congestive heart failure, any of which can occur years after completion of treatment. This "late onset" anthracycline-induced cardiomyopathy is more common than acute cardiotoxicity and may not occur for periods of 15–20 years after therapy. Most survivors exhibit some degree of subclinical disease, and a smaller population eventually develops congestive heart failure. Risk factors associated with the development of cardiomyopathy include mantle radiation, pregnancy, and early age at treatment. Studies are ongoing to determine whether the cardioprotectant, dexrazoxane, can modify short-term as well as long-term cardiotoxicity.[59]

Current monitoring recommendations include an exercise echocardiogram and electrocardiogram every 1–5 years, depending on the age at therapy, total cumulative dose, and presence or absence of mediastinal irradiation. Selective monitoring with various modalities is indicated for those who were treated with anthracyclines when they were younger than 4 years of age or received more than 500 mg/m^2 of drug. Measurements of serum levels of cardiac troponin-T or atrial natriuretic peptide may be useful in assessing early cardiotoxicity.[59,95]

Pulmonary Complications

Late pulmonary toxicity may be the result of either radiotherapy to the lung, TBI, and/or chemotherapy. Asymptomatic radiographic findings or restrictive changes in pulmonary function tests have been reported in more than 30% of patients receiving radiation therapy encompassing a significant volume of the lung.[91]

Chemotherapy is also associated with pulmonary toxicity.[91] Agents such as bleomycin, carmustine, busulfan, and lomustine are well known for their pulmonary toxicity, which is generally dose dependent. Cumulative carmustine doses greater than 600 mg/m^2 result in a 50% incidence of symptomatic pulmonary disease. Bleomycin dosages exceeding 400 mg/m^2 have been associated with interstitial pneumonitis and pulmonary fibrosis. Either condition is exacerbated by any concomitant or subsequent radiation therapy. Busulfan is another agent with marked pulmonary toxicity. This occurs more frequently in patients who have received HSCTs when doses exceeded 500 mg. It should be noted, however, that whereas the majority of pulmonary toxicity seen with these agents is indeed associated with cumulative dosage, there are anecdotal reports of pulmonary toxicity occurring after only one or two doses. The lung damage occurring with any of these agents is usually characterized by irreversible interstitial fibrosis and bronchopulmonary dysplasia.[91] Individuals exposed to any of these risk factors should be strongly counseled to refrain from smoking and to give proper notification to any care provider of their treatment history especially if they require general anesthesia.

Neuroendocrine Complications

Neuroendocrine complications have been documented in 20%–50% of childhood cancer survivors.[94] These result from injury to the hypothalamic-pituitary axis or thyroid gland or to disturbances in growth hormone, adrenocorticotropic hormone, and gonadotropin as well as to secondary and less well-defined effects on bone density and appetite (obesity).

Precocious puberty, delayed puberty, and infertility are all potential consequences of treatment. Precocious puberty is more common in girls and is thought to be the result of CSI causing premature activation of the hypothalamic-pituitary axis. This also results in premature closure of the epiphysis and decreased adult height. Luteinizing hormone analog and growth hormone can be given in an attempt to stop early puberty and allow continued growth.[94]

Gonadal dysfunction in boys can result from radiation to the testes. The highest risk of gonadal dysfunction is in those patients who undergo testicular or abdominal radiation as part of the treatment for ALL or HD or TBI for HSCT. Patients who undergo testicular radiation as part of their ALL treatment, abdominal radiation for HD or TBI for HSCT have the highest risk. Radiation damages both the germinal epithelium, producing azoospermia, and the Leydig cells, causing low testosterone levels. As a result, puberty is delayed. Alkylating agents (e.g., ifosfamide and cyclophosphamide) can also interfere with male gonadal functions, resulting in sterility. Testicular size monitoring, semen analysis, and measurement of testosterone, follicle-stimulating hormone (FSH) and luteinizing hormone (LH) levels need to be done to help identify abnormalities in those at risk. If possible, male adolescents should be offered the option to bank their sperm.[94]

Abdominal radiation treatment fields that include the exposure of the ovaries to radiation can also result in delayed puberty with resulting increases in FSH and LH and a decrease in estrogen level. Girls receiving TBI or CSI have an exceptionally high risk for delayed puberty and premature menopause. In those women at risk, a detailed menstrual history should be obtained, and LH, FSH, and estrogen levels should be monitored as indicated.[94]

To date no studies have confirmed an increased risk of spontaneous abortions, stillbirths, premature births, congenital malformations, or genetic diseases in the offspring of childhood cancer survivors. Women who have received abdominal radiation may develop uterine vascular insufficiency or fibrosis of the abdominal and pelvic musculature or uterus, and their pregnancies should be considered high risk.[94]

In patients with CNS tumors, the prevalence of central endocrinopathy is greater than 70% and is almost always a result of radiation injury to the hypothalamus, thyroid, or gonads. Growth disturbances may result from a lack of growth hormone production or secretion or from hypothyroidism or sex steroid deficiency. Growth hormone secretion is extremely sensitive to external radiation. The development and severity of growth hormone deficiencies are dependent on the dose of radiation.[91] Up to 90% of patients who receive greater than 3000 cGy of radiation to the CNS will show evidence of growth hormone deficiency within 2 years. Approximately 50% of children receiving 2400 cGy will develop growth hormone deficiency.[96]

Children who received mantle radiation for Hodgkin's disease, CSI for brain tumors, or TBI as a condition for bone marrow transplantation are all at risk of developing neuroendocrine deficits. As the dose of radiation gets higher, these problems become more likely.[94] Children who have the greatest risk are those with brain tumors who received more than 3000 cGy of radiation and those who received more that 4000 cGy to the neck region. The average time to develop thyroid dysfunction is 12 months after exposure, but the range is wide, and therefore individuals at risk should be monitored yearly for at least 7 years from completion of therapy.[94]

Bone Complications

The level of bone mineral density has been investigated mainly in survivors of ALL and bone marrow transplantation. Osteoporosis has been observed in approximately 10% of patients at the time of diagnosis of ALL and in a much greater percentage (greater than 65%) during and after therapy. This problem may persist with little or no change for many years after completion of therapy. Risk factors for the development of osteoporosis include prolonged corticosteroid and methotrexate therapy, nutritional deficiencies, cranial irradiation, and a low level of physical activity.[59]

Early intervention may limit the degree of osteoporosis and its associated complications later in life. Physical activity, including weight-bearing exercises, helps prevent or delay the occurrence of osteoporosis and should be encouraged. The use of biphosphonates and calcium supplements in children is currently being studied.

Spinal radiation inhibits vertebral body growth. In 30% of such individuals, standing heights may be less than the fifth percentile. Asymmetrical radiotherapy to the spine may result in scoliosis. Growth should be closely monitored. Follow-up studies should include height, weight, growth velocity, scoliosis examination, and growth hormone testing as indicated.[91]

Acute vascular necrosis is another possible sequela of chemotherapy treatment; it usually develops during therapy and is more common in adolescents than in any other age groups. Major risk factors include systemic corticosteroid therapy. Dexamethasone appears to have more bone toxicity than equivalent doses of prednisone. Clinically significant avascular necrosis has been well documented in adolescent patients with HD and NHL and in children with ALL.[91] Radiation therapy fields encompassing bones, particularly joint areas, may also cause avascular necrosis.

Urinary Complications

Long-term renal side effects have been mostly associated with treatment with cisplatin, alkylating agents, or pelvic radiation. Patients who have received cisplatin may develop abnormal creatinine clearance and have abnormal serum creatinine levels and persistent wasting of magnesium due to chronic tubular dysfunction. Alkylating agents can cause hemorrhagic cystitis, which may be an ongoing problem long after the therapy is complete. Ifosfamide can also cause Fanconi syndrome, which may result in clinical rickets if adequate phosphate replacement is not provided.[93]

Patients seen in long-term follow-up who have received nephrotoxic agents should be monitored with urinalysis, appropriate electrolyte profiles, and serial blood pressures. Urine collection for creatinine clearance or renal ultrasound may be indicated in individuals with suspected renal toxicity.[93] Pelvic radiation can result in abnormal bladder function with dribbling, frequency, and enuresis.

Gastrointestinal Complications

Gastrointestinal complications in cancer survivors commonly include chronic enteritis and fibrotic changes in the liver and the gastrointestinal tract. These problems are more frequently related to radiation therapy. Over time, adhesions or stricture formation, sometimes with obstruction, ulcers, and fistulae may occur.

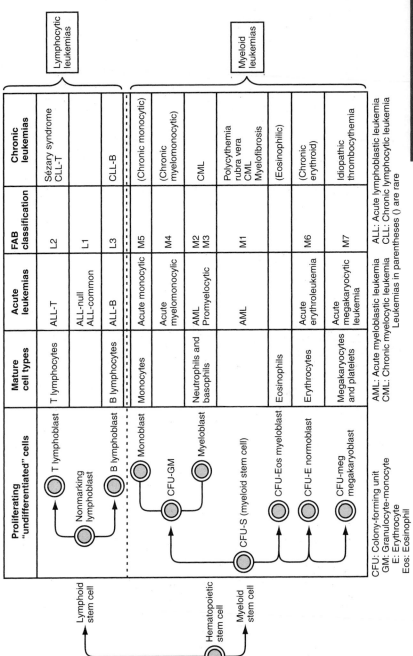

Proliferating "undifferentiated" cells	Mature cell types	Acute leukemias	FAB classification	Chronic leukemias
T lymphoblast	T lymphocytes	ALL-T	L2	Sézary syndrome CLL-T
Nonmarking lymphoblast		ALL-null ALL-common	L1	
B lymphoblast	B lymphocytes	ALL-B	L3	CLL-B
Monoblast	Monocytes	Acute monocytic	M5	(Chronic monocytic)
CFU-GM		Acute myelomonocytic	M4	(Chronic myelomonocytic)
Myeloblast	Neutrophils and basophils	AML Promyelocytic	M2 M3	CML
CFU-S (myeloid stem cell)		AML	M1	Polycythemia rubra vera CML Myelofibrosis
CFU-Eos myeloblast	Eosinophils			(Eosinophilic)
CFU-E normoblast	Erythrocytes	Acute erythroleukemia	M6	(Chronic erythroid)
CFU-meg megakaryoblast	Megakaryocytes and platelets	Acute megakaryocytic leukemia	M7	Idiopathic thrombocythemia

Lymphoid stem cell

Hematopoietic stem cell

Myeloid stem cell

Lymphocytic leukemias

Myeloid leukemias

CFU: Colony-forming unit
GM: Granulocyte-monocyte
E: Erythrocyte
Eos: Eosinophil

ALL: Acute lymphoblastic leukemia
CLL: Chronic lymphocytic leukemia
Leukemias in parentheses () are rare

AML: Acute myeloblastic leukemia
CML: Chronic myelocytic leukemia

Figure 2–1 Classification of leukemias according to cell type and lineage. (Reproduced with permission from Chandrasoma P, Taylor CE. *Concise Pathology*, 3rd ed. Originally published by Appleton & Lange. Copyright © 1998 by The McGraw-Hill Companies, Inc.)

The degree of damage increases with the volume of radiation delivered and concomitant use of dactinomycin as well as anthracyclines. Younger age may exacerbate the problem.[91]

Follow-up should include a history and physical examination to monitor for hepatomegaly, icterus, and malabsorption. Potential adverse consequences of excessive alcohol use and other high-risk behaviors in these patients should be emphasized. Patients who have received hepatotoxic therapy (e.g., methotrexate, mercaptopurine, dactinomycin, and abdominal radiation) should receive post-treatment baseline screening, including bilirubin, transaminases, and synthetic activity including total protein and albumin, as well as fibrinogen, and prothrombin time.[91]

SUMMARY

Providing appropriate health care for survivors of cancer is emerging as one of the major challenges of medicine. The goal for these patients should be to optimize quality of life by addressing the multiple physical and psychosocial impacts of disease and treatment. The Children's Oncology Group has developed risk-based, exposure-related guidelines that were designed for patients who have completed therapy for pediatric cancer. These guidelines provide education on screening, management, and prevention of long-term complications of childhood cancer. Academic settings allow for the establishment of a specialized multidisciplinary follow-up team to care for large number of survivors. Unfortunately, geographic access and local resources make these centers an option for only a limited number of survivors. Regardless of whether such care occurs, finding ways to educate survivors and their local health care providers regarding needed follow-up should be a priority.[91]

CHEMOPROTECTANTS

The toxicity associated with antineoplastic agents results from the nonselective nature of most chemotherapy: tumor and normal host tissue are both targets. As a result of this nonspecificity, attempts to increase treatment intensity are often limited by prolonged and irreversible host toxicity, which can easily result in the situation that treatment is as bad as or worse than the disease. Specific examples of toxicity include cisplatin-related nephrotoxicity, anthracycline-induced cardiotoxicity, and cyclophosphamide-induced hemorrhagic cystitis.[97]

With the significant improvement in survival of patients with pediatric cancer, it has become imperative to focus as much on the toxicity and the prevention of unwanted sequelae of treatment as much as on a cure.[98] Chemoprotectants are now a common part of the treatment program, and their use can ameliorate many of the side effects associated with specific organ toxicities without a compromise in antitumor effect.[97] Among the most commonly used chemoprotectants are dexrazoxane, amifostine, and mesna. All seem to share a common mechanism of limiting/preventing oxidative damage by chemotherapy treatment–associated free radicals.[98]

Dexrazoxane

The anthracycline antibiotics, including doxorubicin, daunorubicin, epirubicin, and others, are widely used agents with clinical activity against a multitude of solid and hematologic malignancies.[99] These agents are associated with cumulative irreversible cardiotoxicity, which limits the total tolerable dose of these agents. Long-term survivors of cancer who received anthracyclines for treatment of their malignancy may be at an increased risk of cardiac morbidity and mortality as a result of their therapy. The cardiac damage caused by the anthracyclines ranges from electrocardiogram changes to severe myocardial damage and congestive heart failure.[99] The dose-toxicity relationship for severe chronic congestive heart failure is 0.14% at cumulative doxorubicin doses of greater than 400 mg/m^2 and increases to 7% at 550 mg/m^2 and to 18% at 700 mg/m^{2}.[97] The cardiotoxic effects of anthracyclines may be related to the generation of reactive oxygen species that react with lipids and other cellular compounds to cause damage to mitochondrial and cellular membranes.[97]

Dexrazoxane is an organ-specific cardioprotective agent that protects against anthracycline-induced cardiac toxicity primarily through its metal-chelating activity in the myocardium. Chelation of free iron and that in iron-anthracycline complexes is suggested to inhibit the formation of cardiotoxic reactive oxygen radicals.[97] Fortunately, there is no apparent effect of dexrazoxane on the antitumor activity of anthracyclines. Its use has not been shown to deter progression-free and overall patient survival. The recommended dose of dexrazoxane with doxorubicin is a 10:1 ratio (300 mg of dexrazoxane to 30 mg of doxorubicin). Because of the short half-life of dexrazoxane, it should be administered 15–30 minutes before the administration of the anthracycline. Thus, delaying the subsequent administration of anthracyclines beyond this time may diminish the protectant effect of dexrazoxane.[99]

To date, dexrazoxane seems to be an extremely safe drug with few adverse effects. Limited studies in children with cancer receiving anthracyclines indicate good tolerance.[99] Yet to be determined is whether dexrazoxane is as effective in preventing the risk of late cardiac toxicity as it is in the early manifestations of this problem.[97]

Amifostine

Cisplatin is an alkylating platinum agent often used in the treatment of a variety of pediatric solid tumors. Nephrotoxicity, manifested as azotemia and electrolyte disturbances, is the primary dose-limiting toxicity. Aggressive hydration with diuresis is the mainstay for minimizing these problems but provides only modest protection in the end.

Amifostine may lessen the severity of renal damage by cisplatin without measurably altering the antitumor effect of cisplatin.[97] Amifostine, an inactive prodrug, appears to be converted to its active free thiol metabolite, WR 2721, in healthy tissue but not in neoplastic tissue.[100,101] It has unique properties in that it provides both radiotherapy and chemotherapy protection. It is approved by the U.S. Food and Drug Administration for use to decrease the cumulative nephrotoxicity associated with administration of cisplatin and seems to be helpful in diminishing radiation-induced mucositis. The ability of amifostine to prevent cisplatin-induced ototoxicity is uncertain.[102]

The exact mechanism of action of amifostine is not well defined. Like dexrazoxane, it seems to be a potent scavenger of reactive oxygen species, and this reduces the DNA-damage caused by free radicals. It also may protect normal tissue against the toxicity of platinum agents and prevents the membrane transport of anthracyclines.[101] Several studies have shown that amifostine may protect granulocytes, erythrocytes, and platelets from the toxicity of chemotherapy.[98]

The recommended dose for administration of amifostine when given with cisplatin is 910 mg/m^2 just before the cisplatin dose, although in adults the effective dosage is 740 mg/m^2. Administration of amifostine requires close patient monitoring. This agent possesses dose-related toxicities of its own, principally hypotension, which is usually evident by the end of its infusion. Because of this effect, patients should refrain from taking any antihypertensive medications within 24 hours of administration. Blood pressures should be checked every 15 minutes until the infusion is completed. Pretreatment with normal saline before infusion is recommended and may diminish the degree of hypotension. Because of the emetogenic potential of amifostine, all patients should receive a 5-hydroxytryptamine$_3$ antagonist before each dose. Administration of dexamethasone and an H_2 antagonist is also a recommended intervention.[102] Because hypocalcemia can occur due to the inhibition of parathyroid hormone, serum calcium concentrations should also be monitored.[97]

When amifostine is given concurrently with radiation, the recommended dose is 200 mg/m^2/day given as a slow intravenous push over 3 minutes 15–30 minutes before each radiation treatment. Hypotension does not occur as frequently with this dose.[102]

Mesna

The traditional oxazaphosphorine alkylating agents, ifosfamide and cyclophosphamide, undergo metabolic activation by the hepatic microsomal enzymes to form phosphoramide mustard and acrolein. Acrolein, which has no antineoplastic activity, is subsequently excreted intact in the bladder to cause hemorrhagic cystitis. Mesna, another thiol scavenger compound, was developed as a specific chemoprotective agent for acrolein-induced hemorrhagic cystitis. It inactivates alkylating metabolites by forming an inert thioether. Mesna is cleared rapidly, does not interfere with the antitumor effects of chemotherapy, and is excreted by the kidney to concentrate in the bladder where it scavenges acrolein.[97] The use of mesna is recommended to decrease the incidence of ifosfamide and cyclophosphamide urothelial toxicity.[102]

The suggested daily dose of mesna is 60% of the total daily dose of cyclophosphamide or ifosfamide. This is typically given as three bolus doses at times of 15 minutes before and 4 and 8 hours after the administration of each cyclophosphamide and ifosfamide dose. If continuous ifosfamide is given, mesna should be given initially as a bolus dose equal to 20% of the total alkylator dose, followed by a continuous infusion equivalent to 40% of the ifosfamide dose continuing for 12–24 hours after completion of the continuous ifosfamide dose. The efficacy of mesna for ifosfamide doses greater than 2.5 g/m^2/day has not been well established.[102]

Oral mesna is now available as a 400-mg tablet. The initial dose is 20% of the total daily ifosfamide dose given intravenously and then 40% of the total alkylator dose orally at 2 and 6 hours after each dose of cyclophosphamide or ifosfamide. The dosing schedule should be repeated on each day that ifosfamide is given.[102] Oral dosing may be less reliable because of nausea/vomiting or delayed absorption. The intravenous form is more reliable.

REFERENCES

1. Gurney JG, Bondy ML. The epidemiology of childhood cancer. In Pizzo PA, Poplack DG, eds. *Principles and Practice of Pediatric Oncology,* 5th ed. Philadelphia: Lippincott Williams & Wilkins; 2006:1–13.
2. Smith MA, Gloeckler LA. Childhood cancer: incidence, survival, and mortality. In Pizzo PA, Poplack, eds. *Principles and Practice of Pediatric Oncology,* 4th ed. Philadelphia: Lippincott Williams & Wilkins; 2002:1–20.
3. Jemal A, Murray T, Ward E, et al. Cancer statistics, 2005. *CA Cancer J Clin* 2005;55:10–30.
4. Young G, Toretsky JA, Campbell AB, Eskenazi AE. Recognition of common childhood malignancies. *Am Fam Physician* 2000;61:2144–2154.
5. Leather HL, Bickert B. Acute leukemias. In DiPiro JT, Talbert RL, Yee GC, et al., eds. *Pharmacotherapy: A Pathophysiologic Approach,* 6th ed. New York: McGraw-Hill; 2005:2485–2511.
6. Campana D, Pui CH. Childhood leukemia. In Abeloff MD, Armitage JO, Niederhuber JE, et al., eds. *Clinical Oncology,* 3rd ed. Philadelphia: Elsevier; 2004:2731–2764.
7. Pui CH, Relling MV, Downing JR. Acute lymphoblastic leukemia. *N Engl J Med* 2004;350:1535–1548.
8. Margolin JF, Steuber CP, Poplack DG. Acute lymphocytic leukemia. In Pizzo PA, Poplack DG, eds. *Principles and Practice of Pediatric Oncology,* 5th ed. Philadelphia: Lippincott Williams & Wilkins; 2006:538–590.
9. Hjalgrim L, Rostgaard K, Schmiegelow K, et al. Age- and sex- specific incidence of childhood leukemia by immunophenotype in the Nordic countries. *J Natl Cancer Inst* 2003;95:1539–1544.

10. Smith MA, Ries LA, Gurney JG, et al. Leukemia. In Ries LA, Smith MA, Gurney JG, et al., eds.: *Cancer Incidence and Survival among Children and Adolescents: United States SEER Program 1975–1995.* Bethesda, MD: National Cancer Institute, SEER Program, 1999:17–34 (NIH Publ. No. 99-4649).

11. McNally R, Rowland D, Roman E, et al. Age and sex distribution of hematologic malignancies in the U.K. *Hematol Oncol* 1997;15:173–189.

12. Faderl S, Jeha S, Kantarjian HM. The biology and therapy of adult acute lymphoblastic leukemia. *Cancer* 2003;98:1337–1354.

13. Golub TR, Arceci RJ. Acute myelogenous leukemia. In Pizzo PA, Poplack DG, eds. *Principles and Practice of Pediatric Oncology,* 5th ed. Philadelphia: Lippincott Williams & Wilkins; 2006:591–644.

14. Taub JW, Konrad MA, Ge Y, et al. High frequency of leukemic clones in newborn screening blood samples of children with B-precursor acute lymphoblastic leukemia. *Blood* 2002;99:2992–2996.

15. Feranando A, Look A. Pathobiology of acute lymphoblastic leukemia. In Hoffman R, Benz E, Shattil S, et al., eds. *Hematology Basic Principles and Practice,* 4th ed. Philadelphia: Elsevier; 2005:1135–1154.

16. Lowenberg B, Downing JR, Burnett A. Acute myeloid leukemia. *N Engl J Med* 1999;341:1051–1062.

17. Kantarjian HM, Faderl S. Acute lymphoid leukemia in adults. In Abeloff MD, Armitage JO, Niederhuber JE, et al., eds. *Clinical Oncology,* 3rd ed. Philadelphia: Elsevier; 2004:2793–2824.

18. Dahl, G, Weinstein, H. Acute myeloid leukemia in children. In Hoffman R, Benz E, Shattil S, et al., eds. *Hematology Basic Principles and Practice,* 4th ed. Philadelphia: Elsevier; 2005:1121–1133.

19. *Tabers Cyclopedic Medical Dictionary,* 17th ed. Philadelphia: FA Davis; 1993:1100.

20. Bürger B, Zimmermann M, Mann G, et al. Diagnostic cerebrospinal fluid examination in children with acute lymphoblastic leukemia: significance of low leukocyte counts with blasts or traumatic lumbar puncture. *J Clin Oncol* 2003;21:184–188.

21. Pui CH, Campana D, Evans WE. Childhood acute lymphoblastic leukaemia: current status and future perspectives. *Lancet Oncol* 2001;2:597–607.

22. Pui C, Boyette J, Relling M. et al. Sex differences in prognosis for children with acute lymphoblastic leukemia. *J Clin Oncol* 1999;17:818–824.

23. Chessells JM, Richards SM, Bailey CC, et al. Gender and treatment outcome in childhood lymphoblastic leukaemia: report from the MRC UKALL trials. *Br J Haematol* 1995;89:364–372.

24. Bhatia S. Influence of race and socioeconomic status on outcome of children treated for childhood acute lymphoblastic leukemia. *Curr Opin Pediatr* 2004;16: 9–14.

25. Pui CH, Sandlund JT, Pei D, et al. Improved outcome for children with acute lymphoblastic leukemia: results of Total Therapy Study XIIIB at St Jude Children's Research Hospital. *Blood* 2004;104: 2690–2696.

26. Macfarlane GJ, Evstifeeva T, Boyle P, et al. International patterns in the occurrence of Hodgkin's disease in children and young adult males. *Int J Cancer* 1995;61:165–169.

27. Stone RM, O'Donnell MR, Sekeres MA. Acute myeloid leukemia. *Hematology (Am Soc Hematol Educ Program)* 2004:1:98–117.

28. Silverman L, Sallans S, Cohen H. Treatment of childhood acute lymphoblastic leukemia. In Hoffman R, Benz E, Shattil S, et al., eds. *Hematology Basic Principles and Practice,* 4th ed. Philadelphia: Elsevier; 2005:1163–1174.

29. Gaynon PS, Trigg ME, Heerema NA, et al. Children's Cancer Group trials in childhood acute lymphoblastic leukemia: 1983–1995. *Leukemia* 2000;14:2223–2233.

30. Schrappe M, Reiter A, Zimmermann M, et al. Long-term results of four consecutive trials in childhood ALL performed by the ALL-BFM study group from 1981 to 1995. Berlin-Frankfurt-Münster. *Leukemia* 2000;14:2205–2222.

31. Hurwitz CA. Substituting dexamethasone for prednisone complicates remission induction in children with acute lymphocytic leukemia. *Cancer* 2000;88:1964–1969.

32. Pui CH, Relling MV, Campana D, et al. Childhood acute lymphoblastic leukemia. *Rev Clin Exp Hematol* 2002;6:161–180.

33. Pui CH, Campana D, Evans WE. Childhood acute lymphoblastic leukaemia—current status and future perspectives. *Lancet Oncol* 2001;2:597–607.

34. Pui CH, Schrappe M, Ribeiro RC, Niemeyer CM. Childhood and adolescent lymphoid and myeloid leukemia. *Hematology (Am Soc Hematol Educ Program)* 2004;1:118–145.

35. Appelbaum FR: Hematopoietic cell transplantation beyond first remission. *Leukemia* 2002;16: 157–159.

36. Wheeler KA, Richards SM, Bailey CC, et al. Bone marrow transplantation versus chemotherapy in the treatment of very high-risk childhood acute lymphoblastic leukemia in first remission: results from Medical Research Council UKALL X and XI. *Blood* 2000;96: 2412–2418.

37. Biondi A, Cimino G, Pieters R, et al. Biological and therapeutic aspects of infant leukemia. *Blood* 2000;96:24–33.

38. de Bont JM, Holt B, Dekker AW, et al. Significant difference in outcome for adolescents with acute lymphoblastic leukemia treated on pediatric vs adult protocols in the Netherlands. *Leukemia* 2004;18:2032–2035.

39. Adams VR, Yee GC. Lymphomas. In DiPiro JT, Talbert RL, Yee GC, et al., eds. *Pharmacotherapy: A Pathophysiologic Approach,*. 6th ed. New York: McGraw-Hill; 2005:2439–2466.

40. Sandlund JT, Downing JR, Crist WM. Non-Hodgkin's lymphoma in childhood. *N Engl J Med* 1996; 334:1238–1248.

41. Pileri SA, Ascani S, Leoncini L, et al. Hodgkin's lymphoma: the pathologist's viewpoint. *J Clin Pathol* 2002; 55:162–176.

42. Harris NL. Hodgkin's lymphomas: classification, diagnosis, and grading. *Semin Hematol* 1999; 36: 220–232.

43. Kraus MD, Haley J. Lymphocyte predominance Hodgkin's disease: the use of bcl-6 and CD57 in diagnosis and differential diagnosis. *Am J Surg Pathol* 2000;24:1068–1078.

44. Schwartz CL. The management of Hodgkin disease in the young child. *Curr Opin Pediatrics* 2003;15:10–16.

45. Hudson M, Onciu M, Donaldson SS. Hodgkin lymphoma. In Pizzo PA, Poplack DG, eds. *Principles and Practice of Pediatric Oncology,* 5th ed. Philadelphia: Lippincott Williams & Wilkins; 2006: 695–721.

46. Carbone PP, Kaplan HS, Musshoff K, et al. Report of the Committee on Hodgkin's Disease Staging Classification. *Cancer Res* 1971;31:1860–1861.

47. Lister TA, Crowther D, Sutcliffe SB, et al. Report of a committee convened to discuss the evaluation and staging of patients with Hodgkin's disease: Cotswolds meeting. *J Clin Oncol* 1989;7:1630–1666.

48. Diehl V, Thomas RK, Re D. Part 11: Hodgkin's lymphoma-diagnosis and treatment. *Lancet Oncol* 2004;5:19–26.

49. Diehl V, Re D, Josting A. Hodgkin's disease: clinical manifestations, staging and therapy. In Hoffman R, Benz E, Shattil S, et al., eds. *Hematology Basic Principles and Practice,* 4th ed. Philadelphia: Elsevier; 2005:1347–1377.

50. Rühl U, Albrecht M, Dieckmann K, et al. Response-adapted radiotherapy in the treatment of pediatric Hodgkin's disease: an interim report at 5 years of the German GPOH-HD 95 trial. *Int J Radiat Oncol Biol Phys* 2001;51:1209–1218.

51. Smith RS, Chen Q, Hudson M, et al. Prognostic factors in pediatric Hodgkin's disease. [Abstract]. *Int J Radiat Oncol Biol Phys* 2001;51 (3 Suppl 1):119.

52. Nachman JB, Sposto R, Herzog P, et al. Randomized comparison of low-dose involved-field radiotherapy and no radiotherapy for children with Hodgkin's disease who achieve a complete response to chemotherapy. *J Clin Oncol* 2002;20:3765–3771.

53. Hennessy BT, Hanrahan EO, Daly PA. Non-Hodgkin lymphoma: an update. *Lancet Oncol* 2004; 5:341–353.

54. Link MP, Weinstein HJ. Non Hodgkin lymphoma in children. In Pizzo PA, Poplack DG, eds. *Principles and Practice of Pediatric Oncology,* 5th ed. Philadelphia: Lippincott Williams & Wilkins; 2006:722–747.

55. Sandlund J, Link M. Malignant lymphomas in childhood. In Hoffman R, Benz E, Shattil S, et al., eds. *Hematology Basic Principles and Practice,* 4th ed. Philadelphia: Elsevier; 2005:1421–1435.

56. Shad A, Magrath I. Non-Hodgkin's lymphoma. *Pediatric Clin North Am* 1997;4:863–890.

57. Harvey DR, Valgus JM, Holdsworth M. Hematologic malignancies. In Koda-Kimble MA, Young LY, Kradjan WA, et al, eds. *Applied Therapeutics: The Clinical Use of Drugs,* 8th ed. Philadelphia: Lippincott Williams & Williams; 2005:90-1–90-42.

58. Sandlund J, Behm F. Childhood lymphoma. In Abeloff MD, Armitage JO, Niederhuber JE, et al., eds. *Clinical Oncology,* 3rd ed. Philadelphia: Elsevier; 2004:2765–2792.

59. Hoelzer D, Gokbuget N, Ottmann O, et al. Acute lymphoblastic leukemia. *Hematology (Am Soc Hematol Educ Program)* 2002:162–192.

60. Blaney SM, Kun LE, Hunter J. Rorke-Adams LB, et al. Tumors of the central nervous system. In Pizzo PA, Poplack DG, eds. *Principles and Practice of Pediatric Oncology,* 5th ed. Philadelphia: Lippincott Williams & Wilkins; 2006:786–864.

61. Ullrich NJ, Pomeroy SL. Pediatric brain tumors. *Neurol Clin* 2003;21:897–913.

62. Heideman RL. Pediatric neuro-oncology: an overview for the general practitioner. *HK J Paediatr* 1998;3:21–28.

63. Maity A, Pruitt A, Judy K, et al. Cancer of the central nervous system. In Abeloff MD, Armitage JO, Niederhuber JE, et al., eds. *Clinical Oncology,* 3rd ed. Philadelphia: Elsevier; 2004:1347–1431.

64. Lee KL, Ma JF, Shortliff LD. Neuroblastoma: management, recurrence, and follow-up. *Urol Clin North Am* 2003;30:881–890.

65. Brodeur GM, Maris JM. Neuroblastoma. In Pizzo PA, Poplack DG, eds. *Principles and Practice of Pediatric Oncology,* 5th ed. Philadelphia: Lippincott Williams & Wilkins; 2006:933–970.

66. Dome JS, Rodriguez-Galindo C, Spunt SL, Santana VM. Pediatric solid tumors. In Abeloff MD, Armitage JO, Niederhuber JE, et al., eds. *Clinical Oncology,* 3rd ed. Philadelphia: Elsevier; 2004:2661–2711.

67. Weinstein JL, Katzenstein HM, Cohn SL. Advances in the diagnosis and treatment of neuroblastoma. *Oncologist* 2003;8:278–292.

68. Wittig JC, Bickels J, Priebat D, et al. Osteosarcoma: a multidisciplinary approach to diagnosis and treatment. *Am Fam Physician* 2002;65:1123–1132.

69. Buckley J, Pendergrass T, Buckley C, et al. Epidemiology of osteosarcoma in childhood: a study of 305 cases by the Children's Cancer Group. *Cancer* 1998;83:1440–1448.

70. Dome JS, Schwartz CL. Osteosarcoma. *Cancer Treat Res* 1997;92:215–251.

71. Ross JA, Davies SM, Potter JD, et al. Epidemiology of childhood leukemia, with a focus on infants. *Epidemiol Rev* 1994;16:243–272.

72. Tucker M, D'angio G, Boice J, et al: Bone sarcomas linked to radiotherapy and chemotherapy in children. *N Engl J Med* 1987;371:588–593.

73. Link MP, Gebhardt MC, Meyers PA. Osteosarcomas. In Pizzo PA, Poplack DG, eds. *Principles and Practice of Pediatric Oncology,* 5th ed. Philadelphia: Lippincott Williams & Wilkins; 2006: 1074–1114.

74. Dagher R, Helman L. Rhabdomyosarcoma: an overview. *Oncologist* 1999;4:34–44.

75. Albano E, Bassal M, Porter C, et al. Neoplastic diseases. In Hay W, Levin M, Sondheimer J, Deterding R, eds. *Current Pediatrics: Diagnosis and Treatment,* 17th ed. http://www.accessmedicine.com/content. aspx?aID=535405=535405.

76. Wexler LH, Meyer WH, Helman LJ. Rhabdomyosarcoma and the undifferentiated sarcomas. In Pizzo PA, Poplack DG, eds. *Principles and Practice of Pediatric Oncology,* 5th ed. Philadelphia: Lippincott Williams & Wilkins; 2006:971–1001.

77. Carvajal R, Meyers P. Ewing's sarcoma and primitive neuroectodermal family of tumors. *Hematol Oncol Clin North Am* 2005;19:501–525.

78. Kennedy JG, Frelinghuysen P, Hoang BH. Ewing sarcoma: current concepts in diagnosis and treatment. *Curr Opin Pediatr* 2003;15:53–57.

79. Winn D, Li F, Robison L, et al: A case-control study of the etiology of Ewing's sarcoma. *Cancer Epidemiol Biomarkers Prev* 1992;1:525–532.

80. Bernstein M, Kovar H, Paulussen M, et al. Ewing sarcoma family of tumors: Ewing sarcoma of bone and soft tissue and the peripheral primitive neuroectodermal tumors. In Pizzo PA, Poplack DG, eds. *Principles and Practice of Pediatric Oncology,* 5th ed. Philadelphia: Lippincott Williams & Wilkins; 2006:1002–1032.

81. Valery P, Williams G, Sleigh, A, et al: Parental occupation and Ewing's sarcoma: pooled and meta-analysis. *Int J Cancer* 2005;115:799–806.

82. Kalapurakal JA, Dome JS, Perlman EJ, et al. Management of Wilms' tumour: current practice and future goals. *Lancet Oncol* 2004;5:37–45.

83. Dome JS, Perlman EJ, Ritchey ML, et al. Renal tumors. In Pizzo PA, Poplack DG, eds. *Principles and Practice of Pediatric Oncology,* 5th ed. Philadelphia: Lippincott Williams & Wilkins; 2006:905–932.

84. Stocker JT. Liver tumors: hepatic tumors in children. *Clin Liver Dis* 2001;5:259–281.

85. Melamud A, Palekar R, Singh A. Retinoblastoma. Am Fam Physician 2006;73:1039–1044.

86. Hurwitz RL, Shields CL, Shields JA, et al. Retinoblastoma. In Pizzo PA, Poplack DG, eds. *Principles and Practice of Pediatric Oncology,* 5th ed. Philadelphia: Lippincott Williams & Wilkins; 2006: 865–886.

87. Castillo BV, Kaufman L. Pediatric tumors of the eye and orbit. *Pediatr Clin North Am* 2003;50: 149–172.

88. Rodriquez-Galindo C, Wilson, MW, Haik GB, et al. Treatment of intraocular retinoblastoma with vincristine and carboplatin. *J Clin Oncol* 2003;21:2019–2025.

89. Honavar SG, Singh AD. Management of advanced retinoblastoma. *Ophthalmol Clin North Am* 2005;18:65–73.

90. Mueller BU, Lopez-Terrada, D, Finegold MJ. Tumors of the liver. In Pizzo PA, Poplack DG, eds. *Principles and Practice of Pediatric Oncology,* 5th ed. Philadelphia: Lippincott Williams & Wilkins; 2006:887–904.

91. Bhatia S, Landier W. Evaluating survivors of pediatric cancer. *Cancer J* 2005;11:340–353.

92. Neglia J, Friedman D, Yasui Y, et al. Second malignant neoplasms in five-year survivors of childhood cancer: childhood cancer survivor study. *J Natl Cancer Inst* 2001;93:618–629.

93. Friedman D, Meadows A. Late effects of childhood cancer therapy. *Pediatr Clin North Am* 2002; 49:1083–1106.

94. Cohen LE. Endocrine late effects of cancer treatment. *Endocrinol Metab Clin North Am* 2005;34: 769–789.

95. Poutanen T, Tikanoja T, Riikonen P, et al. Long-term prospective follow up of cardiac function alter cardiotoxic therapy for malignancy in children. *J Clin Oncol,* 2003;21:2349–2356.

96. Duffner. Long-term effects of radiation therapy on cognitive and endocrine function in children with leukemia and brain tumors. *The Neurologist* 2004;10:293-310.

97. Links M, Lewis C. Chemoprotectants: a review of their clinical pharmacology and therapeutic efficacy. *Drugs* 1999;57:293–308.

98. Bukowsi R. Cytoprotection in the treatment of pediatric cancer: review of current strategies in adults and their application to children. *Med Pediatr Oncol* 1999;32:124–134.

99. Cvetkovic RS, Scott LJ. Dexrazoxane: a review of its use for cardioprotection during anthracycline chemotherapy. *Drugs* 2005;65:1005–1024.
100. Stolarska M, Mylnarski W, Zalewska-Szewszyk B, et al. Cytoprotective effect of amifostine in the treatment of childhood neoplastic diseases—a clinical study including the pharmacoeconomic analysis. *Pharmacol Rep* 2006;58:30–34.
101. Jeremic B. Radiation therapy. *Hematol Oncol Clin North Am* 2004;18:1–12.
102. Schucter LM, Hensley ML, Meropol NJ, et al. 2002 update of recommendations for the use of chemotherapy and radiotherapy protectants: clinical practice guidelines of the American Society of Clinical Oncology. *J Clin Oncol* 2002;20:2895–2903. Available at www.childrensoncologygroup.org

Chapter 1
Management and Treatment of Hematologic Toxicities
Andrea Iannucci and Alexandre Chan

BACKGROUND

Despite recent advances in the identification and development of anticancer drugs that specifically target tumor cells, thereby minimizing toxicity to normal cells, treatment with traditional, cytotoxic chemotherapeutic agents remains a mainstay of standard therapy for many types of cancer. Because these agents are not selectively toxic only to tumor cells, they pose a significant risk of major systemic toxicities to the recipient, including myelosuppression. Myelosuppression, or suppression of normal bone marrow and blood cell production and function, is a major, dose-limiting side effect associated with many chemotherapy agents and regimens. This chapter reviews the incidence and management of hematologic toxicities of chemotherapy agents, focusing on neutropenia, anemia, and thrombocytopenia.

NORMAL HEMATOPOIESIS

Hematopoiesis, or production of blood cells, occurs in the bone marrow. All blood cells arise from a pluripotent stem cell (Figure 3–1). The pluripotent stem cell differentiates into the various lymphoid and myeloid cells. The process of differentiation of stem cells is regulated by hematopoietic growth factors, which are cytokines that bind to specific receptors on blood cell precursors, stimulating growth and differentiation.[1] Table 3–1 describes some of the important growth factors that are involved in hematopoiesis and their effects. Under the influence of hematopoietic growth factors, the pluripotent stem cell differentiates first into myeloid or lymphoid cell precursors. The lymphoid precursors then further differentiate into B and T lymphocytes. Myeloid precursors differentiate again into red blood cells, neutrophils, macrophages, and platelets.

CHEMOTHERAPY EFFECTS

The life span of blood cells is relatively short and because these cells proliferate at a rapid rate, they are susceptible to the cytotoxic effects of traditional chemotherapy agents. Bone marrow toxicity from cytotoxic drugs may result in neutropenia, anemia, and thrombocytopenia. Neutropenia (decreased numbers of neutrophils) and thrombocytopenia (decreased numbers of platelets) are very serious side effects that can put patients at risk for life-threatening infections or bleeding. Anemia (decreased levels of red blood cells) can contribute to symptoms of fatigue and shortness of breath, because of the decreased oxygen-carrying capacity of the reduced number of red blood cells, which has an impact on overall quality of life. Table 3–2 describes the normal life span of circulating blood cells and the expected time to onset of myelosuppression by cytotoxic chemotherapy agents.[2,3] Neutrophils and platelets have the shortest life span, and the myelosuppressive effects of chemotherapy agents on these cell lines are often seen over a period of 7–10 days.[1] The nadir (lowest level) for neutrophils and platelets typically occurs 1–2 weeks after chemotherapy is given, but it may be seen as early as 5 days and as late as 35 days, depending on the specific agent. Complete neutrophil and platelet recovery usually takes approximately 3–4 weeks. Because of the longer life span of the red blood cell, anemia occurs later than other myelosuppressive effects

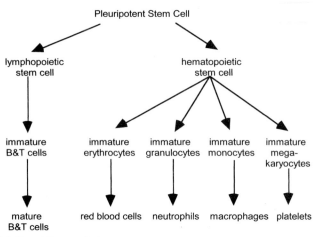

Figure 3–1 **Normal Hematopoiesis**

Table 3–1 **Hematopoietic Growth Factors**

Growth Factor	Effect
Granulocyte colony-stimulating factor (GCSF)	Regulates production of neutrophils
Granulocyte-macrophage colony-stimulating factor (GM-CSF)	Regulates production of neutrophils, eosinophils, and macrophages
Erythropoietin (EPO)	Regulate production of red blood cells
Interleukin-11 (IL-11)	Stimulates proliferation of megakaryocytes and megakaryocyte maturation, resulting in increased platelet production
Thrombopoietin (TPO)	Regulates production of platelets

Data from Mughl TI. Current and future use of hematopoietic growth factors in cancer medicine. *Hematol Oncol* 2004;22:121–134; and Neumega (oprelvekin) prescribing information. Madison, NJ: Wyeth; 2004.

Table 3–2 **Life Span of Blood Cells and Chemotherapy Effects**

	Lifespan	Nadir*	Recovery*
Neutrophils	< 1 day	7–14 days	3–4 weeks
Platelets	1 week	7–14 days	3–4 weeks
Red blood cells	3 months	Delayed, cumulative	Variable

*Measured from the date of initiation of chemotherapy.
Data from Balmer CM, Finley RS. Systemic toxicity. In Finley RS, Balmer CM, eds. *Concepts in Oncology Therapeutics*, 2nd ed. Bethesda, MD: American Society of Health-System Pharmacists; 1998:99–106.

of chemotherapy and tends to be cumulative.[1] Anemia is frequently more debilitating to patients than the other myelosuppressive effects of chemotherapy, and it will often persist through subsequent cycles of treatment.

The chemotherapy drugs that frequently induce myelosuppression as a major dose-limiting toxicity include alkylating agents, nitrosoureas, taxanes, anthracyclines, topoisomerase inhibitors, and many antimetabolite agents. The list of chemotherapy drugs that do not cause significant myelosuppression is relatively short in comparison (Box 3–1).

BOX 3–1 Chemotherapy Drugs Not Commonly Associated with Significant Myelosuppression

Asparaginase
Bleomycin
Cisplatin (doses $\leq$ 50 mg/m^2)
Corticosteroids
Hormonal agents
Methotrexate (with leucovorin rescue)
Tretinoin
Vincristine

Table 3–3 Levels of Hematologic Toxicity

Cell Type	Normal Levels	Grade 1*	Grade 2	Grade 3	Grade 4
Hemoglobin	12–18 g/dL	< LLN–10	< 10–8	< 8–6.5	< 6.5
Neutrophils	3000–7000 cells/mm^3	< LLN–1500	< 1500–1000	< 1000–500	< 500
Platelets	150,000–450,000 cells/microliter	< LLN–75,000	< 75,000–50,000	< 50,000–25,000	< 25,000

*LLN refers to the lower limit of normal within an institution's specific "normal" range.
Data from Common Terminology Criteria for Adverse Events: Blood/Bone Marrow, version March 31, 2003 (published December 12, 2003). Available at http://ctep.cancer.gov/forms/CTCAEv3.pdf. Accessed November 3, 2005.

SUPPORTIVE CARE

Depending on the type of cancer being treated, severe bone marrow suppression may not be an acceptable toxicity of cancer treatment. In general, when one is treating hematologic cancers, such as leukemias and lymphomas, in which the cancer cells may infiltrate the bone marrow or the malignant cell originates in the marrow, myelosuppression is both an expected and desired treatment outcome.[1] However, when one is treating patients with solid tumors such as lung, colorectal, or prostate cancer, administration of myelosuppressive chemotherapy regimens that increase the risk of a potentially life-threatening toxicity is not an acceptable treatment outcome. For many patients, these toxicities (anemia, neutropenia, or thrombocytopenia) may necessitate dose reductions or treatment delays for subsequent cycles of chemotherapy, depending on the duration and severity of the toxicity. The Common Terminology Criteria for Adverse Events (CTCAE) is a system for quantifying the toxic effects of cancer treatment using a grading scale of 1–5, where 1 is the mildest toxicity and 5 is death.[4] Table 3–3 describes the CTCAE definitions for grades 1–4 hematologic toxicities of cancer treatment. Reduction of chemotherapy drug doses may be considered when patients experience moderate to severe (i.e., grade 3–4) toxicities. Although for some tumors (e.g., germ cell tumors and adjuvant treatment for breast cancer) for which chemotherapy is being administered with curative intent, there may be a benefit to maintaining both the initial doses of chemotherapy and the treatment cycle (dose intensification), in an effort to provide the patient with the best treatment outcome.

Administration of hematopoietic growth factors to minimize the effects of neutropenia, anemia, and thrombocytopenia may offer patients an alternative to chemotherapy dose reduction and cycle delays. The remainder of this chapter will focus on the management and prevention of chemotherapy-induced bone marrow toxicities and the therapeutic use of hematopoietic growth factors (Table 3–4).

Table 3–4 **Hematopoietic Growth Factor Products**

Product (Trade Name)	FDA-Approved Oncology Uses	Typical Dose (Subcutaneous Injection)	Formulation	Approximate Cost (AWP)[12]
Darbepoetin (Aranesp)	Chemotherapy-induced anemia	100 mcg once per week	100-mcg vial	$498.75
		200 mcg every 2 weeks	200-mcg vial	$997.50
Epoetin alfa (Epogen; Procrit)	Chemotherapy-induced anemia	40,000 units once per week	40,000-unit vial	$534
Filgrastim (Neupogen)	After myelosuppressive chemotherapy in patients with non-myeloid malignancies After induction/consolidation chemotherapy for AML After bone marrow transplantation Mobilization of hematopoietic progenitor cells Severe, chronic neutropenia	5 mcg/kg once daily (dose rounded to nearest vial size)	300-mcg vial 480-mcg vial	$207.50 $330.60
Pegfilgrastim (Neulasta)	After myelosuppressive chemotherapy in patients with nonmyeloid malignancies	6 mg once per cycle	6-mg prefilled syringe	$2,950
Sargramostim (Leukine)	After induction chemotherapy for AML Mobilization and after bone marrow transplantation of autologous peripheral blood progenitor cells After bone marrow transplantation Bone marrow transplantation failure or engraftment delay	250 mg/m^2 once daily	500-mcg vial	$305.90
Oprelvekin (Neumega)	Prevention of severe thrombo-cytopenia and reduction in the need for platelet transfusions after myelosuppressive chemotherapy in patients with nonmyeloid malignancies	50 mcg/kg once daily	5-mg vial	$288

FDA, U.S. Food and Drug Administration; AWP, average wholesale price; AML, acute myeloid leukemia.

Neutropenia

Neutrophils (granulocytes) are a type of white blood cell responsible for destroying bacteria in the bloodstream and tissues.[1] They are the major infection-fighting cells in the human body. Because of their short life span, neutrophils are exquisitely susceptible to the toxic effects of chemotherapy drugs. Chemotherapy-induced neutropenia is one of the most serious complications of myelosuppressive chemotherapy. Neutropenic cancer patients are extremely vulnerable and prone to infection. Not only are they immunocompromised, but also conditions such as mucositis and the presence of venous access devices lead to disruption of normal protective barriers. In addition, frequent hospitalizations for treatment can expose patients to colonization with resistant organisms. This combination of factors puts neutropenic cancer patients at high risk for developing infections. The occurrence of severe neutropenia and neutropenic infections is associated with increased morbidity, mortality, and treatment-related costs.[5] The two risk factors consistently associated with the development of neutropenic infections are the degree and duration of neutropenia. Lower neutrophil counts and/or a longer duration of neutropenia are associated with higher risks of developing an infection.[6] The degree of neutropenia is determined by the absolute neutrophil count (ANC), which is calculated by multiplying the total number of white blood cells by the total percentage of neutrophils (Box 3–2). The percentage of neutrophils may be reported in the complete blood count as neutrophils alone or as neutrophils and band cells (immature neutrophils).[1] Patients are at high risk for infection when their ANC falls below 500 cells/mm³, but the greatest risk is seen when the ANC is less than 100 cells/mm³. Because of their immunocompromised state, neutropenic patients often cannot mount a normal response to infection, and frequently the only symptom of infection is fever. "Neutropenic fever" is defined as a single temperature spike of greater than 38.3 °C (greater than 101 °F) or a temperature of greater than 38 °C (greater than 100.4 °F) for more than 1 hour, in the presence of severe neutropenia (ANC less than 500 cells/mm³).[6] Neutropenic fever signals the presence of a potential life-threatening infection that requires prompt initiation of antibiotic therapy. Outpatient management of neutropenic fever with oral antibiotics may be an option in some practice settings but only for very carefully selected group of patients who have a high probability of compliance with taking the medication, will follow-up daily, and have access to 24-hour emergency care.[6] Hospitalization including treatment with intravenous antibiotics is the typical management approach for the vast majority of cancer patients who develop a neutropenic fever.

Various strategies have been used to prevent neutropenic infection in cancer patients. Dose reduction of chemotherapy drugs for subsequent cycles of treatment is one option, but this approach is generally not desirable for patients who are being treated with curative intent. Administration of prophylactic antibiotics is another approach. There is emerging evidence to suggest that some cancer patients, particularly those with hematologic malignancies, may benefit from administration of prophylactic antibiotics (typically a fluoroquinolone)[7–9] for prevention of bacterial infections during their period of neutropenia. However, routine administration of prophylactic antibiotics to all cancer patients remains controversial. The practice of prophylactic antibiotic administration is costly and puts patients at risk for infection with resistant organisms. The current guidelines of the Infectious Diseases Society of America[6] (IDSA) and National Comprehensive Cancer Network[10] (NCCN) for management of neutropenic infections advise against routine administration of prophylactic antibiotics to neutropenic cancer patients.

Unlike the management of anemia and thrombocytopenia, transfusion of white blood cells or granulocytes is not an effective means of supporting neutropenic patients. Granulocyte transfusions are occasionally used to support profoundly neutropenic patients through a serious infection, but their use is associated with significant infusion-related toxicity, and the benefits are short-lived.

BOX 3–2   **Calculation of ANC (Absolute Neutrophil Count)**

$$ANC = (total\ WBC) \times (\%\ neutrophils)$$

where WBC is total number of white blood cells from a complete blood count (CBC), and % neutrophils is the percentage of neutrophils (neutrophils + band cells) from the CBC.

The approach that has been most effective in decreasing the risk and incidence of neutropenic infection after myelosuppressive chemotherapy in cancer patients is administration of a hematopoietic colony-stimulating factor (CSF) such as filgrastim or sargramostim. Prophylactic administration of a CSF after myelosuppressive chemotherapy has been shown to decrease the duration and severity of neutropenia. In patients receiving chemotherapy regimens associated with a high incidence of neutropenic infection, administration of a CSF can decrease the occurrence of neutropenic fever by 50%.[11] However, despite the potential benefits of CSF administration, these agents are quite expensive[12] (Table 3–4), and routine administration to all patients receiving myelosuppressive chemotherapy is not practical or cost-effective.[5,11] The American Society for Clinical Oncology (ASCO) Guidelines for the Clinical Use of Colony Stimulating Factors[11] were developed as a means of providing oncology practitioners with practical, evidence-based guidance for the judicious use of these costly agents (Table 3–5).

The ASCO guidelines support the use of CSFs for primary prevention of neutropenic infection in patients receiving myelosuppressive chemotherapy regimens associated with an incidence of neutropenic fever of greater than 40%. This recommendation is based on fact that the additional expense of a CSF is outweighed by the higher potential cost of hospitalization for patients who need inpatient treatment for neutropenic fever. However, the most recent version of the NCCN guidelines for CSF use suggest that with the escalating costs of hospitalization, the benefit of CSF use may now be extended to chemotherapy regimens associated with a 20% incidence of

Table 3–5 ASCO Guidelines for Clinical Use of Colony-Stimulating Factors

Indication	Yes	No
Primary prophylaxis: CSF administered to prevent neutropenic fever after initial and subsequent cycles of chemotherapy with regimens that are associated with ≥ 40% incidence of neutropenic fever.	✓	
Secondary prophylaxis: CSF administered after subsequent cycles of chemotherapy to patients who developed a neutropenic fever or prolonged neutropenia (leading to a delay in therapy) with a prior cycle of the same chemotherapy regimen; recommended for patients with cancers in which maintenance of dose intensity is important for positive outcomes/cure (e.g., germ cell tumors); dose-reduction would be a reasonable alternative for other patients.	✓	
Afebrile neutropenia: CSF administered to patients who develop neutropenia, but not fever, after chemotherapy regimens that did not include prophylactic CSF administration. Prolonged neutropenia leading to a delay in the next scheduled treatment may warrant secondary prophylaxis with a CSF after subsequent chemotherapy cycles (see above).		✓
Febrile neutropenia: CSF administration in combination with appropriate antibiotic and supportive measures as a treatment intervention for management of neutropenic fever is not routinely recommended. However, CSF therapy may be considered in patients who are profoundly neutropenic (ANC < 100/microliter) or have a documented fungal infection and/or pneumonia or sepsis syndrome.		✓
Acute leukemias: CSFs can be safely administered to patients with AML or ALL after initial and consolidation chemotherapy and may provide a clinical benefit in terms of decreasing the duration of neutropenia and/or hospitalization.	✓	
Increase chemotherapy dose intensity: CSF administered after chemotherapy with the goal of increasing dose intensity, dose density or both is not recommended outside of the setting of a clinical trial.		✓
Concurrent chemotherapy and radiotherapy: CSF administered to patients receiving concurrent chemotherapy and radiotherapy is not recommended because of the potential for increasing bone marrow toxicity.		✓

AML, acute myeloid leukemia; ALL, acute lymphoblastic leukemia.
Data from Ozer H, Armitage JO, Bennett CL, et al. 2000 update of recommendations for the use of colony-stimulating factors: evidence-based, clinical practice guidelines. *J Clin Oncol* 2000;18:3558–3585.

neutropenic fever, when assessed purely on the basis of costs.[5] Table 3–6 provides a listing of some commonly used chemotherapy regimens that are associated with a high risk of neutropenic infection.

The ASCO guidelines also support secondary prophylaxis with a CSF in those patients who had developed a neutropenic infection or prolonged neutropenia with a previous cycle of the same chemotherapy regimen and who are expected to benefit from maintaining the dose intensity of their chemotherapy regimen.

Although once controversial because of concerns over possible stimulation of leukemic cell growth, the use of CSFs to prevent neutropenic fever in patients with acute leukemias, including myeloid leukemias, is supported by the ASCO guidelines. Additionally, the use of a CSF for mobilization of peripheral blood progenitor cells for hematopoietic stem cell transplantation is acceptable.

The ASCO guidelines do not support the routine use of CSFs in the management of neutropenic fever for patients who had not received a CSF before. Trials evaluating the efficacy of CSFs in the management of neutropenic fever have not consistently demonstrated a clinical benefit in terms of morbidity, mortality, and survival. However, a recent meta-analysis of clinical trials evaluating the use of CSFs in management of neutropenic fever did suggest a clinical benefit from CSF use in accelerating the time to neutrophil recovery and decreasing the time spent in the hospital.[13] The ASCO guidelines do suggest that certain patients with neutropenic fever may benefit from CSF administration. These include patients with profound neutropenia (ANC less than 100 cells/mm^3), pneumonia, hypotension, sepsis syndrome, invasive fungal infections, and uncontrolled primary cancer.[11]

For treatment of afebrile patients with neutropenia and no signs of infection after myelosuppressive chemotherapy, the ASCO guidelines do not support CSF use. Additionally, the ASCO guidelines advise against using CSFs to increase dose intensity and/or dose density of chemotherapy regimens outside of a clinical trial because data to demonstrate a favorable effect on survival, quality of life, or toxicity are lacking.[11,11a] The use of CSFs administered concurrently with combined modality chemoradiotherapy is also not recommended, because of the potential for increased bone marrow toxicity.

Table 3–6 Chemotherapy Regimens Associated with a High (>20%) Incidence of Neutropenic Fever

Tumor Type	Chemotherapy Regimen
Bladder cancer	TC (paclitaxel, cisplatin)
	MVAC (methotrexate, vinblastine, doxorubicin, cisplatin)
Breast cancer	AC→T (doxorubicin, cyclophosphamide, docetaxel)
	AT (doxorubicin, paclitaxel)
Lymphoma	DHAP (dexamethasone, cisplatin, cytarabine)
	ESHAP (etoposide, methylprednisolone, cisplatin, cytarabine)
Non–small cell lung cancer	VIG (vinorelbine, ifosfamide, gemcitabine)
	DP (docetaxel, carboplatin)
Small cell lung cancer	CAE (cyclophosphamide, doxorubicin, etoposide)
	Topotecan
	TopT (topotecan, paclitaxel)
Ovarian cancer	Topotecan
	Paclitaxel
	Docetaxel
Sarcoma	MAID (mesna, doxorubicin, ifosfamide, dacarbazine)
	AI (doxorubicin, ifosfamide)
Testicular cancer	VIP (vinblastine, ifosfamide, cisplatin)

Data from Myeloid growth factors in cancer treatment, V.2.2005. NCCN Clinical Practice Guidelines in Oncology. Available at: www.nccn.org.

SUPPORTIVE CARE

The ASCO and NCCN guidelines for CSF use are excellent tools to help clinicians make decisions about how to use CSFs in the safest and most cost-effective manner. Ultimately, it is up to the individual practitioner to decide which of his or her patients will benefit the most from CSF use. In considering the evidence as presented in the consensus guidelines, clinicians must also factor in specific patient issues that might influence their decision to use a CSF.[5] Regardless of the chemotherapy regimen being administered, some patients may have additional risk factors for developing infection or experiencing prolonged neutropenia. Patients may also have underlying medical conditions that would increase their risk of morbidity or mortality from a neutropenic infection. Box 3–3 describes some additional risk factors for developing a neutropenic infection that might sway practitioners toward the use of a CSF.

Three CSF products are commercially available in the United States: granulocyte CSF (filgrastim, Neupogen); pegfilgrastim (Neulasta), a pegylated, longer-acting formulation of filgrastim; and granulocyte-macrophage CSF (sargramostim, Leukine) (Table 3–4). Filgrastim and sargramostim are typically administered as a subcutaneous injection once daily, starting 24–72 hours after completion of myelosuppressive chemotherapy and continuing until neutrophil recovery is complete. The ASCO guidelines state that continuing the CSF until the ANC is above 10,000 cells/mm^3 is safe and effective but further suggest that the CSF can be stopped once "clinically adequate" neutrophil recovery is complete.[11] For practical reasons, including patient convenience and drug cost, many institutions establish their own ANC threshold for stopping CSF therapy. In establishing a stopping point for CSF therapy, it is important to consider, that there may be a rebound drop

---

BOX 3–3   Risk Factors for Neutropenic Infection in Cancer Patients

Treatment-Related
Chemotherapy regimen (types of drugs, combination)
Dose-intensity of the regimen
Extensive prior chemotherapy
Concurrent or prior radiotherapy to marrow-producing bones (mediastinum, hips, and long bones)
Previous history of severe neutropenia with similar chemotherapy

Patient-Related
Elderly (age >65 years)
Female sex
Poor performance status
Poor nutritional status
Decreased immune function
Open wounds
Active infection

Disease-Related
Bone marrow involvement of tumor
Advanced or uncontrolled cancer
Hematologic malignancy

Comorbid Medical Conditions
Chronic obstructive pulmonary disease
Heart disease
Diabetes
Liver disease

Data from Hughes WT, Armstrong D, Bodey GP, et al. 2002 guidelines for the use of antimicrobial agents in neutropenic patients with cancer. *Clin Infect Dis* 2002;34:730–751.

in the neutrophil count by as much as 50% after discontinuation of the CSF. Threshold ANC levels should be set at a point high enough that a drop in the ANC after the CSF is stopped would not bring the patient back into the neutropenic range.

Pegfilgrastim is administered as a single injection 24 hours after the end of chemotherapy. The manufacturer advises that pegfilgrastim should not be given within 14 days of the next scheduled cycle of myelosuppressive chemotherapy because of the potential for increased bone marrow toxicity.[14] Because the elimination of pegfilgrastim is mediated by neutrophils, the effects of pegfilgrastim are expected to last only until neutrophil recovery is complete. Thus, the potential for prolonged effects of pegfilgrastim on neutrophil production is self-limited. Occasionally, patients may experience prolonged neutropenia that outlasts the expected duration of effect of pegfilgrastim (approximately 2 weeks). In these patients, administration of daily filgrastim injections until neutrophil recovery is complete may be a reasonable approach to support them through their remaining period of neutropenia.

The therapeutic equivalence of filgrastim and sargramostim is difficult to determine because no large-scale, prospective clinical trials have been performed to compare the clinical efficacy of the two agents.[11] Small prospective and retrospective studies comparing the use of filgrastim and sargramostim in the prevention of neutropenic fever after myelosuppressive chemotherapy have generated mixed results.[15–17] However, the available evidence suggests that these two agents do exhibit similar efficacy in the prevention of neutropenic fever after myelosuppressive chemotherapy.[11] For mobilization of peripheral blood progenitor cells, filgrastim appears to be superior to sargramostim.[11] Studies comparing the use of filgrastim and pegfilgrastim in prevention of neutropenic fever after myelosuppressive chemotherapy have shown the two agents to be equal in terms of safety and efficacy.[18–20]

Selection of a CSF may be determined on the basis of clinical efficacy, institutional formulary availability, and cost. Administration of a CSF after chemotherapy typically costs between $1,500 and $3,000 per cycle, depending on the dose and the total duration of treatment (Table 3–4). Most patients require 7–10 days of CSF therapy before neutrophil recovery is complete. Based on average wholesale pricing, the cost of one dose of pegfilgrastim is equivalent to the costs of approximately 14 300-mcg doses of filgrastim, 9 480-mcg doses of filgrastim, and 10 500-mcg doses of sargramostim.[12] Because of the higher acquisition cost, it is usually not practical or cost-effective to administer pegfilgrastim to hospitalized patients in the inpatient setting. Once per cycle treatment with pegfilgrastim may provide patients with a convenient alternative to daily filgrastim injections in the outpatient setting. However, the convenience is frequently associated with higher drug cost and/or out-of-pocket expenses (e.g., co-payments) for patients.

The side effect profiles of the three CSFs are similar. Bone pain, back pain, and arthralgias are among the most common side effects. Leukocytosis is more common with filgrastim than with pegfilgrastim or sargramostim. Fever, rash, and injection site reactions are more common with sargramostim. Additionally, there is a "first-dose" phenomenon that can occur with sargramostim administration, which is characterized by respiratory distress, hypoxia, flushing, hypotension, syncope, and/or tachycardia.[21] This phenomenon typically occurs with the first dose of sargramostim administered after a cycle of chemotherapy, and it is frequently confused with an anaphylactic or severe hypersensitivity reaction. Management may require symptomatic treatment, but symptoms do not usually recur with subsequent doses within the same cycle of treatment. Overall, CSFs are fairly well tolerated and pose little risk in comparison with the potential benefits for patients receiving myelosuppressive chemotherapy.

SUPPORTIVE CARE

Anemia

Erythropoiesis, or production of red blood cells, is regulated in large part by erythropoietin. Erythropoietin is not stored in the body but is produced in response to low levels of tissue oxygenation in an indirect feedback loop.[1,22] When the kidneys sense hypoxia, erythropoietin production is increased almost immediately.[22a] Erythropoietin stimulates red blood cell formation in the bone marrow. When oxygenation is restored to normal levels, erythropoietin production decreases.[22]

In states of anemia, in which hemoglobin levels are low and tissue oxygenation is decreased, the normal body response is to increase endogenous production of erythropoietin. However, this response seems to be blunted in many cancer patients with anemia.[23] Despite low hemoglobin levels, erythropoietin levels are often disproportionately low relative to the degree of anemia in cancer patients.[25] There are many potential causes of anemia in cancer patients (Box 3–4). Cancer-related factors may include blood loss from disease or surgery, hemolysis, bone marrow infiltration of tumor cells and nutritional deficiencies (e.g., iron, vitamin B_{12}, or folic acid).[1,24,25] Treatment-related factors may include radiation therapy, damage to the bone marrow from extensive prior treatment, and direct myelosuppressive effects of chemotherapy and other medications.[1]

Anemia of chronic disease (ACD) may also contribute to cancer-related anemia.[25] This type of anemia occurs in patients with chronic inflammatory conditions, such as cancer. In ACD, inflammatory cytokines suppress erythropoiesis and inhibit erythropoietin production.[22,25] ACD is characterized by a defect in iron utilization or a "functional iron deficiency." Patients with ACD have adequate stores of iron in the bone marrow, but serum iron levels are low because the body is not able to reuse the iron that is released after normal erythrocyte destruction.[22,25]

Unlike some of the other myelosuppressive effects of chemotherapy, which may not even be noticeable to patients, the signs and symptoms of anemia affect many normal body systems and can be quite debilitating. Cancer patients with anemia may develop symptoms of fatigue, dizziness, impaired cognitive function, shortness of breath, palpitations, menstrual irregularities, and decreased libido. Physical findings include pale skin and mucous membranes, low skin temperature, tachycardia, and edema.[22] Because these effects can interfere with patients' ability to function and perform normal activities, anemia can have a significant impact on cancer patients' overall quality of life.

Given that there are so many potential causes of anemia in cancer patients, a thorough workup must be performed before initiating treatment to identify any reversible causes (e.g., iron or vitamin deficiency). A comprehensive workup of cancer-related anemia includes a complete blood count and review of the peripheral blood smear, red blood cell indices, reticulocyte counts, and serum B_{12} and folic acid levels. Patients must be evaluated for sources of blood loss, and a stool sample should be tested for occult blood. Iron studies, including a serum iron

---

BOX 3–4 Causes of Anemia in Cancer Patients

Myelosuppressive effects of chemotherapy
Blood loss
Hemolysis
Bone marrow infiltration of tumor
Nutritional deficiencies
Anemia of chronic disease

level, transferrin saturation, ferritin levels, and total iron-binding capacity should also be done.[24] Serum ferritin levels less than 100 ng/ml or transferrin saturation levels less than 20% indicate a functional iron deficiency.[25] A hemolysis workup, including lactate dehydrogenase direct and indirect bilirubin levels, and an direct Coombs' test, should also be performed.[25]

Evaluation and workup for chemotherapy-induced anemia typically begins when a patient's hemoglobin level falls below 10 g/dL (or if patients are symptomatic with a hemoglobin level less than 11 g/dL). Although this level of anemia is only considered grade 1 toxicity according to CTCAE criteria (Table 3–3), the consensus guidelines for management of chemotherapy-induced anemia as developed by the ASCO/ American Society of Hematology[24] and the NCCN[25] both recommend initiation of treatment at this level (Table 3–7). Treatment options for chemotherapy-induced anemia include supportive care, red blood cell transfusions, or erythropoietic growth factors. Transfusions provide the most efficient means of correcting the anemia, and patients generally feel rapid symptom relief. However, blood transfusions are a limited resource, are associated with some risk of infection, and take a significant amount of time to obtain and administer.

Epoetin alfa (Epogen, Procrit) was the first recombinant erythropoietic agent marketed in the United States. It was developed in the 1980s when there was great concern about the possible infectious complications from administration of blood products. Several large-scale clinical trials have demonstrated a benefit with the use of erythropoietin in increasing hemoglobin levels, reducing the need for red blood cell transfusions, and providing symptom relief and improved quality of life for patients with chemotherapy-induced anemia.[24–26] A second, longer-acting erythropoietic agent, darbepoetin alfa (Aranesp) has recently become available and has demonstrated comparable efficacy in treatment of chemotherapy-induced anemia.[27–29] Table 3–8 provides dosing information for epoetin alfa and darbepoetin in the treatment of chemotherapy-induced anemia from the NCCN guidelines.[25]

Patients should be evaluated for response to treatment after 4 weeks of epoetin alfa therapy and after 6 weeks of darbepoetin therapy. Doses should be increased if the hemoglobin level has not risen by at least 1 g/dL in that time period.[25] For patients experiencing a very rapid response to erythropoietic growth factor treatment (defined as more than 1 g/dL rise in hemoglobin level in a 2-week period), the dose of epoetin or darbepoetin should be reduced by 25%.[25]

SUPPORTIVE CARE

Table 3–7 **Guidelines for Management of Chemotherapy-Induced Anemia**

When to initiate anemia workup	Hb < 10 g/dL or
	Hb < 11 g/dL with symptoms
Workup	Peripheral blood smear
	RBC indices
	Reticulocyte count
	Iron studies
	Stool for occult blood
Iron support indicated	Ferritin < 100 ng/ml
	Transferrin saturation < 20%
Target Hb level	12 g/dL

Hb, hemoglobin; RBC, red blood cell.
Data from Rizzo JD, Lichtin AE, Woolf SH, et al. Use of epoetin in patients with cancer: evidence-based clinical practice guidelines of the American Society of Clinical Oncology and the American Society of Hematology. *J Clin Oncol* 2002;20:4083–4107; and Cancer and treatment-related anemia, V.2.2005. NCCN Clinical Practice Guidelines in Oncology. Available at: www.nccn.org.

Table 3–8 Erythropoietic Growth Factors for Chemotherapy-Induced Anemia

Guideline	Epoetin Alfa	Darbepoetin
Starting dose options	Subcutaneous injection 150,000 units/kg 3 times per week 40,000 units once per week	Subcutaneous injection 2.25 mcg/kg once per week 3 mcg/kg once every 2 weeks 200 mcg once every 2 weeks
Rapid response: Hb increases by >1 g/dL within 2 weeks	Decrease dose by 25%	Decrease dose by 25%
Hb exceeds target level (>12 g/dL)	Hold therapy, resume at 25% previous dose if Hb drops target	Hold therapy, resume at 25% previous dose if Hb drops target
Delayed response	Hb does not increase by 1 g/dL after 4 weeks; increase dose to: 300,000 units/kg 3 times per week 60,000 units once per week	Hb does not increase by 1 g/dL after 6 weeks; increase dose to: Up to 4.5 mcg/kg once week 5 mcg/kg once every 2 weeks 300 mcg once every 2 weeks

Hb, hemoglobin.
Data from Rizzo JD, Lichtin AE, Woolf SH, et al. Use of epoetin in patients with cancer: evidence-based clinical practice guidelines of the American Society of Clinical Oncology and the American Society of Hematology. *J Clin Oncol* 2002;20:4083–4107; and Cancer and treatment-related anemia, V.2.2005. NCCN Clinical Practice Guidelines in Oncology. Available at: www.nccn.org.

The target hemoglobin level for patients treated with erythropoietic growth factors for chemotherapy-induced anemia is 11–12 g/dL.[24,25] In studies in which quality-of-life improvements with the use of epoetin alfa have been examined, the greatest improvements have been observed with incremental changes in hemoglobin levels from 11 to 12 g/dL.[24,25] However, there does not appear to be any benefit in further normalizing hemoglobin. Studies evaluating the use of epoetin alfa or a similar product, epoetin beta (not available in the United States), to push target hemoglobin levels into the "normal" range have not demonstrated good outcomes in terms of cancer control, patient survival, and/or toxicities of therapy, and this strategy is not recommended.[30,31] If hemoglobin levels rise above 12 g/dL, erythropoietic agents should be held until the hemoglobin level is below 12 g/dL, and then treatment should be resumed with a 25% reduction in the dose. If the hemoglobin level fails to increase after 8–12 weeks of therapy with erythropoietic agents, the agent should be discontinued, and the patient should be managed with transfusion support.[25]

Iron supplementation is an important component of therapy with erythropoietic agents because iron is a required element for red blood cell production. Iron replacement is particularly crucial for patients who are iron deficient at the onset of treatment, but even patients who do not have iron deficiency at initiation of therapy often develop a functional iron deficit with continued use of an erythropoietic agent.[25] One of the most common reasons for treatment failure with erythropoietic growth factors is lack of adequate iron support. Oral iron therapy is generally the most convenient approach for iron supplementation. However, parenteral iron may be required in patients who are intolerant of or unresponsive to oral iron. One drawback to parenteral iron administration in the past was the risk of hypersensitivity reactions with iron dextran (INFed or DexFerrum). Now that there are two additional parental iron products to choose from, ferric gluconate (Ferrlecit) and iron sucrose (Venofer), parenteral iron administration may be a more feasible option. There is also some evidence to suggest that parenteral iron supplementation may be superior to oral iron therapy when combined with erythropoietin in management of chemotherapy-induced anemia.[32] Erythropoietic agents are generally very well tolerated, but their use is associated with some risks. Hypertension and seizures have been reported in some patients receiving erythropoietic agents. Patients should be closely monitored for hypertension, and blood pressure should be under control before treatment is initiated.[25] In early clinical trials with epoetin, in which hematocrit levels were targeted in the normal range, thrombotic events contributed to increased mortality.[25] Product labeling for both epoetin and darbepoetin have recently been revised to encourage prescribers not to allow hemoglobin levels to rise too quickly (greater than 1 g/dL in a 2-week period) or to rise above 12 g/dL in a effort to minimize the risk of thrombosis. Pure red cell aplasia (PRCA) is a rare, antibody-mediated blood disorder that leads to severe anemia.[33] PRCA has been linked primarily to an epoetin alfa product, Eprex (not available in the United States). Worldwide 206 cases of antibody-mediated PRCA have been reported.[33] Any patient who develops a lack of response to erythropoietic agents should be evaluated for possible PRCA, and, if PRCA is confirmed, the agent should be immediately discontinued.[25]

For many cancer patients, anemia is one of the most noticeable and incapacitating of the hematologic toxicities of chemotherapy. Management of anemia with erythropoietic growth factors can provide patients with symptom relief and decrease dependence on transfusion support. When used appropriately, these agents can have a significant, positive impact on a patient's overall well-being and quality of life.

Thrombocytopenia

Thrombocytes, also called platelets, are derived from fragments of the cytoplasm of megakaryocytes, which are platelet precursors in myeloid cell differentiation.[34] In a normal adult, the platelet count can vary between 150,000 and 350,000 cells/microliter. Platelets survive for approximately 10 days on average, and younger platelets usually have greater functional ability. Platelets circulate in humans for approximately 7 days; they are cleared primarily in the spleen and liver by macrophages that recognize phagocytic signals expressed on the platelet surface.

Platelets are the smallest among blood cells, but they play a vital role in the regulation of human hemostasis. They are normally activated when endothelial or vascular damage occurs. Activated platelets then form a hemostatic plug and further release and recruit other blood-borne substances such as fibrinogen and clotting factors to areas of vascular damage.

Thrombocytopenia is a common problem in the management of cancer patients who receive chemotherapy. The mildest grade of thrombocytopenia is defined as a platelet count less than 75,000 cells/microliter (Table 3–4). The most severe level, grade 4 thrombocytopenia, is defined as a platelet count less than 25,000 cells/microliter. Cancer chemotherapy agents exert direct toxicity to the cells of the bone marrow, resulting in suppressed thrombopoiesis.[35] Thrombocytopenia usually begins within 1 week of completion of myelosuppressive chemotherapy (Table 3–2).[36] Certain chemotherapeutic agents, such as gemcitabine, mitomycin, cytarabine, carmustine, and carboplatin, are associated with a higher risk of thrombocytopenia by exerting direct injury to megakaryocytes and other progenitor cells or by inhibiting thrombopoetin.[37]

Thrombopoietin is an endogenous physiologic regulator of platelet production.[38] Natural thrombopoietin is synthesized in the liver and is usually increased in response to reduced numbers of platelets. Most patients who are persistently thrombocytopenic due to chemotherapy have elevated levels of thrombopoietin as the body attempts to increase platelet production.[39]

Bleeding is the major complication from thrombocytopenia, and patients frequently present with evidence of bleeding such as bruising, nose bleeds or epistaxis, and petechiae (Box 3–5). Petechiae are tiny red patches of mucocutaneous bleeding caused by small, unsealed endothelial lesions that occur under the skin. Bleeding time is substantially increased in thrombocytopenic patients. The frequency of bleeding episodes in cancer patients who are thrombocytopenic from myelosuppressive chemotherapy for treatment of lymphomas and other solid tumors is reported to be in the range of 9–15%.[40–42] Approximately one-third of those episodes can be classified as major hemorrhages. The most common sites for major hemorrhages are the nose and pharynxs, gastrointestinal tract, bladder, and lung (Table 3–9). Thrombocytopenia-induced bleeding episodes can potentially be fatal.[41] However, spontaneous bleeding rarely occurs when platelet counts are greater than 20,000 cells/microliter.

Risk factors associated with bleeding during thrombocytopenia are host specific and include a prior history of bleeding, poor bone marrow function, low baseline platelet counts, bone marrow infiltration of tumor cells, and poor performance status.[40,43] There is a direct relationship between platelet nadir and the risk of bleeding: the lower the platelet nadir, the higher the patient's risk of bleeding. When the platelet count drops to less than 20,000 cells/microliter, the frequency of major and minor bleeding episodes nearly doubles (from 5% to 10%), and the rate nearly quadruples when the platelet levels drop to less than 10,000 cells/microliter.[40] Bleeding times are inversely related to platelet counts and peak when the platelet count drops to less than approximately 15,000–20,000 cells/microliter.[44]

Platelet transfusions are used extensively for the prevention and treatment of thrombocytopenic bleeding in patients who receive chemotherapy. It is estimated that approximately 2 million platelet transfusions are given per year in the United States. Patients who are thrombocytopenic from chemotherapy, including patients who receive intensive, high-dose chemotherapy with stem cell support appear to be the largest group of patients who receive platelet transfusions.[45] Comparative studies have shown that either random-donor platelets or platelets from a single donor have similar hemostatic benefits and side effects and produce similar boosts in post-transfusion platelet levels. The ASCO guidelines state that both products can

---

BOX 3–5 Clinical Manifestations of Chemotherapy-Induced Thrombocytopenia

Petechiae (hallmark)
Bruising
Ecchymoses
Epistaxis
Bleeding from mucous membrane
Severe purpura

Table 3–9 **Examples of Major and Minor Bleeding**

Major Bleeding	Minor Bleeding
Nasal bleeding	Bleeding gums
Gastrointestinal hemorrhage	Mild vaginal bleeding
Bladder and vaginal hemorrhage	Bloody urine
Pulmonary hemorrhage	Bloody sputum

Data from Elting, Rubenstein EB, Martin CG, et al. Incidence, cost and outcomes of bleeding and chemotherapy dose modification among solid tumor patients with chemotherapy-induced thrombocytopenia. *J Clin Oncol* 2001; 19:1137–1146.

Table 3–10 Platelet Products

Product	Method of Isolation	Advantages	Disadvantages
Random-donor platelets (contain ~0.5–0.75 × 10^11 platelets cells/unit)	Platelet concentrates from whole blood	Less costly More available	Must be pooled at the time of collection Not leukoreduced at time of collection and requires additional steps
Single-donor platelets (contain ~3 × 10^11 platelet cells/unit)	By apheresis from single donors	Lower risk of alloimmunization Decrease risk of disease transmission	Cost 50%–100% more than an equivalent dose of pooled platelets

be used interchangeably.[46] Table 3–10 describes some of the differences between random-donor platelets, which are obtained from pooled blood donations, and single donor-platelets, which are obtained from a single donor by plasmapheresis.

There are two major reasons for transfusing platelets to thrombocytopenic patients: for prevention or treatment of bleeding. Today, in the United States, prophylactic transfusion of platelets is a common practice to prevent the risk of serious bleeding when the platelet count falls to less than 20,000 cells/microliter.[47] In a recent survey, more than 70% of clinicians indicated that they administer platelet transfusions to patients prophylactically when they anticipate that a patient's platelet count will fall below a certain threshold.[48] Of the hospitals surveyed, 60% used a level of 20,000 cells/microliter as the threshold level for prophylactic platelet transfusion.

Although platelet transfusions are an effective strategy for managing chemotherapy-induced thrombocytopenia, platelets are a limited resource, and because platelets are a blood product, transfusion is associated with some risks. The ASCO guidelines were developed to help guide clinicians through the decision-making process for appropriate utilization of platelet products. The ASCO guidelines recommend that prophylactic platelet transfusion should be administered to patients with thrombocytopenia due to impaired bone marrow function to reduce the risk of hemorrhage when platelet levels fall below a predefined threshold level, depending on the clinical situation (Table 3–11).[46] The recommendations emphasize that the decision to give a patient a transfusion should not depend solely on the platelet count; rather, it should be determined on the basis of specific patient needs. For treatment of active bleeding, platelet transfusions are generally unnecessary in patients with platelet counts greater than 100,000 cells/microliter.[45] However, the optimal threshold platelet count necessitating transfusion for patients who are bleeding is not clear and may vary depending on the patient and the clinical situation.

One unit of whole blood–derived platelet concentrate usually contains approximately 70 billion platelet cells and would be expected to raise the platelet count by as much as 10,000 cells/microliter. This increase is typically achieved within 1–3 hours after transfusion, although not all patients will experience a boost to this degree in their platelet counts. There is a dose-response relationship with platelet transfusion. An empiric way to determine the total dose of platelets required is to give a patient 1 unit of platelet concentrate per 20 kg of body weight.[47] On average, the administration of 6 units of platelets should increase platelet levels by approximately 40,000 cells/microliter. Monitoring of the platelet count 1 hour after transfusion has proven to be an excellent indicator for effective platelet transfusion.[49]

Table 3–11 ASCO Guidelines for Prophylactic Platelet Transfusions for Different Oncologic Conditions

Conditions	Recommended Threshold for Prophylactic Platelet Transfusions	Comments
Acute leukemia	10,000 cells/microliter	Transfusion at higher threshold may be required if patients possess higher risks for hemorrhage or coagulation abnormalities or undergo invasive procedures
Hematopoietic cell transplantation	10,000 cells/microliter	Transfusion at higher threshold may be required if patients possess higher risks for hemorrhage or coagulation abnormalities or undergo invasive procedures
Chronic, stable, severe thrombocytopenia in aplastic anemia or myelodysplasia patient	Reserve platelet transfusions only for episodes of hemorrhage or during times of active treatment	It is observed that patients have minimal or no significant bleeding for long periods of time despite low platelet counts
Solid tumors	Generally at 10,000 cells/microliter; however, at 20,000 cells/microliter under special considerations	Patients with gynecologic, colorectal, or bladder tumors or melanoma may receive radiation therapy and have higher bleeding risks from necrotic tumor sites; ASCO guidelines suggest higher platelet transfusion thresholds (>20,000 cells/microliter) for those patients. Patients with poor performance status who have limited access to health care facilities during thrombocytopenia that is expected to be profound and prolonged should be considered for a higher infusion threshold (>20,000 cells/microliter)
Surgical or invasive procedures including lumbar puncture, liver biopsy, gastrointestinal endoscopy, bronchoscopy, bronchoalveolar lavage, and transbronchial biopsy	40,000–50,000 cells/microliter	Guidelines state that a platelet count of 40,000–50,000 cells/microliter is sufficient to perform major invasive procedures with safety, in the absence of associated coagulation abnormalities. If platelet transfusions are administered before a procedure, a post-transfusion count should be obtained to prove that the target count has achieved.
Bone marrow biopsy and aspirations	20,000 cells/microliter	Guidelines state that biopsies clearly can be performed safely even below this threshold

Data from McCullough J. Transfusion medicine. In Handin RI, Lux SE, Stossel TP, eds. *Blood: Principles and Practice of Hematology.* Philadelphia: JB Lippincott; 2003.

Since the widespread utilization of nucleic acid testing starting in 1999, the risk of transmission of human immunodeficiency virus and hepatitis C virus through transfusions of blood products is extremely low—almost as low as 1 case per 1 million units of blood product transfused.[50] However, there are still public health concerns related to the transmission of other diseases through the blood supply, such as the West Nile virus or Creutzfeldt-Jakob disease, which pose a potential risk to patients receiving blood product support. The development of transfusion "refractoriness" is another major concern with platelet transfusions.

Patients who do not obtain the expected post-transfusion increase in platelet count are considered to be transfusion refractory. The use of modified platelet products such as leukoreduced platelets is associated with a significant reduction of lymphocytotoxic antibody formation that can prevent patients from becoming alloimmunized and decreases the risk of patients' developing refractoriness to platelet transfusions.[51] The ASCO guidelines recommend the use of modified platelet products in patients who are expected to require multiple transfusions, such as those with newly diagnosed acute leukemia. However, leukocyte-poor blood products are costly and should be reserved for use in patients who are at greatest risk for developing refractoriness to platelet transfusions.

Acute systemic reactions to platelet transfusions are common and affect approximately 2% of patients who receive platelets.[52] Clinical manifestations such as rash, wheezing, fever, chills, dyspnea, urticaria, and hypotension are commonly observed. The older the platelet product and the higher the patient's white cell count, the more likely it is that a reaction episode could occur. Premedication with diphenhydramine and acetaminophen does not reduce the incidence of infusion reactions with platelet transfusions.[53]

Various thrombopoietic growth factors have been investigated for the management of chemotherapy-induced thrombocytopenia. Oprelvekin (recombinant interleukin-11, Neumega) is a thrombopoietic growth factor that stimulates the proliferation of hematopoietic stem cells and megakaryocyte progenitors and induces megakaryocytic maturation. Oprelvekin is indicated for the prevention of severe thrombocytopenia and a reduction in the need for platelet transfusions after myelosuppressive chemotherapy in adult patients with nonmyeloid malignancies who are at high risk of severe thrombocytopenia.[3] The use of oprelvekin in 93 cancer patients who had severe chemotherapy-induced thrombocytopenia was studied in a randomized, controlled clinical trial.[54] Patients enrolled in this trial had solid tumors and lymphomas and received either oprelvekin at 50 mcg/kg daily or placebo starting 1 day after chemotherapy, in addition to transfusion support. Subsequent chemotherapy treatment continued during the study period without dose reduction. Patients in the oprelvekin arm received significantly fewer platelet transfusions (30% in oprelvekin group versus 4% in placebo group). Similar efficacy was shown when oprelvekin was studied in breast cancer patients who received chemotherapy treatment and were supported with oprelvekin.[55] Investigators initially believed that oprelvekin could reduce the cost of management of thrombocytopenia by decreasing the need for platelet transfusions. The cost of 6 units of platelets is approximately $300.[56] However, despite the reduction in platelet transfusions with oprelvekin therapy, a recent pharmacoeconomic analysis revealed that oprelvekin does not provide any overall cost savings.[57]

The recommended dose of oprelvekin in adults without severe renal impairment is 50 mcg/kg given once daily subcutaneously as a single injection in the abdomen, thigh, or hip. Patients are encouraged to rotate injection sites while receiving oprelvekin. Dosing should be initiated 6–24 hours after the completion of chemotherapy and should be continued daily until the post-nadir platelet count is greater than 50,000 cells/microliter. Platelet counts should be monitored periodically to assess the optimal duration of therapy. The manufacturer does not recommend doses beyond 21 days per treatment course. Treatment with oprelvekin should be discontinued at least 2 days before the next planned cycle of chemotherapy is started. Oprelvekin is supplied as a vial with lyophilized powder for subcutaneous injection and must be reconstituted before administration. Oprelvekin is stable only for 3 hours once reconstituted. For some patients, the process of reconstituting the drug may be technically challenging.

SUPPORTIVE CARE

Table 3–12 **Side Effects Associated with Oprelvekin**

Side Effects	Clinical Manifestations	Comments
Hypersensitivity reactions and anaphylaxis	Edema of the face, tongue, and larynx, shortness of breath, wheezing, chest pain, hypotension, loss of consciousness, mental status changes, rash, urticaria, flushing, and fever	Hypersensitivity reactions may occur after the first dose or subsequent doses of oprelvekin. Oprelvekin should be discontinued permanently if patients experience allergic or hypersensitivity reactions.
Edema	Fluid retention, weight gain, and dilutional anemia	Fluid balance should be monitored closely. Patients with congestive heart failure or preexisting ascites or pleural effusions should be observed carefully for increasing fluid accumulation. For some patients, water weight gain may cause serious problems that require diuretic or hospitalization. Both fluid retention and dilutional anemia are reversible within several days to a week after discontinuation of oprelvekin.
Cardiovascular events	Transient arrhythmias, pulmonary edema, and stroke have been observed. Arrhythmias were typically brief and converted to sinus rhythm spontaneously or after rate-control drug therapy. Recurrent arrhythmias were observed in patients who were re-challenged with oprelvekin. Strokes have been reported in patients who experienced atrial arrhythmias while receiving oprelvekin.	Patients with a history of congestive heart failure are at high risk for developing atrial arrhythmias and should be monitored closely when receiving oprelvekin. Patients with a history of stroke or transient ischemic attack may also be at increased risk for cardiovascular events.
Papilledema	Papilledema has been reported in 1.5% of patients receiving oprelvekin.	Oprelvekin should be used with caution in patients with preexisting papilledema or with tumors involving the central nervous system because it is possible that papilledema could worsen or develop during treatment.

Data from Neumega (oprelvekin) prescribing information. Madison, NJ: Wyeth; 2004.

Oprelvekin is associated with significant side effects, including hypersensitivity reactions, fluid retention and edema, cardiac arrhythmias, and other cardiovascular events. Table 3–12 provides a detailed listing of some of the side effects and management strategies for oprelvekin.

Oprelvekin is the only commercially available thrombopoietic growth factor. Researchers have focused extensively on the development of recombinant thrombopoietin, not only because of its potential efficacy but also because it is relatively specific in its action to stimulate megakaryocyte growth. In the past decade, two different recombinant thrombopoietin products were developed, namely recombinant human thrombopoietin and **pegylated recombinant human megakaryocyte growth** and development factor (PEG-rHuMGDF). Studies have suggested an almost fivefold increase in platelet counts after the administration of recombinant thrombopoietin.[39] However, there is a lag time of 4–5 days before circulating platelet counts rise after recombinant thrombopoietin administration and often normal platelet recovery in the bone marrow is already underway. In addition, PEG-rHuMGDF was found to be immunogenic and produced neutralizing antibodies, which has limited its clinical usefulness.[58] The utilization of recombinant thrombopoietin seems promising in theory for the management of chemotherapy-induced thrombocytopenia; however, its efficacy in the clinical setting is extremely limited.

Thrombocytopenia is one of the most common complications among cancer patients who receive chemotherapy. To date, platelet transfusions remain the standard of care for the acute management of thrombocytopenia in cancer patients. Recently investigators have identified patients who are at higher risk for bleeding, and guidelines that suggest appropriate transfusion thresholds to prevent bleeding due to thrombocytopenia are in place. The discovery of thrombopoietic growth factors is encouraging; however, the utility of these agents is limited because of significant, intolerable side effects and modest clinical activity.

CONCLUSION

As long as the use of traditional, cytotoxic chemotherapy drugs remains a part of standard cancer treatment, the hematologic toxicities such as neutropenia, anemia, and thrombocytopenia will continue to be contentious side effects. Transfusions of platelets and red blood cells can prevent acute complications from anemia and thrombocytopenia. Administration of hematopoietic growth factors may decrease the incidence and severity of life-threatening neutropenia and neutropenic infections after myelosuppressive chemotherapy. Erythropoietic factors can decrease the need for blood transfusions and provide patients with symptomatic relief from anemia that affects functional ability and quality of life. These interventions to support patients through the myelosuppressive effects of chemotherapy can have an overall positive impact on cancer patient care by allowing patients to successfully complete their therapy.

REFERENCES

1. Balmer CM, Finley RS. Systemic toxicity. In Finley RS, Balmer CM, eds. *Concepts in Oncology Therapeutics,* 2nd ed. Bethesda, MD: American Society of Health-System Pharmacists; 1998:99–106.
2. Mughl TI. Current and future use of hematopoietic growth factors in cancer medicine. *Hematol Oncol* 2004;22:121–134.
3. Neumega prescribing information. Madison, NJ: Wyeth; 2004.
4. Common Terminology Criteria for Adverse Events: Blood/Bone Marrow, version March 31, 2003 (published December 12, 2003). Available at: http://ctep.cancer.gov/forms/CTCAEv3.pdf. Accessed December 7, 2006.
5. Myeloid growth factors in cancer treatment, V.2.2005. NCCN Clinical Practice Guidelines in Oncology. Available at: www.nccn.org/professionals/physician_gls/PDF/myeloid_growth.pdf. Accessed December 7, 2006.
6. Hughes WT, Armstrong D, Bodey GP, et al. 2002 guidelines for the use of antimicrobial agents in neutropenic patients with cancer. *Clin Infect Dis* 2002;34:730–751.
7. Bucaneve G, Micozzi A, Menichetti F, et al. Levofloxacin to prevent bacterial infection in patients with cancer and neutropenia. *N Engl J Med* 2005;353:977–987.
8. Cullen M, Steven N, Billingham L, et al. Antibacterial prophylaxis after chemotherapy for solid tumors and lymphomas. *N Engl J Med* 2005;353:988–998.
9. Gafter-Gvill A, Frase A, Paul M, Leibovici L. Meta-analysis: antibiotic prophylaxis reduces mortality in neutropenic patients. *Ann Intern Med* 2005;142:979–995.
10. Fever and neutropenia, version 1.2005; NCCN Clinical Practice Guidelines in Oncology Available at: www.nccn.org/professionals/physician_gls/PDF/fever.pdf. Accessed December 7, 2006.
11. Ozer H, Armitage JO, Bennett CL, et al. 2000 update of recommendations for the use of colony-stimulating factors: evidence-based, clinical practice guidelines. *J Clin Oncol* 2000;18:3558–3585.
11a. Smith TJ, Khatcheressian J, Lyman GH, et al. 2006 update of recommendations for the use of white blood cell growth factors: an evidence-based clinical practice guideline. *J Clin Oncol* 2006;24(19): 3187-3205.

SUPPORTIVE CARE

12. *Thompson PDR Redbook*, 2004 ed. Montvale, NJ: Medical Economics Company.

13. Clark OAA, Lyman GH, Castro AA, et al. Colony-stimulating factors for chemotherapy-induced febrile neutropenia: a meta-analysis of randomized controlled trials. *J Clin Oncol* 2005;23:4198–4124.

14. Neulasta prescribing information. Thousand Oaks, CA: Amgen.

15. Beverage RA, Miller JA, Kales AN, et al. A comparison of the efficacy of sargramostim (yeast-derived RhuGM-CSF) and filgrastim (bacteria-derived RhuG-CSF) in the therapeutic setting of chemotherapy-induced myelosuppression. *Cancer Invest* 1998;16:366–373.

16. Stull DM, Bilmes R, Kim H, Fichtl R. Comparison of sargramostim and filgrastim in the treatment of chemotherapy-induced neutropenia. *Am J Health-Syst Pharm* 2005;62:83–87.

17. Wong SF, Chan HO. Effects of a formulary change from granulocyte colony-stimulating factor to granulocyte-macrophage colony-stimulating factor on outcomes in patients treated with myelosuppressive chemotherapy. *Pharmacotherapy* 2005;25:372–378.

18. Holmes FA, O'Shaughnessy JA, Vukelja S, et al. Blinded, randomized, multicenter study to evaluate single administration of pegfilgrastim once per cycle versus daily filgrastim as an adjunct to chemotherapy in patients with high-risk stage II or stage III/IV breast cancer. *J Clin Oncol* 2002;20: 727–731.

19. Vose JM, Crump M, Lazarus H, et al. Randomized, multicenter, open-label study of pegfilgrastim compared with daily filgrastim after chemotherapy for lymphoma. *J Clin Oncol* 2003;21:514–519.

20. Green M, Koelbl H, Baselga J, et al. A randomized, double-blind, phase III study evaluating fixed-dose, single administration pegfilgrastim. V. Daily filgrastim in patients receiving myelosuppressive chemotherapy. *Ann Oncol* 2003;14:29–35.

21. Leukine prescribing information. Richmond, CA: Berlex Laboratories.

22. Koeller JM. Clinical guidelines for the treatment of cancer-related anemia. *Pharmacotherapy* 1998; 18:156–169.

22a.Prchal JT. In Lichtman MA, Beutler E, Kipps TJ, Seligsohn U, Kaushansky K, Prchal JT, eds. *Williams Hematology*, ed 7. 2005.

23. Meadowcroft AM, Gilbert CJ, Maravich-May D, Hayward SL. Cost of managing anemia with and without prophylactic epoetin alfa therapy in breast cancer patients receiving combination chemotherapy. *Am J Health-Syst Pharm* 1998;55:1898–1902.

24. Rizzo JD, Lichtin AE, Woolf SH, et al. Use of epoetin in patients with cancer: evidence-based clinical practice guidelines of the American Society of Clinical Oncology and the American Society of Hematology. *J Clin Oncol* 2002;20:4083–4107.

25. Cancer and treatment-related anemia, V.2.2005. NCCN Clinical Practice Guidelines in Oncology. Available at: www.nccn.org.

26. Witzig TE, Silberstein PT, Loprinzi CL, et al. Phase III, randomized, double-blind study of epoetin alfa versus placebo in anemic patients with cancer undergoing chemotherapy. *J Clin Oncol* 2005;23:2606–2617.

27. Schwartzberg LS, Yee LK, Senecal FM, et al. A randomized comparison of every-2-week darbepoetin alfa and weekly epoetin alfa for the treatment of chemotherapy-induced anemia in patients with breast, lung or gynecological cancer. *Oncologist* 2004;9:696–707.

28. Patton J, Reeves T, Wallace J. Effectiveness of darbepoetin alfa versus epoetin alfa in patients with chemotherapy-induced anemia treated in clinical practice. *Oncologist* 2004;9:451–458.

29. Schwartzberg L, Shiffman R, Tomita D, et al. A multicenter retrospective cohort study of practice patterns and clinical outcomes of the use of darbepoetin alfa and epoetin alfa for chemotherapy-induced anemia. *Clin Ther* 2003;23:2781–2796.

30. Henke M, Laszig R, Rube C, et al. Erythropoietin to treat head and neck cancer patients with anemia undergoing radiotherapy: randomized, double-blind, placebo-controlled trial. *Lancet* 2003;362: 1255–1260.

31. Leyland-Jones B, Semiglazov V, Pawlicki M, et al. Maintaining normal hemoglobin levels with epoetin alfa in mainly nonanemic patients with metastatic breast cancer receiving first-line chemotherapy: a survival study. *J Clin Oncol* 2005;23:5960–5972.

32. Auerbach M, Ballard H, Trout JR, et al. Intravenous iron optimizes the response to recombinant human erythropoietin in cancer patients with chemotherapy-related anemia: a multicenter, open-label, randomized trial. *J Clin Oncol* 2004;22:1301–1307.

33. Macdougall I. Antibody-mediated pure red cell aplasia (PRCA): epidemiology, immunogenicity and risks. *Nephrol Dial Transplant* 2005;20(Suppl 4):iv9–iv15.

34. George JN. Platelets. *Lancet* 2000;355:1531–1539.

35. Weaver SJ, Johns TE. Drug-induced hematologic disorders. In DiPiro JT, Talbert RL, Yee GC, et al., eds. *Pharmacotherapy: A Pathophysiologic Approach,* 7th ed. Stamford, CT: Appleton & Lange; 2005:1875–1879.

36. Wang R. Hematologic abnormalities. In Ford MD, Delaney KA, Ling LJ, Erickson T, eds. *Clinical Toxicology,* 1st ed. Philadelphia: WB Saunders; 2001:198–210.

37. Warkentin TE, Kelton JG. Thrombocytopenia due to platelet destruction and hypersplenism. In Hoffman R, Benz EJ, eds. *Hematology: Basic Principles and Practice.* Philadelphia: Elsevier; 2005:2305–2325.

38. Fruchtman SM, Hoffman R. Essential thrombocythemia. In Hoffman R, Benz EJ, eds. *Hematology: Basic Principles and Practice.* Philadelphia: Elsevier; 2005:1277–1296.

39. Kuter DJ, Begley CG. Recombinant human thrombopoietin: basic etiology and evaluation of clinical studies. *Blood* 2002;100:3457–3469.

40. Elting EL, Rubenstein EB, Martin CG, et al. Incidence, cost and outcomes of bleeding and chemo-therapy dose modification among solid tumor patients with chemotherapy-induced thrombocytope-nia. *J Clin Oncol* 2001;19:1137–1146.

41. Belt RJ, Leite C, Hass CD, Stephens RL. Incidence of hemorrhagic complications in patients with cancer. *JAMA* 1978;;239:2571–2574.

42. Dutcher JP, Schiffer CA, Aisner J, et al. Incidence of thrombocytopenia and serious hemorrhage among patients with solid tumors. *Cancer* 1984;53:557–562.

43. Capo G, Waltzman R. Managing hematologic toxicities. *J Support Oncol* 2004;2:65–79.

44. Hartwig JH, Italiano JE Jr. In Handin RI, Lux SE, Stossel TP, eds. *Blood: Principles and Practice of Hematology.* Philadelphia: JB Lippincott; 2003.

45. McCullough J, Steeper TA, Connelly DP, et al. Platelet utilization in a university hospital. *JAMA* 1988;259:2414–2418.

46. Schiffer CA, Anderson KC, Bennett CL, et al. Platelet transfusion for patients with cancer: clinical practice guidelines of the American Society of Clinical Oncology. *J Clin Oncol* 2001;19:1519–1538.

47. McCullough J. Transfusion medicine. In Handin RI, Lux SE, Stossel TP, eds. *Blood: Principles and Practice of Hematology.* Philadelphia: JB Lippincott; 2003.

48. Pisciotto PT, Benson K, Hume H. Prophylactic versus therapeutic platelet transfusion practices in hematology and/or oncology patients. *Transfusion* 1995;35:498–502.

49. Daly PA, Schiffer CA, Aisner J, Wiernik PH. Platelet transfusion therapy: one-hour posttransfusion incre-ments are valuable in predicting the need for HLA-matched preparations. *JAMA* 1980;243:435–438.

50. Stramer SL, Glynn SA, Kleinman SH, et al. Detection of HIV-1 and HCV infections among anti-body-negative US blood donors by nucleic acid amplification testing. *N Engl J Med* 2004;351:760–768.

51. Group TTS: Leukocyte reduction and UV-B irradiation of platelets to prevent alloimmunization and refractoriness to platelet transfusion. *N Engl J Med* 1997;337:1861–1869.

52. Kickler TS. Principles of platelet transfusion therapy. In Hoffman R, Benz EJ, eds. *Hematology: Basic Principles and Practice.* Philadelphia: Elsevier; 2005:2433–2440.

53. Wang SE, Lara PN Jr, Lee-Ow A, et al. Acetaminophen and diphenhydramine as premedication for platelet transfusions: a prospective randomized double-blind placebo-controlled trial. *Am J Hematol* 2002;70:191–194.

54. Tepler I, Elias L, Smith JW, et al. A randomized placebo-controlled trial of recombinant human in-terleukin-11 in cancer patients with severe thrombocytopenia due to chemotherapy. *Blood* 1996;87:3607–3614.

55. Isaacs C, Robert NJ, Bailey FA, et al. Randomized placebo-controlled study of recombinant human interleukin-11 to prevent chemotherapy-induced thrombocytopenia in patients with breast cancer receiving dose-intensive cyclophosphamide and doxorubicin. *J Clin Oncol* 1997;15:3368–3377.

56. Kaushansky K. Thrombopoietin. *N Engl J Med* 1998;339:746–754.

57. Cantor SB, Elting LS, Hudson DV, Rubenstein EB. Pharmacoeconomic analysis of oprelvekin (recombinant human interleukin-1) for secondary prophylaxis of thrombocytopenia in solid tumor patients receiving chemotherapy. *Cancer* 2003;97:3099–3106.

58. Demetri GD. Targeted approaches for the treatment of thrombocytopenia. *Oncologist* 2001;6(Suppl 5):15–23.

SUPPORTIVE CARE

Chapter 2
Management and Treatment of Nausea and Vomiting
Courtney W. Yuen

INTRODUCTION

Chemotherapy-induced nausea and vomiting (CINV) is one of the most feared side effect facing cancer patients.[1–3] Although improvement has been seen throughout the years, patients still shudder at the thought of persistent, uncontrolled nausea and vomiting. Uncontrolled nausea and vomiting can significantly affect one's quality of life, and studies have shown dramatic decreases in the ability to carry on normal day-to-day functions, such as preparing and enjoying meals.[4] The importance of controlling CINV has led to the development of various practice guidelines by both national and international organizations such as the American Society of Clinical Oncology (ASCO),[5] the American Society of Health-System Pharmacists (ASHP),[6] the National Comprehensive Cancer Network (NCCN),[7] and the Multinational Association of Supportive Care in Cancer (MASCC).[8] Despite the fact that the above-mentioned guidelines are based on analysis of published trials, they all have slightly different recommendations. These differences have led to some confusion regarding the optimal therapy for the prevention of CINV. Studies have shown that although these guidelines are available, utilization and adherence by practitioners are minimal at best.[9] Guidelines are established to help assure optimal evidence-based patient care. They also serve as an educational aid to trainees and help contain health care costs by standardizing ordering, preparation, and administration of antiemetic therapy. Understanding the rational behind the guidelines, as well as the pathophysiology of CINV, will allow the practitioners to provide optimal care for the cancer patient.

CINV is generally divided into three phases: acute, delayed, and anticipatory. Acute CINV is defined as nausea and/or vomiting that occurs within 24 hours of chemotherapy administration, with peak activity between 4 and 6 hours after its administration. Acute CINV tends to be very responsive to drug therapy.

Delayed CINV is nausea and vomiting that occurs 24 or more hours after the administration of chemotherapy. Anticipatory nausea and vomiting occurs in about 20% of chemotherapy-treated patients and is associated with emesis before the administration of a cycle of chemotherapy. Delayed nausea can persist for as long as 120 hours after the administration of chemotherapy.[6] It is best characterized by the nausea that is seen after high-dose cisplatin, with peak effects occurring at 48–72 hours and subsiding in another 48–72 hours.[10] Delayed emesis is more difficult to control, with widely variable responses to drug therapy.

Anticipatory nausea can be elicited by a variety of stimuli and usually occurs before the second or subsequent chemotherapy regimen.[11] Patients whose CINV was poorly controlled after they received their initial or previous/chemotherapy are at risk for developing anticipatory nausea or vomiting. It is considered a conditioned or learned response, and there is a strong psychological component to anticipatory nausea and vomiting that does not respond as well as the other types of CINV to drug therapy or prophylaxis. Behavior modification, however, may be beneficial.[6]

The best strategy is to prevent acute nausea and vomiting from occurring in the first place. Patients who have emesis despite receiving prophylactics antiemetics are classified as having breakthrough emesis. Breakthrough nausea and vomiting occurs on the day of chemotherapy, despite appropriate preventative antiemetic therapy. The underlying pathogenesis of refractory or breakthrough nausea and vomiting is unknown.

PHYSIOLOGY

CINV is made up of different components that should be evaluated individually. Nausea is very subjective. It is defined as the conscious recognition of the need to vomit, usually associated with hypersalivation, flushing, and tachycardia. Because it is subjective, it is very difficult to assess, and assessment will usually depend on open communication with the patient.

Vomiting is defined as the oral expulsion of gastric contents. It involves the coordination of the abdominal muscles, diaphragm, and the gastric cardia.[6] Vomiting is initiated by the vomiting center, located in the reticular formation of the medulla. The vomiting center will receive afferent impulses from the chemoreceptor trigger zone (CTZ) or from afferent fibers located in the gastrointestinal tract, cerebral cortex, or vestibular apparatus. Neurotransmitters play a significant role in the stimulation of the vomiting center (see Color Plate 1). More than 30 different neurotransmitters have been found to be involved in the stimulation of the chemoreceptor trigger zone (CTZ); however, only three have been identified as having significant clinical relevance with CINV: dopamine, serotonin, and neurokinase-1 (NK-1).[11]

Dopamine has long been known to stimulate dopamine-2 receptors. Dopamine-2 receptors are located on neurons in the area postrema adjacent to the CTZ. Blocking these receptors has been shown to treat nausea. However, the effectiveness of dopamine 2-receptor blockage has been minimal at best. In early studies, treatment of CINV with a higher dose of dopamine antagonist showed a slightly better response, especially with metoclopramide. It was subsequently found that at higher doses, metoclopramide also blocked serotonin receptors.[12]

Serotonin receptors are found predominately in the gastrointestinal tract. Various studies have showed an exponential increase in serotonin after the administration of single-dose cisplatin.[13] Chemotherapy drugs are thought to stimulate the enterochromaffin cells and, at least in part, form free oxygen radicals, which in turn release serotonin.[14]

Substance P is a peptide neurotransmitter that binds to NK-1 receptors. NK-1 receptors are predominately located in the intestine and nucleus tractus solitarius of the brain. Substance P is localized in the enterochromaffin cells of the intestine with serotonin. In response to stimulation by chemotherapy, substance P is released along with serotonin. Substance P may also be released on its own in response to cytotoxic stimulation of the CTZ.[13,16] In the delayed phase of CIVN, substance P is still present, indicating a potential role in delayed emesis that may be significant.[17]

RISK FACTORS

Various factors, which can be categorized into either patient-specific or treatment-specific, have been associated with a high risk of poorly controlled nausea and vomiting. Patient-specific factors include age younger than 50 years, female sex, and prior exposure to chemotherapy (Table 3–13).[17] Treatment-specific factors include the chemotherapeutic agent used, dosing, route, and method of administration (Table 3–14).[18,19]

In 1997, Hesketh et al.[20] proposed a system of classifying the emetogenic potential of chemotherapy. Agents were divided into five levels of emetogenicity based on their risk of emesis without the use of antiemetic agents (Box 3–6), with agents in level 1 having the least emetogenic potential and agents in level 5 having the most.

The chemotherapy routes, rates of administration, and ages of patients were standardized (i.e., intravenous, short bolus infusions in adults). These authors also proposed a schema for prediction of the emetogenicity of combination therapy (Box 3–7).

Another tool used to grade toxicity is the National Cancer Institute Common Toxicity Criteria. Severity of nausea and vomiting is separated into grades. These grades are used frequently in studies to standardize the rating of nausea and vomiting (Table 3–15).

Table 3–13 **Patient-Specific Risk Factors**

High Risk	Low Risk
Acute Emesis	
Age younger than 50 years	Age older than 50 years
Female	Male
History of prior chemotherapy	History of significant ethanol consumption
	Chemotherapy naïve
Delayed Emesis	
Poorly controlled acute emesis with chemotherapy	
Chemotherapy known to cause delayed emesis (cisplatin, cyclophosphamide, carboplatin, doxorubicin, ifosfamide)	
Anticipatory Emesis	
Poorly controlled emesis with previous chemotherapy regimen	
History of anxiety or depressive disorders	

Table 3–14 **Treatment-Specific Risks**

High Risk	Low Risk
Intravenous	Oral
Bolus	Continuous infusion
High dose	Low dose
High emetic potential agent	Low emetic potential agent

Box 3–6 Chemotherapy Drugs with a High Risk of Producing Emesis

Level 5
Carmustine >250 mg/m^2
Cisplatin >50 mg/m^2
Cyclophosphamide >1500 mg/m^2
Dacarbazine
Mechlorethamine
Streptozocin

Level 4
Carboplatin
Carmustine <250 mg/m^2
Cisplatin <50 mg/m^2
Cyclophosphamide 750–1500 mg/m^2
Cytarabine >1000 mg/m^2
Doxorubicin >60 mg/m^2
Methotrexate >1000 mg/m^2
Oxaliplatin
Procarbazine

Level 3
Cyclophosphamide <750 mg/m^2
Cyclophosphamide (oral)
Doxorubicin 20–60mg/m^2
Epirubicin <90 mg/m^2
Idarubicin
Ifosfamide
Irinotecan
Methotrexate 250–1000 mg/m^2
Mitoxantrone <15 mg/m^2
Temozolomide

Level 2
Capecitabine
Docetaxel
Etoposide
Fluorouracil
Gemcitabine
Methotrexate 50–250 mg/m^2
Paclitaxel
Topotecan

Level 1
Bleomycin
Busulfan
Chlorambucil
2-Chlorodeoxyadenosine
Fludarabine
Hydroxyurea
Methotrexate <50 mg/m^2
Vinblastine
Vincristine
Vinorelbine

Data from UpToDate. August 2005.[21]

Box 3–7 Algorithm for Defining the Emetogenicity of Combination Chemotherapy

Identify the most emetogenic agent in the combination.
  Assess the relative contribution of the other agents to the combination.
  Level 1 agents do not contribute to the emetogenicity.
  Adding one or more Level 2 agents increases the emetogenicity of the combination by one level greater than the most emetogenic agent in the combination.
  Adding a Level 3 or greater agent increases the emetogenicity of the combination by one level per agent.

Table 3–15 **Common Toxicity Criteria (CTC)**

	Grade 1	Grade 2	Grade 3	Grace 4	Grade 5
Nausea	Loss of appetite without alteration in eating habits	Oral intake decreased without significant weight loss, dehydration; IV fluids indicated <24 hours	Inadequate oral caloric or fluid intake, tube feedings or TPN indicated ≥24 hours	Life-threatening consequences	Death
Vomiting	1 episode in 24 hours	2-5 episodes in 24 hours; IV fluids indicated <24 hours	>6 episodes in 24 hours; IV fluids or TPN indicated ≥24 hours	Life-threatening consequences	Death

IV, intravenous; TPN, total parenteral nutrition.
Data from National Cancer Institute Cancer Therapy Evaluation Program (CTEP).

Table 3–16 **Currently Available Serotonin Antagonist and Equivalent Dosing**

Intravenous	Oral
Ondansetron 8 mg IV × 1 dose or 0.15 mg/kg IV × 1 dose	24 mg PO × 1 dose (for highly emetogenic) 8 mg PO bid × 2 doses or 16 mg PO × 1 dose (for moderate emetogenic)
Granisetron 0.01 mg/kg IV (maximum 1 mg) or 1 mg IV × 1 dose	2 mg PO or 1 mg PO 2 times/day × 2 doses
Dolasetron 1.8 mg/kg IV × 1 dose or 100 mg IV × 1 dose	100–200 mg PO × 1 dose
Palonosetron 0.25 mg IV × 1 dose	Not available

IV, intravenous; PO, oral.
Can be used to prevent CINV for all chemotherapy with level 3–5 emetogenicity.
Should be used in combination with corticosteroids.
Oral seratonin antagonists should be administered at least 30 minutes before chemotherapy.

PHARMACOLOGY
Serotonin Antagonist

Serotonin type 3 receptor antagonists (5-hydroxytryptamine 3) are the mainstay of preventing acute CINV. As the name suggests, serotonin antagonists block serotonin type 3 receptors located throughout the gastrointestinal tract and the CTZ. At present, four serotonin antagonists are available in the United States. Ondansetron (Zofran) was the first to be approved by the U.S. Food and Drug Administration

SUPPORTIVE CARE

(FDA) and is perhaps the most well known. Later granisetron (Kytil), dolasetron (Anzemet), and palonosetron (Aloxi) were also approved for use. All agents, except palonosetron, are available as both oral tablets and intravenous solutions. These agents differ slightly from each other, but overall, studies show that all serotonin antagonists tend to be equivalent in efficacy and safety when given in appropriate doses.[22–26] Palonosetron has the highest binding affinity and the longest half-life of approximately 40 hours.[26] One dose of palonosetron should bind serotonin receptors for up to 7 days, and no subsequent dosing should be needed during those 7 days. It is the only serotonin type 3 antagonist that is approved by the FDA for both acute and delayed nausea and vomiting, but as indicated above it is only available as an intravenous injection.

Various studies have been conducted on use of multiple doses versus single doses of the serotonin antagonists. Economic issues have lead investigators to examine whether a single dose would provide the same benefits as multiple doses over the course of a day. Large randomized studies have shown that a single dose is just as effective as multiple doses in a 24-hour period.[27–29] Because the site of serotonin receptor binding is predominately in the gastrointestinal tract, oral administration has been proposed. Theoretically, as long as the serotonin type 3 receptors are blocked by the antagonist before the chemotherapy can stimulate the receptors, oral dosing should be just as effective as intravenous administration. In fact, equivalent oral dosing has been shown to be not only effective but also less costly.[30,31] Table 3–16 shows currently available serotonin antagonist and equivalent dosing.

Neurokinase-1 Receptor Antagonist

Aprepitant (Emend) was the first drug approved by the FDA in this class of antiemetic agents. Substance P is a peptide that is present throughout the brain and the gastrointestinal tract. Substance P sends signals via the NK-1 receptor that induce emesis.[32] When used with both a serotonin antagonist and dexamethasone, it has shown improved prevention of acute and delayed cisplatin-induced nausea and vomiting.[32–34] The current recommended dose of aprepitant is 125 mg orally once on day 1 before chemotherapy followed by 80 mg orally once daily on days 2 and 3. At this time, there are no dosing recommendations for multiple days of chemotherapy. Aprepitant is simultaneously a cytochrome P450 substrate, a moderate inducer and an inhibitor of enzyme 3A4 (CYP3A4), and an inducer of enzyme 2C9 (CYP2C9).[35] Aprepitant can increase the area under the curve of dexamethasone. Doses of dexamethasone should be reduced when used in combination with aprepitant (Table 3–17).[31] Many chemotherapy agents, such as the taxanes, vinca alkaloids, and etoposide are known to be metabolized by CYP3A4, and therefore the combination of aprepitant and agents metabolized by CYP3A4 or CYP2C9 should be used with caution because the effect would be enhanced toxicity of these agents. However, a recent study showed that aprepitant does not affect the pharmacokinetics of docetaxel in cancer patients.[36]

Table 3–17 **Use of Dexamethasone and Aprepitant**

In highly emetogenic chemotherapy	If used with aprepitant
Dexamethasone 20 mg IV/PO	Dexamethasone 12 mg PO or Dexamethasone 10 mg IV

IV, intravenous; PO, oral.

Corticosteroids

Corticosteroids, such as dexamethasone, methylprednisolone, and prednisone, have been used as antiemetics.[37–39] In combination with a serotonin antagonist, steroids are thought to increase antiemetic efficacy.[40–42] Although different steroids have been used, dexamethasone tends to be used most frequently. Doses greater than 20 mg have not been shown to be more effective,[43] but one study did show that doses of less than 20 mg of dexamethasone were inferior as an antiemetic.[44] Corticosteroid use has also been one of the cornerstones of preventing delayed chemotherapy-induced emesis. Before aprepitant, corticosteroids were the only agents that consistently provided some relief from delayed emesis.[45,46] Corticosteroids used in combination with either metoclopramide or a serotonin antagonist have demonstrated equivalent complete control of delayed emesis.[47]

Dopamine Antagonist

One of the more traditional classes of medications used to control emesis is the dopamine antagonist. For CINV, dopamine antagonists such as prochlorperazine (Compazine), promethazine (Phenergan), and metoclopramide (Reglan) are rarely used alone (Table 3–18). These agents tend to be less effective than serotonins antagonists for the control of acute CINV and often are associated with significant side effects such as dystonia, akathisia, sedation, and postural hypotension. More often, they are used for refractory emesis or for patients who are intolerant of serotonin antagonists and corticosteroids.[5]

Table 3–18 Dopamine Antagonists

Drug	Dosage
Metoclopramide	5–20 mg IV/PO every 6 hours
Prochlorperazine	5–10 mg IV/PO every 6 hours
	15–30 mg PO every 12 hours (extended release capsules)
	25 mg PR every 12 hours
Promethazine	12.5–50 mg IV/PO/PR every 6 hours

IV, intravenous; PO, oral; PR, per rectum.

Cannabinoids

Cannabinoids such as tetrahydrocannabinol appear to have antiemetic effects. Dronabinol (Marinol) is a synthetic tetrahydrocannabinol found in the *Cannabis sativa* plant. The mechanism for the prevention of CINV is not known, but the cannabinoid is thought to bind to cannabinoid-1 receptors found in the brain. As with the dopamine antagonists, cannabinoids are rarely used alone for the prevention of CINV. Doses range from 2.5 to 10 mg/m^2 orally every 8 hours. Side effects include drowsiness, sedation, and confusion. Younger patients or patients with a history of marijuana use tend to tolerate the side effects better than older patients.[48]

CONSENSUS GUIDELINES

In the late 1990s, four major health care professional organizations (ASCO, ASHP, MASCC, and NCCN) published their recommendations for the control of CINV. All had similar evidence-based recommendations with slight variations. These variations had probably led to some confusion and contributed to the lack of compliance by practitioners to the guidelines. Thus, in March 2004, the MASCC hosted a meeting of nine oncology organizations from around the world in Perugia, Italy, to obtain a consensus on the prevention of CINV.[49] The conference attendees addressed the issue of CINV as it pertained to highly emetogenic, moderately emetogenic, and low emetogenic chemotherapy and the issue of anticipatory nausea and vomiting.

SUPPORTIVE CARE

Table 3–19 **Highly Emetogenic Chemotherapy**

Acute	Delayed
Serotonin antagonist and Corticosteroid and Aprepitant	Corticosteroid and Aprepitant
• Use to lowest tested fully effective dose • No schedule better than single dose given before chemotherapy • Antiemetic efficacy and adverse effect of these agents are comparable in controlled trials • Intravenous and oral formulations are equally effective and safe • Always give with dexamethasone before chemotherapy	• Delayed nausea and vomiting after cisplatin is a distinct syndrome defined as nausea and vomiting that starts or continues the day after chemotherapy. • Delayed nausea and vomiting have been defined as commencing $\geq$24 hours after chemotherapy; however, more recent observations suggest these syndromes can begin earlier. • All patients receiving cisplatin should receive antiemetics to prevent delayed nausea and vomiting. • Given the dependence of delayed nausea and vomiting on acute antiemetic outcomes, optimal acute antiemetic prophylaxis should be employed.

Table 3–20 **Moderately Emetogenic Chemotherapy**

Acute	Delayed
Serotonin antagonist and Corticosteroid and Aprepitant (only in women receiving anthracycline plus cyclophosphamide).	Use only in patients known to be associated with a significant incidence of delayed nausea and vomiting Corticosteroid or Aprepitant (if used for acute)

Highly Emetogenic Chemotherapy

Although all of the previous guidelines recommended the use of serotonin antagonists and steroids, there were still several factors and principles that were not clearly defined. First of all, aprepitant was not commercially available until 2003, several years after the initial guidelines were published. Since the publication of these guidelines, two randomized studies have shown the benefits of adding aprepitant to a regimen of a serotonin antagonist and corticosteroids to prevent both acute and delayed nausea in patients receiving cisplatin.[32,50] The consensus conference participants agreed that aprepitant should be part of the antiemetic regimen for patients receiving highly emetogenic chemotherapy.[49] Other topics addressed by the consensus conference attendees included the use of a serotonin antagonist for delayed nausea and vomiting. The consensus conference participants did not find that recent studies adding dexamethasone to a serotonin antagonist demonstrated any improvement in the control of delayed CINV.[51–53] The recommendations of the consensus conference for the prevention of acute and delayed emesis induced by highly emetogenic chemotherapy are listed in Table 3–19.

Moderately Emetogenic Chemotherapy

The standard antiemetic therapy for acute emesis in patients receiving moderately emetogenic chemotherapy is the combination of a serotonin antagonist and dexamethasone.[54] This therapy was confirmed at the consensus meeting. However, the meeting attendees also suggested that aprepitant should be added in female patients who are receiving a combination of anthracycline and cyclophosphamide and thus

Table 3–21 Agents for Anticipatory Nausea and Vomiting

Lorazepam	0.5–1 mg PO/IV/SL before chemotherapy
Diazepam	2.5–5 mg PO/IV before chemotherapy

IV, intravenous; PO, oral; SL, sublingual.

have a higher risk of nausea and vomiting. For the prevention of delayed nausea and vomiting in patients receiving moderately emetogenic chemotherapy, the original published guidelines generally recommended the combination of dexamethasone and a serotonin antagonist. Studies, however, failed to show the superiority of the combination over dexamethasone alone.[55] The consensus conference participants therefore recommended using dexamethasone alone in patients with a higher risk of delayed emesis. If aprepitant was indicated for the acute phase of nausea and vomiting, it should be continued for the prevention of delayed nausea and vomiting. A summary of the consensus conference recommendations for the prevention of acute and delayed emesis induced by moderately emetogenic chemotherapy is listed in Table 3–20.

Low or Minimal Emetogenic Chemotherapy
For patients receiving low or minimal emetogenic chemotherapy, there is little evidence to support the use of any antiemetic therapy. However, it was also recognized that accurate assessment of CINV attributable to low or minimal emetogenic chemotherapy is not well documented. The consensus conference attendees did recommend the use of a single dose of 8 mg of oral dexamethasone in these patients.[56]

Anticipatory Nausea and Vomiting
Anticipatory nausea and vomiting is considered a conditioned response. If nausea and vomiting are well controlled initially, the risk of a patient's developing anticipatory nausea and vomiting decreases. Patient characteristics, such as age younger than 50 years or susceptibility to motion sickness, can predict the occurrence of anticipatory nausea and vomiting.[57] A benzodiazepine, such as lorazepam, is effective in reducing anticipatory nausea and vomiting (Table 3–21), but its efficacy tends to decrease with subsequent chemotherapy cycles.[49]

CONCLUSION
There have been many advances in the prevention of CINV; however, there is still much to learn. Although we have identified mechanisms for acute and delayed CINV, we still do not know what causes breakthrough refractory CINV. To date, there are no guidelines or consensus on how to treat breakthrough refractory CINV. We also do not know whether other factors contribute to acute and delayed CINV. Various professional organizations have attempted to use evidence-based trials to guide practice, but, as always, clinical judgment will play a major role in adherence to these guidelines.

REFERENCES
1. Coates A, Abraham S, Kaye SB, et al. On the receiving end—patient perception of the side-effects of cancer chemotherapy. *Eur J Cancer Clin Oncol* 1983;19:203–208.
2. de Boer-Dennert M, de Wit R, Schmitz PI, et al. Patient perceptions of the side-effects of chemotherapy: the influence of 5HT3 antagonist. *Br J Cancer* 1997;76:1055–1061.
3. Griffin AM, Butow PN, Coates AS, et al. On the receiving end: V. Patient perceptions of the side effects of cancer chemotherapy in 1993. *Ann Oncol* 1996;7:189–195.
4. Lindley CM, Hirsch JD, O'Niell CV, et al. Quality of life consequences of chemotherapy induced emesis. *Qual Life Res* 1992;1:331–340.
5. Gralla RJ, Osoba D, Kris G, et al. Recommendation for the use of antiemetics: evidence based clinical practice guidelines. *J Clin Oncol* 1999;17:2971–2994.

SUPPORTIVE CARE

6. American Society of Health System Pharmacists. ASHP guidelines on the pharmacologic management of nausea and vomiting in adult and pediatric patients receiving chemotherapy or radiation therapy or undergoing surgery. *Am J Health-Syst Pharmacist* 1999;56:729–764.

7. NCCN Clinical Practice Guidelines in Oncology, V.1.2005. Antiemesis. NCCN 2005. Available at www.nccn.org/professionals/physician%5Fgls/PDF/antiemesis.pdf. Accessed December 7, 2006.

8. Koeller JM, Aapro MS, Gralla RJ, et al Antiemetic guidelines: creating a more practical treatment approach. *Support Care Cancer* 2002;10:519–522.

9. Roila F, De Angelis V, Patoia L, et al. Prevention of Cisplatin-induced delayed emesis: still unsatisfactory. Italian Group for Anti-emetic Research. *Support Care Cancer* 2000;8:229–232.

10. Kris MG, Gralla RJ, Clark RA, et al. Incidence, course, and severity of delayed nausea and vomiting following the administration of high-dose cisplatin. *J Clin Oncol* 1985;3:1379–1384.

11. Morrow GR; Roscoe JA; Kirshner JJ, et al. Anticipatory nausea and vomiting in the era of 5-HT3 antiemetics. *Support Care Cancer* 1998;6:244–247

12. Gralla RJ, Itri LM, Pisko SE, et al. Antiemetic efficacy of high-dose metoclopramide: randomized trials with placebo and prochlorperazine in patients with chemotherapy-induced nausea and vomiting. *N Engl J Med* 1981;305:905–909.

13. Hesketh PJ, Gandara DR. Serotonin antiemetic antagonist: a new class of antiemetic agents *J Natl Cancer Inst* 1991;83:613–620.

14. Andrews PLR, Naylor RJ, Joss, RA. Neuropharmacology of emesis and its relevance to anti-emetic therapy. *Support Care Cancer* 1998;6:197–203.

15. Hesketh PJ, Van Belle SM, Aapro M, et al. Differential involvement of neurotransmitters through the time course of cisplatin-induced emesis as revealed by therapy with specific receptor antagonist. *Eur J Cancer* 2003;39:1074–1080.

16. Stahl SM. The ups and downs of novel antiemetic drugs, part 1: substance P, 5-HT, and the neuropharmacology of vomiting. *J Clin Psychiatry* 2003;64:498–499.

17. Pollera CF, Giannarelli D. Prognostic factors influencing cisplatin-induced emesis. definition and validation of a predictive logistic model. *Cancer* 1989;64:1117–1122.

18. Oliver IN, Simon RM, Aisner J. Antiemetic studies: a methodological discussion. *Cancer Treat Rep* 1986;70:55.

19. Jordon NS, Schauer PK, Schauer A, et al. The effect of administration rate on cisplatin-induced emesis. *J Clin Oncol* 1985;3:559–561

20. Hesketh PJ, Kris MG, Grunberg SM, et al. Proposal for classifying the acute emetogenicity of cancer chemotherapy. *J Clin Oncol* 1997;115:103–109.

21. Prevention and treatment of chemotherapy-induced nausea and vomiting. http://www.UpToDate.com. Accessed December 14, 2005.

22. Ruff P, Paska W, Goedhals L, et al. Ondansetron compared with granisetron in the prophylaxis of cisplatin-induced acute emesis: a multi-centered double-blind, randomized, parallel-group study. *Oncology* 1994;51:113–118.

23. Navari R, Gandara D, Hesketh P, et al. Comparative clinical trial of granisetron and ondansetron in the prophylaxis of cisplatin-induced emesis. *J Clin Oncol* 1995;13:1242–1248.

24. Hesketh PJ, Navari R, Grote T, et al. Double blinded, randomized comparison of the antiemetic efficacy of intravenous dolasetron mesylate and intravenous ondansetron in the prevention of acute cisplatin-induced emesis in patients with cancer. *J Clin Oncol* 1996;14:2232–2249.

25. Audhuy B, Cappelaere P, Martin M, et al. A double blinded randomized comparison of the anti-emetic efficacy of two intravenous doses of dolasetron mesylate and granisetron in patients receiving high-dose cisplatin chemotherapy. *Eur J Cancer* 1996;807–813.

26. Grunberg SM, Koeller JM. Palonosetron: a unique 5HT-3 receptor antagonist for the prevention of chemotherapy-induced emesis. *Expert Opin Pharmacother* 2003;4:2297–2303.

27. Beck TM, Hesketh PJ, Madajeqicz S, et al. Stratified, randomized double-blinded comparison of intravenous ondansetron administered as multidosing regimen versus two single dose regimens in the prevention of cisplatin-induced nausea and vomiting. *J Clin Oncol* 1992;10:1969–1975.

28. Ettinger DS, Eisenberg PD, Fitts D, et al. A double blind comparison of the efficacy of two dose regimens of oral granisetron in preventing acute emesis in patient receiving moderately emetogenic chemotherapy. *Cancer* 1996:78;144–151.

29. Harman GS, Omura GA, Ryan K, et al. A randomized, double-blinded comparison of single dose and divided multiple dose dolasetron for cisplatin-induced emesis. *Cancer Chemother Pharmacol* 1996:38; 323–328.

30. Perez EA, Hesketh P, Sandbach J, et al. Comparison of single dose oral granisetron versus intravenous ondansetron in the prevention of nausea and vomiting induced by moderately emetogenic chemotherapy; a multicenter, double-blind, randomized parallel study. *J Clin Oncol* 1998;16:754–760.

31. Gralla R, Narvari RM, Hesketh PJ, et al. Single dose granisetron has equivalent antiemetic efficacy to intravenous ondansetron for highly emetogenic cisplatin-based chemotherapy. *J Clin Oncol* 1998;16: 1568–1573.

32. Hesketh PJ, Grunberg SM, Gralla RJ, et al. The neurokinin 1 antagonist aprepitant for the prevention of chemotherapy-induced nausea and vomiting: a multinational, randomized, double-blind placebo

controlled trial in patients receiving high dose cisplatin—the Apreipant Protocol 052 Group *J Clin Oncol* 2003;21:4112–4119.

33. de Wit R, Herrstedt J, Rapoport B, et al. The oral NK1 antagonist aprepitant, given with standard antiemetics provides protection against nausea and vomiting over multiple cycles of cisplatin based chemotherapy; a combined analysis of two randomized, placebo controlled phase III clinical trials. *Eur J Cancer* 2004;40:403–410.

34. Chawla SP, Grunberg SM, Gralla RJ, et al. Establishing the dose of oral NK1 antagonist aprepitant for the prevention of chemotherapy-induced nausea and vomiting. *Cancer* 2003;97:2290–2300.

35. Shadle CR, Lee Y, Majumdar AK, et al. Evaluation of potential inductive effects of aprepitant on cytochrome P450 3A4 and 2C9 activity. *J Clin Pharmacol* 2004;44:215–223.

36. Nygren P, Hande K, Petty KJ, et al. Lack of effect of aprepitant on the pharmacokinetics of docetaxel in cancer patients. *Cancer Chemother Pharmacol* 2005;55:609–616.

37. Aapro MS, Plezia PM, Alberts DS, et al. Double blind cross-over study of the antiemetic efficacy of high dose dexamethasone versus high dose metoclopramide. *J Clin Oncol* 1984;2:466–471.

38. Lee B. Methylprednisolone as an antiemetic. *N Engl J Med* 1981;304:486–498.

39. Morrow G, Laughner J, Bennett J. Prevalence of nausea and vomiting and other side effects in patients receiving Cytoxan, methotrexate and fluorouracil (CMF) therapy with and without prednisone [abstract C-408]. *Proc Am Soc Clin Oncol* 1984;3:105.

40. Roila F, Tonato M, Cognetti F, et al. Prevention of cisplatin induced emesis: a double blind, multi-centered randomized crossover study comparing ondansetron and ondansetron plus dexamethasone. *J Clin Oncol* 1991;9:675–678.

41. Hesketh PJ, Harvey WH, Harker WG, et al. A randomized double-blind comparison of intravenous ondansetron alone and in combination with intravenous dexamethasone in the prevention of nausea and vomiting associated with high-dose cisplatin *J Clin Oncol* 1994;12:596–600.

42. Carmichael J, Bessel EM, Harris AL, et al. Comparison of granisetron alone and granisetron plus dexamethasone in the prophylaxis of cytotoxic-induced emesis. *Br J Cancer* 1994;70:1161–1164.

43. Kris MGF, Gralla RJ, Tyson LB et al. Improved control of cisplatin-induced emesis with high dose metoclopramide and with combinations of metoclopramide, dexamethasone and diphenhydramine, results of consecutive trials in 255 patients. *Cancer* 1985;55:527–534.

44. Italian Group for Antiemetic Research. Double blind, dose finding study of four intravenous doses of dexamethasone in the prevention of cisplatin induced acute emesis. *J Clin Oncol* 1998;16: 2937–2942.

45. Kris MG, Gralla RJ, Tyson LB, et al. Controlling delayed vomiting: double-blind, randomized trial comparing placebo, dexamethasone alone, and metoclopramide plus dexamethasone in patients receiving cisplatin. *J Clin Oncol* 1989;7:108–114.

46. Roila F, Boschetti E, Tonato M. Predictive factors of delayed emesis in cisplatin treated patient and the antiemetic activity and tolerability of metoclopramide or dexamethasone: a randomized single blind study. *Am J Clin Oncol* 1991;14:238–242.

47. Italian Group for Antiemetic Research. Ondansetron versus metoclopramide both combined with dexamethasone, in the prevention of cisplatin-induced delayed emesis. *J Clin Oncol* 1997;15:124–130.

48. Vinciguerra V, Moore T, Brennan E. Inhalation marijuana: an antiemetic for cancer chemotherapy. *NY State J Med* 1988;88:525–527.

49. The Antiemetic Subcommittee of the Multinational Association of Supportive Care in Cancer (MASCC). Prevention of chemotherapy and radiotherapy induced emesis: results of the 2004 Perugia International Antiemetic Consensus Conference. *Ann Oncol* 2006;12:20–28.

50. Poli-Bigelli S, Rodrigues-Pereira B, Carides AD, et al. Addition of the neurokinin 1 receptor antagonist aprepitant to standard antiemetic therapy improves control of chemotherapy-induced nausea and vomiting: results from a randomized double-blind, placebo controlled trial in Latin America. *Cancer* 2003;97:3090–3098.

51. De Wit R, Schmitz PIM, Verweij J, et al. Analysis of cumulative probabilities show that the efficacy of 5-HT3 antagonist prophylaxis is not maintained. *J Clin Oncol* 1996;14:644–651.

52. De Wit R, van der Berg H, Burghouts J, et al. Initial high antiemetic efficacy of granisetron with dexamethasone is not maintained over repeated doses. *Br J Cancer* 1998;77:1487–1491.

53. DeMulder PH, Seynaeve C, Vermorken JB, et al. Ondansetron compared with high dose metoclopramide in prophylaxis of acute and delayed cisplatin induced nausea and vomiting: a multicentered, randomized, double blind, crossover study. *Ann Intern Med* 1990;113:834–840.

54. Herrstedt J, Koeller JM Roila F, et al. Acute emesis: moderately emetogenic chemotherapy. *Support Care Cancer* 2005;13:97–103.

55. Italian Group for Antiemetic Research. Dexamethasone alone on in combination with ondansetron for the prevention of delayed nausea and vomiting induced by chemotherapy. *N Engl J Med* 2000;342:1554–1559.

56. Tonato M, Clark-Snow R, Osoba D, et al. Emesis induced by low or minimal emetic risk chemotherapy. *Support Care Cancer* 2005;13:109–111.

57. Morrow GR. Clinical characteristics associated with the development of anticipatory nausea and vomiting in cancer patients undergoing chemotherapy treatment. *J Clin Oncol* 1984;2:1170–1176.

Chapter 3
Management and Treatment of Mucositis
Monica Lee

Mucositis is a common and debilitating complication of radiotherapy and cancer chemotherapy. It occurs in about 40% of patients receiving standard chemotherapy, in 75%–85% of patients receiving high-dose chemotherapy before stem cell transplantation, and in more than 50% patients undergoing radiation to the head or neck or the pelvis or abdomen.[1,2] Although mucositis may affect any mucosal membrane, including the gastrointestinal tract, the focus of this chapter will be on oral mucositis.

Severe mucositis may delay the patient's next cycle of chemotherapy or result in a dose reduction, thus limiting the efficacy of therapy. There is also a major economic impact associated with mucositis. Sonis et al.[3] reported in a study of 92 patients undergoing hematopoietic stem cell transplantation that worsening of oral mucositis resulted in significantly longer hospital stays, with an average increase in hospital charges of $43,000 for patients with ulcerative mucositis.

THE COURSE OF ORAL MUCOSITIS
Typically, starting 5–7 days after the initiation of chemotherapy, mucositis may present as erythema of the tongue or buccal mucosa, tenderness or pain in the mouth, or severe ulceration involving the soft palate, ventrum of the tongue, floor of the mouth, and buccal mucosa.[2,4] The severity of mucositis peaks approximately 7–10 days after chemotherapy is given. It can be so severe that patients are unable to tolerate solid food or liquids and require systemic analgesics for pain control and total parenteral feeding to prevent malnutrition. Healing occurs within 2–3 weeks, usually coinciding with marrow recovery, and when it is not complicated by infection or graft-versus-host disease in patients undergoing allogeneic transplantation.[4]

Pathogenesis
The process of mucosal injury is described as having five phases: initiation, up-regulation with generation of messengers, signaling and amplification, ulceration with inflammation, and eventually healing (see Color Plate 2). Most recent research suggests that mucosal injury is a multistep process, involving not only the epithelium but also deeper tissue and vessels.

In the initial phase, chemotherapy or radiation causes direct DNA damage and cellular dysfunction in basal epithelial cells and in the underlying submuscosa. Chemotherapy and radiation also generate reactive oxygen species in phase 2, which can damage cells directly, initiating a cascade of events in the submuscosa by activating transcription factors such as nuclear factor-κB. As a result, phase 3 begins when there is an increase in the production of cytokines such as tumor necrosis factor-α and interleukins (interleukin-1β and -6). These inflammatory cytokines stimulate cells in the submuscosa through positive feedback mechanisms that amplify the signaling cascades and cause further mucosal destruction. The ulcerative phase of oral mucositis leads to loss of mucosal integrity, resulting in the appearance of lesions. This loss of integrity of the mucosal membranes provides a portal of entry for bacteria, viruses, and fungi. Bacterial cell wall products can also stimulate immune cells to produce cytokines that cause further inflammation. In the final phase of oral mucositis, signaling from the submuscosa stimulates migration of healthy epithelial cells, which leads to renewal of epithelial proliferation, differentiation, and eventually restoration of mucosal integrity.[5]

Grading Oral Mucositis

There have been many clinical trials designed to evaluate the efficacy of different modalities to either manage or prevent cancer therapy–induced oral mucositis. The data from these trials are often conflicting and difficult to interpret because of the different oral mucositis grading scales used to evaluate the results among studies.[4,6] Currently, there are no standard scales to grade the severity of oral mucositis. The most commonly used grading scales for mucositis management are based on the World Health Organization's (WHO) oral toxicity scale (Table 3–22) or the National Cancer Institute's (NCI) Common Toxicity Criteria (CTC), version 3 (Table 3–23).[4,7]

Table 3–22 Mucositis Grading Systems: WHO Oral Toxicity Scale

| | GRADE | | | | |
	0	1	2	3	4
Signs and symptoms	No symptoms	Sore mouth, no ulcers	Sore mouth with ulcer, but able to eat normally	Liquid diet only	Unable to eat or drink

Table 3–23 Mucositis Grading Systems: Common Toxicity Criteria (NCI-CTC Version 3)

| | GRADE | | | | |
	1	2	3	4	5
Mucositis (clinical examination)	Erythema of the mucosa	Patchy ulcerations or pseudomembranes	Confluent ulceration or pseudomembranes; bleeding with minor trauma	Tissue necrosis: significant spontaneous bleeding, life-threatening consequences	Death
Mucositis (functional/ symptomatic)	*Upper aerodigestive tract:* Minimal symptoms, normal diet; minimal respiratory symptoms but not interfering with function *Lower GI sites:* Minimal discomfort, intervention not indicated	*Upper aerodigestive tract:* Symptomatic but can eat and swallow modified diet; respiratory symptoms interfering with function but not interfering with ADL *Lower GI sites:* Symptomatic, medical intervention indicated but not interfering with ADL	*Upper aerodigestive tract:* Symptomatic and unable to adequately aliment or hydrate orally; respiratory symptoms interfering with ADL *Lower GI sites:* Stool incontinence or other symptoms interfering with ADL	Symptoms associated with life-threatening consequences	Death

GI, gastrointestinal; ADL, activities of daily living.
Note: Mucositis/stomatitis (functional/symptomatic) may be used to indicate mucositis of the upper aerodigestive tract caused by radiation, chemotherapy agents, or graft-versus-host disease.

Recently, a panel of experts including nurses, dentists, and physicians developed another new assessment scale called the Oral Mucositis Assessment Scale (OMAS). The OMAS is designed as a research tool for the clinical trial setting (Table 3–24). It requires more time and examiner experience than the other grading systems. It measures ulceration on a 0–3 scale and erythema on a 0–2 scale and evaluates pain, difficulty swallowing, and the impact on food intake.[6]

Risk Factors

Chemotherapy regimens containing antimetabolites, antitumor antibiotics, plant alkaloids, and taxanes (Table 3–25) or radiation treatment to the head and neck have high potential to cause mucositis. Other than therapy-related risks, there are a variety of patient-related factors that appear to increase the potential for

Table 3–24 Oral Mucositis Assessment Scale

Location	Ulceration/Pseudomembranes*				Erythema†		
Upper lip	0	1	2	3	0	1	2
Lower lip	0	1	2	3	0	1	2
Right cheek	0	1	2	3	0	1	2
Left cheek	0	1	2	3	0	1	2
Right ventral and lateral tongue	0	1	2	3	0	1	2
Left ventral and lateral tongue	0	1	2	3	0	1	2
Floor of mouth	0	1	2	3	0	1	2
Soft palate	0	1	2	3	0	1	2
Hard palate	0	1	2	3	0	1	2

*Ulceration/Pseudomembrane: 0 = no lesion; 1 = <1 cm^2; 2 = 1–3 cm^2; 3 = >3 cm^2.
†Erythema: 0 = none; 1 = not severe; 2 = severe.

Table 3–25 Chemotherapeutic Regimens with High Potential to Cause Grade 3–4 Oral or Gastrointestinal Mucositis

Occurring in ≥50% of Patients	Occurring in ≥30% of Patients	Occurring in ≥10% of Patients
Anthracycline + docetaxel + 5-fluorouracil	Paclitaxel + XRT	Anthracycline + cyclophosphamide
Docetaxel + XRT	Docetaxel + 5-fluorouracil	Anthracycline + taxane
Paclitaxel + 5-fluorouracil + XRT	Oxaliplatin + XRT	Anthracycline + cyclophosphamide + docetaxel
Paclitaxel + platinum + XRT	5-Fluorouracil + platinum + XRT	Anthracycline + docetaxel + platinum
Adult BMT with TBI	Stem cells transplant: myeloma	Docetaxel alone
	5-Fluorouracil + taxane + leucovorin	Docetaxel + platinum + XRT
	5-Fluorouracil CIV + irinotecan + XRT	Platinum + XRT
	Irinotecan alone	Platinum + taxane + gemcitabine
	Irinotecan + 5-fluororacil + leucovorin + platinum	Platinum + methotrexate + leucovorin
		5-Fluorouracil CIV ± XRT
		5-Fluorouracil CIV + platinum
		5-Fluorouracil + leucovorin
		5-Fluorouracil + mitomycin C
		Irinotecan + taxane

XRT, radiation; TBI, total body irradiation; CIV, continuous intravenous infusion.
Data from Sonis ST, Elting LS, Keefe D, et al. Perspectives on cancer therapy-induced mucosal injury. *Cancer* 2004;100(9 Suppl):1995–2025.

SUPPORTIVE CARE

Box 3–8 Risk Factors Contributing to Mucositis

Age younger than 20 years old or elderly
Exposure to alcohol and tobacco
Periodontal disease
Ill-fitting dentures
Poor nutritional status
Dehydration

Data from Köstler WJ, Hejna M, Wenzel C, Zielinski CC. Oral mucositis complicating chemotherapy and/or radiotherapy options for prevention and treatment. *CA Cancer J Clin* 2001;51:290–315; and Grosenwald SL, Frogge MH, Goodman M, Yarbro CH. *Cancer Symptom Management*. Sudbury, MA: Jones and Bartlett Publishers; 1996:308–321.

Box 3–9 Prophylactic Measures: Goal Is to Maintain Good Oral Hygiene

Oral Care
Brush with soft-bristle toothbrush after each meal and at bedtime
Remove and clean dentures every night
Avoid commercial mouthwashes that contain alcohol
Use bland rinses (see Table 3–26)
Stop smoking

Dietary Hints
Avoid hot and spicy foods
Cook solid foods until they are tender
Eat soft, bland foods, or even a liquid or pureed diet
Avoid extremes in temperature; eat most food at room temperature
Avoid acidic food such as tomatoes or citrus fruits
Avoid alcohol

Data from Ruberstein EB, Peterson DE, Schubert M, et al. Clinical practice guidelines for the prevention and treatment of cancer therapy-induced oral and gastrointestinal mucositis. *Cancer* 2004:100(9 Suppl): 2026–2046; and Köstler WJ, Hejna M, Wenzel C, Zielinski CC. Oral mucositis complicating chemotherapy and/or radiotherapy options for prevention and treatment. *CA Cancer J Clin* 2001;51:290–315.

Table 3–26 Mouthwashes and Bland Rinses

Mouthwashes and Rinses	Ingredient	Direction
0.9% saline solution	1 tsp of table salt in 1 L of warm water	Swish and spit after each meal and at bedtime
Sodium bicarbonate (baking soda) solution	2 tbsp of baking soda in 1 L of warm water	Swish and spit after each meal and at bedtime
Saline and bicarbonate combination	½ tsp of table salt and 2 tbsp of baking soda in 1 L of warm water	Swish and spit after each meal and at bedtime

---

development of mucositis after chemotherapy or radiotherapy. They are summarized in Box 3–8.

MANAGEMENT OF ORAL MUCOSITIS

There are no standardized guidelines for treatment or prophylaxis of oral mucositis. Measures for prevention and treatment of mucositis are primarily supportive and include good oral hygiene (Box 3–9), rinses (Table 3–26), mouthwashes, and analgesia with topical anesthetics and systemic analgesics.[6,8]

Good oral hygiene helps prevent mucosal irritation and has been shown to reduce the incidence and complications of mucositis, including infection. Regular, gentle brushing with a soft toothbrush and a fluoride-based toothpaste and flossing to reduce oral bacteria colonization and any foreign substances that may cause gum or mucosal irritation. In patients with preexisting gum irritation or those who have a risk of thrombocytopenic hemorrhage, the use of cotton swabs or sponges rather that a toothbrush is recommended.

Patients with poor oral hygiene are more likely to develop mucositis than patients with good oral hygiene. Poor oral hygiene may be indicated by the presence of dental caries and periodontal and pulpal disease, and other sources of irritation to the gums or mucous membranes, such as ill-fitting prostheses and wearing of orthodontic devices (e.g., partials, dentures, retainers, and braces).

Chlorhexidine is a broad-spectrum topical antiseptic wash that is used to reduce plaque, gingivitis, the risk of dental caries, and oropharyngeal candidiasis. There are conflicting data on the use of this agent to reduce or prevent mucositis. Until more data are available, chlorhexidine is not recommended for use in either chemotherapy- or radiation-associated mucositis.[1]

Dry mouth (xerostomia) is also associated with increased bacterial colonization on dental surfaces. The patient's medication list should be evaluated, and medications that cause dry mouth such as tricyclic antidepressants, oxybutynin, or antihistamines should be avoided, if possible. Dry mouth can be relieved by sugar-free drops or chewing gum, alkaline saline solutions, low-dose pilocarpine, or salivary substitutes. The use of saline or sodium bicarbonate (baking soda) rinses is often recommended for this purpose (Table 3–26).

Lifestyle habits such as good nutrition and smoking cessation are also important for oral care. The patient should avoid spicy or acidic foods as they tend to aggravate mucosal ulcers. Rough foods such as potato chips or crusty breads may cause tears or bruising of the buccal mucosa. Chewing large pieces of food may also cause irritation. Alcohol may cause mucosal inflammation and irritation as does smoking.

Pain is the most common symptom associated with mucositis. Also worrisome in the patient with mucositis is the possibility of infection. Mouthwashes that contain antihistamines, anesthetics, and antifungal agents or local anesthetics agents (Table 3–27) or coating agents (Table 3–28) can be used for mild pain, whereas systemic analgesia is used for moderate to severe pain control. Topical analgesics such as 2% viscous lidocaine, benzocaine (Hurricaine, Orajel), and dyclonine HCl (Dyclone) provide relief by numbing the affected area. The patient should be advised to be careful when chewing or eating while using these agents. Accidental biting of the numb areas may occur without the patient's feeling it. Relief with these topical analgesics is short, so they may need to be combined with other pain-relieving agents. Mucosal barriers or coating agents may also be used for mild pain relief. They coat the ulcer or mucosa and act as a barrier from foreign substances. As with

SUPPORTIVE CARE

Table 3–27 Topical Anesthetics

Drug	Form	Direction
Lidocaine	2% viscous liquid	15 mL to swish and expectorate every 6 hours as needed
Benzocaine (Hurricane, Orajel)	Spray, gel, or liquid	Apply to affected area as needed
Dyclonine HCl (Dyclone)	0.5% or 1% topical solution	5–10 mL to swish and spit 3–4 times daily as needed

Note: Do not eat for 60 minutes after application to minimize aspiration risk.

Table 3–28 Mucosal Barrier and Coating Agents

Name	Ingredient/Recipe	Direction
Magic mouthwash	Mylanta, viscous lidocaine 2%, diphenhydramine elixir in a 1:1:1 ratio	Swish 5 mL every 2–4 hours to maximum 12 doses/24 hr.
Hydroxypropyl methylcellulose (Zilactin, Zilactin-B)	Hydroxypropylcellulose, benzocaine (Zilactin-B)	Use every 4–6 hours or as needed. Dry the affected area. Apply a thin coat of Zilactin and allow 30–60 seconds for the gel to dry into a film.
Sucralfate suspension	1 g/10 mL	Swish and swallow or expectorate 10 mL 4 times/day.
Cyanoacrylate mucoadherent film (Orabase Soothe-N-Seal)	2-Octyl cyanoacrylate	Use as needed. Provides relief up to 6 hours.
Gelclair	One Gelclair packet (15 mL) and 40 mL of water. Stir mixture well and use at once	Swish for at least 1 minute or as long as possible to coat. Gargle and spit out. Use 3 times a day or as needed. Do not drink or eat for at least 1 hour after treatment.

Table 3–29 Antifungal Agents

Drug	Dosage	Direction
Nystatin suspension	100,000 units/mL	5 mL; swish for 3–5 minutes and expectorate every 4–6 hours
Nystatin troche	200,000 units	Dissolve in mouth, keep in contact with tongue for 3–5 minutes, 4-5 times/day for up to 14 days
Clotrimazole troche	10 mg	Dissolve in mouth, keep in contact with tongue for 3–5 minutes, 5 times daily
Fluconazole (Diflucan)	100 mg	Take two tablets on day 1, then 100 mg daily for 14 days
Amphotericin B	100 mg/mL	1 mL 4 times/day; swish for 3 minutes and swallow or expectorate

the topical analgesics, the duration of relief with mucosal barrier or coating agents may be short-lived, and thus they are commonly used in combination with other treatments.

For moderate to severe pain that is not controlled by topical agents, systemic pain control is required. Analgesics in the form of acetaminophen, hydrocodone/ acetaminophen (Vicodin), and other opioids are often used for moderate to severe pain. Aspirin-containing products or nonsteroidal anti-inflammatory products, which can increase the risk of bleeding, should be avoided. Opioids may be in the form of oral, intravenous, bolus, continuous infusion, or patient-controlled analgesia. Pain medications such as hydromorphone, fentanyl, or morphine delivered via patient-controlled analgesia are recommended for patients undergoing hematopoietic stem cell transplantation.[1]

Despite good oral care and other prophylaxis measures, some patients develop oral infections. The most common oral infection is fungal infection caused by *Candida albicans*,[2] which can be treated with antifungal agents such as clotrimazole troches or nystatin suspension (Table 3–29). Candidiasis presents as mucosal erythema, white plaques, and, rarely, ulceration. It may cause a burning sensation or a change in taste and extend to the esophagus. Herpes simplex virus reactivation, which can worsen and prolong the course of mucositis, is common in patients undergoing hematopoietic stem cell transplant.

Oral herpes, also known as cold sores, present as grouped, small vesicles that, after rupturing, leave behind painful ulcers. Such infections can be treated with antiviral medications such as acyclovir, famciclovir, or valacyclovir. Gram-negative bacterial infections are also common and have serious sequelae when untreated. Broad-spectrum antibiotics are usually initiated when there is a suspicion of bacterial infection. Although infections with fungal, viral, and bacterial agents are all common, mucositis prophylaxis measures are only common with fungal and viral infections.

Cryotherapy is often used for 5-fluorouracil therapy and has been shown to prevent oral mucositis.[9] Ice chips are held in the mouth for a total of 30 minutes starting 5 minutes before 5-fluorouracil bolus injection. Theoretically, this causes vasoconstriction of mucosal blood vessels and prevents full exposure to chemotherapy during peak levels after administration.

Emerging Strategies

With the improved understanding of the pathogenesis of mucositis, targeted therapy to manage mucositis has been developed.

Palifermin. Palifermin (Kepivance), a recombinant human keratinocyte growth factor (KGF), is the only agent so far approved (in 2005) by the U.S. Food and Drug Administration (FDA) for the prevention of severe oral mucositis in patients with hematologic malignancies receiving myelotoxic therapy requiring hematopoietic stem cell support. Palifermin works by binding to keratinocyte growth factor receptors and stimulating epithelial cell proliferation, differentiation, and up-regulation of cytoprotective mechanisms.[10] In a phase III, randomized, placebo-controlled trial of 212 patients undergoing stem cell transplantation; the incidence of grade 3 or 4 mucositis was 63% in the palifermin group and 98% in the placebo group ($P < 0.001$). The duration of grade 3/4 mucositis was shortened in patients treated with palifermin (6 days versus 9 days, $P < 0.001$). Fewer patients treated with palifermin experienced grade 4 mucositis compared with those who received placebo (20% versus 62%, $P < 0.001$). Palifermin was associated with a significant reduction in patient-reported soreness of the mouth and throat compared with placebo (area under the curve score, 29.0 versus 46.8, $P < 0.001$). The incidences of use of total parenteral nutrition and narcotics were also reduced in the group of patients treated with palifermin.[11] Palifermin is currently in phase III clinical studies to investigate its safety and efficacy for oral mucositis in patients with solid tumors receiving localized radiation with or without chemotherapy.

Specific information about palifermin is as follows.

- *Preparation*: Palifermin should be reconstituted with 1.2 mL of sterile water for injection to yield a final concentration of 5 mg/mL. Do not shake.
- *Storage*: Refrigerate at 2–8 °C.[10]
- *Stability*: The reconstituted solution may be stored refrigerated in its carton for up to 24 hours. Before injection, palifermin may be allowed to reach room temperature for a maximum of 1 hour but should be protected from light. Do not freeze.[10]
- *Dosage and Administration*: The dose is 60 mcg/kg per day, administered as an intravenous bolus for 3 consecutive days before and 3 consecutive days after myelotoxic chemotherapy and/or total body irradiation for a total of six doses.[10] The first three doses should be administered before myelotoxic therapy, with the third dose administered 24–48 hours before the myelotoxic therapy. The last three doses should be administered after myelotoxic therapy; the first of these doses should be administered after, but on the same

day of hematopoietic stem cell infusion and at least 4 days after the most recent palifermin administration.

- *Adverse Reactions*: The incidence of adverse reactions, including rash, pruritus, erythema, fever, pain, tongue thickness, tongue discoloration, oral/perioral dysesthesia, arthralgia, hypertension, proteinuria, and reversible elevation of lipase and amylase levels, is ≥5% higher than that with placebo.[10]

AES-14. AES-14 (Saforis) is another agent for the prevention and reduction of the severity of oral mucositis in patients undergoing chemotherapy that was recently granted fast track status (in 2003) by the FDA. AES-14 is an enhanced-uptake L-glutamine in a proprietary vehicle, which can deliver 100 times more L-glutamine to epithelial cells.[12] It is hypothesized that anthracycline-based chemotherapy regimens cause depletion of L-glutamine, which leads to oral mucositis. L-Glutamine is an essential amino acid that facilitates wound repair and the rebuilding of tissues. In the past, there has been conflicting data about the efficacy of L-glutamine possibly due to poor solubility and limited uptake by cells. Data from a phase III, multicenter, placebo-controlled, double-blind, crossover study of AES-14 demonstrated its effectiveness in treatment of oral mucositis due to anthracycline-based chemotherapy in 2,064 women with breast cancer. AES-14 reduced the incidence of clinically relevant oral mucositis by 22% ($P = 0.026$) and also significantly reduced the duration of oral mucositis ($P = 0.48$) compared with placebo. Interestingly, AES-14 has a statistically significant carryover benefit in treatment cycle 2 in the group of patients who received AES-14 during the first treatment cycle and placebo in treatment cycle 2: 18% fewer patients experienced oral mucositis when treated with the drug followed by placebo compared with patients who received placebo first and then crossed over to AES-14 ($P = 0.027$). There were no significant adverse events reported in either group.[13] Approximately 5% of patients had dry mouth and less than 9% had nausea. AES-14 was administered as an oral suspension, and each dose was 5 mL, swished for 30 seconds and then swallowed, three times daily. The total dose was 7.5 g/day.[13]

CONCLUSION

Oral mucositis is a clinically significant and debilitating complication in patients with cancer. Strategies to prevent and treat mucositis are continually being developed and use different agents with different mechanisms of action, based on the patient's needs and clinical response. Recent progress in understanding the complexity of the process of oral mucositis provides research opportunities for potential targeted therapies. Palifermin is the first agent approved by the FDA on the basis of this approach, and other therapies are in various stages of development.

REFERENCES

1. Ruberstein EB, Peterson DE, Schubert M, et al. Clinical practice guidelines for the prevention and treatment of cancer therapy-induced oral and gastrointestinal mucositis. *Cancer* 2004;100(9 Suppl): 2026–2046.
2. Karthaus M, Rosenthal C, Gasner A. Prophylaxis and treatment of chemo- and radiotherapy-induced oral mucositis—are there new strategies? *Bone Marrow Transplant* 1999;24:1095–1108.
3. Sonis ST, Oster G, Fuchs H, et al. Oral mucositis and the clinical and economic outcomes of hematopoietic stem-cell transplantation. *J Clin Oncol* 2001;19:2201–2205.
4. Scully C, Epstein J, Sonic S. Oral mucositis: a challenging complication of radiotherapy, chemotherapy, and radiochemotherapy. Part 2: diagnosis and management of mucositis. *Head Neck* 2004;26:77–84.
5. Sonis ST, Elting LS, Keefe D, et al. Perspectives on cancer therapy-induced mucosal injury. *Cancer* 2004;100(9 Suppl):1995–2025.
6. Sonis ST, Eilers JP, Epstein JB, et al. Validation of a new scoring system for the assessment of clinical trial research of oral mucositis induced by radiation or chemotherapy. *Cancer* 1999;85:2013–2113.
7. Peterson DE, Cariello A. Mucosal damage: a major risk factor for severe complications after cytotoxic therapy. *Semin Oncol* 2004;31(8 Suppl):35–44.

8. Sharma R, Tobin P, Clarke SJ. Management of chemotherapy-induced nausea, vomiting, oral mucositis and diarrhoea. *Lancet Oncol* 2005;6:93–102.

9. Cassinu S, Fedeli A, Fedeli SL, Catalano G. Oral cooling(cryotherapy), an effective treatment for the prevention of 5-fluorouracil-induced stomatitis. *Eur J Cancer B Oral Oncol* 1994;30B:234–236.

10. Kepivance (palifermin) prescribing information. Thousand Oaks, CA: Amgen; 2005.

11. Spielberger E, Stiff P, Bensinger W, et al. Palifermin for oral mucositis after intensive therapy for hematologic cancers. *N Engl J Med* 2004:351:2590–2598.

12. Report from the Chicago Supportive Oncology Conference: experimental L-glutamine agent shown effective in OM. *J Support Oncol* 2005;3:414.

13. Peterson DE. Phase III study: AES in patients at risk for mucositis secondary to anthracycline-based chemotherapy. In *Proceedings from the 40th Meeting of the American Society of Clinical Oncology*; 2004:Abstract 8008.

SUPPORTIVE CARE

Chapter 4
Management and Treatment of Diarrhea and Constipation
Maureen A. Cannon and Theresa A. Moran

INTRODUCTION
The goal of administering chemotherapy to patients with cancer is to destroy malignant cells. Unfortunately, despite advances in attempts to target only malignant cells and spare nonmalignant ones, current chemotherapeutic agents cannot distinguish between rapidly growing cancer cells and rapidly growing normal cells and ultimately affect both. Because of this, the majority of side effects associated with chemotherapy (anorexia, mucositis, nausea, vomiting, and diarrhea or constipation), are found in the organs with the fastest growing cells, including the gastrointestinal tract, the bone marrow (neutropenia, thrombocytopenia, and anemia), and the skin (alopecia). In this chapter we will discuss the side effects diarrhea and constipation.

NORMAL BOWEL PHYSIOLOGY
The physiology and function of normal bowel are complex and essential to the maintenance of adequate nutrition, fluid and electrolyte balance, and ultimately a healthy body. These involve motor functions of specialized organs (pancreas, liver, gallbladder, stomach, and small and large intestines) and muscle groups, input from the brain, spinal cord, and sympathetic, parasympathetic, and enteric divisions of the autonomic nervous system and somatic motor systems, and enteric neural control of motor movements to achieve gastric motility (wall movement). When these integrated systems work in harmony, the outcome is efficient digestion and absorption of nutrients, including carbohydrates, fat, protein, fat-soluble and water-soluble vitamins, electrolytes, bile salts, and water.[1] Constipation and diarrhea occur when the systems are not working as planned.

Muscles
The smooth muscles of the digestive tract are generally organized in distinctive layers, longitudinal and circular, and are responsible for exerting contractile forces on the contents of the lumen. They are innervated by the enteric nervous system. Calcium, either as an influx from the outside of the muscle cells or as a release from inside the cell itself, is important for excitation-contraction coupling. Therefore, anything that interferes with the function of these muscles, either slowing the contractile force down (e.g., opioids) or speeding it up (e.g., metoclopramide), has consequences.[2]

Nerves
The innervation of the digestive tract controls not only muscle contraction but also secretion and absorption across the mucosal lining and blood flow inside the walls of the intestines. Depending on the type of neurotransmitter released, the neurons can activate or inhibit muscle contraction, affecting secretion of water, electrolytes, and mucus into the lumen and the absorption of these elements from the lumen. The amount and distribution of blood flow between the muscle layers and mucosa are also controlled by nerves.[1]

Sensory nerves transmit information on the state of the gut to the brain. Sensory transmission accounts for the sensations of discomfort (fullness), abdominal pain, and chest pain (heartburn).[1]

The sympathetic, parasympathetic, and enteric nervous systems make up the divisions of the autonomic nervous system that innervate the digestive tracts. Autonomic signals to the gut are carried from the brain and spinal cord by sympathetic and parasympathetic nervous pathways.[3]

The end result of the muscle and nerves working together is the propulsion of ingested food, liquids, gastrointestinal secretions, and sloughed cells from the mucosa through the digestive tract. This movement is accomplished at a sufficient rate for efficient digestion and absorption and ultimately elimination of the residue.

Digestion and Absorption

Most of the digestive enzymes/acids are released in the upper portion of the gastrointestinal tract (salivary glands in the mouth, parietal cells in the stomach, pancreatic enzymes by the pancreas, and bile salts by the liver/gallbladder). Hydrochloric acid, bile salts, and pancreatic enzymes all contribute to the digestion of food and liquids, breaking them down into absorbable components. Nearly all of the dietary nutrients and approximately 95%–98% of the water and electrolytes that enter the upper small intestine are absorbed in both an active and passive process. This results in the movement of electrolytes, water, and metabolic substrates into the blood for distribution and use throughout the body.[4]

Any disruption in the function of the muscles or nerves or any change in the lining of the gastrointestinal tract, changing the quality or quantity of digestive enzymes released, has an impact on the absorption of nutrients and affects all other organs.[4]

CONSTIPATION

Normal bowel function is defined as what is usual and/or typical for each individual and, therefore, varies greatly. For some, normal bowel function may be a bowel movement twice a week; for others, it may be several times per day. Because of this variation, assessment of bowel function must be made in the context of any variation from the individual's norm to determine whether a problem exists.[5]

One definition of constipation is a decrease in the motility of the large intestine, resulting in a prolonged fluid absorption time.[6,7] As a result of this prolonged transit time, the stool dehydrates, and propulsion through the large intestine becomes difficult, often requiring straining and force.[8]

Incidence

It is estimated that 25%–45% of all cancer patients experience constipation at some point, although the percentage is probably closer to 100%, as even healthy individuals experience constipation from time to time.[9–11] It is more common in elderly patients and is estimated that 35% of patients undergoing chemotherapy will experience severe constipation.[12] Of interest, constipation occurs in 1 of 6 people who stop smoking.[13]

Pathophysiology

Constipation can be attributed to a change in the strength of contractions within the intestine, poor muscle tone in the colon, and/or a neurological change in sensation relating to the large intestine, rectum, or anus.[7] Weak contractions or poor muscle tone will not sufficiently push fecal material through the colon to the rectum; conversely, strong contractions clamp down and block the flow of stool. Changes in sensation due to surgery, radiation therapy, tumor, fissures, or prolonged desensitization of nerves that occurs when defecation is delayed contribute to constipation. Additionally, medications that are neurotoxic (Table 3–30 and Box 3–10) or that affect specific receptors and/or the direct mechanical effect of

Table 3–30 **Specific Chemotherapy Drugs Associated with Constipation**

Drug	Mechanism
Vinorelbine tartrate (Navelbine)	Semisynthetic vinca alkaloid derived from vinblastine; used to treat non–small cell lung cancer and breast cancer; up to 29% of patients will experience constipation; the incidence increases in those who have received prior vinca alkaloid treatment or abdominal radiation
Thalidomide (Thalomid)	Antiangiogenic agent inhibits tumor necrosis factor-α; used to treat multiple myeloma; causes mild constipation in 3%–30%
Vinblastine (Velban)	Plant alkaloid; used to treat lymphomas and testicular cancer; patients may experience abdominal cramping
Vincristine (Oncovin, Vincasar, Leurocristine)	Vinca alkaloid used to treat multiple malignancies; *dose-limiting toxicity:* abdominal pain, obstipation, and paralytic ileus
Vindesine (Eldisine, desacetylvinblastine amide sulfate)	Experimental vinca alkaloid used to treat lung cancer and leukemia; causes less severe neurotoxicity

Data from Skidmore-Roth L. *Mosby's 2006 Nursing Drug Reference.* St. Louis, MO: Mosby, 2006.

SUPPORTIVE CARE

Box 3–10 Antiemetics Causing Constipation

Palonosetron (Aloxi)
Granisetron (Kytril)
Ondansetron (Zofran)
Dolasetron (Anzemet)

All of the above are 5-hydroxytryptamine 3 antagonists that block serotonin.
Data from Skidmore-Roth L. *Mosby's 2006 Nursing Drug Reference.* St. Louis, MO: Mosby; 2006

---

the tumor or tumor-related processes (e.g., ascites or compression by the tumor itself) can also cause constipation. Opioids are perhaps some of the most well-recognized medications that cause constipation, and, as a result, a bowel regimen is generally started at the same time as narcotics are started. For other causes of constipation, see Box 3–11.[7,14]

Assessment

Assessment begins with a thorough history of the patient's usual and current bowel habits, including the frequency of bowel movements, the character and volume of the stool, use of laxatives and other measures to enhance bowel function, and the date of the last bowel movement. Any symptoms the patient is experiencing should be documented, including changes in bowel habits or incomplete bowel movements, straining or the passage of hard stool, and streaking of blood on stool. In addition, the patient may complain of loss of appetite, feeling full, indigestion, nausea, vomiting, oozing of liquid stool, or a feeling of rectal fullness. Furthermore, the patient may report abdominal distention, pain, and severe flatus.[5,10]

On examination, the abdomen may be distended and tender to palpation, hyper- or hypoactive bowel sounds may be heard, and a palpable abdominal mass may be present. On rectal examination, there may be poor rectal tone or stool in the vault, and an impaction may be felt. Evaluation for fissures, hemorrhoids, or other lesions should also be done. If a bowel obstruction is suspected, a kidney-ureter-bladder radiograph may show dilated loops of bowel; if the bowel is perforated, this same examination may show free air in the abdomen. A computed tomography scan of the abdomen may show a transition point, that is, a point where the bowel appears

---

Box 3–11 Causes of Constipation

Dietary Changes
Low fiber
Reduced fluid intake

Pharmacologic Therapies
Chemotherapeutic neurotoxic agents
Antiemetics (5-hydroxytryptamine 3 receptor antagonists)
Anticholinergics
Narcotic analgesics
Diuretics
Antacids containing aluminum or calcium
Anticonvulsants
Tricyclic antidepressants
Antihypertensives
Calcium and iron supplements
Phenothiazines
Nonsteroidal anti-inflammatory drugs

Complications of Cancer
Ascites
Hypercalcemia
Hypokalemia
Obstruction of the bowel by tumor
Spinal cord compression: T8 through L3 nerves innervate the bowel

Hospitalization
Lack of privacy within the hospital
Altered timing in bowel routine
Use of bedpans
Reduced mobility and exercise

Related Conditions
Addison's disease
Cushing's syndrome
Diabetes mellitus
Hypothyroidism
Hyperthyroidism
Lead poisoning
Excessive laxative use
Depression
Stress: sympathetic nervous system is stimulated, which causes a decrease in gastrointestinal motility
Sigmoid spasm

Adapted from Pace J. Symptom management. In Miaskowski C, Buschel P, eds. *Oncology Nursing: Assessment and Clinical Care.* St. Louis, MO: Mosby; 1999.

---

distended above, and normal, or "deflated" below. In the case of a partial bowel obstruction, the transition point may be more subtle. If a perforation is present, the patient may be febrile and show signs of sepsis.

If untreated or unrecognized, the complications of constipation can be very serious and include bowel obstruction, obstipation, nausea, vomiting, anorexia, lethargy, trauma to the rectum and anus, urinary retention, and cognitive impairment. The goals for patient care are prevention and early intervention.[5,7,15]

Management

In most patients constipation can be prevented. Preventative measures are listed in Box 3–12. However, because preventative measures are often overlooked, treatment is frequently necessary. Preventative measures include patient education,

> **Box 3–12 Preventative Measures**
>
> - Encourage fluid intake—Unless contraindicated patients should drink 8–10 glasses of fluid per day, and warm fluids promote movement of stool through the gastrointestinal tract.[12]
> - Limit intake of fluids that promote diuresis such as caffeinated beverages (coffees, teas, and sodas) and grapefruit juice.[12]
> - Encourage exercise—Exercise stimulates the gastrointestinal tract, promoting passage of stool.[8]
> - Encourage a high-fiber diet—High-fiber diets cause water to be drawn into the stool by osmosis, keeping the stool soft and facilitating movement of stool through the intestines. The bulk of fiber causes dilation of the intestine thus promoting defecation. High-fiber foods include corn, raisins, popcorn, dates, vegetables, fruits, and whole grains in any form.[25]
> - Teach diaphragmatic breathing and abdominal muscle exercises—These help increase the tone of the muscles used in defecation.[12]
> - Encourage patients to follow the urge to defecate as soon as possible.
> - Provide privacy.
> - Assist patient in formulating a daily bowel program.[25]
> - Initiate a prophylactic bowel regimen for all patients who are taking opioid pain medication and for those patients receiving therapy with the potential to cause constipation.[20]
> - Instruct the patient to notify his or her doctor if he or she has not had a bowel movement in 3 days.[25]

SUPPORTIVE CARE

nonpharmacologic measures, and pharmacologic therapies such as laxatives and stool softeners. If practical, an exercise program should be encouraged because exercise is known to stimulate peristalsis. Glycerin suppositories or other lubricants may help ease defecation, and the use of comfortable commodes and privacy, whenever possible, are helpful. See Table 3–31 for classifications of laxatives and stool softeners. There have been no studies performed to compare the efficacy of various laxatives; therefore, personal experience or preference is acceptable in recommending or prescribing these agents. For patients with soft stools that are difficult to expel, a laxative is appropriate. For patients with frequent hard stools, softening agents would be beneficial. Patients with opioid-induced constipation often require both a laxative and a stool softener. In addition, recent studies have suggested that naloxone administered orally to patients with refractory opioid-induced constipation may to beneficial.[16–18] Naloxone works by binding to the opioid receptors within the enteric wall, antagonizing the constipating effects.

Other methods for relieving constipation include enemas and manual disimpaction. These methods can be very painful and should be used only when pharmacologic interventions are not effective and should never be used for patients who are thrombocytopenic and neutropenic.

Dietary changes may also help prevent constipation, but their usefulness in treating severe constipation is unclear. Increasing fiber and water intake can be helpful in preventing constipation. As mentioned earlier, exercise is also useful.[5,18]

Nursing Care

Nurses are in a prime position both to help prevent constipation and to recognize the signs and symptoms for early intervention. Documenting the patient's normal bowel routine, assessing for risk factors of constipation, and educating the patient and family members about preventative measures and treatment strategies are all roles for the nurse. Providing comfort measures, such as glycerin suppositories, water-soluble lubricants, topical anesthetics, systemic analgesics, or antispasmodics, during painful bowel movements, enemas, or disimpactions is important. In the patient with severe constipation, the anal area should be assessed for hemorrhoids, tears, and fissures. Thought should also be given to the patient's home situation. Is the patient able to give himself or herself a suppository? Is there a

Table 3–31 **Medications Used to Manage Constipation**

Category	Mechanism of Action	Example	Onset	Comment
Bulk forming	Absorbs water, increases bulk, stimulates peristalsis	Metamucil	Within 24 hr	Contraindicated in patients with abdominal pain, nausea and vomiting in patients suspected of having appendicitis, biliary tract obstruction or acute hepatitis; take with fluids
Stimulants	Increases peristalsis by irritating colon wall and stimulating enteric nerves	Cascara, senna	Within 12 hr	Causes melanosis coli, most widely abused in laxatives; should not be used in patients with impaction or obstipation
Stool softeners and lubricants	Lubricate intestinal tract and soften feces, making hard stool easier to pass; do not affect peristalsis	Mineral oil, dioctyl sodium Colace	Softeners up to 72 hr and lubricants up to 8 hr	Can block absorption of fat soluble vitamins, which may increase risk of bleeding in patients on anticoagulants
Saline and osmotic solutions	Cause retention of fluid in intestinal lumen caused by osmotic effect	Magnesium salts: magnesium citrate; milk of Magnesia Sodium phosphates: Fleet enema, phospho-soda, lactulose Polyethylene glycol-saline solutions: Go-LYTELY	15 min–3 hr	Magnesium-containing products may cause hypermagnesemia in patients with renal insufficiency

caregiver? Does the caregiver need to be educated about prevention of constipation? Does the patient need a bedside commode or raised toilet seat or other assistive devices? Preventing constipation by recognizing early symptoms and intervening before it becomes a severe problem improves patient quality of life and as such should be a goal for all nurses.[19]

DIARRHEA

Diarrhea is defined both subjectively and objectively as an increase in the liquidity and frequency of stools.[20] For patients with cancer, it may be a symptom of the cancer itself (e.g., bowel obstruction or carcinoid syndrome), a symptom of an infection (*Salmonella, Campylobacter,* or *Shigella* species or *Clostridium difficile*), or a side effect of certain chemotherapeutic agents. It can occur acutely, within 24–48 hours of a stimulus and last for 1–2 weeks, or, in some patients, the onset may be delayed, and the symptoms may last as long as 3 weeks.[10,21,22] Whatever the cause, diarrhea is a serious complication and needs to be addressed quickly. In this chapter, our focus will be on chemotherapy-induced diarrhea.

Box 3–13 Other Causes of Diarrhea

Diagnosis of carcinoid tumor
Graft-versus-host disease
Anxiety and stress
Radiation therapy to the abdomen, pelvis, lower thoracic, and lumbar spine
Alcohol abuse
Laxative abuse
Tube feedings
Medication side effect
Travel
Use of alternative therapies
Immunocompromise
Malabsorption
Parasites
Infection
Dietary causes
Abdominal surgeries
Chemotherapy regimens containing 5-fluorouracil or irinotecan
Spinal cord compression

Data from Brown K, Esper P, Kelleher L, et al., eds. *Chemotherapy and Biotherapy Guidelines and Recommendations for Practice.* Pittsburgh, PA: Oncology Nursing Society; 2005; and Ackley B. Diarrhea. In Ackley B, Ladwig B, eds. *Nursing Diagnosis and Handbook: A Guide to Planning Care.* St. Louis, MO: Mosby; 2006:443–450.

Incidence

Diarrhea is listed as a side effect of multiple chemotherapeutic agents. It is estimated that up to 90% of patients who receive chemotherapy and/or radiation therapy will develop diarrhea.[23] Up to 80% of patients who receive 5-fluorouracil and irinotecan develop diarrhea during their course of treatment.[24]

The severity of diarrhea is often associated with the dose, route, medication combination, and administration schedule of the chemotherapy agent.[25] Box 3–13 lists additional causes for development of diarrhea.[26]

Pathophysiology

The gastrointestinal tract receives 9 L of fluid per day from ingestion, including saliva and gastric, biliary, pancreatic, and intestinal secretions. The majority of these secretions are absorbed by the small intestine (7.5 L/day), and the colon absorbs the remaining fluid, leaving approximately 200 mL or less per day to be excreted via the stool. In patients with cancer, diarrhea may be caused by a number of pathophysiologic factors.[4,26,27]

Secretory diarrhea is associated with neuroendocrine tumors and with intestinal inflammation. It is characterized by hypersecretion caused by endogenous stimulators, producing a disturbance in the transport of water and electrolytes through the intestinal wall. Fluids accumulate in the intestinal lumen, and patients typically present with large-volume, watery stool that persists despite no oral intake.[27]

Exudative diarrhea is the result of excess amounts of blood, protein, or mucus in the intestinal lumen due to an alteration in the integrity of the intestinal lumen, which may result from radiation colitis, ulcers, colonic malignancies, infection, or inflammation. The patient will usually report variable stool volume with frequent stools.[27]

Dysfunctional intestinal motility can also cause diarrhea. It may be the result of slower transit times, which allow bacterial overgrowth or increased motility causing reduced absorption. It can be caused by surgical resection and is commonly associated with inflammatory conditions. Frequent small semisolid or liquid stools of variable volume and frequency are the consequence.[27]

Chemotherapy-induced diarrhea is characterized by a series of events starting from mitotic arrest of intestinal epithelial crypt cells, followed by superficial necrosis and extensive inflammation of the bowel wall. There is oversecretion of intestinal water and electrolytes as a result of cytokine release and other substances from the intestinal epithelial cells. Inflammation of the bowel wall promotes the release of prostaglandins, leukotrienes, cytokines, and free radicals that contribute to the secretion of intestinal fluid and electrolytes. Chemotherapeutic agents also cause destruction of brush-border enzymes responsible for carbohydrate and protein digestion, resulting in further gut-wall secretion and decreased reabsorption. Patients usually experience frequent watery semisolid stools.[8,25,27,28] Chemotherapeutic agents associated with diarrhea are listed in Box 3–14.

Osmotic diarrhea is caused by the consumption of a substance that increases the osmotic activity of the intestine and an increase in the amount of water that enters the colon. This results in a rate of absorption that is disproportionate. Large-volume, watery stool results and usually resolves with withdrawal of the causative agent, which can include fruits, certain medications, and nonabsorbed carbohydrates. Osmotic diarrhea can also be seen after pancreatic resection.[27]

Patients with pancreatic insufficiency due to either large pancreatic tumors or surgical resection of part of the intestine can also develop malabsorptive diarrhea. In these patients, the integrity of the mucosal membrane is disrupted or there are enzymatic changes. Unabsorbed osmotically active substances enter the bowel lumen and exert a direct stimulatory effect. Diarrhea associated with lactose intolerance, celiac sprue, or short gut syndrome is osmotic diarrhea. Large-volume, foul-smelling, steatorrhea-type stool is typical. Any or all of these factors can contribute to diarrhea experienced by the patient with a malignancy, and all need to be assessed when a patient presents with diarrhea as a major complaint.[27]

Assessment

A patient diary may be helpful in assessing the patient with diarrhea. Onset, frequency, and duration of diarrhea, stool consistency, and any interventions used should be listed. In addition, quality-of-life tools may be useful in assessing the impact of diarrhea on the patient. Obtaining the primary diagnosis, comorbid conditions, prior therapy, and current medications, including herbal and vitamin supplements, as well as usual bowel patterns, diet, weight loss, and travel are essential for a thorough assessment of the patient. Coexisting signs and symptoms should also be assessed, including fever, dizziness, malaise, nausea and vomiting, bloating, cramping, malnutrition, and hydration status. The patient should be asked about nocturnal diarrhea to assess the extent and severity of the problem. In addition, a medication history should be obtained, because if the patient's diarrhea is severe enough, oral medications may not be absorbed.[5,27,28]

On physical examination the patient may be orthostatic, hypovolemic and/or dehydrated. Hypovolemia and/or dehydration may cause poor skin turgor, and an oral examination may reveal dry mucous membranes. The patient may have tachycardia and report dizziness when changing positions; orthostatic vital signs should be assessed.

A thorough abdominal assessment and examination of the perianal or periostomal area to assess skin integrity are essential. Bowel sounds may be hyperactive, and the patient's abdomen may be tender to palpation.

Laboratory evaluation should include a complete blood count, electrolyte values, and stool analysis. The patient may be acidotic or, if severely hypovolemic/dehydrated, may show signs of a contraction alkalosis.

Box 3–14 Chemotherapeutic Agents Associated with Diarrhea

Alkylating Agents
Amsacrine
Ifosfamide
Nitrogen mustard
Nitrosureas
Streptozocin
Oxaliplatin
Dacarbazine
Procarbazine

Antimetabolites
Azacytidine
Cytarabine
Fludarabine
5-Fluorouracil capecitabine
Gemzar
Hydroxyurea
Mercaptopurine
Methotrexate
Mitoguazone
Pemetrexed
Pentostatin
Raltitrexed
Thioguanine
Uracil

Antitumor Antibiotics
Actinomycin D
Daunorubicin
Doxorubicin
Epirubicin
Idarubicin
Mithramycin

Mitotic Spindle Agents
Abraxane
Taxol
Taxotere
Vinblastine

Topoisomerase Inhibitors
Irinotecan
Topotecan
Etoposide
Teniposide

Monoclonal Antibodies
Avastin
Erbitux
Rituxan

Other Agents
Anagrelide
Asparaginase
Darbepoetin alfa
Epoetin alfa
Gefitinib
Mitotane
Octreotide
Velcade

For agents in *italics* diarrhea is a dose-limiting toxicity.

SUPPORTIVE CARE

The National Cancer Institute Common Toxicity Criteria (NCI-CTC) is the most commonly used standardized method for assessing the severity of treatment-induced diarrhea. According to these criteria, diarrhea is divided into five grades based on the number of loose stools per day and the associated symptoms and nature of the diarrhea (Table 3–32). It should be mentioned that the NCI-CTC grading system does not take into account quality-of-life information.

Gastrointestinal and Vascular Syndrome

During the late 1990s through 2002, Irinotecan, 5-fluorouracil, and leucovorin (IFL) was one of the primary regimens for the treatment of metastatic colorectal cancer. In 2001 the North Central Cancer Treatment Group coordinated Intergroup Trial N9741 to compare irinotecan-based therapy with oxaliplatin-based therapy. The data were reviewed by an external data monitoring committee, who noted and reported on an unexpected number of deaths within the first 60 days of study entry, the majority of which occurred on the IFL arm of the study.[29] At the same time, the Cancer and Leukemia Group B (CALGB) was accruing participants on another study involving irinotecan. Because of the reported deaths, CALGB elected to review their data and found 19 deaths within the first 60 days (14 on the IFL arm and 5 on the 5-fluorouracil/leucovorin arm). CALGB concluded that all the deaths were related to either a gastrointestinal syndrome or a vascular syndrome.[30]

The gastrointestinal syndrome was defined by the presence of watery diarrhea, nausea, vomiting, anorexia, abdominal cramping, and sepsis. These symptoms were associated with severe dehydration, fever, neutropenia, and electrolyte abnormalities. The vascular syndrome was defined as an acute, fatal myocardial infarction, pulmonary embolus, or cerebrovascular event associated with recent use of chemotherapy. Recognition of these syndromes prompted further analysis of appropriate management of treatment-induced diarrhea.[30–32]

Treatment

In 1998 an expert panel published guidelines to manage treatment-induced diarrhea.[33] The need for these guidelines grew out of the lack of consistent evidence-based recommendations in the literature for the management of treatment-induced

Table 3–32 **Common Toxicity Criteria for Diarrhea**

Adverse Event	0	1	2	3	4	5
Diarrhea	None	Increase of <4 stools/day over baseline; mild increase in ostomy output compared with baseline	Increase of 4–6 stools/day over baseline; IV fluids indicated <24 hr; moderate increase in ostomy output compared with baseline; not interfering with activities of daily living	Increase of ≥7 stools/day over baseline; incontinence; IV fluids ≥24 hr hospitalization; severe increase in ostomy output compared with baseline; interfering with activities of daily living	Life-threatening consequences (e.g., hemodynamic collapse)	Death

Data from Cancer Therapy Evaluation Program: Common Toxicity Criteria for Adverse Events, version 3.0. Available at http://ctep.cancer.gov/forms/CTCAEv3.pdf. Accessed December 7, 2006.

diarrhea. The panel reviewed and reissued the guidelines in 2002. They recommended that treatment-induced diarrhea be categorized as either uncomplicated or complicated. Complicated diarrhea is described as grade 3 or 4 diarrhea or lower-grade diarrhea with multiple other symptoms. Uncomplicated diarrhea is grade 1 or 2 diarrhea without any other exacerbating signs or symptoms.[32,33]

Initial management of uncomplicated diarrhea includes dietary modifications (initiation of a lactose-free diet and elimination of high-osmolar dietary supplements). The patient is instructed to keep a diary of episodes of diarrhea and severity as well as accompanying symptoms. Loperamide is started at a 4-mg dose followed by 2 mg every 4 hours or after every unformed stool but not to exceed 16 mg/day. If the diarrhea improves or resolves, the patient should continue the dietary restrictions and may discontinue the loperamide 12 hours after the last diarrheal stool. If the diarrhea persists for longer than 24 hours, the dose of loperamide is increased to 2 mg every 2 hours, and use of oral antibiotics should be considered. If the diarrhea persists for longer than 48 hours, loperamide should be discontinued and another agent such as octreotide, oral budesonide, or tincture of opium should be started. Of note, octreotide has been found to be effective after the failure of loperamide.[34] Table 3–33 lists the classifications of antidiarrheal agents and their mechanism of action.

Patients with complicated diarrhea are generally admitted to the hospital. The guidelines recommend that octreotide be started at a dose of 100–150 mcg 3 times/day with dose escalation to 500 mcg until the diarrhea is controlled. In addition, intravenous fluids should be initiated. Further workup should include stool cultures, a complete blood count, and electrolyte assessment. Stool cultures for the presence of fecal leukocytes, blood, *Clostridium difficile, Salmonella, Shigella, Escherichia coli,* and *Campylobacter* should be obtained. If the patient has a significant history of travel or a comorbid condition such as human immunodeficiency virus, stool cultures for ova and parasites should also be obtained.[33]

As a result of the independent review of the Intergroup trial, describing the gastrointestinal and vascular syndromes, the guidelines also recommended more stringent assessment of patients receiving combination regimens. There should be at least weekly evaluation during the first cycle of chemotherapy. Particular attention must be paid to elderly patients, who have a greater risk of hypovolemia/dehydration and may need more aggressive intervention. Furthermore, although these recommendations

SUPPORTIVE CARE

Table 3–33 **Mechanism of Action of Antidiarrheal Agents**

Classification	Action
Intraluminal agents	Decrease water absorption, increase the bulk of the stool, and protect the lining of the intestine. Examples include activated charcoal, mucilloid preparations, psyllium, kaolin and pectate.
Intestinal transit inhibitors	Slow peristalsis and increase fluid absorption. Examples are anticholinergic agents such as atropine sulfate and scopolamine, opiate agonists such as diluted tincture of opium and synthetic opioids such as diphenoxylate and loperamide.
Antisecretory agents	Inhibit secretion of hormones such as serotonin and motilin, slowing transit time and balancing electrolyte and water regulation in the intestine. An example is octreotide.
Bismuth subsalicylate	Decreases inflammation of the intestinal lining and decreases the hypermotility of the gastrointestinal tract. An example is Pepto Bismol.

Modified from Ippoliti C. Antidiarrheal agents for the management of treatment-related diarrhea in cancer patients. *Am J Health-Syst Pharm* 1998;55:1573–1580.

were necessitated because of the side effects of an irinotecan-based combination therapy, capecitabine, oxaliplatin, and 5-fluorouracil also have a high risk of inducing diarrhea.[33]

In addition, patients should avoid dairy products, high-fat content and spicy foods, alcohol, and caffeine. Consumption of bananas, rice, applesauce, and toast (BRAT diet) can be helpful. A clear liquid diet to allow for bowel rest may also be of benefit. Although a small study showed that glutamine was beneficial for treatment-induced diarrhea, other data are conflicting, suggesting that more research is needed.[33]

Herbal supplements such as milk thistle, aloe, saw palmetto, Siberian ginseng, and plantago seed can all contribute to diarrhea and should to be discontinued. Other supplements, such as coenzyme Q10, vitamin C at high doses, and the beverage green tea also cause diarrhea and should be discontinued as well.[27]

Nursing Care

As a potentially life-threatening side effect of some chemotherapeutic agents, diarrhea must be assessed and treated quickly, especially in elderly patients. Nurses are pivotal in this process, first by educating the patient and family members about diarrhea and its possible complications and then by making sure that any diarrhea the patient is experiencing is reported accurately. Having the patient keep a diary can be helpful. The patient should know the importance of hydration and dietary modification and, most importantly, should know when to seek medical attention. Fever, dizziness, excessive thirst, bloody stools, intense cramping, or refractory diarrhea are all symptoms that require attention. The patient and family members should be instructed on the proper use of any antidiarrheal medications along with skin care of the perianal area. The use of Tucks medicated pads or baby wipes after bowel movements is usually less irritating than the use of toilet paper. Barrier agents such as zinc oxide may be useful in protecting the area. If fissures, hemorrhoids, or breakdowns occur, the appropriate management should be instituted.[5,15,35]

CONCLUSION

The symptoms of constipation and diarrhea are serious side effects of certain chemotherapeutic agents, surgery, radiation therapy, adjunctive medications, and/or the tumor itself. Recognizing these symptoms early and intervening as quickly and as effectively as possible improve quality of life for the patient.

REFERENCES

1. Wood J. Neurogastroenterology and gastrointestinal motility. In Rhoades R, Tanner G, eds. *Medical Physiology,* 2nd ed. Philadelphia, PA: Lippincott Williams & Wilkins; 2003 pp 449-480.
2. Wood J, Alpers D, Andrews P. Fundamentals of neurogastroenterology. *Gut* 1999;45:1–44.
3. Costa M, Brookes S, Hennig G. Anatomy and physiology of the enteric nervous system. *Gut* 2000;47 (Suppl 4):12–15.
4. Tso P. Gastrointestinal secretion, digestion and absorption. In Rhoades R, Tanner G, eds. *Medical Physiology,* 2nd ed. Philadelphia: Lippincott Williams & Wilkins; 2003 pp. 481-513.
5. Wilkes G, Barton-Burke M. Constipation. In *Nursing Drug Handbook.* Boston, MA: Jones & Bartlett; 2005:924–938.
6. Guyton AC. *Textbook of Medical Physiology,* 7th ed. Philadelphia, PA: WB Saunders; 1986.
7. Paice J. Symptom management. In Miaskowski C, Buschel P, eds. *Oncology Nursing: Assessment and Clinical Care.* Portland, OR: Mosby, 1999, pp 275-304.
8. Merkle J. *Handbook of Physiology,* 2nd ed. Philadelphia, PA: Lippincott Williams & Wilkins; 2005.
9. Sykes N. Current approaches to the management of constipation. *Cancer Surv* 1994;21:137–146.
10. Wright P, Thomas S. Constipation and diarrhea: the neglected symptoms. *Semin Oncol Nurs* 1995;11: 289–297.
11. Vainio A, Auvinen A. Prevalence of symptoms among patients with advanced cancer: an international collaborative study. *J Pain Symptom Manage* 1996;12:3–10.
12. Tuchmann L. Constipation. In Gates R, Fink R, eds. *Oncology Nursing Secrets.* Philadelphia, PA: Hanley & Belfus, 1997; 216–225.

13. Hajek P, Gillison F, McRobbie H. Stopping smoking can cause constipation. *Addiction* 2003;98: 1563–1567.
14. Patt R. Cancer pain management: an essential component of comprehensive cancer care. In Rubin P, Williams J, eds. *Clinical Oncology: A Multidisciplinary Approach for Physicians and Students,* 8th ed. Philadelphia: WB Saunders; 2001:864–892.
15. Bisanz A. Managing bowel elimination patterns in patients with cancer. *Oncol Nurs Forum* 1997;24: 679–688.
16. Sykes N. An investigation of the ability of oral naloxone to correct opioid-related constipation in patients with advanced cancer. *Palliat Medicine* 1996;10:135–144.
17. Culpeper-Morgan J, Inturrisi C, Portenoy R, et al. Treatment of opioid-induced constipation with oral naloxone: a pilot study. *Clin Pharmacol Ther* 1992;52:90–95.
18. Curtiss C. Constipation. In Yarbro C, Frogge M, Goodman M, eds. *Cancer Symptom Management.* Boston, MA: Jones & Bartlett; 1999:508–521.
19. Ackley B. Constipation. In Ackley B, Ludwig B, eds. *Nursing Diagnosis and Handbook, A Guide to Planning Care.* St. Louis, MO: Mosby; 2006:353–360.
20. Ackley B. Diarrhea. In Ackley B, Ludwig B, eds. *Nursing Diagnosis and Handbook, A Guide to Planning Care.* St. Louis, MO: Mosby; 2006:443–450.
21. Rutledge D, Engelking C. Cancer related-diarrhea: selected findings of a national survey of oncology nurse experiences. *Oncol Nurs Forum* 1998;25:861–878.
22. Wilkes G, Barton-Burke M. Diarrhea. In Wilke, G, Barton-Burke, M, eds. *Oncology Nursing Drug Handbook,* Boston, MA: Jones & Bartlett; 2005:939–949.
23. Tuchmann L. Diarrhea. In Gates R, Fink R, ed. *Oncology Nursing Secrets.* Philadelphia, PA: Hanley & Belfus; 1997:226–233.
24. Benson A, Ajani J, Catalano R, et al. Recommended guidelines for the treatment of cancer treatment-induced diarrhea. *J Clin Oncol* 2004;22:2918–2926.
25. Polovich M, White J, Kelleher L, eds. *Chemotherapy and Biotherapy Guidelines and Recommendations for Practice,.* 2nd ed. Pittsburgh, PA: Oncology Nursing Society; 2005.
26. Prommer E, Casciato D. Supportive care. In Casciato D, ed. *Manual of Clinical Oncology.* Philadelphia, PA: Lippincott Williams & Wilkins; 2004:102–129.
27. O'Brien B, Kaklamani, V, Benson A. The assessment and management of cancer treatment-related diarrhea. *Clin Colorectal Cancer* 2005;4:375–381.
28. Engelking C. Diarrhea. In Yarbro C, Frogge M, Goodman M, eds. *Cancer Symptom Management.* Boston, MA: Jones & Bartlett; 2003.
29. Goldberg R, Sargent D, Morton R, et al. A randomized controlled trial of fluorouracil plus leucovorin, irinotecan and oxaliplatin combinations in patients with previously untreated metastatic colorectal cancer. *J Clin Oncol* 2004;22:23–30.
30. Rothenberg M, Meropol N, Poplin E, et al. Mortality associated with irinotecan plus bolus fluorouracil/leucovorin: summary findings of an independent panel. *J Clin Oncol* 2001;19:3801–3807.
31. Prudden J. *Clinical Consequences and Prophylaxis of Chemotherapy-Induced Diarrhea* [oncology special edition monograph]. McMahon Publishing Group, New York, 2001.
32. Camptosar (irinotecan) prescribing information. New York, NY: Pfizer Oncology, 2004.
33. Wadler S, Benson A, Engelkin C, et al. Recommended guidelines for the treatment of chemotherapy-induced diarrhea. *J Clin Oncol* 1998;16:3169–3178.
34. Barbounis V, Koumakis G, Vassilomanolakis M, et al. Control of irinotecan-induced diarrhea by octreotide after loperamide failure. *Support Cancer Care* 2001;9:258–260.
35. Hogan C. The nurse's role in diarrhea management. *Oncol Nurs Forum* 1998;25:879–886.

Chapter 5
Management and Treatment of Bone Disease
Tammy J. Rodvelt

The word *skeleton* conjures up images of inanimate, dusty, dry bones akin to what one would find at an anthropologic dig, on display in a museum, or on a vestment worn to a masquerade ball. Indeed, the word skeleton is derived from the Greek word *skeletos*, which means "dried up or withered." Bones, however, hardly meet the criteria of a dead, inert substance. Much of what makes up bony tissue is unambiguously living. Mature bone is constructed from inorganic elements or minerals, deposited on a framework of organic support material. A frequently quoted analogy is to envision an ordinary kitchen sponge dipped in plaster and left to dry.[1] The porous sponge is a surrogate for the organic support material, and the plaster is analogous to the deposited inorganic bone minerals.

The inorganic component of bone, or the plaster, is predominately made up of minute crystals of calcium phosphate in the form of the mineral hydroxyapatite. Historically, because of the properties of calcium and phosphorus, bone has revealed much of our current knowledge of prehistoric entities. This is due to the fact that calcium and phosphorus are inorganic components that resist decomposition even after death has occurred. Other lesser constituents include magnesium, sodium, carbonate, and water. This inorganic component of bone is also called cortical bone. The organic portion of bone, or the sponge, is called osteoid. A specialized type of collagen fiber, type I collagen, makes up 90%–95% of osteoid.[2] Various proteins originating from the serum constitute the remaining 5%–10% (albumin, α_2-HS glycoproteins, α-carboxyglutamic acid proteins, osteonectin, osteopontin, sialoproteins, and thrombospondin). This inner spongy organic component of bone is called trabecular bone. Structurally, the hydroxyapatite crystals line up beside the collagen fibers. This association results in the characteristic strength and hardness attributed to bone. This concept is proven by the following experiment: If bone were demineralized, the remaining spongy collagen component would retain the shape of the bone, but the bone would be flexible, much like a tendon. Conversely, if the collagen and proteoglycans were removed from bone, again the shape would be maintained, owing to the hard inorganic deposits, but the bone would be quite brittle and subject to easy breaking.

Although the exact number of bones varies from person to person, depending on age and genetic variability, the average number of bones in the human adult skeleton is approximately 206. Bone is adaptable in carrying out various functions including mechanical support, vital organ protection, movement, hemopoiesis, and mineral storage. Calcium and phosphorus are by far the most prevalent minerals found in the human body. There are 1–2 kg of calcium and 1 kg of phosphorus present in the average adult[3]; 99% of that calcium and 85% of the phosphorus are stored in the skeleton and teeth. In addition to providing rigidity to bone, both calcium and phosphorus are critical and indispensable in other bodily functions and reactions. Calcium is a requirement for muscle contraction and the transportation of ions and nutrients across plasma membranes and is involved in the blood clotting cascade. Phosphorus is an absolute necessity for the activities of the nucleic acids DNA and RNA and in the process of ATP utilization.

NORMAL BONE PHYSIOLOGY

To better comprehend the mechanisms of bone disease, a general understanding of normal bone physiology must first be attained. Bone is recognized as being in a dynamic state. In other words, it is continually being built up and broken down. This process is called bone remodeling. Bone remodeling ensures the structural integrity of the skeletal framework and maintains mineral homeostasis. There are three types of cells involved in bone remodeling: osteoblasts, osteocytes, and osteoclasts. Osteoblasts arise from the mesenchymal cells. They are cuboidal cells that line up on the surface of bone. They synthesize and secrete osteoid that is then deposited on the existing bony surface. As new bone mineral is annexed and deposited on the osteoid, the osteoblasts eventually become surrounded and encased by mineralized bone and then lose their ability to produce further osteoid. Osteoblasts that have ceased producing osteoid become resting cells and are henceforth termed osteocytes. These osteocytes, some of which are deeply embedded in bone, are living cells that require nutrients, ions, hormones, and other substances. These necessary substances travel from nearby blood vessels through a network of channels called canaliculi that traverse deep into bone.

The third cell type involved in bone remodeling is the osteoclasts, which develop from monocyte-macrophage precursor cells. Osteoclasts are also located on the surface of bone. They are larger than osteoblasts and are multinucleated. Their function is the polar opposite of that of osteoblasts. Instead of building bone, osteoclasts break down or resorb bone, creating an erosion cavity or crater. Although their mechanism is not yet completely understood, osteoclasts are theorized to secrete certain acids and proteolytic enzymes. The function of the acid is to increase the solubility of the mineral component of bone, where as the proteolytic enzymes break down the osteoid component. Once bone resorption has begun, and erosion cavities are forged, a reversal process ensues. Mononuclear cells amass at the crater and prepare the surface for bone replacement. Stimulatory signals are then sent out, which in turn activate osteoblasts to synthesize new osteoid and replace or repair the recently resorbed bone. Thus, a cycle of normal bone remodeling is established (see Color Plate 3). In normal bone, this process encompasses approximately 120 days. It is estimated that the entire human skeleton is remodeled over the course of about 10 years. A mnemonic device to help one remember the function of these bone cells is: "Blasts build bone and clasts create craters."

Healthy bone is maintained by a homeostatic mechanism. Several hormones are intimately involved in the bone remodeling schema and have a complex relationship in the regulation of homeostasis and overall bone health. In general, normal bone remodeling in the healthy adult demonstrates essentially equal and parallel activity between the osteoblasts and osteoclasts. The delicately balanced interplay between osteoblasts and osteoclasts is orchestrated by different hormonal influences including parathyroid hormone, 1,25-hydroxyvitamin D_3, calcitonin, growth hormone, insulin-like growth factor, and the gonadal steroids (estrogen and androgen).[4] Any deficiency or malfunctioning in these hormones quickly upsets the meticulous balance between these two opposing forces, creating a diseased state.

Where the cycle of bone remodeling is initiated—with osteoblasts or osteoclasts—is dependent on what physiologic factor, physical stressor, or metabolic malfunction has occurred. For example, when the brain senses a low serum calcium level, the parathyroid gland is stimulated to release parathyroid hormone, which in turn activates the osteoclasts. This process frees calcium ions from the bone, which then move into the circulation to restore the critical calcium balance in the serum. At the same time, parathyroid hormone also induces increased synthesis of calcitriol. Calcitriol enables additional calcium to be absorbed from the gut and increases the retrieval of calcium in the kidneys before urinary excretion. If this metabolic process is allowed to proceed unchecked, calcium levels in the serum will eventually surpass their critical point, and a hypercalcemic state will develop. The body normally monitors and prevents this situation by activating a negative-feedback mechanism. Once appropriate calcium levels are achieved in the serum, the thyroid gland is stimulated to increase secretion of calcitonin. The presence of calcitonin serves to deactivate the activity of the osteoclasts, thus decreasing calcium loss from the bones. Secondarily, calcitonin leads to a decrease in the synthesis of calcitriol, which in turn causes a decrease of calcium in the serum by absorbing less calcium from the gut and allowing calcium to be excreted through the urine. Any excess calcium in the serum is once again stored in the bone via the activity of the osteoblasts. See Tables 3–34 and 3–35 for other systemic and local factors regulating osteoblasts and osteoclasts.[5]

A second example is the application of orthodontic braces to crooked teeth. The physical stress caused by the tightening of the braces stimulates osteoblastic activity, thus literally reshaping the sockets of the individual teeth. A right-handed tennis player will always build more bone in the right arm than in the left. These examples illustrate the concept that more bone is automatically built in areas under stress. Thus,

Table 3–34 Factors Influencing Osteoclasts

Stimulatory	Inhibitory
Systemic Factors	**Systemic Factors**
Parathyroid hormone	Corticosteroids
1,25-Hydroxyvitamin D_3	Prostaglandin E_2
Thyroxine	
Local Factors	**Local Factors**
Interleukin-6	Transforming growth factor–β
Interleukin-1	Osteoprotegerin
T Cells	**T Cells**
Interleukin-17	Interleukin-4
Colony stimulating factors	Interleukin-18
Prostaglandins	Interferon-γ

Data from Roodman GD. Mechanisms of bone metastasis. *N Engl J Med* 2004;350:1655–1664.

Table 3–35 Factors Influencing Osteoblasts

Stimulatory	Inhibitory
Systemic Factors	**Systmeic Factors**
Parathyroid hormone	Corticosteroids
Prostaglandins	
Cytokines	
Local Factors	
Bone morphogenetic protein	
Transforming growth factor–β	
Insulin-like growth factor	
Fibroblast growth factor	
T Cells	
Platelet-derived growth factor	

Data from Roodman GD. Mechanisms of bone metastasis. *N Engl J Med* 2004;350:1655–1664.

weight-bearing activities are extraordinarily important for strengthening bone. Bone strength is determined by its density. Bone density refers to how densely packed the bone crystals are. The weightlessness of space travel presents a significant problem for the bone health of space travelers. Without the force of gravity, there is no weight or stress placed on the bones, especially the major joints. This leads to a muting of osteoblast activity and the development of microfractures. These microfractures accumulate and eventually allow a major fracture to occur. Even on the gravity-laden Earth, microfractures are constantly developing, but in a normal healthy adult the activity of the osteoclasts and osteoblasts are in harmony, and the microfractures are knitted back together without the individual even knowing they have occurred.

Normal bone remodeling is described as *coupled and balanced* (Figure 3–2 *A*).[6] This means that new bone is synthesized in the appropriate location and proportion to the amount of old bone that was previously resorbed. In other words, the activity of both osteoclasts and osteoblasts are equivalent, and there is no net gain or loss of bone. When normal bone remodeling goes awry because of extrinsic factors, three alternative scenarios can then potentially develop, as illustrated by Theriault[6] (Figure 3–2*B–D*).

In the first abnormal scenario (Figure 3–2*B*), the remodeling process is defined as *coupled but imbalanced*. In this situation, there is excessive osteoclastic activity. The activity of the osteoblasts fails to meet the activity of the osteoclasts and there is a net loss of bone.

In the second abnormal scenario (Figure 3–2*C*), the remodeling process is *uncoupled but balanced*. The activities of the osteoblasts and osteoclasts are equivalent but rather disorganized. Therefore, there is no net gain or loss of bone. However, abnormal bone is still present. There are areas of bone that have been inappropriately built up along with areas that have inappropriately decreased amounts of bone.

In the final scenario of abnormal bone remodeling, the process is described as *uncoupled and imbalanced* (Figure 3–2*D*). Here, the osteoblasts exhibit excessive

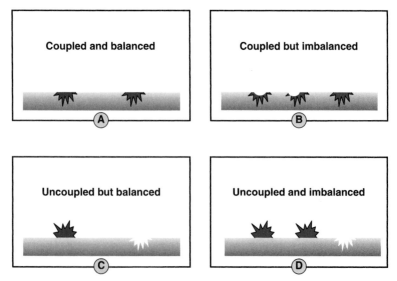

Coupled and balanced

(A)

Coupled but imbalanced

(B)

Uncoupled but balanced

(C)

Uncoupled and imbalanced

(D)

Figure 3–2 Normal *(A)* versus abnormal bone remodeling *(B–D)*.

activity, resulting in bone formation at locations where there has been no or little bone resorption. The outcome is an abnormal net gain of bone.

BONE DISEASES

Multiple diseases of bone have been documented, including Paget's disease, rickets, and osteonecrosis of the bone, to name a few. In the remainder of this chapter, however, I will focus on the three most commonly occurring bone problems in patients with cancer. These problems are bony metastases and the ensuing risk of pathologic fracture and spinal cord compression, hypercalcemia, and osteoporosis. All three of these disorders contribute to increasing the overall morbidity and mortality of individuals battling cancer. A better understanding of how these disorders develop and progress allows one to be a more effective caregiver and to administer appropriate treatments and adequate support, which will improve the individual's overall quality of life and perhaps even their quantity of life.

Bony Metastases

Cancer can develop almost anywhere in the body, including the bones. Bone tumors are classified as either primary or metastatic. Primary bone cancer is not very common. The American Cancer Society[7] estimated that only 2,760 new cases of primary cancer in the bone and joints would be diagnosed in 2006 in the United States. Metastatic bone cancer or secondary cancer originates in another organ and then travels or metastasizes to the bone by way of the circulatory system the lymphovascular system and sometimes by direct extension from the primary tumor or even another metastasis. Although bone metastases are considerably more common than primary bone tumors, the actual incidence is not accurately known. Although any cancer has the potential to develop bone metastases, certain cancers have a higher predilection for developing bone metastases. Carcinoma-type solid tumors tend to have a higher incidence of bone metastases than other tumor types. Carcinomas are malignant neoplasms that have an epithelial origin as opposed to sarcomas, which have a mesenchymal origin, or neoplasms of the hematopoietic system. Examples of epithelial-derived carcinomas are adenocarcinoma, squamous cell carcinoma, and transitional cell carcinoma. The overall incidence of bone metastasis in the United States by tumor type is shown in Table 3–36.[8]

The incidence of bone metastases in children is less common than that in adults. The predominant cancers associated with bone metastases in children are

Table 3–36 **U.S. Incidence of Bone Metastases in Descending Order of Frequency**

Overall	Women	Men
Breast	Breast	Prostate
Prostate	Uterus	Lung
Lung	Colon	Bladder
Colon	Stomach	Stomach
Stomach	Rectum	Rectum
Bladder	Bladder	Colon
Uterus		
Rectum		
Thyroid		
Kidney		

Data from Peh WCG, Muttarak M. *Bone metastases.* Available at /www.emedicine.com/radio/topic88.htm. Retrieved December 7, 2006.

SUPPORTIVE CARE

neuroblastoma and the leukemias. When bone metastases are discovered in children, they tend to be widespread throughout the skeleton, whereas in adults, a different pattern emerges. The spread of cancer cells into the bone, or seeding, initially begins in the red marrow. Red marrow is the principal organ that forms blood cells. It follows then that the red marrow is an area in the body with ample vasculature and high blood flow. In children, the bones contain only red marrow, thus explaining the widespread nature of bone metastases among the young. As children normally mature into adolescents and adults, the red marrow is eventually replaced by fat-storing yellow marrow in the shafts of the long bones. In adults, the red marrow persists in the ribs, sternum, vertebrae, skull, and bones of the pelvis. Although bone metastases can occur anywhere in the adult skeleton, the typical distribution of bone metastases in the adult is predominantly in the axial skeleton followed by any other residual red marrow–containing bones (i.e., the pelvic girdle).

The development of metastases is a continuous process, and the major contributing cause of treatment failure, morbidity, and mortality. The formation of metastatic lesions in both bones and soft tissue can begin quite early in the growth and development of the primary tumor. These lesions tend to increase in frequency and number with prolonged tumor duration and overall tumor burden. As the disease advances, metastases can originate from either the primary tumor or other metastases or both. Fortunately, the formation of metastatic lesions is an inefficient process. Although many times large numbers of individual tumor cells and clusters of tumor cells called emboli are shed from a tumor and pass into the vasculature, very few ultimately land at a distant site and then grow into metastatic foci. In fact, Stetler-Stevenson and Kleiner[9] demonstrated by injecting highly metastatic tumor cells intravenously into laboratory animals that only 0.01% actually formed tumors. The inefficiency by which cancer spreads is due to a highly complex, interdependent, and tightly controlled cascade of events.[9] Each of the eight steps (Box 3–14) is rate limiting, so failure to complete one step in the cascade disrupts the whole process. Research in the scientific community has upheld the fact that the various steps involved in metastatic formation are similar for all tumor types.

The first step in the metastatic cascade is *oncogenesis,* otherwise known as tumorigenesis. This occurs after the initial transformation to a neoplastic state has been accomplished at the primary site. The normal healthy cells that have now been converted into malignant tumor cells undergo cellular proliferation and further genetic

---

Box 3–14 Metastatic Cascade

1. Oncogenesis
2. Angiogenic switch
3. Clonal dominance
4. Survival in the circulation
5. Tumor arrest
6. Extravasation and growth
7. Secondary angiogenic switch
8. Evasion of the immune response

Data from Stetler-Stevenson WG, Kleiner DE Jr. Molecular biology of cancer: invasion and metastases. In DeVita VT Jr, Hellman S, Rosenberg SA, eds. *Cancer: Principles and Practice of Oncology.* Philadelphia, PA: Lippincott Williams & Wilkins; 2001:123–136.

changes. What develops is a malignant cellular population that is heterogenous in nature, in that the individual cells possess varying degrees of metastatic potential.

The second step in the metastatic cascade is *angiogenic switch*. The immediate microenvironment of the primary tumor initially supports its continued growth. However, as the tumor continues to expand and grow, reliance on the nearby, neighboring vasculature becomes insufficient, and the cells in the central interior of the mass become hypoxic. The angiogenic switch is then thrown, and the tumor begins to secrete its own angiogenic factors that enable the tumor to synthesize its own directly connected vasculature system. The turning on of the angiogenic switch also functions to remove, or at least suppress, angiogenesis inhibitors. Vascularization of the tumor is directly associated with an almost immediate and dramatic increase of metastatic potential because the tumor now has direct access to the vascular highway, which can potentially carry tumor cells and emboli to other distant sites in the body. When a primary tumor develops in an already very highly vascularized area, it is also possible for the tumor to commandeer those existing vessels in addition to creating new vessels via angiogenesis.

Clonal dominance is the third step in the metastatic cascade. As the tumor cells continue to undergo genetic mutations, there is eventually a selection of tumor cell clones that exhibit both a distinct growth advantage and have an invasive property or phenotype. These two characteristics allow a sequence of critical steps to proceed. First, tumor cells with an invasive phenotype are able to down-regulate cell-to-cell adhesion. Secondly, these cells are capable of altering the expression of the trans-membrane protein, integrin, which is present in the extracellular matrix (ECM), thus altering attachment of the tumor cells to the ECM. Finally, the tumor cells proteolytically alter the ECM. In other words, the invasive tumor cells are able to detach from the primary tumor, create defects in the ECM, including the basement membrane, and then invade the stroma. The previously developed tumor blood vessels that formed in response to the angiogenic switch are not of good quality and are easily penetrated by these invasive tumor cells. Nearby lymphatic channels that are generally thin-walled are also readily penetrated by the invasive malignant cells. The tumor cell population now has an easy ingress to the systemic circulation. *Survival in the circulation* is the fourth step. Tumor cells and emboli that have made it to the systemic circulation now must encounter and maintain viability against numerous immunologic and hemodynamic challenges.

The fifth step in the development of metastatic disease is *tumor arrest*. Once tumor cells have successfully traveled through the lymphatic or circulatory system, they eventually arrest, or stop. The cessation of their movement is caused by the cells becoming lodged and trapped in the tiny capillary vessels, by sticking to lymphatic or capillary endothelial cells, or by adhering to exposed basement membrane.

Extravasation and growth is the next step. It is known that in most cases, tumor cells and emboli extravasate or pass through the lymphatic or capillary wall before proliferating. They first migrate through the local environment to a locale that is favorable for their ongoing growth. These metastatic tumor cells then enter a dormant state or respond to growth factors and proceed to proliferate. Poor growth after extravasation is a major deterrent to the metastatic cascade.

The seventh step in the metastatic process is essentially a repeat of the second step: a *secondary angiogenic switch*. The newly formed metastases are also dependent on the blood supply for maintenance and growth. As the metastatic foci increase in size, the demand for blood increases. The mechanism of angiogenesis is again switched on and the burgeoning tumor develops a network of new vasculature. This sets up a domino effect in the sense that the metastases themselves are now capable of metastasizing by initiating a new metastatic cascade.

SUPPORTIVE CARE

The eighth and final step in the metastatic cascade is *evasion of the immune response*. These tumor cells must avoid being detected and eradicated by immune-mediated responses. The immune system is capable of directing either a nonspecific or targeted approach against the malignant cells. Active research is currently ongoing to better understand and manipulate this particular event.

Once bony metastases are established, they are categorized as either osteoblastic or osteolytic and represent the two dysregulation extremes of the normal bone remodeling process. Osteoblastic lesions are those related to the excessive formation of bone. In this type of lesion, the activity of the osteoblasts is greater than the activity of the osteoclasts, and bone piles up on top of itself, resulting in a net gain of bone. In a model put forth by Mundy[10] tumor cells produce multiple factors such as fibroblast growth factors, bone morphogenic proteins, platelet-derived growth factor, and transforming growth factor–β, which stimulate osteoblast activity, resulting in subsequent bone formation. In addition, proteases, such as prostate-specific antigen, for example, can release insulin-like growth factor, which, in turn, deactivates an osteolytic factor called parathyroid hormone–related peptide (PTHrP), critical in turning on osteoclasts.[10] By failing to turn on the osteoclasts, bone formation is further promoted.

The opposite is observed with osteolytic lesions, in which there is dissolution of bone. The bone erodes away, leaving craters. Here, the activity of the osteoclasts surpasses the activity of the osteoblasts, and there is a net loss of bone. Again, a hypothesis by Mundy[10] illustrates the details of the process. Tumor cells secrete PTHrP, which as previously mentioned, is important in stimulating osteoclast precursors to mature and proceed with osteolysis. The PTHrP down-regulates osteoprotegerin (OPG) and stimulates osteoblasts to release receptor activator of nuclear factor-κB ligand (RANKL). RANKL activates osteoclast precursors, which leads to crater formation by the osteoclasts. Bone-derived growth factors are subsequently released, which then return to the tumor cell surface, signaling it to continue production of PTHrP. A vicious cycle of osteoclastic activity is thus established.

Patients may present with osteoblastic, osteolytic, or even mixed metastatic lesions, but trends do occur in certain cancers. For example, patients with prostate cancer have predominantly blastic metastases, although they also exhibit increased bone resorption within these osteoblastic lesions. On the other hand, individuals with breast or renal cell carcinoma tend to have predominantly lytic metastases, but up to 15%–20% of breast cancer patients also have documented osteoblastic lesions.[11] Only multiple myeloma has lesions of a purely lytic nature. Early detection and aggressive management of metastatic disease is the primary goal to maintain and maximize an individual's functioning and overall quality of life. Although pain is the principle presenting symptom of bone metastases, one may have metastases without any aches or pain at all. Schaberg and Gainor[12] reported that 36% of study patients with known spinal metastases did not complain of bone pain. In an earlier study by Galasko and Sylvester,[13] only 66% of patients with a known history of malignancy and back pain were actually determined to have bony metastases. Thus, surveillance imaging becomes necessary to monitor for the progression of disease.

The current gold standard for evaluating bony metastases is the bone scan. Bone scanning utilizes technetium-99m (^{99m}Tc) diphosphonate. ^{99m}Tc is a radioactive metal produced from the fission products of uranium and nuclear fuel and has a half-life ($T_{1/2}$) of 6.049 hours.[14] ^{99m}Tc diphosphonate is a radioactive, but nontoxic, substance commercially used as a medical tracer. It is delivered through the body intravenously and eventually binds to functioning osteoblasts. Initially, radioactive uptake is bodywide, and 3–4 hours must pass between infusion and imaging to reduce the background of the soft tissue while capturing the activity still remaining in the skeletal structure. ^{99m}Tc diphosphonate is cleared via renal excretion. Approximately 50% of the tracer is cleared in the first 2–4 hours, and 80% is excreted in the first 24 hours.[15] Less than 1% remains after 48 hours. Impaired renal function will impede the quality of the scan as background activity will be cleared at a slower rate. In ordering diagnostic tests, one should allow a minimum of 48 hours to pass between a bone scan and other tests with radioactive labeling.

When one is evaluating a bone scan film or reading a bone scan report, it is important to pay attention to the descriptors of the lesions. The significance of increased intensity of a lesion is sometimes misinterpreted to equate to progressive disease. In fact, the opposite is true. In the absence of new lesions, increased intensity indicates that the metastatic focus has become static, which is indicative of osteoblasts engaged in vigorous repair. Clinically, this is termed a *flare reaction* and is a representation of either stable or regressing disease.[16] An increase in the size of a lesion should lead one to suspect progressive disease, but an increase in the absolute number of lesions is the hallmark of tumor load expansion and thus defines progressive disease. Normally, a bilateral renal outline should be visible on the film as the ^{99m}Tc diphosphonate is cleared by the kidneys. This outline is readily visible in patients with no bone metastases or mild to moderate bone metastases. In patients with very advanced disease in which a majority of the skeleton has metastatic involvement, the renal outline disappears, and the term *superscan* is used. This simply means that nearly all of the ^{99m}Tc diphosphonate has been taken up by the bones, and therefore very little of this substance has been filtered through the kidneys. The development of a superscan is a poor prognostic factor.

The bone scan is a very sensitive test. It can detect lesions as small as 5 mm. However, it is not a specific test in that it can also detect other nonmalignant bone activity. Other situations that cause increased bone labeling include any condition exhibiting increased osteoblastic activity, such as normal juvenile skeletal growth, bone repair, healing fractures, and arthropathies. Inexperienced observers may have difficulty distinguishing true metastatic lesions from common degenerative or post-traumatic changes. A careful history may help to delineate prior traumatic injuries, whereas observing for symmetrical uptake may prove useful in specifying certain arthritic changes. Many times a questionable metastasis can only be proven or disproven with serial scanning or by follow-up diagnostic tests. Conventional x-rays are routinely used in the attempt to answer such questions. X-rays also have their limits though, as 30%–50% of the bone mineral must be affected for the lesion to be noticeable on the film. Therefore, a positive x-ray finding can verify the presence of a metastatic lesion, but a negative x-ray finding does not necessarily negate the presence of metastatic foci. Other scanning techniques that are useful in elucidating metastatic lesions include magnetic resonance imaging (MRI), fluorodeoxyglucose positron emission tomography (FDG-PET), and occasionally computed tomography (CT) scans. Although the bone scan is a very useful tool, it is an imperfect diagnostic test for evaluating the full extent of bony metastatic lesions. A bone scan provides a map of osteoblastic lesions only, leaving any osteolytic lesions hidden and off the radar. If a repair process has been set in motion by the osteoblasts and secondary bone formation has occurred at the site of a lytic lesion, then the ^{99m}Tc diphosphonate may still be able to detect the osteolytic lesion by binding the osteoblasts. Other scanning methods may need to be used if osteolytic lesions are suspected. Further scanning should be considered in any patient who presents with pain and a negative bone scan. Although MRI and in some cases FDG-PET scans exhibit greater accuracy and provide earlier detection of these bony lesions, their high cost and limited access currently prevent them from being routine techniques in many settings. As the cost of these diagnostic tests decreases, their routine use will undoubtedly increase. Currently, the cost of MRI is estimated to be two to three times that of a standard bone scan, whereas FDG-PET costs approximately 8 times the cost of a bone scan. CT scans are considered superior to x-rays in defining metastatic lesions; however, they are used less frequently in the search for bone lesions because they are relatively insensitive to intramedullary lesions, and they have the basic disadvantage of limited skeletal coverage.[8]

The treatment of bone metastases is palliative in nature. Generally speaking, systemic therapy, such as hormonal therapy, immunotherapy, antiangiogenesis therapy, or chemotherapy, is started to treat the cancer throughout the body, regardless of its location. In addition, aggressive pain management is a priority. Bisphosphonates are sometimes given in conjunction with standard antineoplastic therapy. Bisphosphonates are known to bind to bone and inhibit osteoclast activity. All bisphosphonates have the general molecular formula shown in Figure 3–3.

R^1 and R^2 differentiate drugs within this class. R^1 determines binding affinity to bone, and R^2 determines the potency of osteoclast inhibition. There are currently three generations of bisphosphonates, and potency has been augmented with each subsequent generation. Pamidronate disodium (Aredia) is a second-generation bisphosphonate and therefore has moderate potency. Zoledronic acid (Zometa) is a third-generation bisphosphonate and is currently the most potent drug FDA approved drug in this class. Pamidronate disodium has been the standard of care for patients with osteolytic lesions from breast cancer and multiple myeloma. However, zoledronic acid has recently emerged as the new standard of care, not only for lesions from breast cancer and multiple myeloma, but also for lesions from all solid tumors. When a bisphosphonate is required, therapy with zoledronic acid should be initiated. Zoledronic acid has shown safety and efficacy equal to or superior than that of pamidronate disodium in every population tested to date.[11] Pamidronate disodium may still be useful in patients who are intolerant of zoledronic acid. Some patients who have experienced worsening renal dysfunction with zoledronic acid may tolerate pamidronate disodium.

Although the exact mechanism is not completely understood, the primary pharmacologic action of zoledronic acid is to function as an osteoclastic bone resorption inhibitor.[17] This blockade of resorption occurs in both bone and cartilage. In vitro studies have shown that zoledronic acid both inhibits the activity of osteoclasts and induces apoptosis of individual osteoclastic cells. In a neoplastic setting, tumors secrete certain chemical signals that in turn stimulate osteoclasts and mobilize the release of skeletal calcium. Zoledronic acid has been shown to impede this process by limiting the capacity of tumor cells to invade and adhere

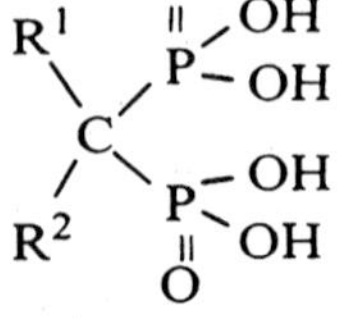

Figure 3–3 **General molecular formula of bisphosphonates.**

to the bone. Zoledronic acid is approved to treat the osteolytic lesions associated with multiple myeloma and for the treatment of documented bone metastases from solid tumors. Given in these settings, it has been shown to slow the progression of pain, decrease the incidence of skeletal-related events (SRE), and delay the onset of SREs. SREs are further described in Box 3–15.[18]

Zoledronic acid should be administered with caution as renal dysfunction may develop or progress to full renal failure requiring dialysis. There have been reports of renal dysfunction after the first dose, but it may occur at any time. Therefore, doses of zoledronic acid should never exceed the maximum recommended dose of 4 mg, and the infusion time should never be less than 15 minutes. Factors that potentially increase the risk for renal dysfunction include baseline renal insufficiency, repetitive cycles of zoledronic acid or other bisphosphonates, dehydration, and use of other nephrotoxic drugs. All patients undergoing therapy with zoledronic acid should have serum creatinine assessment before each infusion. Renal deterioration is defined as follows:

Increase of 0.5 mg/dL for patients with normal baseline serum creatinine

Increase of 1.0 mg/dL for patients with an abnormal baseline serum creatinine

If renal deterioration is observed, drug should be held. If the creatinine level subsequently returns to within 10% of baseline, the patient may be re-challenged with caution and close observation. Patients with mild to moderate renal impairment require reduced doses based on creatinine clearance. Creatinine clearance should be calculated using the Cockcroft-Gault formula as shown below. The following equation will determine the glomerular filtration rate (GFR) or creatinine clearance[19]:

GFR (mL/min) = (140 − age) × weight (kg) × (0.85 for females)/72 × serum creatinine

Table 3–37 shows dosage adjustments for patients with renal insufficiency and the corresponding volume to be used during preparation of drug for infusion.

SUPPORTIVE CARE

Box 3–15 Skeletal-Related Events (SRE)

Pathologic fracture
Spinal cord compression
Radiation therapy to treat bone pain, pathologic fracture, or spinal cord compression
Surgery to bone
A change in antineoplastic therapy for bone pain

Data from Massaro AM. Zoledronic acid: a bisphosphonate for hypercalcemia of malignancy and osteolytic metastases. *Cancer Pract* 2002;10:219–221.

Table 3–37 Dosage Adjustments for Patients with Renal Insufficiency

Baseline Creatinine Clearance (mL/min)	Dose (mg)	Volume (mL)
>60	4.0	5.0
50–60	3.5	4.4
40–49	3.3	4.1
30–39	3.0	3.8

Data from Zometa (zoledronic acid) prescribing information. East Hanover, NJ: Novartis Pharmaceutical Corporation; 2005.

Another significant potential side effect is osteonecrosis of the jaw. Osteonecrosis of the jaw has been reported in patients receiving bisphosphonate therapy, including zoledronic acid.[20] Many of these patients were undergoing treatment for cancer and were concomitantly receiving chemotherapy, radiation therapy, and/or corticosteroid therapy. According to Marx et al.,[21] most incidents of osteonecrosis of the jaw were associated with tooth extraction (37.8%), advanced periodontitis (28.6%), spontaneous development (25.2%), periodontal surgery (11.2%), dental implants (3.4%), and root canal surgery (0.8%). In addition, many of these patients also had evidence of local infection, occasionally progressing to osteomyelitis. Common signs and symptoms include a "heavy jaw" sensation, pain, edema, halitosis resulting from superimposed infection, loose teeth, discharge, and exposed bone, which can be sharp and spiculated. If osteonecrosis is suspected or diagnosed, the patient should be referred to an oral surgeon. Surgical intervention may actually worsen the situation; however, minimal bony debridement may be necessary to remove sharp edges of bone. Intermittent or continuous antibiotic therapy may be of benefit along with 0.12% chlorhexidine gluconate oral rinses. Patients should be encouraged to maintain excellent oral hygiene routines and to immediately report any suspicious symptoms. A complete dental examination is strongly recommended before institution of therapy.[22]

If skeletal pain is a presenting symptom of metastases, aggressive management and a multimodality approach should ensue. Obviously, the use of nonopioid and opioid analgesia along with other accepted pain-relieving mechanisms should be immediately instituted. The new development of skeletal pain is probably an indicator of progressive disease, and thus a change in systemic therapy may be warranted. If a patient is not already receiving bisphosphonate therapy, it should be considered. Pain originating from bone metastases is classified as either biologic pain or mechanical pain. Biologic pain occurs when there is periosteal irritation, pressure from mass effect within the bone, or stimulation of intraosseous nerves by either direct tumor contact or by chemical mediators such as cytokines. Mechanical pain occurs when there is decreased bone strength and increased stiffness. This pain eventually progresses with activity. Initially, most metastatic bone pain is sharp and intermittent in nature and then progresses to a more constant pain. There are four goals that are generally accepted in managing patients with painful bony metastases: pain relief, preservation and restoration of function, skeletal stabilization, and local tumor control.[23]

When pain increases in severity or becomes difficult to control with standard analgesia, radiation therapy should be considered. Uncontrolled pain obviously has a negative and detrimental impact on an individual's quality of life and therefore requires prompt attention and action. External beam radiotherapy is a useful tool for treating locally isolated or clustered lesions. In addition to relieving pain and restoring activity, radiotherapy suppresses local tumor growth. This is especially important in the treatment of an impending pathologic fracture or impending spinal cord compression. Radiation also plays a critical role in the treatment of recognized spinal cord compression and postsurgical repair of pathologic fractures. Gross reduction of the tumor and pain relief can begin almost immediately for radiosensitive tumors, but it should be understood that there is variability in the response curve: 70% of patients will experience some degree of pain relief within 10–14 days, and up to 90% achieve relief within 3 months.[24] Some tumors, such as renal cell carcinomas, are less radiosensitive but may still have at least a partial response to the treatment. A few malignancies, such as germ cell tumor and lymphoma, are exquisitely responsive to chemotherapy. Radiation should be reserved for chemotherapy failures in these patients. It is controversial whether nonpainful solitary bone metastases should be treated. If the lesion is indeed a solitary one, then radiation to this lesion may provide cure. The great unknown, however, is the theoretical possibility of micrometastases, tiny cells or clusters of cells that have metastatic potential and are lying dormant elsewhere in the body waiting for growth factors and other chemical and hormonal mediators to be turned on. Treatment should be guided by individualized decision making.

Palliative radiation for the treatment of bone metastases can be delivered by external beam or via systemic routes. Treatment with external beam radiation begins with a planning stage. Imaging is used to direct the radiation field and to set up blocking of vital organs. Radiation portals are tightly defined to avoid overtreatment and repetitive irradiation. Careful planning also minimizes toxicity. There is great variability and debate over the optimal dosing and fractionation.[23] In some institutions a single dose of 800 cGy is administered, whereas in other institutions 300 cGy is used over the course of 10 days. Responses with both regimens have been similar. High-dose therapy, up to 4000 cGy, has been used in some situations. This dose is usually reserved for patients with potentially longer survival times.

Systemic radiotherapy can also be very effective and should be considered when a patient reports multiple sites of painful bone metastases. Generally, administration of external beam radiotherapy simultaneously to multiple locations or to large portions of the body is considered too toxic. Systemically delivered radiation allows comprehensive coverage of the entire skeleton. The mechanism behind intravenously administered radionuclides includes a radioactive carrier that travels through the circulation and has an affinity for either the tumor or more often the bone matrix. The two most commonly used substances are strontium-89 (^{89}Sr) and samarium-153 (^{153}Sm). ^{89}Sr is the most widely used. It travels to the bone and binds to the calcium component. Areas of bone exhibiting high osteoblastic activity are areas undergoing active calcification and therefore ^{89}Sr is especially useful for treating osteoblastic lesions. As the isotope degrades, short-acting radiation is released into the local environment of the bone. Response rates range from 51%–91%.[23] Patients with prostate cancer, which is a predominantly osteoblastic disease, have an 80% response rate.[23] ^{89}Sr emits only low energy β-particles and is therefore considered safer and better tolerated than higher energy isotopes. It has a half-life of 52.7 days. On the other hand, ^{153}Sm emits both β- and γ-particles and has a half-life of only 1.95 days, thereby delivering higher dose intensity.[14] The significantly shorter half-life allows quicker recovery as well. Re-treatment with ^{153}Sm is typically safe after 8 weeks, whereas retreatment with ^{89}Sr is deemed safe after 12 weeks.

As with any treatment modality, radiopharmaceuticals have potential side effects. Both ^{89}Sr and ^{153}Sm are myelosuppressive. Significantly depressed blood counts have been observed with both agents. All patients should have close monitoring of blood counts, and heavily pretreated patients may require transfusion support. It is generally recommended that neither agent be used simultaneously with standard chemotherapy as both modalities affect the bone marrow and lower blood cell productivity. Studies using ^{153}Sm in combination with radiosensitizing doses of chemotherapy are ongoing.[25] A general guideline is to start or resume standard chemotherapy 4–6 weeks after treatment with ^{153}Sm and 6–8 weeks after treatment with ^{89}Sr or whenever blood counts have recovered adequately. Heavily pretreated patients may have protracted recovery times. Any systemic radionuclide therapy can cause an acute exacerbation of pain. This is generally termed a *flare response* and is noted in approximately 10%–15% of treated patients. The flare typically manifests within 48 hours of initial treatment, and the patient may require additional analgesia.[26]

Table 3–38 **Radiation Source and Corresponding Dose**

Average Dose to U.S. Public	
All sources	360 mrem/yr
Natural sources	300 mrem/yr
Medical uses	53 mrem/yr
Nuclear power plant	<0.1 mrem/yr
Occupational Limit for Radiation Workers	5000 mrem/yr
Radiation Doses	
Chest x-ray	8 mrem
Head/neck x-ray	20 mrem
Head and body CT scan	1100 mrem

Data from Brooke Buddemeier, Lawrence Livermore National Laboratory, 2006.

Many patients raise concerns about radiation exposure. In addition to actual radiation therapy, patients are exposed to radiation through a myriad of medical procedures and diagnostic tests. It has been well documented that radiation is a known carcinogen and mutagen. The reassuring fact, however, is that lower levels of radiation are considered a rather weak carcinogen and mutagen.[27] Although the development of a secondary cancer after exposure to radiation is possible, the path to full-blown cancer is a long and complicated one. When a genetic mutation occurs, the cell can undertake maneuvers to arrest or correct most errors in DNA replication. For those errors that are not corrected, a series of further mutations must occur over the course of 20–40 years before a malignancy is fully developed. In counseling patients, one must weigh the cost-benefit analysis of increased exposure to radioactivity when discussing and deciding on treatment options. This is especially important in young adults and children. Table 3–38 illustrates data on typical radiation exposures.

Pathologic Fractures. As stated earlier, there are two major complications of advancing bone metastases: pathologic fracture and spinal cord compression. A pathologic fracture occurs when a bone undergoes a reduction of its weight-bearing capacity. These fractures do not necessarily occur as a result of a fall or other traumatic event. A metastatic, disease-laden bone may break merely when a patient takes a step, coughs, or rolls over in bed. Destructive osteolytic lesions are the type of metastases most frequently associated with pathologic fractures, although fractures are also noted in osteoblastic disease in which disorganized bone remodeling has reduced the strength of the bone. Therefore, it follows that the majority of pathologic fractures occur in patients with a higher prevalence of osteolytic lesions. Women with breast cancer have the highest incidence of pathologic fractures followed by patients with kidney, lung, and thyroid cancer.[28] Patients with prostate cancer, with its predominantly osteoblastic metastases also have a notable incidence of pathologic fractures.

The initial and most optimal method to treat a pathologic fracture is surgery followed by radiotherapy. Although some fractures might be deemed minor and ordinarily could heal with nonoperative therapy, most orthopedic surgeons usually recommend internal fixation for both major and minor fractures because the presence of tumor and its continued growth at the fracture site will impede and overwhelm the normal healing process. Therefore, the intent of surgery is not to aid in full and complete healing of the fracture; rather, the goal is to provide a mechanism for immediate weight bearing and swift return of function and activity. Prosthetic hardware is routinely used in combination with a stabilization agent that acts as bone glue or cement. Polymethyl methacrylate is frequently used as the stabilization agent. Surgical intervention might be contraindicated in certain clinical situations, e.g., the presence of infection or sepsis, low blood counts, other comorbid conditions, or a preterminal or imminently terminal state. In any of these scenarios, secondary modes of treatment must be considered, including external fixation, casting, bracing, and even amputation.

The diagnosis of an impending pathologic fracture is an area of scientific debate. Multiple studies have been done in an attempt to develop criteria that would provide guidance on risk stratification. The results are largely controversial. Mirels[29] stated two observations: that routine radiographs are typically inadequate to diagnose an impending fracture and that CT scanning is a more accurate diagnostic tool. He also delineated between "pain" and "functional pain," where functional pain is pain that worsens with weight bearing. Increased pain with weight bearing suggested decreased structural integrity. In Mirels' work, the presence of functional pain was the most significant indicator of impending bone fracture. Radiation therapy should be pursued if an impending fracture is suspected. In a patient with continued functional pain after radiation therapy, prophylactic fixation should be considered.

Spinal Cord Compression. The second major complication of advancing bone metastases is spinal cord compression. Metastases frequently migrate from the primary tumor and other metastases and take up residence in the spinal column. The preferred landing zone in the vertebrae is the highly vascularized marrow of the posterior vertebral body. The high number of vertebral metastases is largely attributed to a network of valveless, low-pressure, high-volume vertebral veins called Batson's plexus. This network of veins has direct communication with the pelvic venous plexus, providing an easy and communicable route for the metastases to travel. The most common mechanism of spinal cord compression is the application of pressure by a tumor to the thecal sac surrounding the cord. The source of this pressure may be by indentation, displacement, or partial to complete encasement. There are multiple paths by which a spinal cord compression may develop. Continued tumor growth in the vertebral body obliterates the marrow space and eventually spills over into the epidural space, impinging on the cord. In addition, continued tumor growth leads to bone destruction that may culminate with collapse of the vertebral body. The collapse may displace the cord, and fragments of bone may now be in position to invade the epidural space and thecal sac. The neural foramen is a third path for tumor progression. This route is usually seen in advancing paraspinous masses and from metastatic para-aortic lymph nodes. The epidural and subarachnoid spaces may also be seeded by tumor and compress the cord. The final potential pathway, which is significantly less common, is development of intramedullary spinal cord metastases. This type of metastasis also arrives at the cord through the circulation and grows within the parenchyma of the cord, causing internal compression (see Color Plate 5). Compression to accessory structures such as nerve roots and blood vessels can occur from invasion of tumor through the neural foramen or from associated edema.[30]

In the microenvironment, the most commonly upheld theory used to explain the pathophysiology of spinal cord compression is vascular in nature. Invasion of tumor into the epidural space leads to venous stasis due to compression of the epidural venous plexus. Subsequently, hypoxia develops. Released cytokines and other mediators such as vascular endothelial growth factor (VEGF) and prostaglandin E_2 increase vascular permeability, resulting in an expansion of water content and increased specific gravity of the cord. Increased vascular permeability leads to local edema of the interstitial spaces, which then correspondingly apply

SUPPORTIVE CARE

pressure to the neighboring arterioles, further impeding the flow of blood. Patients may begin to have symptoms of weakness and sensory impairment at this stage. If the compression is not treated, and the event is allowed to further advance, pressure begins to build in the intramedullary arterioles due to the increasing edema. Vascular permeability also results in edema of the cord itself. Simultaneously, the actively growing tumor applies extrinsic, mechanical compression to the cord. The event terminates with arrested capillary blood flow causing local ischemia and ultimately infarction.[31]

The most common location of spinal cord compression is the thoracic spine followed by the lumbar spine and the cervical spine. Pain occurring in combination with any of the following symptoms should raise suspicion for cord compression and warrant further workup: weakness, loss of balance, numbness, paresthesias, paresis, and dysfunction of bowel and/or bladder. Pain may be present for days to months before diagnosis. Pain is universally localized to the site of the compression but may also radiate if nerve roots or the cauda equina is involved. The local pain is usually dull and aching but progressive in nature, whereas the radicular pain is more often sharp and shooting. Pain with thoracic cord compressions is typically described as band-like pressure. Pain with compressions of the lumbar or cervical spine tends to be radicular in nature. Weakness is eventually noticed, and difficulty with balance and motor skills ensues. As ischemia in the cord continues to progress, paresis becomes unavoidable, and there is a complete loss of sensory and motor function below the level of the compression. The speed with which these events transpire can be variable and influence the individual patient's outcome. Work completed by Rades et al.[32] demonstrated that patients experienced more significant improvement of their neurologic functioning after treatment if their neurologic deficits began more than 14 days before treatment versus less than 14 days before treatment. In a separate cohort, only 6% of patients with severe neurologic deficits undergoing treatment within 48 hours experienced meaningful improvement. This work, among other studies, has given rise to the premise that more gradually occurring compressions have a higher likelihood of reversal and recovery.

Spinal cord compression is an oncologic emergency, and prompt treatment is necessary to potentially arrest or reverse paralysis and other neurologic deficits. Any patient with signs and symptoms of acute spinal cord compression or impending spinal cord compression should undergo diagnostic evaluation including a history, a physical examination with a careful, detailed neurologic examination, and radiographic imaging. The history should include the onset, quality, and location of pain as well as a detailed description of other motor or sensory dysfunction. The patient should be asked to point to the site of pain, and then gentle percussion of this area can quickly ascertain the expected location of the compression. Flexor and extensor muscular strength should be tested in the extremities along with appropriate reflexes. Sensory evaluation should include pin prick testing and a rectal examination to assess anal sphincter tone. MRI is the radiographic procedure of choice and should be used routinely to diagnose spinal cord compression. The specificity and sensitivity for MRI are exceptionally high, and the diagnostic accuracy rate is 95%.[33] Multiple sites of impingement do occur, so it is important to image the entire spine. Although spinal cord compression is rarely a fatal development, treatment should be started immediately to prevent or reverse paralysis. Numerous researchers have demonstrated that life expectancy is decreased when a loss of ambulation evolves. Even in a patient with terminal disease, the development of paralysis is a devastating event and should be avoided at all costs.

The cornerstone of spinal cord compression treatment has historically been corticosteroid and radiation therapy. The corticosteroids used include dexamethasone

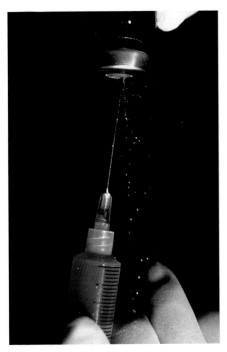

Color Plate 1. Chemotherapy exposure during the preparation of doxorubicin. This illustrates the aerosolization when excessive air pressure is injected into a chemotherapy vial. Copyright mel davis & associates, www.meldavis.com.au.

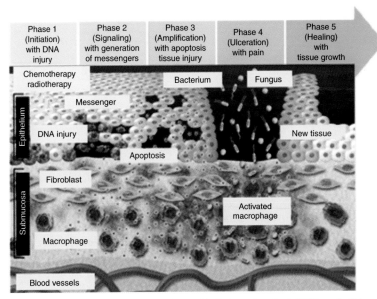

Color Plate 2. Oral mucosa and phases of mucositis. Redrawn from Sonis ST. The pathobiology of mucositis. Nat Rev Cancer. 2004;4:277-284.

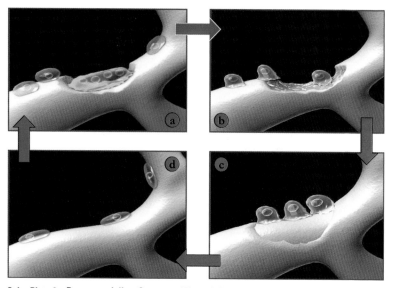

Color Plate 3. **Bone remodeling.** Courtesy of Novartis Pharmaceuticals, Zometa Slide Kit.

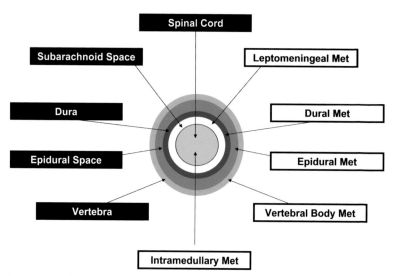

Color Plate 4. **Cross-sectional diagram of vertebral column structures and corresponding metastases.**

and methylprednisolone. At the tissue level, dexamethasone lowers the free water content, reduces prostaglandin E_2 levels, and decreases the specific gravity of the cord. These actions delay the onset of paralysis and begin to improve pain and neurologic deficits while the patient is awaiting further workup and the start of radiotherapy. Surprisingly, no standard schedule, dosing, or tapering guidelines are available. Various researchers have examined high-dose versus low-dose regimens and have found no significant benefit of one over the other in regard to neurologic recovery. Higher doses of steroids do offer the advantage of increased pain control. One conventionally accepted regimen is dexamethasone 10 mg intravenously every 6 hours with the institution of radiation therapy as directed by the radiation oncologist. If there is no neurologic improvement in the first 4–8 hours, the dose should be titrated accordingly. Once a stable dose is achieved, it should be maintained for 48 hours. The dosing should then be changed to 4–8 mg orally every 6 hours and tapered every 3–4 days. If neurologic deterioration is noted after a dose reduction, the prior dose should be resumed until the patient's radiation has progressed further, at which point the taper can resume. Patients without any neurologic dysfunction could be considered for treatment without corticosteroids. More recently, Patchell et al.[34] compared direct decompressive surgical resection followed by radiotherapy with radiotherapy alone. A significantly higher percentage of patients in the surgical arm (84%) were able to walk after treatment than in the radiotherapy alone arm (57%). Of patients who were paralyzed at study entry, significantly more patients in the surgery arm regained their ability to walk (62% versus 19%). In addition, the need for corticosteroids and opioid analgesics was also significantly reduced in the surgical arm. Therefore, a new standard of care will likely emerge, favoring decompressive surgical resection followed by radiation.

The presentation, management, and treatment of spinal cord compression in children differ from those in adults. In children, motor weakness routinely accompanies pain, and the incidence of motor weakness has been reported to be as high as 82%–100%. Most tumors causing spinal cord compression in children invade the spinal column through the neuroforaminal opening. In addition to applying pressure to the cord, compression is also applied to the nerve roots. These tumors are traditionally characterized as "dumbbell tumors" on MRI reports owing to their characteristic shape. Childhood cancers most frequently associated with spinal cord compression include neuroblastoma, Ewing's sarcoma, Wilms' tumor, lymphoma, and soft tissue and bone sarcomas. Unlike adult malignancies, these tumor types tend to be very chemosensitive and, therefore, chemotherapy is frequently used as the treatment of choice. Chemotherapy allows children to avoid the potential hazards of spinal surgery and lowers the potential risk for future secondary cancers that could be caused by radiation exposure. As with the adult population, however, surgical intervention does play a role, especially in patients in whom severe neurologic deficits are observed. In the realm of soft tissue and bone sarcomas, surgical intervention via laminotomy or laminectomy followed by chemotherapy or radiation provided significantly greater ambulatory outcomes over chemotherapy or radiation alone.[35]

For responsible decision making in the overall management of metastatic bone pain, pathologic fracture, and spinal cord compression, the patient's estimated life expectancy must be acknowledged as patients with these disorders frequently have advanced cancer. Patients with a prolonged life expectancy should be offered aggressive treatment. For patients with very limited life expectancy or for those who are in imminent danger of dying, travel back and forth to the hospital for radiation treatments or surgical intervention may do more harm than good. In this situation, titrating doses of narcotic pain medications administered and managed through a professional hospice organization may be more optimal and will provide comfort and care for the patient to palliate symptoms. The conventional guideline is that patients should undergo surgical intervention for pathologic fractures of weight-bearing bones if their life expectancy is greater than 1 month. For non–weight-bearing bones, surgery should generally be pursued if the patient's life expectancy is greater than 3 months. Of course, these statements are only guidelines, and all decision-making should include the wishes of the patient.

Hypercalcemia

Patients with cancer may also be confronted with metabolic problems associated with the bone. The most common metabolic disorder is hypercalcemia of malignancy. Although the incidence in adults is only 10%–20%, it is a potentially fatal occurrence and is categorized as an oncologic emergency requiring prompt attention and treatment.[36] Hypercalcemia can also develop in children, but at the much lower rate of 0.5%–1%.[37] Certain cancers have a higher predilection for development of hypercalcemia. The highest incidence occurs in non–small cell lung cancer and breast cancer. It is reported at an intermediate level for multiple myeloma, head and neck cancer, kidney cancer, and the lymphomas and leukemias and is relatively uncommon in colon, prostate, and small cell lung cancer.[38]

Hypercalcemia can occur in both a malignant and nonmalignant form. Causes of nonmalignant hypercalcemia are mentioned here solely to assist with the differential diagnosis, but the remainder of this discussion will focus on hypercalcemia of malignancy (Box 3–16).[39]

Hypercalcemia of malignancy is primarily a direct result of accelerated osteoclastic bone resorption. As the abnormal resorption of bone proceeds, increasing amounts of calcium are mobilized and move into the bloodstream. This accelerated

---

Box 3–16 Potential Causes of Nonmalignant Hypercalcemia

Endocrine and Metabolic Diseases
Primary hyperparathyroidism
Hyperthyroidism
Pheochromocytoma
Osteopetrosis
Infantile hyperphosphatasia
Familial hypercalcemia

Infectious Diseases
Tuberculosis
Coccidioidomycosis
HIV

Renal Insufficiency

Granulomatous Disease
Sarcoidosis
Berylliosis

Dietary and Drug-Related
Vitamin D intoxication
Vitamin A intoxication
Overuse of calcium supplements
Lithium therapy
Milk-alkali syndrome

Data from Warrell RP. Metabolic emergencies. In De Vita, VT Jr, Hellman S, Rosenberg SA, eds. *Cancer: Principles and Practice of Oncology.* Philadelphia, PA: Lippincott Williams & Wilkins; 2001:2633–2645.

state develops in response to multiple biochemical factors released or activated by the neoplastic cells. Patients with hypercalcemia of malignancy traditionally present with symptoms and characteristics of parathyroid hormone (PTH) overstimulation. It had historically been theorized that malignant tumors were an ectopic source of PTH. However, Simpson et al.[40] debunked this theory by demonstrating the absence of PTH mRNA in nonparathyroid tumors. A few years later, a substance termed *parathyroid hormone-related peptide (PTHrP)* was purified.[41] This novel protein had biologic properties very similar to those of PTH, shared several homologous amino acids with PTH, and bound to PTH receptors. Currently, PTHrP is accepted as the most common mediator of hypercalcemia of malignancy.

PTHrP is known to be normally distributed throughout the body. It has been isolated in tissues such as the brain, kidneys, parathyroid gland, skin, atria, uterus, and breast. The current understanding of this protein is that it appears to play a role in calcium transport and developmental biology. It normally functions in the local environment and is not released into the general circulation. Patients with malignant solid tumors have been found to have elevated circulating blood levels of PTHrP.[42] These increased levels are especially evident in patients with squamous cell carcinomas. PTHrP is directly produced by malignant cells. As was discussed earlier, Mundy[10] stated that PTHrP down-regulates OPG and stimulated osteoblasts to release RANKL. RANKL activates osteoclast precursors to fully functional osteoclasts. The osteoclasts then embark upon active bone resorption. Bone-derived growth factors are subsequently released, which then return to the tumor cell surface, signaling it to continue production of PTHrP. As the osteoclasts continue to cause the release of excessive amounts of calcium into the bloodstream, a cascade of events will ensue. Patients initially become symptomatic with gastrointestinal symptoms and polyuria. A state of progressive dehydration develops, and the glomerular filtration rate decreases. This, in turn, leads to increased renal resorption of calcium, setting up a vicious cycle of worsening hypercalcemia.

In addition to PTHrP, other less frequently occurring factors are related to hypercalcemia of malignancy. These are evidenced by the fact that elevated serum levels of PTHrP are only noted in 30%–50% of hypercalcemic breast cancer patients.[43] In addition, the majority of hypercalcemic patients with hematologic cancers, such as multiple myeloma and lymphoma, have not demonstrated significantly elevated levels of PTHrP. Other factors involved in the development of a hypercalcemic state have not been well characterized. Factors of interest that potentially play a role and may warrant further research include vitamin D_3, the prostaglandins, numerous cytokines including interleukin-6 and -1, tumor necrosis factor, and tumor-derived hematopoietic colony-stimulating factors.[39]

Hypercalcemia of malignancy is defined as a serum calcium level of 11 mg/dL or greater (or 1–1.6 mg/dL above the upper limit of normal for the given laboratory). One must be aware, however, that the total serum calcium level may not accurately reflect the true severity of hypercalcemia, if a low serum albumin level is also present. Serum calcium has a high affinity for albumin, and therefore the serum calcium level can fluctuate significantly with increases and decreases in the level of serum albumin. Ideally, the optimal method of detecting and diagnosing hypercalcemia of malignancy is to follow ionized calcium levels. Frequently, however, this test is not commonly or rapidly available in most institutions. Indeed, the concept of following ionized calcium is itself controversial as some experts purport that it provides no advantage over total calcium except in research applications. Alternatively, a more prevalent practice is to calculate the corrected serum calcium level when hypoalbuminemia is observed. Several equations have been developed to calculate the corrected calcium level. The units used to measure

SUPPORTIVE CARE

calcium levels globally include mg/dL, mEq/L, or mmol/L. Most U.S. laboratories use the standardized units of mg/dL. A commonly used equation that gives the corrected calcium in mg/dL is the modified Orell equation[44,45]:

Corrected calcium (mg/dL) = serum calcium (mg/dL) + 0.8 [4 − serum albumin (g/dL)]

Example 1: Cancer patient with serum calcium = 10.7 mg/dL and serum albumin = 2.1 g/dL

Corrected calcium = 10.7 + 0.8 (4 − 2.1)

Corrected calcium = 12.22 mg/dL

The above calculation is accepted as being relatively accurate except for use in patients with multiple myeloma with evidence of elevated serum paraproteins. In these patients, measuring the ionized calcium concentration may be necessary.

Symptoms of hypercalcemia of malignancy (Table 3–39) are variable and depend largely on how abruptly the situation develops. At one extreme, a patient with only a mild to moderately elevated serum calcium level may present in an obtunded state if the increase was sudden and acute. At the other extreme, patients with chronic hypercalcemia, such as that seen with parathyroid carcinoma, may have quite high calcium levels with relatively few symptoms. The most frequently reported symptoms are fatigue, lethargy, polyuria, constipation, and nausea. All of these symptoms are relatively nonspecific, but an evaluation of the serum calcium and albumin levels is recommended, as polyuria and nausea, which may progress to vomiting, lead to rapid dehydration that exacerbates the hypercalcemia.

Treatment of the underlying malignant disease serves as prophylaxis for the prevention of hypercalcemia of malignancy, but when this maneuver fails, further therapy is necessary. Optimal management is to reduce the serum calcium level by decreasing bone resorption. Patients with hypercalcemia are frequently dehydrated. Prior recommendations for the treatment of hypercalcemia included very vigorous hydration. Fluid replacement should be used, but only to restore euvolemia, because excessive overhydration may cause fluid overload. In addition, fluid replacement alone is rarely sufficient to correct the hypercalcemia. In theory, the loop diuretic furosemide increases urinary calcium excretion, but there has been no evidence to date to prove a benefit for its routine use in this clinical setting, and it may lead to further dehydration. The use of furosemide should be limited to balancing fluid intake and output in fully rehydrated patients. Thiazide diuretics increase renal calcium absorption and their use is therefore contraindicated. Use of drugs that inhibit renal blood flow such as nonsteroidal anti-inflammatory drugs and histamine H_2-receptor antagonists is discouraged. Furthermore, supplementation with calcium, vitamin D, vitamin A, and other retinoids should be discontinued. A low calcium diet is recommended.[39]

Mild hypercalcemia (corrected calcium level less than 12 mg/dL) that is asymptomatic and expected to respond to antineoplastic therapy may require only

Table 3–39 Clinical Manifestations of Hypercalcemia of Malignancy

Constitutional	Fatigue, dehydration, anorexia, weight loss, pruritus, polydipsia
Cardiac	Bradycardia, prolonged P-R interval, shortened Q-T interval, wide T wave, arrhythmias
Gastrointestinal	Nausea, vomiting, constipation, obstipation, ileus
Genitourinary	Polyuria, renal insufficiency
Neuromuscular	Lethargy, muscle weakness, hyporeflexia, confusion, agitation, psychosis, seizure, obtundation, coma

Data from Warrell RP. Metabolic emergencies. In De Vita VT Jr, Hellman S, Rosenberg SA, eds. *Cancer: principles and Practice of Oncology.* Philadelphia, PA: Lippincott Williams & Wilkins; 2001:2633–2645.

fluid replacement and close observation. Patients who are symptomatic or those who may have a slow or questionable response to cancer therapy should undergo treatment for hypercalcemia and ancillary treatment for the associated symptoms. Many clinicians today opt to treat hypercalcemia early on with bisphosphonates. As discussed earlier, bisphosphonates function as osteoclast inhibitors and therefore decrease bone resorption. Zoledronic acid has again emerged as the bisphosphonate drug of choice for the treatment of hypercalcemia of malignancy.[46] The maximum recommended dose for the treatment of hypercalcemia of malignancy is 4 mg intravenously over at least 15 minutes. Repeat dosing should occur no more frequently than every 7 days if the calcium level has not adequately returned and remained in the normal range. Moderate to severe hypercalcemia (corrected calcium level equal to or greater than 12 mg/dL) should automatically be treated with fluid replacement first, quickly followed by zoledronic acid. A corrected calcium level of greater than 15 mg/dL may evoke coma and cardiac arrest and warrants immediate attention and care. Adequate hydration should always be maintained before every dose of zoledronic acid, and renal function should be carefully monitored. Deterioration of renal function should be fully evaluated before subsequent infusions, and dose adjustments may be necessary (Table 3–37). Calcium, phosphorus, and magnesium levels should also be monitored. Pamidronate should be used as second-line therapy for patients intolerant of zoledronic acid. The maximum recommended dose for the treatment of moderate hypercalcemia of malignancy (corrected calcium level of 12–13.5 mg/dL) is 60–90 mg administered intravenously over 2–24 hours. The maximum recommended dose for severe hypercalcemia of malignancy (corrected calcium of level greater than 13.5 mg/dL) is 90 mg intravenously over 2–24 hours. Although the 2-hour infusion time is acceptable, longer infusion times may diminish the risk for renal toxicity. If a patient has baseline renal insufficiency, a prolonged infusion time should be considered.

Other agents approved for the treatment of hypercalcemia of malignancy include gallium nitrate, calcitonin, oral phosphorus, plicamycin, and corticosteroids. Gallium nitrate functions as a potent bone resorption inhibitor.[47] Its disadvantages include nephrotoxicity and a prolonged infusion time: 100–200 mg/m^2 per day infused over 24 hours for up to 5 days. Patients usually require hospitalization for the infusion and for monitoring, as the calcium-lowering effect continues even after the drug is stopped. Conversely, the hypocalcemic effect of calcitonin is rather weak with only a 30% response rate.[48] Because of its low response rate, calcitonin is not recommended for use as a single agent or for routine use in combination with bisphosphonates for the treatment of mild to moderate hypercalcemia. The use of calcitonin is most advantageous in the setting of acute severe hypercalcemia in combination with a bisphosphonate. Calcitonin has a rapid onset of action of 1–4 hours and can therefore quickly begin lowering serum calcium levels in these critically ill patients. The onset of action of the bisphosphonates is approximately 24–48 hours. Calcitonin should definitely be used in combination with bisphosphonates as its effect peaks at around 48 hours and then diminishes despite continued administration.[48] Although corticosteroids have historically been used in combination with calcitonin, Warrell et al.[48] demonstrated a lack of benefit in patients whose baseline cancer was not responsive to steroid therapy. Corticosteroids, plicamycin, and oral phosphorus all have response rates in the 5%–30% range.[39] These agents are significantly inferior to zoledronic acid and are not recommended for routine front-line use.

Supportive care for both the patient and family should be undertaken. The development of hypercalcemia of malignancy has a significant impact on the patient's quality of life, is potentially life-threatening, and is an overall poor prognostic indicator. Prompt recognition and treatment are crucial. Guidelines for the management of hypercalcemia of malignancy are listed in Box 3–17.

More recent work has shown new promise for the treatment of hypercalcemia of malignancy. The protein RANKL is known to be secreted by osteoblasts and activates osteoclast precursors into fully mature osteoclasts. It is also known that OPG is an inhibitor of RANKL. Morony et al.[49] demonstrated that infusions of OPG into two hypercalcemic mouse models inhibited RANKL and resulted in a more rapid reversal of hypercalcemia than did zoledronic acid or pamidronate. It was also shown that the rapidity and duration of the RANKL suppression were significantly higher in the OPG group than in either the pamidronate or zoledronic acid group and that OPG caused a greater reduction of other markers of bone resorption than the bisphosphonates. It was observed, however, that eventually hypercalcemia returned despite ongoing RANKL suppression by OPG. The authors theorized that the use of bisphosphonate therapy (such as zoledronic acid) in combination with RANKL inhibition therapy (such as OPG) may be a rational approach to treating hypercalcemia of malignancy and warrants further investigation.

Box 3–17 Hypercalcemia of Malignancy Management Guidelines

Correct dehydration with 0.9% normal saline IV
Manage fluid status with furosemide 20–40 mg IV every 12 hours PRN
Monitor intake and output
Monitor closely for fluid overload
Initiate bisphosphonate therapy
1. Zoledronic acid 4 mg IV over 15 minutes (see Table 3–37 for renal dosing)
2. Pamidronate 60–90 mg IV over 2–24 hours (if intolerant of zoledronic acid)
3. Gallium nitrate 100–200 mg/m² per day continuous IV up to 5 days (if intolerant of bisphosphonates)
For acute severe hypercalcemia
1. Calcitonin 2–8 units/kg subcutaneously or IM every 6–12 hours in combination with bisphosphonate
Follow laboratory values
1. Calcium, magnesium, phosphorus
2. Albumin
3. Blood urea nitrogen and creatinine
4. Electrolytes
5. Digoxin level if applicable
6. Consider parathyroid hormone to rule out coexisting hyperparathyroidism
Baseline electrocardiogram and consider telemetry
Discontinue thiazide diuretics, nonsteroidal anti-inflammatory drugs, histamine H₂-receptor antagonists
Discontinue calcium, vitamin D, vitamin A
Order low calcium diet
Antiemetics for nausea and vomiting
Management of mental status changes
1. Protect from injury
2. Mini Mental Status Exam
3. Haloperidol 0.5–5 mg IV 2–4 times PRN daily for agitation or confusion
4. Lorazepam 0.5–2 mg IV every 4–6 hours PRN for sedation
Standard bowel regimen for constipation
Maintain mobility if possible
Ongoing pain management
Provide patient and family support, education, and counseling
1. Disease state and symptoms
2. Emotional and psychosocial support
3. Treatment goals
4. Discharge planning

IV, intravenous; PRN, as needed; IM, intramuscular.

Table 3–40 **Level of Care Guidelines**

Outpatient	Inpatient
Serum calcium <12 mg/dL	Serum calcium ≥12 mg/dL
No significant nausea	Nausea or vomiting
Able to ingest fluids	Dehydration
Fatigue	Altered mental status
Normal renal function	Renal insufficiency
Stable cardiac rhythm	Cardiac arrhythmia
Mild constipation	Obstipation or ileus
Available supervision	Lives alone
Access to health care	Limited access to health care

Data from Warrell RP. Metabolic emergencies. In De Vita VT Jr, Hellman S, Rosenberg SA, eds. *Cancer: principles and practice of oncology.* Philadelphia, PA: Lippincott Williams & Wilkins; 2001:2633–2645.

The decision on whether to treat hypercalcemia on an inpatient or outpatient basis is dependent on the patient's symptoms, the value of the corrected calcium level, the patient's social situation, and the speed of evolution of the clinical picture. For example, a patient with a slowly rising calcium level may experience a sudden increase with the onset of emesis. A decision that should also be considered in very advanced clinical situations is not to treat the hypercalcemia. If a patient has no further options for the treatment of his or her cancer or has chosen not to undergo any further therapy, providing supportive care through hospice may be the treatment of choice. Untreated hypercalcemia progresses to painless loss of consciousness, coma, cardiac arrest, and death. This clinical course may be preferable to some patients, especially those who have no other treatment options for their cancer and may be suffering from prolonged intractable pain and other difficult to control symptoms of their cancer. The criteria listed in Table 3–40 can be used as a guide for decision making.[39]

Osteoporosis

The final topic to be discussed briefly in this chapter is osteoporosis. Osteoporosis is characterized as a condition with both decreased bone mass and decreased bone density. Abnormal spaces develop in the bone, producing a porous environment that leads to bone fragility and increased risk of fractures even with minimal stress or trauma. During this reduction of bone mass, equal losses of both the mineral component and the organic matrix are seen. Because there is a net decrease in the amount of bone, it follows that bone resorption is occurring at a faster rate than bone formation. In other words, the activity of the osteoclasts outweighs the activity of the osteoblasts.

The prevalence of osteoporosis is significant. According to the National Osteoporosis Foundation,[50] 10 million people in the United States are affected by osteoporosis, of which 8 million (80%) are women and the remaining 2 million (20%) are men. Furthermore, an additional 34 million people are estimated to have decreased bone mass (osteopenia) and are at risk of developing osteoporosis. The list of potential risk factors for osteoporosis is long and multifactorial. The more commonly occurring risk factors are summarized in Box 3–18.

It has been well documented that certain therapies used in the treatment of cancer result in unintended bone loss and treatment-related osteoporosis. In both men and women, the hypothalamic-pituitary-gonadal axis plays an important role in regulating hormonal balance and thus maintaining normal bone metabolism. Manipulation of the hypothalamic-pituitary-gonadal axis is an avenue for treating certain cancers such as prostate and breast cancer. For men with prostate cancer, who have not been cured

---

Box 3–18 Risk Factors for Osteoporosis

Advancing age
Female sex
Estrogen deficiency in women
   1. Naturally occurring menopause
   2. Surgically induced menopause
   3. Medically induced menopause
Testosterone deficiency in men
   1. Naturally occurring with age
   2. Orchiectomy (surgical castration)
   3. Medically induced castration
Osteopenia
Fracture after age 50
Family history of osteoporosis
   1. Higher risk with fracture history in primary relative
Low lifetime calcium intake/deficiency
Vitamin D deficiency
Thin body habitus or small skeletal structure
Physical inactivity
Tobacco and alcohol use
Certain chronic medical conditions
Certain medications (i.e., corticosteroids, chemotherapy, and others)
Caucasian and Asian more than African American and Hispanic

Data from National Osteoporosis Foundation. About osteoporosis: fast facts. Available at www.nof.org/osteoporosis/diseasefacts.htm. Accessed December 7, 2006.

---

with either primary surgery or radiation therapy, the cornerstone of therapy is lifelong androgen suppression. This is accomplished with luteinizing hormone-releasing hormone (LHRH) agonists, frequently in combination with anti-androgens. LHRH agonists stop testosterone production from the testicles by interrupting the production of luteinizing hormone at the level of the hypothalamus. For women with breast cancer, hormonal manipulation is also often the treatment of choice. LHRH agonists are used in women to purposely suppress ovarian function and stop production of estrogen from the ovaries. A common mode of therapy in breast cancer is selective estrogen replacement modulators (SERMS), such as raloxifene and tamoxifen. SERMS are hormonal treatments that are protective to the bone and have been shown to increase bone mineral density. The aromatase inhibitors anastrozole, letrozole, and exemestane are another group of hormonal agents used in the treatment of breast cancer. These agents have been shown to cause bone loss. The aromatase inhibitors are only recommended in women who have already gone through menopause.[51]

Surgical resection of the gonads is another starting point in the development of osteoporosis. Bilateral orchiectomy results in complete testosterone ablation of the testicles. This is a desired effect in a patient with prostate cancer but places the patient at future risk for osteoporosis. Patients with testicular cancer usually require only unilateral orchiectomy. Typically, the remaining testicle produces sufficient testosterone to prevent osteoporosis. It is possible, but less common, for a patient to have bilateral disease requiring bilateral orchiectomy. These patients are at risk for the development of osteoporosis. The normal presence of testosterone has not been linked to testicular cancer progression and is not contraindicated. The risk of osteoporosis can be significantly decreased in these patients by initiating testosterone replacement therapy. Obviously, women who have undergone surgical resection of the ovaries undergo abrupt menopause and are thus at increased risk of developing osteoporosis. Estrogen replacement therapy is usually contraindicated in these women. Although primary pituitary cancer is not common, surgical resection of this important gland would have a profound systemic effect on the entire endocrine system and bone metabolism.

Cytotoxic chemotherapy plays a role in the development of osteoporosis as well. Chemotherapy may induce premature ovarian failure and concomitant estrogen deficiency. CMF (cyclophosphamide, methotrexate, and fluorouracil) therapy, for example, has a higher likelihood of permanently shutting down the ovaries than do doxorubicin-containing regimens. Radiation directly aimed at the gonads or ineffectively blocked gonads during radiation treatment increases a patient's risk of osteoporosis owing to the damage sustained to the gonadal tissue, which results in a reduction or cessation of hormonal production. Radiation treatment to bones causes osteonecrosis and reduces the overall numbers and function of osteoblasts. The use of glucocorticoids can independently result in treatment-related osteoporosis.[52]

Osteoporosis is clinically diagnosed with bone mineral density (BMD) testing. Although multiple techniques have been developed to measure BMD, the one used most frequently is dual-energy x-ray absorptiometry (DEXA), which measures the density of bone centrally in the spine, hip, or total body. Peripheral DEXA (pDEXA) measures the density of the wrist, heel, or finger. Most experts believe that pDEXA is not adequate to diagnose osteoporosis in the axial skeleton, where bone loss is more likely to occur and is potentially more debilitating.[50] pDEXA is also considered unsuitable to measure response to treatment. The most common use of pDEXA is as a screening tool at a health fair, for example. To prevent interference of contrast dye, most hospitals and treatment centers recommend that DEXA scans be performed before or 5 days after the following diagnostic tests: barium swallow, upper gastrointestinal tract series, small bowel series, barium enema, intravenous pyelogram, and CT scans using oral and/or intravenous contrast material. A more accurate test of BMD is the quantitative computed tomography (QCT) scan. Although considered more accurate than DEXA, the instrument used to perform this type of scan is not available in most institutions. Furthermore, the World Health Organization (WHO) has developed standardized criteria for interpreting the DEXA scan[50a] (Table 3–41), and, at present, there are no accepted standardized criteria for interpreting the QCT scan. It is important to recognize that the WHO criteria were developed for Caucasian women. The same criteria are extrapolated for use in men and non-Caucasian women, but no studies have been done to verify accuracy. The BMD is statistically compared to two norms: "young normal" and "age-matched." The young normal comparison is called the T-score. The T-score is the difference between the measured BMD and the mean BMD of a young adult. The T-score is referred to as a standard deviation (SD) above or below the mean. This number shows the amount of bone present compared with that of a young adult of the same gender with peak bone mass. The

SUPPORTIVE CARE

Table 3–41 WHO Criteria for DEXA Scan Interpretation in Women*

Normal	T-score > -1 SD below the young adult mean
Osteopenia	T-score -1 to -2.5 SD below the young adult mean
Osteoporosis	T-score < -2.5 SD below the young adult mean
Established osteoporosis	T-score < -2.5 SD below the young adult mean with a history of one or more fractures

*Values extrapolated for interpreting BMD results in males and non-Caucasian females.
Data from National Osteoporosis Foundation. About osteoporosis: fast facts. Available at www.nof.org/osteoporosis/diseasefacts.htm. Accessed December 7, 2006.

age-matched comparison is the Z-score. This number reflects the amount of bone present in other people of similar age, size, and gender. The T-score is the value used for diagnosis.[50]

An alternative method to view and understand the WHO criteria is to map out the t-score on a number line schematic diagram (Figure 3–4), where (x) designates osteoporosis, (*) indicates osteopenia, and (#) represents normal BMD. The number (0) represents the young normal mean.

The most significant complication of osteoporosis is fracture. The National Osteoporosis Foundation[50] estimates that one in two women and one in four men older than age 50 will have an osteoporosis-related fracture in his or her remaining lifetime. Sites of frequently occurring fracture are the hip, spine, wrist, and ribs, but by far the most common fracture site is the spine. Vertebral fractures result in severe back pain, loss of height, and spinal deformities such as kyphosis or stooped posture. The rate of hip fractures in women is two to three times higher than that in men; however, the 1-year mortality rate is nearly twice as high for men.[50] Generally speaking, the risk of fracture doubles for every SD below the young adult mean. For example, if a woman's T-score is −2 SD, she has a 4 times greater risk of fracture than her young adult counterpart.

As with most medical conditions, prevention is the key. Most women have reached their maximal skeletal mass at approximately age 20, whereas men usually continue to build bone mass until around age 30. The best defense against osteoporosis is to build strong bones during childhood and adolescence and then maintain them into adulthood. Consuming a balanced diet with adequate amounts of calcium and vitamin D, along with weight-bearing exercise, is the optimal method of building and maintaining bones. In addition to the other well-recognized adverse effects of cigarette smoking, it has also been shown to have detrimental effects on bone mass.[53]

When cancer therapy is expected to increase the risk of osteoporosis or induce osteoporosis, additional therapy is warranted. Fortunately, medications are now available to slow down or arrest bone loss and in some cases to even help to restore bone density. It is generally recommended that individuals perform weight-bearing exercises and start or continue calcium and vitamin D supplementation, although the efficacy of these modalities has come under scrutiny more recently.

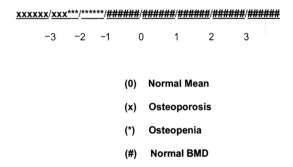

T-score of −2.1 = BMD 2.1 SD below young normal mean = osteopenia

xxxxxx/xxx***/******/#####/#####/#####/#####/#####

    −3   −2   −1   0   1   2   3

(0)   **Normal Mean**

(x)   **Osteoporosis**

(*)   **Osteopenia**

(#)   **Normal BMD**

Figure 3–4 Number line schematic diagram for interpreting BMD results.

Table 3–42 **Bisphosphonate Dosing for the Treatment of Osteoporosis**

Generic Name	Trade Name	Dose
Alendronate	Fosamax	5–10 mg PO daily or 70 mg PO weekly
Risedronate	Actonel	5 mg PO daily or 35 mg PO weekly
Ibandronate	Boniva	2.5 mg PO daily or 150 PO mg monthly
Zoledronic acid	Zometa	Proposed dosing pending FDA approval: 4 mg IV every 3 months

PO, oral; IV, intravenous; FDA, U.S. Food and Drug Administration.
Data from Actonel (risedronate). Available at http://www.actonel.com/prescribinginformation.jsp; Boniva (ibandronate) prescribing information. Nutley, NJ: Roche Therapeutics Inc.; 2005; Fosamax (alendronate) prescribing information. Whitehouse Station, NJ: Merck & Co., Inc.; 2000; Zometa (zoledronic acid) prescribing information. East Hanover, NJ: Novartis Pharmaceuticals Corporation; 2005.

Several drugs within the bisphosphonate family are useful in the treatment of osteoporosis. They have been shown to slow down osteoclastic activity and reduce fracture rates. Alendronate, ibandronate, and risedronate are all approved for the treatment of osteoporosis in women. Only alendronate is approved for use in men. Although pamidronate and zoledronic acid are not currently approved for the treatment of osteoporosis, both are used to protect the bones in other clinical situations as previously described. Trials have been completed demonstrating the efficacy of zoledronic acid in increasing BMD in the hip and spine during androgen deprivation therapy for nonmetastatic prostate cancer.[54] As of the writing of this chapter, the U.S. Food and Drug Administration is considering approval of zoledronic acid for the treatment of osteoporosis. Table 3–42 illustrates dosing guidelines for treatment of osteoporosis.

To prevent side effects, it is recommended that patients take all oral bisphosphonate preparations with a full glass of water (not seltzer) 30 minutes (60 minutes for ibandronate) before eating. In addition, patients should remain in an upright position for at least 30 minutes after ingesting the drug to minimize the risk for esophageal irritation. Once bisphosphonate therapy is discontinued, gradual bone loss will resume. Other side effects are similar to those described earlier for bisphosphonates.[55–58]

Hormone replacement therapy (HRT) in women has been shown to reduce bone loss and increase bone density; however, long-term use of HRT has been shown to increase the risk of breast cancer. HRT is contraindicated in patients who already have breast cancer. As stated earlier, SERMS (tamoxifen and raloxifene) do possess activity in treating osteoporosis, but they are less effective than the bisphosphonates.

SUPPORTIVE CARE

CONCLUSION

The bones play a very important role in the health and well-being of patients with cancer. Knowledge pertaining to the mechanism of bone disease and its subsequent treatment is imperative to adequately support and care for these patients. In addition, it assists care providers in helping patients achieve what all patients desire and strive for: an enhanced quality of life and dignity in both life and death.

REFERENCES

1. Rhoades R., Pflanzer R. Calcium, phosphate, and bone metabolism. In Rhoades R, Pflanzer R, eds. *Human Physiology*. Fort Worth, TX: Saunders College Publishing; 1992:910–935.
2. Prockop DJ, Ala-Kokko L. Inherited disorders of connective tissue. In Kasper DL, Braunwald E, Fauci AS, et al., eds. *Harrison's Principles of Internal Medicine*. New York, NY: McGraw-Hill; 2005: 2324–2331.
3. Holick MF, Krane SM, Potts JT Jr. Calcium, phosphorus, and bone metabolism: calcium-regulating hormones. In Fauci AS, Braunwald E, Isselbacher KJ, eds. *Harrison's Principles of Internal Medicine*. New York, NY: McGraw-Hill; 1998:2214–2227.

4. Peavy DE. Calcium, phosphate, and bone metabolism. In Rhoades R, Pflanzer R, eds. *Human Physiology*. Fort Worth, TX: Saunders College Publishing; 1992:910–935.

5. Roodman GD. Mechanisms of bone metastasis. *N Engl J Med* 2004;350:1655–1664.

6. Theriault RL. Pathophysiology of cancer treatment-induced bone loss. Symposium conducted at The Evolving Role of Bisphosphonates for Cancer Treatment-Induced Bone Loss Meeting, Chicago, IL; May 2003.

7. American Cancer Society. Cancer Facts & Figures 2005. Available at www.cancer.org/docroot/MED/content/MED_1_1_Most-Requested_Graphs_and_Figures_2005.asp. Accessed December 7, 2006.

8. Peh WCG, Muttarak M. Bone metastases. Available at www.emedicine.com/radio/topic88.htm. Retrieved December 7, 2006.

9. Stetler-Stevenson WG, Kleiner DE Jr. Molecular biology of cancer: invasion and metastases. In DeVita VT Jr, Hellman S, Rosenberg SA, eds. *Cancer: Principles and Practice of Oncology*. Philadelphia, PA: Lippincott Williams & Wilkins; 2001:123–136.

10. Mundy GR. Metastasis to bone: causes, consequences, and therapeutic opportunities. *Nat Rev Cancer* 2002;2:584–593.

11. Rosen L, Harland SJ, Oosterlinck W. Broad clinical activity of zoledronic acid in osteolytic to osteoblastic bone lesions in patients with a broad range of solid tumors. *Am J Clin Oncol* 2002;25(6 Suppl 1):19–24.

12. Schaberg J, Gainor BJ. A profile of metastatic carcinoma of the spine. *Spine* 1985;10:19–20.

13. Galasko, CS, Sylvester BS Back pain in patients treated for malignant tumors. *Clin Oncol* 1978;4:273–283.

14. Emsley, J. The elements. Oxford: Clarendon Press; 1989:184-185.

15. Conte FA, Bushberg JT. Essential science of nuclear medicine. In Brant WE, Helms, CA, eds. *Fundamentals of Diagnostic Radiology*. Baltimore, MD: Williams & Wilkins; 1994:1134–1151.

16. Pollne JJ, Witztum KF, Ashburn WL. The flare phenomenon of radionuclide bone scan in metastatic prostate cancer. *AJR Am J Roentgenol* 1984;142:773–776.

17. Sahni M, Guenther HL, Fleisch H, et al. Bisphosphonates act on rat bone resorption through the mediation of osteoblasts. *J Clin Invest* 1993;91:2004–2011.

18. Massaro AM. Zoledronic acid: a bisphosphonate for hypercalcemia of malignancy and osteolytic metastases. *Cancer Pract* 2002;10:219–221.

19. Cockcroft D, Gault M. Prediction of creatinine clearance from serum creatinine. *Nephron* 1976; 16:31–41.

20. Marx RE. Pamidronate (Aredia) and zoledronate (Zometa) induced avascular necrosis of the jaws: a growing epidemic. *J Oral Maxillofac Surg* 2003;61:1115–1117.

21. Marx RE, Sawatari Y, Fortin M, Broumand V. Bisphosphonate-induced exposed bone (osteonecrosis/osteopetrosis) of the jaws: risk factors, recognition, prevention, and treatment. *J Oral Maxillofac Surg* 2005;63:1567–1575.

22. Damato K, Gralow J, Hoff A, et al. *Expert Panel Recommendations for the Prevention, Diagnosis, and Treatment of Osteonecrosis of the Jaws* (ONC-9551); 2004.

23. Brown HK, Healey JH. Metastatic cancer to the bone. In DeVita VT Jr, Hellman S, Rosenberg SA, eds. *Cancer: Principles and Practice of Oncology*. Philadelphia, PA: Lippincott Williams & Wilkins; 2001:123–136.

24. Allen KL, Johnson TW, Hibbs GG. Effective bone palliation as related to various treatment regimens. *Cancer* 1976:37:984–987.

25. Widmark A, Modig H, Johansson M, et al. TAXSAM: a new chemo-radiation regimen for bone metastases in hormone refractory prostate cancer. Presented at the Prostate Cancer Symposium; 2006: Abstract 221.

26. Housten SJ, Rubens RD. The systemic treatment of bone metastases. *Clin Orthop Relat Res* 1995;312:95–104.

27. Buddemeier B. Understanding radiation and its effects. (Publ. No. UCRL-PRES-149818-REV-2). Available at www.nuc.berkeley.edu/news/Sci_teachers_workshop/understanding_radiation.ppt. Retrieved February 26, 2006.

28. Higinbotham NL, Marcove RC. The management of pathological fractures. *J Trauma* 1965;5:792–798.

29. Mirels H. Metastatic disease in long bones: a proposed scoring system for diagnosing impending pathologic fractures. *Clin Orthop Relat Res* 1989;249:256–264.

30. Byrne TN. Spinal cord compression from epidural metastases. *N Engl J Med* 1992;327:614–619.

31. Fuller BG, Heiss JD, Oldfield EH. In DeVita VT Jr, Hellman S, Rosenberg SA, eds. *Cancer: Principles and Practice of Oncology*. Philadelphia, PA: Lippincott Williams & Wilkins; 2001:2617–2633

32. Rades D, Blach M, Nerreter V, et al. Metastatic spinal cord compression: influence of time between onset of motoric deficits and start of irradiation on therapeutic effect. *Strahlenther Onkol* 1999;175:378–381.

33. Li KC, Poon PY. Sensitivity and specificity of MRI in detecting malignant spinal cord compression and in distinguishing malignant from benign compression fractures in vertebrae. *Magn Reson Imaging* 1988;6:547–556.

34. Patchell RA, Tibbs BA, Regine WF, et al. Direct decompressive surgical resection in the treatment of spinal cord compression caused by metastatic cancer: a randomized trial. *Lancet* 2005:366:643-648.

35. Klein SL, Sanford RA, Muhlbauer MS. Pediatric spinal epidural metastases. *J Neurosurg* 1991;74: 70–75.
36. Bilezikian JP. Management of acute hypercalcemia. *N Engl J Med* 1992;326:1196–1203.
37. Kerdudo C, Aerts I, Fattet S, et al. Hypercalcemia and childhood cancer: a 7-year experience. *J Pediatr Hematol Oncol* 2005;27:23–27.
38. Vassilopoulou-Sellin R, Newman B, Taylor SH, Guinee VF. Incidence of hypercalcemia in patients with malignancy referred to a comprehensive cancer center. *Cancer* 1993;71:1309–1312.
39. Warrell RP. Metabolic emergencies. In De Vita, VT Jr, Hellman S, Rosenberg SA, eds. *Cancer: Principles and Practice of Oncology*. Philadelphia, PA: Lippincott Williams & Wilkins; 2001:2633–2645.
40. Simpson EL, Mundy GR, D'Souza SM, et al. Absence of parathyroid hormone messenger RNA in nonparathyroid tumors associated with hypercalcemia. *N Engl J Med* 1983;309:325–330.
41. Moseley JM, Kubota M, Diefenbach-Jagger J, et al. Parathyroid hormone-related protein purified from a human lung cancer cell line. *Proc Natl Acad Sci* 1987;84:5048–5052.
42. Rankin W, Grill V, Martin TJ. Parathyroid hormone-related protein and hypercalcemia. *Cancer* 1997;80(8 Suppl):1564–1571.
43. Bucht E, Rong H, Pernow Y, et al. Parathyroid hormone-related protein in patients with primary breast cancer and eucalcemia. *Cancer Res* 1998;58:4113–4116.
44. Orell DH. Albumin as an aid to the interpretation of serum calcium. *Clin Chim Acta* 1971;35:483–489.
45. Endres DB, Rude RK. Mineral and bone metabolism. In Burtis CA, Ashwood ER, eds. *Tietz Textbook of Clinical Chemistry*. Philadelphia, PA: WB Saunders; 1999:1395–1406.
46. Major P, Lortholary A, Hon J, et al. Zoledronic acid is superior to pamidronate in the treatment of hypercalcemia of malignancy: a pooled analysis of two randomized, controlled clinical trials. *J Clin Oncol* 2001;19:558–567.
47. Hall TJ, Chambers TJ. Gallium inhibits bone resorption by a direct effect on osteoclasts. *J Bone Miner Res* 1990;8:211–216.
48. Warrell RP, Jar IR, Frisone M, et al. Gallium nitrate for acute treatment of cancer-related hypercalcemia; a randomized, double-blind comparison to calcitonin. *Ann Intern Med* 1988;108:669–674.
49. Morony S, Warmington K, Adamu S, et al. The inhibition of RANKL causes greater suppression of bone resorption and hypercalcemia compared with bisphosphonates in two models of humoral hypercalcemia of malignancy. *Endocrinology* 2005;146:3235–3243.
50. National Osteoporosis Foundation. About osteoporosis: fast facts. Available at www.nof.org/osteoporosis/diseasefacts.htm. Accessed March 6, 2006.
50a. WHO Study Group. Assessment of fracture risk and its application to screening for postmenopausal osteoporosis. WHO Technical Report. Series no. 843. Geneva: WHO 1994:1-129.
51. Lester J, Dodwell D, McCloskey E, Coleman R. The causes and treatment of bone loss associated with carcinoma of the breast. *Cancer Treat Rev* 2005;31:115–142.
52. Kendall PH. Steroid osteoporosis. *Proc R Soc Med* 1960;53:206–207.
53. Hannan MT, Felson DT, Dawson-Hughes B, et al. Risk factors for longitudinal bone loss in elderly men and women: the Framingham osteoporosis study. *J Bone Miner Res* 2000;15:710–720.
54. Smith JR, Eastham J, Gleason DM, et al. Randomized controlled trial of zoledronic acid to prevent bone loss in men receiving androgen deprivation therapy for nonmetastatic prostate cancer. *J Urol* 2005;169: 2008–2012.
55. Actonel (risedronate) prescribing information. Procter & Gamble Pharmaceuticals. Available at www.actonel.com/global/Actonel_PIL.pdf.jsp.
56. Boniva (ibandronate) prescribing information. Nutley, NJ: Roche Therapeutics Inc.; 2005.
57. Fosamax (alendronate) prescribing information. Whitehouse Station, NJ: Merck & Co., Inc.; 2000.
58. Zometa (zoledronic acid) prescribing information. East Hanover, NJ: Novartis Pharmaceuticals Corporation; 2005.

SUPPORTIVE CARE

Chapter 6
Management and Treatment of Cancer Pain
Patrick T. Wong

Pain is one of the most common and most feared symptoms of cancer. More than 9 million patients worldwide experience cancer pain. Estimates of cancer patients experiencing pain vary widely, from 14% to 100%.[1] It has been stated that about half of terminally ill patients experience pain during their last 48 hours of life.[2] The World Health Organization estimated that 25% of cancer patients die with unrelieved pain.[3]

PATHOPHYSIOLOGY AND TERMINOLOGY OF PAIN
Cancer pain is complex and can be defined by several physiologic processes. Pain normally results when noxious stimuli activate nociceptors that begin pain transmission. Transmission of this signal is carried by various nerve fibers and transmitted to the central nervous system in the dorsal horn of the spinal cord by numerous interacting neurotransmitters. This signal is ultimately received in the brain and perceived as pain.[4,5]

These pain signals are modulated via many pathways. Endogenous opioid neurotransmitters (e.g., enkephalins and endorphins) activate receptors (e.g., μ, δ, and κ) that can mitigate the perception of pain. Receptors, such as N-methyl-D-aspartate (NMDA) receptors, can diminish the responsiveness of μ receptors. Inflammation causes the release of cytokines such as prostaglandins that enhance certain pain transmission. There are many other neurotransmitters and cytokines that affect this system. Abnormalities and malfunctions of this process can lead to spontaneous or inappropriate transmission of pain.[2,4,5] Terminology associated with pain is listed in Table 3–41.

DIAGNOSIS AND EVALUATION OF CANCER PAIN
Diagnosis and assessment of cancer pain are critical for identifying both physical and psychological factors that might affect a patient's pain intensity, quality, character, and response to treatment. Successful treatment of a patient's cancer can often provide both rapid and long-lasting pain relief and may even prevent further complications such as bone fractures or spinal cord compression. Understanding the underlying cause of pain can often lead to treatment tailored to that specific condition. For example, pain requiring physical therapy, pain from infectious causes, and pain from autoimmune diseases all can have unique assessments and therapies. Pain from mucositis can be approached with local therapies (refer to Unit 3, Chapter 3) and bone pain from metastases can be treated with bisphosphonates.[6]

A thorough workup of cancer pain should be performed and should include a pain history, pain rating score, review of cancer extent and current disease status, diagnostic tests if necessary, and medication history.[7] Most patients report more than one site of pain. Thus, a physical examination along with a pain history is important. In addition, a careful history of prior analgesic interventions must be included in the pain workup. Validated pain questionnaires such as the Brief Pain Inventory and McGill Pain Questionnaire that can help to fully assess pain and can track progress are available.[8] At minimum, the five factors of pain (PQRST)[5] should be assessed:

Table 3–41 Pain Terminology

Pain Terminology	Comments
Acute pain	Sudden onset that declines over a short amount of time; quickly resolves after stimulus is treated, healed, or removed
Allodynia	Condition in which non-noxious stimuli produce pain
Chronic pain	Pain that can range from mild to severe and persists or progresses over a long period of time
Hyperalgesia	More potent and prolonged painful response to the same stimuli
Neuropathic pain	From abnormal processing of sensory inputs
Nociception	Transmission of noxious stimuli that produces the sensation of pain
Somatic pain	From skin, bone, joint, muscle, or connective tissue; its location is usually distinct
Visceral pain	From internal organs; location and character can be difficult to define or referred as originating from another location

Data from Baumann TJ. Pain management. In Dipiro JT, Talbert RL, Yee GC, et al., eds. *Pharmacotherapy: A Pathophysiologic Approach*, 6th ed. New York: McGraw-Hill; 2005; Miaskowski C, Cleary J, Burney R, et al. *Guideline for the Management of Cancer Pain in Adults and Children*. APS Clinical Practice Guideline Series, No. 3. Glenview, IL: American Pain Society; National Comprehensive Cancer Network, Inc. Adult Cancer Pain V.2.2005. Available at: www.nccn.org/professionals/physician_gls/PDF/pain.pdf. Accessed December 8, 2006; and *NCI Thesaurus*. Available at: http://nciterms.nci.nih.gov/NCIBrowser/Dictionary.do. Accessed December 8, 2006.

P: palliative/provocative factors—What makes pain better/worse?

Q: quality—What is the character of the pain?

R: region—Where is the pain located and what is the pattern of pain radiation?

S: severity/intensity—What is the severity/intensity on a pain rating scales?

T: temporal—What happens to the pain over time, how long does it last, and what is the maximum intensity, frequency, and daily variation?

A quick and common way to monitor patients with pain is with a numerical rating scale. Patients are asked to rate their pain on a 0–10 scale, with 0 meaning that the patient has no pain and 10 meaning that the patient is experiencing the worst possible pain. Pain, as a whole, has been considered under-assessed, and regulatory agencies such as the Joint Commission on Accreditation of Healthcare Organizations require pain assessments appropriate to the individual's condition. Thus, cancer patients should have a pain assessment at every encounter.[9]

TREATMENT GUIDELINES AND PHARMACOLOGIC MANAGEMENT OF CANCER PAIN

Treatment guidelines have been developed to standardize care for patients with cancer pain. The World Health Organization developed a pain "ladder" or algorithm for the treatment of cancer pain, which is based on a stepwise approach of analgesic potency (Figure 3–5). Step 1 pain (lowest pain level) should be treated with nonopioids such as acetaminophen or nonsteroidal anti-inflammatory drugs (NSAIDs). For step 2 pain (moderate levels of pain), mildly potent opioids, such as codeine, are incorporated. Lastly, step 3 pain (severe pain) is managed with the most potent opioids, such as morphine and its analogs (e.g., oxycodone and methadone). Therapy can begin at any step, depending on the patient's clinical condition. Coanalgesics, also known as adjuvants, can also be used at any step to lessen pain.[10]

Other organizations such as the American Pain Society and the National Comprehensive Cancer Network have sought to improve cancer pain care. Their guidelines offer sophisticated algorithms based on a patient's pain intensity, depending on a numerical rating scale score to recommend specific doses of opioids for oral or intravenous administration. For example, patients reporting a pain score of 7–10 would be considered to have a "pain emergency" and would immediately be treated

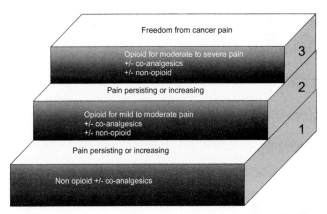

Figure 3–5 WHO pain ladder. (From World Health Organization. Cancer pain relief: with a guide to opioid availability, 2nd ed. Geneva, 1996. Available at: http://libdoc.who.int/publications/9241544821.pdf. Accessed December 8, 2006.)

with potent opioids on the basis of a different algorithm than patients reporting a pain score of 5–6. These guidelines also offer comprehensive assessment and management strategies beyond pharmacologic treatments.[3,11]

Treatment must be tailored to the particular patient on the basis of a careful comprehensive pain assessment. However, ultimately treatment will commonly be administered around-the-clock because cancer pain often has a chronic component. It is important to understand the duration of the effect of the analgesic used to develop a rational interval for the around-the-clock administration. Long-acting analgesics that need to be administered no more frequently than two to three times a day are desired to provide convenience to the patient and improve compliance. A short-acting analgesic should always be provided as needed for breakthrough pain. Pain in the majority of cancer patients will not be adequately treated with only short-acting analgesics. The frequent use of short-acting analgesics (e.g., more than three doses per day) means that the long-acting analgesic dose may need to be increased.[3,12,13]

Opioid Analgesics
Cancer pain is commonly treated with opioids that are full agonists (Table 3–42). Other drug classes such as acetaminophen, NSAIDs, and mixed and partial opioid agonists have a ceiling effect to their analgesia. This means that after a certain threshold, increasing the dose will only increase side effects without improving analgesia. Full agonist opioids will generally continue to provide more analgesia with escalating doses.[4]

There are many factors in the selection of an opioid. Opioids differ from one another in terms of relative potency, pharmacokinetics, pharmacodynamics, side effect profiles, cost, and formulation availability.

All opioids share varying degrees of common side effects. These include respiratory depression, somnolence, constipation, hypotension, nausea, histamine reactions, urinary retention, delirium, and the potential for dependence. Patients develop tolerance to these side effects at different times and at different degrees. Respiratory depression is usually the first side effect patients develop tolerance to, and many patients never develop tolerance to the constipation caused by opioids.[3,13,14]

Table 3–42 Selected* Oral Full Agonist Opioids

Generic Name	Brand Name	Formulation	Strengths	Comments	Schedule
APAP/codeine	Tylenol with Codeine #3	Tablet	300 mg/30 mg	Immediate release (BTP)	C-III
	Tylenol with Codeine #4	Tablet	300 mg/60 mg		C-III
	Capital and Codeine	Suspension	120 mg/ 12 mg/5 mL		C-V
APAP/ hydrocodone	Norco	Tablet	325 mg/5 mg 325 mg/7.5 mg 325 mg/10 mg	Immediate release (BTP)	C-III
	Vicodin, Lortab	Tablet	500 mg/5 mg		
	Vicodin ES, Lortab	Tablet	500 mg/7.5 mg		
	Lortab Elixer	Elixer	500 mg/7.5 mg/ 15 mL		
APAP/ oxycodone	Percocet, Endocet	Tablet	325 mg/2.5 mg 325 mg/5 mg 325 mg/7.5 mg 325 mg/10 mg	Immediate release (BTP)	C-II
	Roxicet	Liquid	325 mg/5 mg/ 5 mL		
Codeine		Tablet	30 mg 60 mg	Immediate release (BTP)	C-II
Fentanyl	Actiq	Oral Transmucosal Unit Dose (Lollipop)	200 mcg 400 mcg 600 mcg 800 mcg 1200 mcg 1600 mcg	Immediate release (BTP); only for highly opioid tolerant; second unit can be used 15 minutes after first unit finished if still in pain	C-II
	Duragesic	Patch	12.5 mcg/hr 25 mcg/hr 50 mcg/hr 75 mcg/hr 100 mcg/hr	Apply new patch every 72 hours	
Hydromor- phone	Dilaudid	Tablet	2 mg 4 mg 8 mg	Immediate release (BTP)	C-II
	Dilaudid	Liquid	1 mg/1 mL		
	Dilaudid	Suppository	3 mg		
Levorphanol	Levo- Dromoran	Tablet	2 mg	Long half-life, dosed 3–4 times/day	C-II
Meperidine	Demerol	Tablet	50 mg 100 mg	Immediate release (BTP); risk of seizures with renal impairment	C-II
		Liquid	50 mg/5 mL		
Methadone		Tablet	5 mg 10 mg	All formulations are immediate release with long half-life; treat as if sustained release; some local laws may restrict once daily dosing for drug detoxification programs; for cancer pain dose 2-3 times/day	C-II
		Tablet dispers- able	40 mg		
		Suspension	1 mg/1 mL 2 mg/1 mL 10 mg/1 mL		

Table 3–42 Selected* Oral Full Agonist Opioids—cont'd

Generic Name	Brand Name	Formulation	Strengths	Comments	Schedule
Morphine	MSIR	Tablet	15 mg 30 mg	Immediate release (BTP)	C-II
	RMS	Suppository	5 mg 10 mg 20 mg 30 mg	Immediate release (BTP)	
	Avinza	Tablet	30 mg 60 mg 90 mg 120 mg	Dosed once daily; alcohol use interferes with control release mechanism and can lead to life-threatening overdose	
	Kadian	Tablet	20 mg 30 mg 50 mg 60 mg 100 mg	Dosed 2 times/day	
	MS Contin	Tablet	15 mg 30 mg 60 mg 100 mg 200 mg	Dosed 2 times/day	
	Oramorph	Tablet	15 mg 30 mg 60 mg 100 mg	Dosed 2 times/day	
	Roxanol	Suspension	2 mg/1 mL 4 mg/1 mL 20 mg/1 mL	Immediate release (BTP)	
Oxycodone	OxyIR, Roxicodone	Tablet	5 mg	Immediate release (BTP)	C-II
	Roxicodone	Tablet	15 mg 30 mg		
	OxyContin	Tablet	10 mg 20 mg 40 mg 80 mg 160 mg	Dosed 2 times/day	
	OxyFast, Roxicodone	Liquid	1 mg/1 mL 20 mg/1 mL	Immediate release (BTP)	

BTP, should be used as needed for breakthrough pain.
*Other combinations, strengths, formulations may exist.
Data from U.S. Department of Health and Human Services, Food and Drug Administration. *Approved Drug Products with Therapeutic Equivalence Evaluations,* 26th ed. Available at: www.fda.gov/cder/orange/obannual.pdf. Accessed December 8, 2006; and Title 21 Volume 9 Code of Federal Regulations (CFR) section 1308; last revised April 1, 2006. Available at: www.gpoaccess.gov/cfr/index.html. Accessed December 8, 2006.

SUPPORTIVE CARE

Many patients report allergies to opioids, but true immunoglobulin E–mediated (IgE-mediated) hypersensitivity reactions are rare. All opioids have the potential to cause histamine release that can manifest as a pruritic rash, which often responds to antihistamines. Opioids with relatively low potency such as morphine tend to cause this reaction more commonly than more potent opioids such as fentanyl. If a patient is suspected of having a true allergy to one opioid, it is prudent to rechallenge with an opioid from a different chemical class if necessary.[3,5] Chemical classes of some widely used opioids are as follows:

Phenanthrene derivatives: codeine, hydrocodone, hydromorphone, morphine, oxycodone

Phenylpiperidine derivatives: fentanyl, meperidine

Diphenylheptane derivative: methadone

Some opioids have unique side effects. Meperidine has a high potential to cause seizures in patients with renal insufficiency because of the accumulation of the toxic metabolite normeperidine. For this reason, this drug should not routinely be used for treatment of chronic pain.[3] Intravenous methadone has a potential to prolong the QT interval and may not be a good option for patients treated for cardiac arrhythmias.[15]

Naloxone can be used in emergencies to reverse the effects of opioids when necessary. Be aware that large boluses, such as 2 mg, will completely reverse analgesia and may precipitate immediate withdrawal. For opioid-induced respiratory depression in patients with cancer pain, the American Pain Society suggests beginning naloxone at 0.02 mg intravenously every 2 minutes and titrating to the minimal dose to reverse respiratory depression while not completely reversing analgesia. Repeat doses will be needed because of the relatively short duration of action of naloxone (about 20 minutes), especially in patients who took long-acting opioids.[3]

Constipation is an adverse effect that is frequently undertreated. Opioid receptors are found in the gastrointestinal (GI) tract and work to slow peristalsis. Constipation from opioids can lead to ileus or treatment failure from patients who stop taking their opioids to avoid this side effect. All patients receiving chronic doses of opioids should be given stimulant laxatives prophylactically to maintain normal bowel function (Table 3–43). A common mistake is to only give stool softeners or fiber, which alone will usually not be adequate to treat opioid-induced constipation. Some patients and clinicians fear serious adverse effects or dependence with chronic laxative use; however, clinical evidence does not suggest that chronic use of laxatives poses significant health risks.[16]

Some patients may benefit from orally administered naloxone if conventional laxatives fail.[17,18] However, there is a risk of systemic reversal of analgesia and opioid withdrawal from orally administered naloxone.[19] Drugs currently under development, such as alvimopan, are designed to counter the effects of opioids on peristalsis while minimizing analgesic antagonism.[20]

Patients may need to change from one opioid to another, which is also known as "rotating opioids," for a variety of reasons including intolerable side effects, cost of medications, and route restrictions. Because there is incomplete cross-tolerance between opioids, some clinicians rotate opioids for a better response. However, there is also incomplete cross-tolerance to the side effects, and patients should be closely monitored for respiratory depression and sedation when their opioid treatment is being rotated. Equianalgesic tables such as the one shown in Table 3–44 have been developed to approximate the dose of an opioid to provide analgesia similar to that of another.

Equianalgesic tables are largely based on single-dose studies in the postoperative setting and do not account for incomplete cross-tolerance or accumulation from chronic dosing. Also, equianalgesic ratios are not always bidirectional. For example, studies suggest use of a higher ratio when morphine is converted to hydromorphone than when hydromorphone is converted to morphine.[21] Furthermore, decreased hepatic or renal function can affect the dosing of opiates. For example, reduced hepatic function will reduce conversion of hydrocodone to its more active metabolites, and renal insufficiency will cause accumulation of morphine metabolites and increase the

Table 3–43 Bowel Regimen Medications

Generic Name	Brand Name Examples	Usual Adult Starting Dose	Formulations and Strengths	Comments
Docusate	Colace, D-S-S	50–500 mg/day PO in 1–4 divided doses	Capsule: 50 mg 100 mg, 240 mg, 250 mg Liquid: 150 mg/15 mL; 60 mg/15 mL	Stool softener; will not stimulate peristalsis; should not be lone agent for opioid bowel regimen
Senna (Sennosides)	Senokot, Ex-Lax	~15 mg sennosides/day PO in 1–2 divided doses	Tablet: 8.6 mg (Senokot); 15 mg (Ex-Lax) Syrup: 8.6 mg/5 mL; 33.3 mg/1 mL	
Bisacodyl	Dulcolax	5–10 mg/day PO/PR	Tablet: 5 mg Suppository: 10 mg Enema: 10 mg/30 mL	Must swallow tablets whole (do not cut, crush, or chew)
Lactulose	Enulose, Kristalose	10–20 g/day PO in 1–2 divided doses	Syrup: 10 gm/15 mL Crystal packets for reconstitution: 10 g, 20 g	Crystals for reconstitution more costly but less sweet tasting
Polyethylene glycol 3350	MiraLax, Glycolax	17 g/day PO dissolved in 8 oz water	Powder for reconstitution: 255 g, 527 g Powder packet for reconstitution: 17 g	
Magnesium citrate		120–240 mL PO once with 8 oz water	Liquid: 290 mg/5 mL	Caution: may result in life-threatening electrolyte abnormalities
Naloxone	Narcan	Doses vary in case studies/case series; given PO and PR	Must be compounded	Variable oral absorption; may precipitate opioid withdrawal

PO, orally; PR, insert rectally.
Data from Baumann TJ. Pain management. In Dipiro JT, Talbert RL, Yee GC, et al., eds. *Pharmacotherapy: A Pathophysiologic Approach.* 6th ed. New York: McGraw-Hill; 2005: Chap.; U.S. Department of Health and Human Services, Food and Drug Administration. *Approved Drug Products with Therapeutic Equivalence Evaluations,* 26th ed. Available at: www.fda.gov/cder/orange/obannual.pdf. Accessed December 8, 2006; Miaskowski C, Cleary J, Burney R, et al. *Guideline for the Management of Cancer Pain in Adults and Children.* APS Clinical Practice Guideline Series, No. 3. Glenview, IL: American Pain Society; 2005; Maheswaran AM, ed. *Mosby's Drug Consult,* 16th ed. St. Louis, MO: Mosby; 2006; and O'Mahony S, Coyle N, Payne R. Current management of opioid-related side effects. *Oncology (Williston Park)* 2001;15:61–73, 77.

Table 3–44 Equianalgesic Table*

Medication	PO Equianalgesic Dose	IV Equianalgesic Dose
Codeine	200 mg	130 mg
Fentanyl (patch; see specific fentanyl patch chart)	Actiq; titrate from starting doses based on manufacturer's recommendations	0.1 mg (100 mcg)
Hydrocodone	30 mg	N/A
Hydromorphone	7.5 mg	1.5 mg
Meperidine	300 mg	75 mg
Methadone	See specific methadone chart	
Morphine	30 mg	10 mg
Oxycodone	20 mg	N/A

IV, intravenous; PO, oral.

*Equianalgesic ratios are usually derived from single-dose studies; refer to text.

Data from Anderson R, Saiers JH, Abram S, et al. Accuracy in equianalgesic dosing. conversion dilemmas. *J Pain Symptom Manage* 2001;21:397–406; Baumann TJ. Pain management. In Dipiro JT, Talbert RL, Yee GC, et al., eds. *Pharmacotherapy: A Pathophysiologic Approach*, 6th ed. New York: McGraw-Hill; 2005: Chap. 58; Miaskowski C, Cleary J, Burney R, et al. *Guideline for the Management of Cancer Pain in Adults and Children*. APS Clinical Practice Guideline Series, No. 3. Glenview, IL: American Pain Society; 2005; National Comprehensive Cancer Network, Inc. Adult Cancer Pain V.2.2005. Available at: www.nccn.org/professionals/physician_gls/PDF/pain.pdf. Accessed December 8, 2006; and Pereira J, Lawlor P, Vigano A, et al. Equianalgesic dose ratios for opioids. a critical review and proposals for long-term dosing. *J Pain Symptom Manage* 2001;22:672–687.

Table 3–45 Conservative Fentanyl Equianalgesic Table

Oral Morphine Daily Dose Equivalent (mg/day)	Fentanyl Patch Dose (mcg/hr)
60–134	25
135–224	50
225–314	75
315–404	100

From Duragesic (fentanyl) package insert. Titusville, NJ: Janssen Pharmaceutica; 2005.

side effects of morphine.[22] These tables also do not take into account pharmacokinetic and pharmacodynamic variability such as onset and duration of analgesia. For example, intravenous fentanyl has an immediate onset of action and a duration of analgesia of 30–60 minutes compared with immediate-release oral morphine, which has an onset of about 60 minutes and duration of analgesia of about 4 hours.

Recommendations for converting from a long-acting opioid to a fentanyl patch vary widely. The U.S. Food and Drug Administration–approved labeling suggests a conservative approach as is seen in Table 3–45. Others convert every 50 mg of morphine equivalent per day to a 25 mcg/hr patch. However, a more aggressive equianalgesic table for fentanyl patches has been developed and had been approved for labeling in Germany (Table 3–46). Fentanyl patches are designed to last 72 hours. The patch strength, but not the frequency, should be increased if patients require frequent breakthrough pain medication throughout the dosing interval. However, some patients will require changing fentanyl patches every 48 hours if there is a significant increase in use of breakthrough pain medications at the end of a dosing interval.[12]

Methadone is a long-acting opioid that is gaining favor and acceptance as a front-line opioid for cancer pain. Its property of NMDA inhibition may improve its analgesic efficacy, especially for neuropathic pain. In addition, methadone is considerably less expensive than other opioid analgesics. However, dosing titration of methadone is difficult because its initial analgesic duration is considerably shorter than its pharmacokinetic half-life. Furthermore, drugs that induce or

Table 3–46 **Aggressive Fentanyl Equianalgesic Table**

Oral Morphine Daily Dose Equivalent (mg/day)	Fentanyl Patch Dose (mcg/hr)
0–90	25
91–150	50
151–210	75
211–270	100

From Skaer TL. Practice guidelines for transdermal opioids in malignant pain. *Drugs* 2004;64:2629 (Table III).

Table 3–47 **Methadone Equianalgesic Table (Use When Converting to Methadone)**

Oral Morphine Daily Dose Equivalent (mg/day)	Oral Morphine : Oral Methadone Ratio
<30	2:1
30–89	4:1
90–299	8:1
300–599	12:1
600–999	15:1
≥1000	17:1

Data from Anderson R, Saiers JH, Abram S, et al. Accuracy in equianalgesic dosing. conversion dilemmas. *J Pain Symptom Manage* 2001;21:397–406; Manfredi PL, Houde RW. Prescribing methadone, a unique analgesic. *J Support Oncol* 2003;1:216–220; and Pereira J, Lawlor P, Vigano A, et al. Equianalgesic dose ratios for opioids. a critical review and proposals for long-term dosing. *J Pain Symptom Manage* 2001;22:672–687.

inhibit hepatic cytochrome P450 isoenzymes may also affect this half-life. Patients can be easily given an inappropriately high dose of methadone, which may not be evident until the patient's body has accumulated the drug for several days. Methadone also has a dose-dependent ratio of equianalgesia to other opioids. Patients whose condition is stable with high doses of opioids require relatively lower doses of methadone than a simple equianalgesic table may calculate. Table 3–47 may be used as a guideline for determining starting doses when changing from other opioids to methadone. This table should not be used when converting methadone to other opioids.[21–23]

Many patients are fearful of the addiction potential of opioid analgesics. Some effective agents, such as methadone, may be associated with the stigma of maintenance therapy for narcotic abuse. Patients may exhibit aberrant drug-seeking behavior when instead they are being inadequately treated for pain or having withdrawal symptoms from opioid dependence, also referred to as pseudoaddiction. Patients should be reassured of the differences between addiction, which is a neurobiologic disease, and physical dependence, which is a physiologic process that requires careful tapering of opioids.[24]

Nonsteroidal Anti-inflammatory Drugs

NSAIDs have been a mainstay for mild to moderate pain and effective for pain due to inflammation, such as bone pain from metastases (Table 3–48). However, most NSAIDs have the unattractive side effect profile of increasing the chances for gastrointestinal bleeding, a reduction in renal function, and diminished platelet function. These side effects are a direct result of the main mechanism of action of NSAIDs, which is the inhibition of cyclooxygenase (COX), which leads to the reduction of proinflammatory prostaglandins. These prostaglandins also are involved in maintaining a protective barrier from acid in the GI mucosa and providing adequate renal blood flow. COX-1 isoenzyme is thought to be the primary isoenzyme involved in producing prostaglandins with these beneficial processes, whereas COX-2 is implicated with painful inflammation.[25]

SUPPORTIVE CARE

Table 3-48 Nonsteroidal Anti-Inflammatory Drugs

Medication	Brand Name	Strengths/Forms Available	Usual Starting Doses	Comments
Celecoxib	Celebrex	Capsules: 100 mg, 200 mg, 400 mg	200 mg 2 times/day PRN	Also used to prevent formation of colonic polyps in familial adenomatous polyposis; questionable cardiovascular safety.
Diclofenac	Cataflam, Voltaren	Immediate release: 50 mg Delayed release: 25 mg, 50 mg, 75 mg Extended release: 100 mg	100–150 mg/day in divided doses	
Diclofenac + Misoprostol	Arthrotec	Capsules: 50 mg + 200 mcg; 75 mg + 200 mcg	Low dose capsule: 2–4 capsules/day in divided doses High dose capsule: 1 capsule 2 times/day	Pregnancy Category X
Diflunisal	Dolobid	Tablets: 250 mg, 500 mg	500–1500 mg/day in 2–3 divided doses	
Etodolac	Lodine	Immediate release capsules: 200 mg, 300 mg Immediate release tablets: 400 mg, 500 mg Extended release tablets: 400 mg, 500 mg, 600 mg	200–1000 mg/day in divided doses	Maximum daily dose = 1000 mg
Fenoprofen	Nalfon	Capsules: 200 mg, 300 mg Tablets: 600 mg	200 mg every 4–6 hours as needed	Maximum daily dose = 3200 mg
Flurbiprofen	Ansaid	Tablets: 50 mg, 100 mg	100 mg 2 times/day	Maximum daily dose = 300 mg
Ibuprofen	Motrin, Advil	Chewable tablets: 50 mg, 100 mg Tablets: 200 mg, 400 mg, 600 mg, 800 mg Suspension 100 mg/5 mL, 40 mg/1 mL	200–400 mg every 6 hours as needed	Maximum daily dose = 3200 mg (OTC max dose = 1200 mg)
Indomethacin	Indocin	Capsules: 25 mg, 50 mg Sustained release capsules: 75 mg Suspension: 25 mg/5 mL	50–150 mg/day in divided doses	Maximum daily dose = 200 mg IV formulation for patent ductus arteriosus in neonates, not for pain management
Ketoprofen	Oruvail	Capsule: 50 mg, 75 mg Extended release capsule: 100 mg, 150 mg, 200 mg	25–50 mg every 6 hours as needed	Maximum daily dose = 300 mg

Drug	Brand	Dosage forms	Dose	Maximum
Ketorolac	Toradol	Injection solution: 15 mg/1 mL, 30 mg/1 mL, 60 mg/2 mL, 300 mg/10 mL; Tablets: 10 mg	60 mg IM as single dose or 30 mg IV as single dose or 30 mg IV every 6 hours; can continue as oral therapy 10 mg every 4–6 hours as needed	Maximum daily dose = 120 mg IV, 40 mg PO; Maximum duration of total (IV + PO) therapy = 5 days/course
Mefenamic acid	Ponstel	Capsules: 250 mg	500 mg × 1 dose then 250 mg every 6 hours as needed	
Meloxicam	Mobic	Tablets: 7.5 mg, 15 mg; Suspension: 7.5 mg/5 mL	7.5 mg/day	Maximum daily dose = 15 mg
Nabumetone	Relafen	Tablets: 500 mg, 750 mg	1000 mg/day in divided doses	Maximum daily dose = 2000 mg
Naproxen	Aleve, Anaprox, Naprosyn	Tablet as sodium: 220 mg, 275 mg, 550 mg; Tablet as naproxen: 250 mg, 375 mg 500 mg; Controlled release tablets: 375 mg, 500 mg	500 mg × 1 dose then 250 mg every 6–8 hours as needed	Maximum daily dose = 1250 mg (OTC maximum dose = 600 mg) 220 mg naproxen sodium equivalent to 200 mg naproxen
Oxaprozin	Daypro	Tablets: 600 mg	600–1200 mg/day	Maximum daily dose = 26 mg/kg up to 1800 mg
Piroxicam	Feldene	Capsules: 10-20 mg	10–20 mg/day	
Sulindac	Clinoril	Tablets: 150 mg, 200 mg	200 mg 2 times/day	Maximum daily dose = 400 mg
Tolmetin	Tolectin	Capsules: 400 mg; Tablets: 200 mg, 600 mg	400 mg 3 times/day	Maximum daily dose = 2000 mg

IV, intravenously; IM, intramuscularly; OTC, over the counter; PO, orally; PRN, as needed.

Data from U.S. Department of Health and Human Services, Food and Drug Administration. *Approved Drug Products with Therapeutic Equivalence Evaluations*, 26th ed. Available at: http://www.fda.gov/cder/orange/obannual.pdf. Accessed May 13, 2006; and Maheswaran AM, ed. *Mosby's Drug Consult*, 16th ed. St. Louis, MO: Mosby Inc.; 2006.

SUPPORTIVE CARE

Celecoxib is an NSAID specific for COX-2 and has a proven safer GI side effect profile. However, large clinical trials of this and COX-2 inhibitors have shown increased cardiovascular mortality from myocardial infarctions, stroke, and heart failure.[26,27] It is currently not fully understood whether this cardiovascular effect includes the COX-nonspecific NSAIDs.[28] It is further unclear whether newer-generation NSAIDs that are more selective for COX-2 than traditional NSAIDs but are not completely specific (e.g., meloxicam) are either any safer in terms of gastrointestinal or cardiovascular side effects. Prophylactic prostaglandin supplementation[29] and concomitant proton-pump inhibitors[30] have also been used to decrease GI side effects.

Salicylates such as aspirin have limited use in pain management because of their strong antiplatelet properties and the potential to cause salicylic toxicities such as tinnitus, which can be irreversible.

Ketorolac is the only parenteral NSAID available for analgesia that is useful in acute pain. However, ketorolac has been implicated in many cases of GI hemorrhage, and its use should be limited to a maximum of 5 days per course. Its use is also contraindicated in patients with a history of GI bleeding episodes, peptic ulcer disease, or renal failure and in those receiving other concomitant NSAIDs.[31]

Acetaminophen can be used to treat mild to moderate pain. It has an excellent safety profile at usual doses; however, large doses result in accumulation of toxic metabolites, which can lead to fulminant hepatic failure. Because of this possibility, the maximum daily dose of acetaminophen should not exceed 4 g in patients with normal hepatic function. Patients with reduced hepatic function and patients using concomitant hepatotoxic substances such as regular ethanol should restrict use to 2 g/day. Acetaminophen is often combined with opioids and is present in many over-the-counter cough and cold products. Patients should be educated to add up acetaminophen amounts from all sources to avoid toxicity.

Coanalgesics

Some medications that were developed for indications other than pain such as anticonvulsants and antidepressants are considered coanalgesics or adjuncts (Table 3–49). They are frequently used to treat neuropathic pain syndromes and can also be used effectively to treat some types of pain that cannot be treated by opioids alone.

Anticonvulsants such as gabapentin are being used increasingly as first-line therapy for neuropathic pain. Gabapentin has been shown to be effective as first-line therapy for cancer-related neuropathic pain.[32] In one trial, 45% of patients receiving gabapentin had a one-third reduction in their pain scores.[33] Second-line anticonvulsants including lamotrigine, pregabalin, and topiramate have not been studied as extensively and have a higher incidence of severe side effects than gabapentin does. Lidocaine has been used topically and is approved for postherpetic neuralgia. It may also be a good option for patients with localized neuropathic pain.[2,34]

Tricyclic antidepressants (TCAs) have efficacy similar to that of gabapentin but have a less desirable side effect profile. They can cause arrhythmias, orthostatic hypotension, sedation, and classic anticholinergic symptoms such as dry mouth, urinary retention, constipation, and tachycardia. The most experience is with amitriptyline; however, secondary amine TCAs, such as nortriptyline and desipramine, have shown fewer anticholinergic side effects. Use should generally be avoided in patients with severe cardiac disease.[34]

Table 3–49 Coanalgesics

Generic Name	Brand Name	Usual Adult Starting Dose	Comments
Amitriptyline	Elavil	25 mg PO daily at bedtime	TCA: use caution in patients with cardiovascular disease
Capsaicin	Various (e.g., Zostrix)	Apply to affected area 3–4 times/day	Questionable efficacy, ensure adequate patient education on application precautions
Desipramine	Norpramin	25–50 mg PO every hour of sleep	TCA: use caution in patients with cardiovascular disease
Duloxetine	Cymbalta	60 mg PO once daily	Avoid in patients with liver disease
Gabapentin	Neurontin	100–300 mg/day PO in 1–3 divided doses	Patients may need titration to high doses (3600–5400 mg/day divided 3 times/day in certain cases)
Ketamine	Ketalar	Doses vary in case studies/case series	Schedule III; off-label use studied in patients with intractable pain with other established treatments and high-dose narcotics; may reverse opioid tolerance and subsequently cause severe respiratory depression; better tolerated if given with benzodiazepine (less delusions); not commercially available as PO formulation
Lamotrigine	Lamictal	25 mg PO every day in absence of drug interactions	May cause life-threatening rash, careful with drug-drug interactions
Lidocaine	Lidoderm	1–3 patches to affected area 12 hours on followed by 12 hours off	
Nortriptyline	Pamelor	10–25 mg every hour of sleep	TCA: use caution in patients with cardiovascular disease
Pregabalin	Lyrica	150 mg/day PO in 2–3 divided doses	Schedule V
Tramadol	Ultram	25–50 mg/day PO in 1–4 divided doses	May lower seizure threshold; slow titrations to maximum dose 50 mg PO 4 times/day decrease GI side effects; has μ agonist and SSRI pharmacologic properties
Tramadol/APAP	Ultracet (combination of 37.5 mg of tramadol and 325 mg of APAP per tablet)	See tramadol	
Venlafaxine	Effexor (available as immediate release or 24-hour extended release)	75 mg/day PO in 1-3 divided doses depending on formulation	

PO, oral; SSRI, selective serotonin reuptake inhibitor.

Data from U.S. Department of Health and Human Services, Food and Drug Administration. *Approved Drug Products with Therapeutic Equivalence Evaluations*, 26th ed. Available at: www.fda.gov/cder/orange/obannual.pdf. Accessed December 8, 2006; and Maheswaran AM, ed. *Mosby's Drug Consult*, 16th ed. St. Louis: Mosby Inc.; 2006.

SUPPORTIVE CARE

Tramadol is a partial μ receptor agonist with selective serotonin reuptake inhibitory properties and has shown efficacy for neuropathic pain. However, tramadol may lower the seizure threshold, and, thus, its use may be limited in patients already receiving other opioids and antidepressants. Serotonin-norepinephrine reuptake inhibitors such as venlafaxine and duloxetine have shown efficacy in mitigating neuropathic pain syndromes, and duloxetine is approved to treat diabetic neuropathy.

Ketamine is frequently used as a dissociating anesthetic; however, its properties as an NMDA antagonist have been shown to be useful in cancer pain management in small studies. It has been particularly useful in patients who do not receive adequate pain control despite really high doses of opioids and for end-of-life treatment in patients with terminal crescendo pain. Ketamine can reverse some of the tolerance to opioids, so empiric dose reductions of opioids are sometimes used to avoid potential severe respiratory or central nervous system depression. Low doses of parenteral ketamine compounded for the oral route have also been studied in patients with pain that is refractory to extremely high doses of opioids with great success. Patients should be receiving a benzodiazepine prophylactically to prevent the hallucinatory side effects of ketamine.[35–37]

Capsaicin is a topical cream derived from chili peppers. Frequent application has been shown to deplete substance P, a neurotransmitter associated with pain syndromes. Patients need to be cautious when applying capsaicin and not allow the drug to come in contact with sensitive areas such as the eyes. Its role in cancer pain is somewhat limited by its topical route and by inconsistent results in studies.[3]

Many cancer patients may benefit from nonpharmacologic treatment of pain (Table 3–50). For example, pancreatic cancer patients with refractory abdominal pain may benefit greatly from celiac plexus blocks.[38] Palliative surgical procedures can be done for many indications after careful risk/benefit assessments. Radiation is also used frequently in palliation. Radiopharmaceuticals such as strontium-89 and samarium-153 have been used effectively to treat pain caused by bone disease.[39] Complementary therapies such as acupuncture have shown efficacy for cancer pain relief.[40] A multidisciplinary approach is essential to effectively treat many cancer patients with refractory pain.

Table 3–50   Examples of Nonpharmacologic Treatments

Nonpharmacologic Treatments	Comments
Acupuncture	Clinical evidence is limited, but low potential for adverse effects
Neurolytic blocks	Example: celiac plexus block for visceral pain in pancreatic cancer patients
Radiation	Typically shorter duration (less fractions) than conventional radiation therapy
Radiopharmaceuticals	Onset of analgesia 1 week; maximal effect 3–4 weeks; duration can last months
Surgery	Examples include curative intent, stabilizing orthosurgery, and neurosurgery, relieving obstruction

Data from Alimi D, Rubino C, Pichard-Leandri E, et al. Analgesic effect of auricular acupuncture for cancer pain: a randomized, blinded, controlled trial. *J Clin Oncol* 2003;21:4120–4126; Finlay IG, Mason MD, Shelley M. Radioisotopes for the palliation of metastatic bone cancer: a systematic review. *Lancet Oncol* 2005;6:392-400; Miaskowski C, Cleary J, Burney R, et al. *Guideline for the Management of Cancer Pain in Adults and Children,* APS Clinical Practice Guideline Series, No. 3. Glenview, IL: American Pain Society; 2005; and Staats PS, Hekmat H, Sauter P, et al. The effects of alcohol celiac plexus block, pain, and mood on longevity in patients with unresectable pancreatic cancer: a double-blind, randomized, placebo-controlled study. *Pain Med* 2001;2:28–34.

REFERENCES

1. Patrick DL, Ferketich SL, Frame PS, et al. National Institutes of Health State-of-the-Science Conference Statement: symptom management in cancer: pain, depression, and fatigue, July 15-17, 2002. *J Natl Cancer Inst Monogr* 2004;No. 32:9–16.
2. Fine PG, Miaskowski C, Paice JA. Meeting the challenges in cancer pain management. *J Support Oncol* 2004;2(6 Suppl. 4):5–22.
3. Miaskowski C, Cleary J, Burney R, et al. *Guideline for the Management of Cancer Pain in Adults and Children.* APS Clinical Practice Guideline Series, No. 3. Glenview, IL:American Pain Society; 2005.
4. Gutstein HB, Akil H. Opioid analgesics. In Brunton LL, ed. *Goodman and Gilman's The Pharmacological Basis of Therapeutics,* 11th ed. New York: McGraw-Hill; 2006: Chap. 21.
5. Baumann TJ. Pain management. In Dipiro JT, Talbert RL, Yee GC, et al., eds. *Pharmacotherapy: A Pathophysiologic Approach,* 6th ed. New York: McGraw-Hill; 2005: Chap. 58.
6. Heidenreich A, Hofmann R, Engelmann UH. The use of bisphosphonate for the palliative treatment of painful bone metastasis due to hormone refractory prostate cancer. *J Urol* 2001;165:136–140.
7. Vogel CL, Yanagihara RH, Wood AJ, et al. Safety and pain palliation of zoledronic acid in patients with breast cancer, prostate cancer, or multiple myeloma who previously received bisphosphonate therapy. *Oncologist* 2004;9:687–695.
8. Jensen MP. The validity and reliability of pain measures in adults with cancer. *J Pain* 2003;4:2–21.
9. Joint Commission on the Accreditation of Healthcare Organizations. JCAHO Requirements. Available at: www.jointcommission.org/Standards/Requirements. Accessed December 8, 2006.
10. World Health Organization. Cancer pain relief: with a guide to opioid availability, 2nd ed. Geneva, 1996. Available at: http://libdoc.who.int/publications/9241544821.pdf. Accessed December 8, 2006.
11. National Comprehensive Cancer Network, Inc. Adult cancer pain, V.2.2005. Available at: www.nccn.org/professionals/physician_gls/PDF/pain.pdf. Accessed December 8, 2006.
12. Skaer TL. Practice guidelines for transdermal opioids in malignant pain. *Drugs* 2004;64:2629–2638.
13. Cherny NI. The pharmacologic management of cancer pain. *Oncology (Williston Park)* 2004;18: 1499–1515.
14. O'Mahony S, Coyle N, Payne R. Current management of opioid-related side effects. *Oncology (Williston Park)* 2001;15:61–73, 77.
15. Kornick CA, Kilborn MJ, Santiago-Palma J, et al. QTc interval prolongation associated with intravenous methadone. *Pain* 2003;105:499–506.
16. Muller-Lissner SA, Kamm MA, Scarpignato C, et al. Myths and misconceptions about chronic constipation. *Am J Gastroenterol* 2005;100:232–242.
17. Meissner W, Schmidt U, Hartmann M, et al. Oral naloxone reverses opioid-associated constipation. *Pain* 2000;84:105–109.
18. Reisner L, Koo PJ. Pain and its management. In Koda-Kimble MA, Young LY, Kradjan WA, et al., eds. *Applied Therapeutics: The Clinical Use of Drugs,* 8th ed. Philadelphia: Lippincott Williams & Wilkins; 2005.
19. Thomas MC, Erstad BL. Safety of enteral naloxone and i.v. neostigmine when used to relieve constipation. *Am J Health-Syst Pharm* 2003;60:1264–1267.
20. Gonenne J, Camilleri M, Ferber I, et al. Effect of alvimopan and codeine on gastrointestinal transit: a randomized controlled study. *Clin Gastroenterol Hepatol* 2005;3:784–791.
21. Anderson R, Saiers JH, Abram S, et al. Accuracy in equianalgesic dosing. conversion dilemmas. *J Pain Symptom Manage* 2001;21:397–406.
22. Pereira J, Lawlor P, Vigano A, et al. Equianalgesic dose ratios for opioids. a critical review and proposals for long-term dosing. *J Pain Symptom Manage* 2001;22:672–687.
23. Manfredi PL, Houde RW. Prescribing methadone, a unique analgesic. *J Support Oncol* 2003;1: 216–220.
24. Kirsh KL, Whitcomb LA, Donaghy K, et al. Abuse and addiction issues in medically ill patients with pain: attempts at clarification of terms and empirical study. *Clin J Pain* 2002;18(4 Suppl.):S52–S60.
25. Burke A, Smyth E, FitzGerald GA. Analgesic-antipyretic and antiinflammatory agents; pharmacotherapy of gout. In Brunton LL, ed. *Goodman and Gilman's The Pharmacological Basis of Therapeutics,* 11th ed. New York: McGraw-Hill Companies; 2006: Chap. 26.
26. Solomon SD, McMurray JJ, Pfeffer MA, et al. Cardiovascular risk associated with celecoxib in a clinical trial for colorectal adenoma prevention. *N Engl J Med* 2005; 352:1071–1080.
27. Bresalier RS, Sandler RS, Quan H, et al. Cardiovascular events associated with rofecoxib in a colorectal adenoma chemoprevention trial. *N Engl J Med* 2005;352:1092–1102.
28. Konstantinopoulos PA, Lehmann DF. The cardiovascular toxicity of selective and nonselective cyclooxygenase inhibitors: comparisons, contrasts, and aspirin confounding. *J Clin Pharmacol* 2005;45:742–750.
29. Valentini M, Cannizzaro R, Poletti M, et al. Nonsteroidal antiinflammatory drugs for cancer pain: comparison between misoprostol and ranitidine in prevention of upper gastrointestinal damage. *J Clin Oncol* 1995;13:2637–2642.
30. Chan FK, Hung LC, Suen BY, et al. Celecoxib versus diclofenac and omeprazole in reducing the risk of recurrent ulcer bleeding in patients with arthritis. *N Engl J Med* 2002;347:2104–2110.

31. Toradol (ketorolac) prescribing information. Nutley, NJ: Roche; 2002.

32. Caraceni A, Zecca E, Bonezzi C, et al. Gabapentin for neuropathic cancer pain: a randomized controlled trial from the Gabapentin Cancer Pain Study Group. *J Clin Oncol* 2004;22:2909–2917.

33. Ross JR, Goller K, Hardy J, et al. Gabapentin is effective in the treatment of cancer-related neuropathic pain: a prospective, open-label study. *J Palliat Med* 2005;8:1118–1126.

34. Guay DR. Adjunctive agents in the management of chronic pain. *Pharmacotherapy* 2001;21: 1070–1081.

35. Slatkin NE, Rhiner M. Ketamine in the treatment of refractory cancer pain: case report, rationale, and methodology. *J Support Oncol* 2003;1:287–293.

36. Pasero C, McCaffery M. Pain control: ketamine: low doses may provide relief for some painful conditions. *Am J Nurs* 2005;105:60–64.

37. Bell RF, Eccleston C, Kalso E. Ketamine as adjuvant to opioids for cancer pain: a qualitative systematic review. *J Pain Symptom Manage* 2003;26:867–875.

38. Staats PS, Hekmat H, Sauter P, et al. The effects of alcohol celiac plexus block, pain, and mood on longevity in patients with unresectable pancreatic cancer: a double-blind, randomized, placebo-controlled study. *Pain Med* 2001;2:28–34.

39. Finlay IG, Mason MD, Shelley M. Radioisotopes for the palliation of metastatic bone cancer: a systematic review. *Lancet Oncol* 2005;6:392–400.

40. Alimi D, Rubino C, Pichard-Leandri E, et al. Analgesic effect of auricular acupuncture for cancer pain: a randomized, blinded, controlled trial. *J Clin Oncol* 2003;21:4120–4126.

A Guide to Clinically Relevant Drug Interactions in Oncology*

Masha S. H. Lam and Robert J. Ignoffo

INTRODUCTION

Articles on drug interactions with anticancer drugs have appeared in the literature with increasing frequency, and this trend will continue as the list of new anticancer drugs and other ancillary medications used concurrently in the treatment of cancer patients expands. It is estimated that in North America drug interactions occur in about 3%–5% of patients treated with even a few drugs and is higher yet for those treated with a greater number of drugs.[1] In oncology, the incidence of drug-drug interactions is likely to be higher than the estimates reported because of the use of concurrent drugs along with complex chemotherapy regimens. Furthermore, a high proportion of cancer patients are elderly, a risk factor known to increase the risk of adverse drug interactions. In many instances, drug interactions are intentional (enhancement of positive outcomes) and provide a rationale for certain combinations of drugs.[2] Thus, drug interactions observed in cancer patients may be classified as positive (beneficial) or negative (adverse). Combinations of drugs intended to enhance the antitumor response (a synergistic effect) or decrease toxicities produce positive drug interactions that are considered desirable. An undesirable or negative drug interaction occurs when one drug (cytotoxic or otherwise) decreases the antitumor effect of the cytotoxic drug or may have no effect on antitumor activity but causes a significant increase in toxicities. Occasionally, a clinician may not be aware that a negative drug interaction has even occurred.

In this chapter, we highlight negative drug interactions in oncology that have been or are likely to result in harm to the patient, either in the form of enhanced toxicity or diminished antitumor response, survival, or quality of life.

METHODS AND RESULTS

Our literature search strategy was as follows. First we listed all the anticancer drugs that are currently available in the United States (Table 4–1). Then we selected English-language review articles, references from retrieved articles, case reports, and clinical trials identified from a MEDLINE (1966–December 2006) literature search for inclusion in this review. Key search terms included "drug interactions," "oncology," "anticancer drug," "drug metabolism," "antineoplastic agent," "toxicities," "pharmacokinetic interactions," and "pharmacodynamic interactions." Information from both drug package inserts and from the MedWatch online Web site[3] from 1996 through December 2006 were also used in some cases as sources of drug interactions that may never have been published.

Table 4–2 lists anticancer drugs that have been reported to have clinically relevant drug-drug interactions along with the purported mechanism, the subsequent effects, and recommendations for monitoring or treating harmful interactions.[4–256]

DISCUSSION

Drug-drug interactions associated with anticancer drugs may be separated into the following categories: pharmacokinetic, pharmacodynamic, or pharmaceutic interactions.[257]

*Parts of the text and tables used in this chapter were originally published in the following publication: (c) [2003] Edward Arnold (Publishers) Ltd. [*Journal of Oncology Pharmacy Practice* 2003; 9(2-3): 45-85] (www.hodderarnoldjournals.com).

DRUG INTERACTIONS

Table 4–1 Generic and Brand Names of Chemotherapy and Other Cancer-Related Drugs

Generic Name	Brand Name	Generic Name	Brand Name
Abarelix	Plenaxis	Granisetron	Kytril
Aldesleukin (recombinant interkeulin-2; rIL-2)	Proleukin	Hydroxyurea	Hydrea
		Ibritumomab tiuxetan	Zevalin
Alemtuzumab	Campath	Idarubicin	Idamycin
Alitretinoin	Panretin	Ifosfamide	Ifex
Altretamine	Hexalen	Imatinib mesylate	Gleevec
Amifostine	Ethyol	Interferon alfa-2a	Roferon-A
Aminoglutethimide	Cytadren	Interferon alfa-2b	Intron-A
Anastrozole	Arimidex	Irinotecan	Camptosar
Aprepitant	Emend	Lenalidomide	Revlimid
Arsenic trioxide	Trisenox	Letrozole	Femara
Asparaginase	Elspar	Leuprolide acetate depot	Lupron depot
Azacytidine	Vidaza	Levamisole	Ergamisol
Bexarotene	Targretin	Leucovorin calcium	Wellcovorin
Bevacizumab	Avastin	Lomustine	CeeNu
Bicalutamide	Casodex	Mechlorethamine	Mustargen
Bleomycin	Blenoxane	Medroxyprogesterone acetate	Provera
Bortezomib	Velcade		
Busulfan	Myleran	Megestrol	Megace
Capecitabine	Xeloda	Melphalan	Alkeran
Carboplatin	Paraplatin	Mercaptopurine	Purinethol
Carmustine	BiCNU	Mesna	Mesnex
Cetuximab	Erbitux	Methotrexate	Mexate, Folex
Chlorambucil	Leukeran	Methylprednisolone	Solu-Medrol
Cisplatin	Platinol	Mitomycin-C	Mutamycin
Cladribine	Leustatin	Mitoxantrone	Novantrone
Clofarabine	Clolar	Nelarabine	Arranon
Cyclophosphamide	Cytoxan	Nilutamide	Nilandron
Cytarabine	Cytosar-U	Paclitaxel (Nanoparticle albumin-bound)	Abraxane
Dacarbazine	DTIC-Dome		
Dasatinib	Sprycel	Octreotide	Sandostatin; Sandostatin LAR
Dactinomycin	Cosmegen		
Daunorubicin	Cerubidine	Ondansetron	Zofran
Daunorubicn (liposomal)	DaunoXome	Oprelvekin (Interleukin-11)	Neumega
Darbepoetin alfa	Aranesp	Oxaliplatin	Eloxatin
Decitabine	Dacogen	Paclitaxel	Taxol
Denileukin diftitox	Ontak	Palifermin	Kepivance
Dexamethasone	Decadron	Palonosetron	Aloxil
Dexrazoxane	Zinecard	Pamidronate	Aredia
Docetaxel	Taxotere	Panitumumab	Vectibix
Dolasetron	Anzemet	Pegfilgrastim	Neulasta
Doxorubicin	Adriamycin	Pemetrexed	Alimta
Doxorubicin HCl liposomal injection	Doxil	Pentostatin	Nipent
		Porfimer	Photofrin®
Epirubicin	Ellence	Prednisone	Deltasone
Erlotinib	Tarceva	Procarbazine	Matulane
Estramustine	Emcyt	Rasburicase	Elitek
Etoposide	VePesid	Rituximab	Rituxan
Exemestane	Aromasin	Sorafenib	Nexavar
Filgrastim	Neupogen	Streptozocin	Zanosar
Floxuridine	FUDR	Sunitinib	Sutent
Fludarabine	Fludara	Tamoxifen	Nolvadex
Fluorouracil	Adrucil	Temozolomide	Temodar
Fluoxymesterone	Halotestin	Teniposide	Vumon
Flutamide	Eulexin	Testolactone	Teslac
Fulvestrant	Faslodex	Thalidomide	Thalomid
Gemcitabine	Gemzar	Thioguanine	Tabloid thioguanine
Gemtuzumab ozogamicin	Mylotarg		
Geftinib	Iressa	Thiotepa	Thioplex
Goserelin acetate	Zoladex	Topotecan	Hycamtin

Generic Name	Brand Name	Generic Name	Brand Name
Toremifene citrate	Fareston	Vinblastine	Velban
Tositumomab Iodine I-131	Bexxar®	Vincristine	Oncovin
Trastuzumab	Herceptin	Vinorelbine	Navelbine
Tretinoin	Vesanoid	Vorinostat	Zolinza
Trimetrexate	Neutrexin®	Zoledronic acid	Zometa
Triptorelin pamoate	Trelstar Depot		

Pharmacokinetic Interactions

Pharmacokinetic interactions involve one drug altering the absorption, distribution, metabolism, or excretion of another drug. These interactions may often result in changes in serum concentrations at an equivalent dose of the drugs that may lead to clinically unfavorable consequences. Interpatient variability may further complicate the pharmacokinetic profile of many anticancer agents, which may ultimately affect patient responses to treatment as well as toxicity profile.[258] For example, high doses of cyclophosphamide and carmustine as are used in the bone marrow transplant setting can decrease absorption of oral digoxin in the tablet form by 20%–45%.[50] Substitution of either an intravenous or a liquid form of digoxin should be considered to avoid inadequate gut absorption of the drug with high-dose chemotherapy. Similarly, the concurrent use of broad-spectrum antibiotics may alter the gut microbial flora and decreased gut absorption of oral methotrexate.[188]

A decrease in protein binding may result from malnutrition, disease processes, or even some drugs that damage liver function. Although several anticancer agents that are highly protein bound would be expected to interact with drugs that compete for the same protein-binding sites, no clinically relevant interactions have been reported. In contrast, the concurrent use of warfarin and bicalutamide, both of which are highly protein bound, may reduce protein binding of warfarin and result in a greater anticoagulant effect.[29] Another anticancer drug, asparaginase, indirectly alters protein binding by inhibiting hepatic protein synthesis including lowering of serum albumin as well as other metabolic changes in liver function.[259] A significant increase in unbound teniposide has been reported in children with acute lymphocytic leukemia.[27]

Several investigators have suggested that wide pharmacokinetic variability is probably the most important mechanism responsible for oncologic drug interactions. In most instances, drug interactions involving hepatic metabolism either increase or decrease the area under the curve (AUC) of the cytotoxic agent and/or the interacting agent because of an effect on drug clearance. Several anticancer drugs such as cyclophosphamide, ifosfamide, busulfan, epipodophyllotoxin, vinca alkaloids, irinotecan, taxanes, and hormonal agents (tamoxifen, aromatase inhibitors, and toremifene) are known to be metabolized by the cytochrome phosphorylase (CYP) 3A4 isoenzyme system.[262,263,274,277,278,282,283,286,288,290,293,294] Many clinically significant drug interactions involving the CYP system have been reported in the literature.[91,92,110,116,138,145–149,152,156,158–161,163,219,220,234,235,241,243,245,250–253] Potent CYP 3A4 inhibitors such as itraconazole, erythromycin, and grapefruit juice can significantly increase serum drug levels of vinca alkaloids that can lead to an increased risk of severe neurotoxicity.[245,251–253,255] Rodman et al.[116] found that concomitant use of enzyme-inducing anticonvulsants such as phenytoin or phenobarbital increased etoposide clearance by 170%. Murry et al.[158] recently reported a case in which concomitant phenytoin administration resulted in a marked decrease in AUC for irinotecan (63%) and for SN-38 (60%). SN-38, the major active metabolite of irinotecan

Table 4-2 Drug Interactions between Anticancer Agents and Other Drugs[4-256]

Anticancer Agent	Concurrent Use with	Effect	Possible Mechanisms of Action if Any	Management Options	Ref.
Aldesleukin (IL-2)	Corticosteroids	↓ antitumor efficacy of aldesleukin	Dexamethasone inhibits release of aldesleukin-induced tumor necrosis factor → opposing pharmacologic effects of aldesleukin.	Avoid concurrent use if possible; if dexamethasone is used as an antiemetic, use of other alternatives is recommended.	4
	Dacarbazine	May ↓ efficacy of dacarbazine	↓ AUC of dacarbazine due to ↑ its volume of distribution	Clinical significance is difficult to assess because both drugs used in melanoma setting.	5
All-*trans*-retinoic acid (ATRA)	Protease inhibitors[a]	↑ toxicity of protease inhibitors	Aldesleukin induces formation of IL-6 inhibits protease inhibitor metabolism via CYP 3A4 → ↑ AUC by 75% (e.g., indinavir).	May need to adjust doses of protease inhibitors when aldesleukin is started or stopped.	6
	Ketoconazole (may apply to other potent CYP 3A4 inhibitors[b])	May ↑ AUC of ATRA transiently on day 1 but did not maintain the increased ATRA levels over time (after 14 days of ketoconazole therapy) → ↑ risk of toxicity including LFT results elevation and vomiting	Increased AUC of ATRA is possibly due to ↓ metabolism of ATRA via inhibition of CYP 3A4 by ketoconazole single dose; however, unclear why chronic daily administration of ketoconazole did not maintain increased levels of ATRA; may be due to the fact that induction of capacity-limited elimination process for ATRA could account for the ↓ in plasma drug concentrations within several days of initiation of drug administration, and not weeks to months after.	Monitor risk of excessive toxicities when ketoconazole is added to ATRA; however, dosing adjustment (reduction) of ATRA is not recommended.	7–9
	CYP 3A4 inducers[c]	May ↑ metabolism of ATRA → ↓ therapeutic efficacy of ATRA	Because of potent induction of hepatic metabolism of ATRA via CYP 3A4	Avoid combination use if possible, especially in situation where disease can be cured, e.g., acute promyelocytic leukemia. Recommend use of non-enzyme-inducing anticonvulsants.	10
Altretamine	Cimetidine	↑ altretamine toxicity	Inhibit altretamine metabolism via P450 isozymes → ↑ T$_{1/2}$ and lethal dose seen in one animal study	Avoid use of cimetidine. May use other histamine H2 blockers (e.g., ranitidine).	11
	Phenobarbital (may apply to other CYP 3A4 inducers[c])	↓ antitumor efficacy	↑ metabolism of altretamine via CYP 450	Avoid use of combination if possible or use other non-enzyme-inducing anticonvulsants.	12

Aminoglutethimide	Dexamethasone	↓ biological activity of dexamethasone → may ↓ antitumor effect, efficacy in cerebral edema, or antiemetic effects	↓ elimination $T_{1/2}$ by twofold and ↑ clearance of dexamethasone via induction of hepatic metabolism via P450 enzymes	Dose of dexamethasone may need to be ↑ to achieve adequate therapeutic response (e.g., used in reducing cerebral edema or for antitumor or antiemetic purposes).	13
	Medroxyprogesterone	↓ antitumor efficacy	↑ metabolism via P450 enzymes	Clinical significance may be minimal as both drugs are rarely given concomitantly in clinical practice nowadays.	14
	Tamoxifen	↓ [tamoxifen] → may ↓ antitumor efficacy of tamoxifen	↑ metabolism via P450 enzymes	Clinical significance may be minimal as both drugs are rarely given concomitantly in clinical practice nowadays.	15
	Theophylline	↓ theophylline efficacy	↑ theophylline clearance by 32% due to induction of hepatic metabolism by P450 enzymes	Monitor for bronchodilatory response, and check theophylline level as clinically indicated.	16
	Warfarin			See Table 4-7	17, 18
Aprepitant	Cyclophosphamide	Autoinduction of cyclophosphamide by aprepitant was reduced by 23% and exposures to active metabolite of 4-hydroxycyclophosphamide was reduced by 5%; 50% inhibitory concentration of aprepitant for inhibition of cyclophosphamide was within therapeutic range	Inhibit bioactivation of high-dose cyclophosphamide (1500 mg/m²/day for 4 days) via CYP 3A4 and/or 2B6	Interaction between aprepitant and high-dose cyclophosphamide is clinically negligible.	19
	Oral steroids (dexamethasone and methylprednisolone), intravenous methylprednisolone	↑ AUC of steroids by 2.2- to 2.5-fold → ↑ risk of infection; increase AUC of steroids by 1.3-fold	Possibly due to ↓ metabolism of dexamethasone via inhibition of CYP 3A4 by aprepitant	Doses of oral steroids are recommended to ↓ by 40%–50% (e.g., oral dexamethasone decreased from 20 to 12 mg or from 8 to 4 mg) and monitor for ↑ incidence of infection.	20, 21

Continued

DRUG INTERACTIONS

Table 4-2 Drug Interactions between Anticancer Agents and Other Drugs[1–256]—cont'd

Anticancer Agent	Concurrent Use with	Effect	Possible Mechanisms of Action if Any	Management Options	Ref.
Aprepitant—cont'd	Midazolam (or other CYP 3A4 substrates[d] such as docetaxel)	Coadministration of midazolam and 125/80 mg aprepitant ↑ midazolam AUC by 2.3-fold on day 1 and by 3.3-fold on day 5; $T_{1/2}$ of midazolam ↑ from 1.7 to 3.3 hrs on both day 1 and day 5; however, other studies did not show clinically significant interactions between midazolam or docetaxel with aprepitant given at 125/80 mg administered over days 1–3.	Aprepitant transiently affects metabolism of midazolam via both induction and inhibition of CYP 3A4.	Clinically relevant interaction may not be of importance; monitor closely for any side effects and efficacy.	22–24
	Tolbutamide (may apply to other CYP 2C9 substrates[e])	↓ AUC of tolbutamide by 15%–28%	Possibly due to ↑ metabolism of tolbutamide or phenytoin via CYP 2C9 induced by aprepitant	Clinical significance is unknown; monitor blood sugar as clinically indicated.	20, 23
	Thiotepa	Formation clearance of thiotepa by aprepitant was reduced by 33% and exposures to active metabolite of tepa was ↓ by 20%; 50% inhibitory concentration of aprepitant for inhibition of thiotepa was within therapeutic range.	Inhibits hepatic metabolism of high-dose thiotepa (120 mg/m²/day for 4 days) via CYP 3A4 and/or 2B6	Interaction between aprepitant and high-dose thiotepa is clinically negligible.	19
	Warfarin	34% ↓ in S-warfarin trough concentrations on days 5–8; INR ↓ with a mean maximum decrease on day 8 of 11% after completion of the aprepitant regimen.	Possibly due to ↑ metabolism of warfarin via induction of CYP 2C9 by aprepitant	INR should be closely monitored during the 2-week period (particularly at 7–10 days) after initiation of the aprepitant dosage regimen (3 days) with each chemotherapy cycle.	20, 25
Asparaginase	Methotrexate	Administration of asparaginase before or concurrently with methotrexate may ↓ methotrexate efficacy.	Asparaginase inhibits protein synthesis and prevents cell entry into S phase→ ↓ methotrexate efficacy.	Administer asparaginase shortly after methotrexate or 9–10 days before methotrexate.	26
	Teniposide	Increase in unbound teniposide → ↑ bone marrow toxicity	Asparaginase ↓ production of albumin→ ↓ protein binding of teniposide.	Monitor for drug toxicity; dosage of teniposide may need to be adjusted.	27

	Vincristine	Administration of asparaginase concurrently with or before vincristine ↑ risk of neurotoxicity of vincristine.	Possibly due to ↓ vincristine metabolism from the effects of asparaginase on hepatic function	Administer vincristine before asparaginase.	28
Bicalutamide					
Bleomycin	Warfarin			See Table 4-7	29
	Cisplatin (when accumulated doses of cisplatin >300 mg/m² have been given)	↑ risk of pulmonary toxicity	Cisplatin may delay bleomycin elimination due to ↓ GFR.	Monitor renal function and adjust dose of bleomycin according to CrCl (see Table 4-4); monitor closely for signs and symptoms of pulmonary toxicities and perform pulmonary function tests as clinically indicated.	30–32
Bortezomib	CYP 3A4 inhibitors[b]	May ↑ risk of myelosuppression and peripheral neuropathy	Possibly due to ↓ metabolism of bortezomib via CYP 3A4	Monitor for ↑ incidence of myelosuppression, peripheral neuropathy.	33, 34
	CYP 3A4 inducers[c]	Significantly ↑ metabolism of bortezomib → ↓ therapeutic efficacy of bortezomib	Because of potent induction of hepatic metabolism of bortezomib via CYP 3A4	No published guidelines for dosing adjustment for bortezomib; use non–enzyme-inducing anticonvulsants if possible and monitor for clinical efficacy of bortezomib.	33, 34
	CYP 2C19 inhibitors[f]	May ↑ risk of myelosuppression and peripheral neuropathy	Possibly due to ↓ metabolism of bortezomib via CYP 2C19	Avoid concomitant use if possible; monitor for ↑ incidence of myelosuppression, peripheral neuropathy.	33, 34
	CYP 2C19 inducers[g]	Significantly ↑ metabolism of bortezomib → ↓ therapeutic efficacy of bortezomib	Due to potent induction of hepatic metabolism of bortezomib via CYP 2C19	Avoid concomitant use if possible; monitor for clinical efficacy of bortezomib.	33, 34
Busulfan	Cyclophospha-mide (when cyclophospha-mide given <24 hrs after the last dose of busulfan)	↑ incidence of venous occlusive disease and mucositis; also ↓ efficacy of cyclophosphamide	Administration of cyclophosphamide <24 hrs after busulfan → ↓ clearance and ↑ elimination $T_{1/2}$ of cyclophosphamide, also ↓ exposure to active metabolite of 4-hydroxycyclophosphamide	Administer cyclophosphamide at least 24 hrs after the last dose of busulfan.	35

Continued

DRUG INTERACTIONS

Table 4-2 Drug Interactions between Anticancer Agents and Other Drugs[4-256]—cont'd

Anticancer Agent	Concurrent Use with	Effect	Possible Mechanisms of Action if Any	Management Options	Ref.
Busulfan—cont'd	Fosphenytoin or phenytoin	May ↓ [busulfan] by ≥15%	Due to induction of glutathione-S-transferase	Phenytoin has been commonly used in transplant settings to prevent high-dose busulfan-induced seizures. Therapeutic level of busulfan used in transplant setting is wide (typical target AUC is 900–1300 μmol/L/min or Cp_{ss} range of ~600–900 ng/mL), clinically relevant interactions may not be of significance. Monitor busulfan levels as clinically indicated.	36
	Itraconazole (may apply to other potent CYP 3A4 inhibitors)[b]	May ↑ busulfan toxicities such as venous occlusive disease or pulmonary fibrosis	↓ busulfan clearance by up to 25% and ↑ busulfan AUCs >1500 μmol/L/min in some patients due to inhibition of CYP 3A4 metabolism.	Monitor clinical toxicity such as venous occlusive disease and pulmonary toxicity in transplant settings; monitoring of busulfan level may be considered to ensure its AUC <1500 μmol/L/min to avoid excessive toxicity.	37
	Thioguanine	↑ risk of hepatic nodular regenerative hyperplasia of the liver, esophageal varices, and portal hypertension	Unknown	Monitor LFTs, signs/symptoms of liver toxicities (portal hypertension, esophageal varices, ascites, splenomegaly, and gastrointestinal bleeding). *Note:* Clinical significance may be minimal as combination of both drugs is rarely used in CML.	38
Capecitabine	Phenytoin	May ↑ phenytoin levels → ↑ toxicity	Interference with metabolism of phenytoin via CYP 2C9	Monitor phenytoin levels closely and adjust the doses as needed.	39
Carboplatin	Warfarin	See Table 4-7			39–41
	Paclitaxel	↓ incidence of thrombocytopenia was observed in patients receiving combination of carboplatin and paclitaxel compared with those who received carboplatin alone.	Unknown; no changes in pharmacokinetics of either drug were seen in the study.	Drug selection depends on different cancer settings and different toxicity profiles (e.g., carboplatin used alone in ovarian cancer has been shown to achieve overall survival similar to that with the combination of carboplatin and paclitaxel but with a lower nonhematologic toxicity profile).	42–45

Carmustine	Phenytoin	May ↓ phenytoin concentrations to as low as 50%	Unclear; may be due to changes of hepatic metabolism and protein replacement	Monitor for seizure activities and phenytoin levels closely to adjust doses as needed to maintain phenytoin therapeutic levels.	46
	Cimetidine	Increase bone marrow suppression and antitumor effect	Cimetidine impaired carmustine clearance by inhibition of metabolism via CYP P450 isozymes.	Avoid use of cimetidine; may use other histamine-H2 blockers (e.g., ranitidine).	47–49
	Digoxin	↓ digoxin serum level → may ↓ efficacy	High-dose carmustine ↓ absorption of digoxin tablet by 45%.	Substitute liquid form for digoxin tablet; monitor for heart rate, CHF symptoms, and check digoxin levels as clinically indicated.	50
	High-dose etoposide in transplant setting	↑ risk of liver toxicity (toxicity occurred 1–2 mos after initiation of treatment without improving tumor response)	Possible additive effects	Avoid use of this combination as no improved tumor response was observed but toxicity was increased.	51
	Phenobarbital (chronic oral administration)	↓ antitumor effects of carmustine in animal model	Possibly due to induction of a change in liver enzymes from chronic oral administration of phenobarbital → ↑ clearance of carmustine. *Note:* No interaction was observed between carmustine and phenytoin, dexamethasone, or methylprednisolone in the study.	Avoid use of this combination; phenytoin may be used as anticonvulsant alternative.	52
Cisplatin	Aminoglycosides or loop diuretics	↑ risk of ototoxicites when cisplatin was given early during the course of treatment with aminoglycosides.	Augmented auditory damage	Treatment with cisplatin should wait until the completion of aminoglycoside therapy; monitor auditory function closely.	53–55
	Anticonvulsants (phenytoin, valproic acid, carbamazepine)	↓ serum concentration of anticonvulsant drugs → ↑ risk of seizures	Possibly due to ↓ absorption or metabolism rate of anticonvulsants by cisplatin	Monitor for seizure activity and anticonvulsant levels closely and adjust the doses of anticonvulsants as needed to maintain therapeutic levels.	56, 57
	Bleomycin (when accumulated dose of cisplatin >300 mg/m² has been given)	↑ risk of pulmonary toxicity	Cisplatin may delay bleomycin elimination due to ↓ GFR.	Monitor renal function and adjust dose of bleomycin according to CrCl (see Table 4-4); monitor closely for signs and symptoms of pulmonary toxicities and perform pulmonary function tests as clinically indicated.	30–32

Continued

DRUG INTERACTIONS

Table 4-2 Drug Interactions between Anticancer Agents and Other Drugs[4-256]—cont'd

Anticancer Agent	Concurrent Use with	Effect	Possible Mechanisms of Action if Any	Management Options	Ref.
Cisplatin—cont'd	Docetaxel (when docetaxel was given after cisplatin)	More profound myelosuppression observed; concomitant use ↑ risk of peripheral neuropathy	Sequential infusion of docetaxel after cisplatin leads to ↓ docetaxel clearance; possible additive effects.	Give docetaxel first, followed by cisplatin; monitor closely for ↑ signs and symptoms of neuropathy.	58–60
	Ifosfamide	↑ risk of neurotoxicity, hematotoxicity, and tubular nephrotoxicity of ifosfamide	Cisplatin-induced renal damage → impaired clearance of ifosfamide metabolites → ↑ toxicities	Monitor renal function and adjust dose of ifosfamide based on CrCl; provide vigorous hydration and give mesna for uroprotection.	61–63
	Lithium	Serum lithium concentrations ↓ by 64% during the first course of cisplatin was reported	Unclear, but may be due to changes in lithium renal clearance induced by cisplatin	The changes in serum lithium concentrations were of clinical insignificance, and the effect became less pronounced during the consecutive courses in the report; continue to monitor lithium levels closely if clinically indicated.	64
	Paclitaxel infused over 24 hrs (when paclitaxel infused over 24 hrs was given after cisplatin)	Caused more profound neutropenia	Administration of cisplatin before paclitaxel ↓ paclitaxel clearance by 25%.	Administer paclitaxel followed by cisplatin.	65
	Rituximab or other known nephrotoxic agents (e.g., aminoglycosides, amphotericin B, cyclosporine, tacrolimus)	↑ risk of developing renal failure	Additive insult to the kidneys	Monitor for renal function closely (before, during, and after administration); hydrate with at least 2 L of fluid, and replenish potassium and magnesium if deficient before administration of both agents.	66–69

Continued

Drug	Interacting drug				Reference
	Topotecan	↓ topotecan clearance and subclinical renal toxicity induced by cisplatin	When topotecan dose was given at >0.75 mg/m^2 on days 1–5 plus cisplatin dose at >50 mg/m^2, the sequence of cisplatin given on day 1 before topotecan caused more severe bone marrow suppression than the alternate sequence in which cisplatin was given on day 5. ↑ incidence of grade III and IV granulocytopenia	Administer cisplatin on day 5 after topotecan if dose of topotecan >0.75 mg/m^2 plus cisplatin >50 mg/m^2 are given, with the aid of granulocyte CSFs.	70
	Vinorelbine	Possibly additive effects		Monitor CBC closely.	71
Cyclophosphamide	Aprepitant (as a CYP 3A4 inhibitor and 2B6 inhibitor)	Aprepitant inhibits bioactivation of high-dose cyclophosphamide (1500 mg/m^2/day for 4 days) via CYP 3A4 and CYP 2B6; both hydroxylation and dechloroethylation pathways of cyclophosphamide metabolism via CYP 2B6 and 3A4 were inhibited by aprepitant → no significant net increase in AUC of hydroxyl metabolite was observed.	Autoinduction of cyclophosphamide by aprepitant was reduced by 23% and exposures to active metabolite of 4-hydroxycyclophosphamide was reduced only by 5%; 50% inhibitory concentration of aprepitant for inhibition of cyclophosphamide was within therapeutic range	Interaction between aprepitant and high-dose cyclophosphamide is clinically negligible.	19
	Busulfan (when cyclophosphamide given <24 hrs after the last dose of busulfan)	Administration of cyclophosphamide <24 hrs after busulfan → ↓ clearance and ↑ elimination $T_{1/2}$ of cyclophosphamide, also ↓ exposure to active metabolite of 4-hydroxycyclophosphamide	↑ incidence of venous occlusive disease and mucositis; also ↓ efficacy of cyclophosphamide	Administer cyclophosphamide at least 24 hrs after the last dose of busulfan.	35
	CYP 3A4 inhibitors[b]	CYP 3A4 inhibitors may ↑ serum concentration of active metabolite of cyclophosphamide → ↑ antitumor effects and toxicities of cyclophosphamide	CYP 3A4 inhibitors may allow more drug to undergo 4-hydroxylation → ↑ the formation of active metabolites, hydroxycyclophosphamide and subsequent phosphoramide mustard.	Clinical interactions between CYP 3A4 inhibitors and cyclophosphamide may not be of importance because only 10% of parent drug of cyclophosphamide undergoes dechloroethylation pathways via CYP 3A4; monitor closely for possible higher incidence of clinical toxicities of cyclophosphamide.	72, 73

DRUG INTERACTIONS

Table 4-2 Drug Interactions between Anticancer Agents and Other Drugs[4-256]—cont'd

Anticancer Agent	Concurrent Use with	Effect	Possible Mechanisms of Action if Any	Management Options	Ref.
Cyclophosphamide—cont'd	CYP 3A4 inducers[c]	↑ rate of biotransformation to an active metabolite, 4-hydroxycyclophosphamide by 2- to 3-fold but no increase in total amounts of metabolites	Induction of metabolism of cyclophosphamide via CYP 3A4	Clinically relevant interactions may not be significant because total amount of metabolites formed was not altered.	72, 74
	CYP 2B6 inhibitors[h]	May ↓ serum concentration of active metabolite → ↓ antitumor effects and toxicities of cyclophosphamide	Inhibition of CYP 2B6 may ↓ the formation of active metabolite, 4-hydroxycyclophosphamide, from the parent drug via hydroxylation. Note: CYP 2B6–inhibiting effect by the normal doses of ritonavir has not shown to be complete and caused clinical relevant interactions.	Clinical significance is unclear and may be a dose-dependent phenomenon; monitor closely for clinical efficacy of cyclophosphamide.	72
	CYP 2B6 inducers[i]	May ↑ serum concentration of active metabolite → ↑ antitumor effects and toxicities of cyclophosphamide	Induction of hydroxylation pathway of cyclophosphamide metabolism via CYP 2B6 by phenobarbital may ↑ active metabolite, 4-hydroxycyclophosphamide.	Clinical significance is unclear and may be dose-dependent; monitor closely for ↑ incidence of clinical toxicities of cyclophosphamide.	69, 74
	Cimetidine	↑ bone marrow toxicity of cyclophosphamide	Concomitant use with cimetidine in animal studies ↑ $T_{1/2}$ and AUC of cyclophosphamide active metabolite via mechanisms other than P450 inhibition.	Avoid cimetidine and use other histamine H2 blocker, e.g., ranitidine	75, 76
	Digoxin	↓ digoxin level → may ↓ its efficacy	High-dose cyclophosphamide ↓ absorption of digoxin tablet by 45%.	Substitute liquid form for digoxin tablet to monitor heart rate and for CHF symptoms, and check digoxin levels as clinically indicated.	47
	Paclitaxel (when paclitaxel was infused over 24 or 72 hrs before cyclophosphamide)	↑ severity of neutropenia, thrombocytopenia, and mucositis	Unknown as no pharmacokinetic parameters were altered for either drugs with sequential administration of both	Administer cyclophosphamide first, followed by paclitaxel.	77, 78
	Pentostatin	Concomitant use with high-dose cyclophosphamide in bone marrow setting resulted in fatal cardiac toxicity.	Possibly due to interference with adenosine metabolism to cyclophosphamide	Avoid this combination outside clinical trials.	79

Drug	Interacting Agent	Effect	Mechanism	Management	Ref.
Cytarabine	Trastuzumab	↑ cardiac toxicities have been reported	Possible additive effects	Monitor closely for cardiac function.	80
	Digoxin	↓ digoxin serum level→ ↓ efficacy	High-dose cytarabine ↓ absorption of digoxin tablet by 45%.	Substitute liquid form for digoxin tablet; monitor for HR, CHF symptoms, and digoxin levels as clinically indicated.	50
Dacarbazine	Aldesleukin (IL-2)	May ↓ efficacy of dacarbazine	↓ AUC of dacarbazine because of ↑ its volume of distribution	Clinical significance difficult to assess because both drugs are used in melanoma setting.	5
Darbepoetin alfa	Thalidomide	Thalidomide ↑ the thromboembolic risk of darbepoetin alfa in patients with myelodysplastic syndrome.	Additive thrombogenic effect	Careful clinical observation is warranted, and thrombosis prophylaxis should be considered	81
Dasatinib	CYP 3A4 inhibitors[b]	May ↑ AUC of dasatinib → ↑ toxicities such as neutropenia	Inhibits hepatic metabolism of dasatinib via CYP 3A4	Monitor for clinical efficacy/toxicities, and adjust doses as needed.	82
	CYP 3A4 inducers[c]	May ↓ AUC of dasatinib → ↓ clinical efficacy of dasatinib	Induces hepatic metabolism of dasatinib via CYP 3A4	Monitor for clinical efficacy/toxicities, and adjust doses as needed.	82
	Gastric acid suppressants (H2 blockers, proton pump inhibitors)	Long-term suppression of gastric acid secretion ↓ dasatinib exposure → ↓ clinical efficacy of dasatinib.	Long-term use of gastric acid suppressants may interfere with absorption of dasatinib.	Concomitant use of H2 blockers or PPIs with dasatinib is not recommended. If antacid therapy is needed, the antacid dose should be administered at least 2 hrs before or 2 hrs after the dose of dasatinib.	82
	CYP 3A4 substrates with a narrow therapeutic index	Coadminister dasatinib with CYP 3A4 substrates with a narrow therapeutic index may ↑ AUC of CYP 3A4 substrates → ↑ toxicities	Inhibits hepatic metabolism of simvastatin via CYP 3A4 by dasatinib.	Monitor adverse effects of CYP 3A4 substrates with a narrow therapeutic index.	82
	Warfarin	See Table 4-7			82
Daunorubicin	Trastuzumab	↑ cardiac toxicities with trastuzumab	Possible additive effects	Monitor closely for cardiac function and signs/symptoms of cardiac toxicities.	80
Dexamethasone	CYP 3A4 inhibitors[b]	May ↑ adrenal-suppressive effects	May ↑ levels of dexamethasone due to inhibiting hepatic metabolism via CYP 3A4	Plasma cortisol level monitoring may be required; monitor for clinical toxicities and ↑ incidence of infection with long-term use.	83
	CYP 3A4 inducers[c]	May ↓ adrenal-suppressive effects or ↓ activity in ↓ing cerebral edema	May ↓ levels of dexamethasone → due to inducing hepatic metabolism via CYP 3A4	If used in ↓ing cerebral edema/inflammation, dose of dexamethasone may need to be ↑.	84–86

Continued

DRUG INTERACTIONS

Table 4-2 Drug Interactions between Anticancer Agents and Other Drugs[4-256]—cont'd

Anticancer Agent	Concurrent Use with	Effect	Possible Mechanisms of Action if Any	Management Options	Ref.
Dexamethasone—cont'd	Interleukin-2	↓ antitumor efficacy of interleukin-2	Dexamethasone inhibits release of interleukin-2–induced tumor necrosis factor → opposing pharmacologic effects of interleukin-2.	Avoid concurrent use if possible; if dexamethasone is used as an antiemetic, use of other alternatives is recommended.	4
	Irinotecan	↑ irinotecan clearance → ↓ clinical efficacy.	Possibly due to potential ↑ biliary excretion of the drug and its metabolite SN-38 or induction of metabolism of irinotecan via CYP 3A4	Monitor antitumor effect and ↑ dose of irinotecan may be required if combined use cannot be avoided (e.g., brain tumor). If dexamethasone is used as an antiemetic, use of other alternatives is recommended.	87
	Lenalidomide	↑ risk of deep venous thrombosis in patients with multiple myeloma	Possibly additive thrombogenic activity of lenalidomide	Closely monitor for signs and symptoms of DVT and PEs. In patients with history of VTE, anticoagulation should be considered as secondary prophylaxis.	88
	Thalidomide	↑ risk of DVT → 15% in patients with multiple myeloma compared with those receiving thalidomide monotherapy	Unknown; possibly additive thrombogenic activity of thalidomide	Closely monitor for signs and symptoms of DVT and PEs. In patients with history of VTE, anticoagulation should be considered as secondary prophylaxis.	89
Docetaxel	Aprepitant	One pharmacokinetic study did not show clinically significant interactions between docetaxel and aprepitant given at 125/80 mg administered over days 1–3.	Aprepitant transiently affects metabolism of docetaxel via both induction and inhibition of CYP 3A4, but did not cause any statistically or clinically significant changes in docetaxel pharmacokinetics.	Clinically relevant interaction is not of importance.	20
	Cisplatin	Higher incidence of profound myelosuppression; ↑ risk of peripheral neuropathy	Sequential infusion of docetaxel after cisplatin may lead to ↓ docetaxel clearance; possibly additive effects	Recommend giving docetaxel followed by cisplatin; monitor patient closely for ↑ signs/symptoms of neurotoxicity.	58–60
	Doxorubicin	Administration of docetaxel after doxorubicin compared with docetaxel given alone → AUC of docetaxel ↑ by 50%–70% → may ↑ clinical efficacy as well as toxicities.	Possibly due to interference at hepatic microsomal enzyme level	Monitor closely for ↑ incidence of clinical toxicities, including bone marrow suppression, neurotoxicity, myalgia, and fatigue.	90

Ketoconazole (may apply to other potent CYP 3A4 inhibitor[b])	Clearance of docetaxel by ↓ 49% → ↑ risk of severe myelosuppression	Because of ↓ metabolism of docetaxel via P450 CYP 3A4	Dose reduction by 50% is suggested if docetaxel has to be administered together with potent inhibitors of CYP 3A4; monitor for ↑ incidence of myelosuppression, peripheral neuropathy, myalgias, and fatigue.	91, 92
Topotecan	Administration of topotecan on days 1–4 and docetaxel on day 4 compared with same regimen except docetaxel given on day 1 ↑ incidence of neutropenia.	Because of 50% ↓ in docetaxel clearance possibly inhibition of hepatic metabolism of docetaxel by topotecan via CYP 3A4	Give docetaxel on day 1 and topotecan on days 1–4	93
Vinorelbine	Sequential administration of docetaxel after vinorelbine → ↑ vinorelbine plasma level → ↑ severity of neutropenia compared with alternate sequence.	Plasma level of vinorelbine ↑ due to its lower drug clearance. No difference in changes of C_{max}, clearance, or AUC of docetaxel between two different sequence schedules	Administer docetaxel first, followed by vinorelbine.	94
Doxorubicin · High-dose cyclosporine	↑ AUC of doxorubicin by 48% and the AUC of doxorubicinol by 443%, doxorubicin clearance ↓ by 37% → ↑ profound myelosuppression; neurotoxicity has also been observed.	Cyclosporine interferes with P-glycoprotein in normal tissues and to selectively inhibit the cytochrome P-450 enzyme system.	↓ dose of doxorubicin may be required to avoid excessive myelosuppression; monitor for sign/symptoms of ↑ neurotoxicity (confusion, headaches, coma, and seizures).	95, 96
Mercaptopurine	Doxorubicin ↑ risk of hepatotoxicity of mercaptopurine.	Possibly due to previous treatment with mercaptopurine	Monitor LFTs and signs/symptoms of liver toxicity during and after concurrent therapy.	97, 98
Paclitaxel	↑ risk of neutropenia, stomatitis, and cardiomyopathy	Sequential infusion over 24 hrs followed by 48 hrs continuous infusion doxorubicin → ↓ doxorubicin clearance → possibly due to competition for biliary excretion of both agents.	Doxorubicin should be given before paclitaxel; cumulative doxorubicin doses should also be limited to 360 mg/m² when used concurrently with paclitaxel.	99–101
Streptozocin	↑ $T_{1/2}$ of doxorubicin and ↓ doxorubicin clearance → ↑ risk of leukopenia and thrombocytopenia.	Possibly due to inhibition of hepatic metabolism of doxorubicin	↓ dose of doxorubicin if streptozocin and doxorubicin are used concomitantly.	102

Continued

DRUG INTERACTIONS

Table 4-2 Drug Interactions between Anticancer Agents and Other Drugs[4-256]—cont'd

Anticancer Agent	Concurrent Use with	Effect	Possible Mechanisms of Action if Any	Management Options	Ref.
Doxorubicin—cont'd	Thalidomide	↑ risk of DVT >6-fold in patients with multiple myeloma compared with those receiving chemotherapy without doxorubicin.	Unknown; possibly additive thrombogenic activity of doxorubicin	Avoid use of this combination outside clinical trials.	89, 103, 104
	Sorafenib	Sorafenib ↑ AUC of doxorubicin by 21% → may ↑ risk of doxorubicin toxicity	Unknown	The clinical significance of this interaction is not known; caution is advised when these two agents are coadministered. Patients should be monitored for signs of doxorubicin toxicity	105
	Trastuzumab	↑ 4 times risk of cardiac toxicities compared with trastuzumab used alone	Possibly additive effects	Avoid use of this combination outside clinical trials.	80
	Valspodar (PSC-833)	↓ clearance of doxorubicin and its active metabolite → ↑ doxorubicin toxicities	Possibly due to blockade of the multidrug resistance glycoprotein	↓ in doxorubicin dose up to 75% may be required when used with valspodar	106, 107
Epirubicin	Cimetidine	↑ mean AUC of epirubicin by 50% → ↑ plasma clearance of epirubicin by 30% → ↑ risk of epirubicin toxicities	Possibly due to inhibition of hepatic metabolism by cimetidine	Cimetidine should be avoided during epirubicin therapy or use of other histamine H2 blockers.	108
	Paclitaxel	Sequential administration of paclitaxel followed by epirubicin ↑ AUC and ↓ clearance of epirubicin by 37% and 25%, respectively compared with alternate sequence → more prolonged neutropenia.	Possibly due to (1) altered distribution of epirubicin in plasma and (2) inhibition of P-glycoprotein transporter in normal tissues by Cremophor, the vehicle of paclitaxel formulation → ↓ elimination of epirubicin	Epirubicin should always be given before paclitaxel in clinical practice.	109
Erlotinib	Ketoconazole (may apply to other potent CYP 3A4 inhibitors[b])	↑ AUC of erlotinib by 67% → may ↑ risk of toxicity	Inhibit hepatic metabolism of erlotinib via CYP 3A4	Avoid concurrent use of potent CYP 3A4 inhibitors. If concurrent use cannot be avoided, dose reduction of erlotinib dose should be considered.	110

Drug	Interacting agent	Effect	Mechanism	Recommendation	Reference
	Rifampicin (may apply to other CYP 3A4 inducers^c)	↑ clearance of erlotinib by 3-fold and ↓ AUC of erlotinib by 67%	Induce hepatic metabolism of gefitinib via CYP 3A4	Avoid concurrent use of potent CYP 3A4 inducers. If concurrent use cannot be avoided, erlotinib dose may need to be increased in the absence of a severe adverse drug reaction.	110
Estramustine	Calcium and dairy products	↓ therapeutic efficacy of estramustine	↓ absorption of estramustine due to formation of calcium-phosphate complex	Take estramustine 1 hr before or 2 hrs after dairy products or calcium supplements.	111
	High-dose carmustine in transplant setting	↑ risk of liver toxicity (toxicity occurred 1–2 mos after initiation of treatment without improving tumor response)	Possible additive effects	Avoid this combination as no improved tumor response was observed, but toxicity was increased.	51
Etoposide	High-dose cyclosporine IV (5–21 mg/kg/day; cyclosporine level >2000 ng/mL)	80% ↑ in AUC and 38% ↓ in clearance of etoposide → ↑ leucopenia and other toxicities	Because of inhibition by cyclosporine of the multidrug transporter P-glycoprotein in normal tissues	↓ dose of etoposide by 40% in children and by 50% in adults with concurrent use of high-dose cyclosporine.	112–115
	CYP 3A4 inducing anticonvulsants (phenytoin, phenobarbital)	Significantly ↑ etoposide clearance to 170% in pediatrics → ↓ therapeutic efficacy of etoposide	Due to potent induction of hepatic metabolism of etoposide via CYP 3A4	Use other anticonvulsants without properties of CYP 3A4 induction, if possible.	116
	Valspodar (PSC-833)	Concurrent use with → ↓ clearance of etoposide by 40%–60% → ↑ etoposide toxicity. See Table 4-7	Due to inhibition by cyclosporine of the multidrug transporter P-glycoprotein in normal tissues	↓ etoposide dose up to 66% may be required when used with valspodar.	117–119
Fludarabine	Warfarin		Unknown	Avoid concurrent use of both drugs outside clinical trials.	120, 121
	Pentostatin	Severe or fatal pulmonary toxicity has been reported.			122, 123
Fluorouracil	Cimetidine (oral)	↑ risk of fluorouracil toxicity	↑ AUC of fluorouracil possibly due to inhibition of hepatic metabolism and hepatic blood flow	Use of other histamine H2 blockers such as ranitidine or famotidine	124
	Hydroxyurea	High incidence of neurotoxicity (21%). No antitumor responses were observed in the study.	Possibly due to an inability to convert fluorouracil to the active metabolite and an accumulation of neurotoxins	Avoid use of this combination!	125

Continued

DRUG INTERACTIONS

Table 4-2 Drug Interactions between Anticancer Agents and Other Drugs[4-256]—cont'd

Anticancer Agent	Concurrent Use with	Effect	Possible Mechanisms of Action if Any	Management Options	Ref.
Fluorouracil—cont'd	Leucovorin	↑ cytotoxic effects but also ↑ incidence of toxicities	↑ cytotoxicity to tumor cells by maximizing binding between thymidylate synthase-fluorouracil complex	Commonly used together for ↑ cytotoxic activities; monitor for ↑ myelosuppression, diarrhea, and hand-foot syndrome.	126
	Levamisole	↑ cytotoxic but also ↑ incidence of hepatotoxicity and neurotoxicity.	Antiphosphatase activity of levamisole may ↑ fluorouracil cytotoxicity.	Monitor for ↑ myelosuppression, diarrhea, hand-foot syndrome, neurotoxicity, and signs/symptoms of hepatotoxicity.	127
	Methotrexate	↓ cytotoxic effect of methotrexate when fluorouracil is given before methotrexate.	Conversion of reduced folates to dihydrofolate is blocked.	Give methotrexate before fluorouracil.	128
	Metronidazole	↑ risk of fluorouracil toxicity by 27% (bone marrow suppression, oral ulceration, nausea, vomiting). No ↑ in antitumor activity was observed.	Due to ↓ fluorouracil clearance	Avoid concurrent use if possible.	129
	Phenytoin	↑ phenytoin levels	Fluorouracil ↓ metabolism of phenytoin by inhibiting CYP 2C9.	Monitor phenytoin levels closely during discontinuation of fluorouracil therapy.	130
	Thalidomide	↑ risk of venous thromboembolism	Unknown; possibly due to increased vascular endothelial damage by fluorouracil → initiate thalidomide-mediated thrombosis	Avoid use of this combination as no improved tumor response was observed between fluorouracil, gemcitabine, and thalidomide.	131
Flutamide	Warfarin	See Table 4-7			132–136
Gefitinib	Warfarin	See Table 4-7			137
	Itraconazole (may apply to other potent CYP 3A4-inhibitors)[b]	↑ AUC of gefitinib doses of 250 and 500 mg by 78% and 61%, respectively → may ↑ risk of toxicity	Inhibit hepatic metabolism of gefitinib via CYP 3A4	Avoid concurrent use of potent CYP 3A4 inhibitors. In the study, the authors suggested that since gefitinib is known to have a good tolerability profile, a dosage reduction is not recommended.	138
	Metoprolol (may apply to other CYP 2D6 substrates)[j]	↑ AUC of metoprolol by 35%, but no apparent change in the safety profile of metoprolol was reported in the study.	Inhibit hepatic metabolism of metoprolol via CYP 2D6 by gefitinib	Clinically relevant drug interactions between gefitinib and CYP 2D6 substrates may be not significant because gefitinib is a weak CYP 2D6 inhibitor, and no dosing adjustment is required.	138
	Rifampin (may apply to other potent CYP 3A4 inducers)[c]	↓ AUC of gefitinib by 83%	Induce hepatic metabolism of gefitinib via CYP 3A4	Avoid concurrent use of potent CYP 3A4 inducers. If concurrent use cannot be avoided, a gefitinib dose increase to 500 mg daily should be considered in the absence of a severe adverse drug reaction.	138

Drug	Interacting agent	Effect	Mechanism	Management	Reference
Gemcitabine	Warfarin	See Table 4-7			139
Hydroxyurea	Warfarin	See Table 4-7			140
	Didanosine and/or stavudine	May ↑ risk of pancreatitis and severe peripheral neuropathy	Due to hydroxyurea ↑ action of nucleoside analogs → potentiating intracellular toxicity of didanosine or stavudine such as pancreatitis	Monitor closely for signs/symptoms of pancreatitis and check lipase/amylase level as clinically indicated; monitor for signs/symptoms of peripheral neuropathy (tingling, numbness, and nerve pain).	141
	Fluorouracil	Associated with high incidence of neurotoxicity (21%). No antitumor responses were observed in the study.	Possibly due to an inability to convert fluorouracil to the active metabolite and an accumulation of neurotoxins	Avoid use of this combination.	125
Ifosfamide	Cisplatin	↑ risk of neurotoxicity, hematotoxicity, and tubular nephrotoxicity of ifosfamide	Cisplatin-induced renal damage → impaired clearance of ifosfamide metabolites → ↑ toxicities.	Monitor renal function and adjust dose of ifosfamide based on CrCl; provide vigorous hydration and give mesna for uroprotection.	61–63
	Ketoconazole (CYP 3A4 inhibitors[b])	May ↓ levels of 4-hydroxyifosfamide, active metabolite of ifosfamide	Due to inhibition of hepatic conversion to active metabolites	Monitor for clinical efficacy/toxicities.	142
Ifosfamide	Rifampin (CYP 3A4 inducers[c])	↑ rate of biotransformation of ifosfamide to 4-hydroxyifosfamide (active metabolite) → but no change in AUC of hydroxyifosfamide; ↑ rate of bio-transformation of ifosfamide to (S)-ifosfamide which in turns generates (R)-3-dechlorethyl-ifosfamide via N-dechlorethylation → ↑ risk of neurotoxicity	Due to increased clearance of ifosfamide via induction of CYP 3A4 and CYP 2B6	Clinical drug interaction is probably of minimal significance.	142
Imatinib	Warfarin	See Table 4-7			143
	CYP 3A4 inhibitors[b]	May ↑ AUC of imatinib → ↑ toxicities such as neutropenia	Inhibits hepatic metabolism of imatinib via CYP 3A4	Monitor for clinical efficacy/toxicities, and adjust doses as needed.	144, 145
	CYP 3A4 inducers[c]	May ↓ AUC of imatinib → ↓ clinical efficacy of imatinib	Induces hepatic metabolism of imatinib via CYP 3A4	Monitor for clinical efficacy/toxicities, and adjust doses as needed.	144, 146–149

Continued

DRUG INTERACTIONS

Table 4-2 Drug Interactions between Anticancer Agents and Other Drugs[4–256]—cont'd

Anticancer Agent	Concurrent Use with	Effect	Possible Mechanisms of Action if Any	Management Options	Ref.
Imatinib—cont'd	CYP 2C9 substrates[e]	May ↑ levels of the interacting drugs → ↑ risk of toxicities	Imatinib is a moderate CYP 2C9 inhibitor → inhibit hepatic metabolism.	Monitor for clinical efficacy/toxicities, and adjust doses as needed	144, 150
	CYP 2D6 substrates[f]	May ↑ levels of the interacting drugs → ↑ risk of toxicities	Imatinib is a moderate CYP 2D6 inhibitor → inhibit hepatic metabolism.	Monitor for clinical efficacy/toxicities, and adjust doses as needed	144, 150
	Cyclosporine (or other CYP 3A4 substrates[d])	↑ AUC of cyclosporine by 20%–23%	Inhibits hepatic metabolism of cyclosporine via CYP 3A4 by imatinib	Clinical drug interaction may not be clinically significant; monitor closely for cyclosporine levels toxicities, and adjust doses as needed.	151
	Simvastatin and other statins (atorvastatin, cerivastatin, lovastatin)	Coadministration of imatinib (400 mg daily) at steady state with simvastatin (40 mg) ↑ the exposure (C_{max} and AUCs) of simvastatin significantly by 2- to 3-fold	Inhibits hepatic metabolism of simvastatin via CYP 3A4	Monitor creatine kinase and BUN/Scr and for signs of muscle weakness or lethargy	152
	Warfarin	See Table 4-7			144, 150
Interferon alfa	Theophylline	100% ↑ in theophylline level → ↑ risk of theophylline toxicity, especially in those who are fast metabolizers of theophylline.	Unknown; interferons may inhibit activity of hepatic P450 enzymes.	Monitor clinical response and theophylline toxicities; may adjust dose of theophylline and monitor theophylline level as clinically indicated.	153
	Zidovudine	↑ risk of hematologic toxicity	Additive hematologic effects	Dose reduction of interferon alfa or discontinuation may be required when used with zidovudine.	154
Irinotecan	Atazanavir	Combination may result in ↑ plasma concentrations of irinotecan and ↑ irinotecan toxicities (diarrhea and bone marrow suppression).	Inhibition of UGT 1A1–mediated irinotecan metabolism by atazanavir	Coadministration of atazanavir and irinotecan is not recommended. If concomitant use cannot be avoided, monitor the patient for signs and symptoms of irinotecan toxicity.	155
	Dexamethasone	↑ irinotecan clearance → ↓ clinical efficacy.	Possibly due to potential ↑ biliary excretion of the drug and its metabolite SN-38 or induction of metabolism of irinotecan via CYP 3A4	Monitor antitumor effect; ↑ dose of irinotecan may be required if combined use cannot be avoided (e.g., brain tumor). If dexamethasone is used as an antiemetic, use of other alternatives is recommended.	87

Continued

Drug	Interacting Drug	Effect	Mechanism	Management	Reference
	Ketoconazole (may apply to other potent CYP 3A4 inhibitors[b])	↑ AUC of SN-38 by 109% → ↑ toxicity of irinotecan.	Inhibits metabolism of irinotecan via CYP 3A4	Dose reduction of irinotecan by 50%–75% is recommended when coadministered with potent CYP-3A4 inhibitors.	156
	Nicotinamide	Intratumoral uptake of irinotecan and its active metabolite SN-38 decreased significantly between 19% and 43%; plasma levels of irinotecan and SN-38 increase and decrease, respectively, after nicotinamide exposure.	Conversion of irinotecan to its active metabolite SN-38 by carboxylesterase is inhibited by nicotinamide.	Clinical significance is unclear; avoid concomitant use if possible and monitor clinical efficacy and toxicity of irinotecan.	157
	Phenytoin (may apply to other potent CYP 3A4 inducers[c])	↓ AUC of irinotecan and SN-38 by 63% and 60%, respectively.	Due to potent induction of hepatic metabolism via CYP 3A4	If enzyme-inducing anticonvulsants need to be used, dose of irinotecan needs to be ↑, probably by 50%. Otherwise, consider use of other non–enzyme-inducing anticonvulsants to avoid this significant drug interaction.	158–161
	Tacrolimus (FK 506)	SN-38 glucuronidation was reduced for up to 12 hrs after irinotecan infusion → increased severity of diarrhea in transplant patients.	An increase in systemic exposure to unbound SN-38 might account for diarrhea.	Dose reduction of starting dose of irinotecan may need to be considered in patients receiving tacrolimus.	162
	Sorafenib	Sorafenib ↑ AUC of irinotecan and its active metabolite SN-38 by 26%–42% and 57%–120%, respectively.	Sorafenib inhibits the UGT1A1 pathway-mediated metabolism of irinotecan and its metabolite SN-38.	Although the clinical significance of this interaction is not known, caution is advised if irinotecan and sorafenib are coadministered; monitor for signs of irinotecan toxicity.	105
Ketoconazole	CYP 3A4 substrates[d]	Significantly ↑ AUC of 3A4 substrates → may ↑ efficacy but also toxicities of substrates	Due to potent inhibition of CYP 3A4 by ketoconazole	Dose reduction of starting dose of CYP 3A4 substrates may need to be considered in patients receiving ketoconazole concomitantly.	163
Letrozole	Tamoxifen	↓ 38% of [letrozole] → may ↓ efficacy of letrozole.	Possibly due to an induction of letrozole-metabolizing enzymes by tamoxifen	Avoid use of this combination outside clinical trials.	164

DRUG INTERACTIONS

Table 4-2 Drug Interactions between Anticancer Agents and Other Drugs[4-256]—cont'd

Anticancer Agent	Concurrent Use with	Effect	Possible Mechanisms of Action if Any	Management Options	Ref.
Levamisole	Fluorouracil	↑ cytotoxic but also ↑ incidence of hepatotoxicity and neurotoxicity	Antiphosphatase activity of levamisole may ↑ fluorouracil cytotoxicity.	Monitor for ↑ myelosuppression, diarrhea, hand-foot syndrome, neurotoxicity, and signs/symptoms of hepatotoxicity.	127
	Rifampicin	↓ clinical efficacy of rifampicin	Levamisole displaces rifampicin from protein binding sites → ↑ free fraction of rifampicin by 3 times → ↑ its clearance.	Avoid use of combination if possible.	165
Lenalidomide	Dexamethasone	↑ risk of DVT in patients with multiple myeloma	Possibly additive thrombogenic activity of lenalidomide	Closely monitor for signs and symptoms of DVT and PEs. In patients with history of VTE, anticoagulation should be considered as secondary prophylaxis.	88
	Digoxin	Coadministration of digoxin and lenalidomide resulted in a 14% increase in digoxin C_{max}; however, digoxin AUC was not significantly affected.	Unknown	If these two agents are coadministered, monitor digoxin plasma levels periodically, based on clinical judgment and standard clinical practices.	166
Lomustine	Cimetidine	↑ bone marrow suppression	Possibly due to inhibition of lomustine metabolism	Avoid use of cimetidine or use other histamine H2 blockers (e.g., ranitidine).	167
	Phenobarbital	↓ efficacy of lomustine	Induction of hepatic metabolism via P450 enzymes	Avoid use of combination or ↑ the dose of lomustine; monitor clinical efficacy.	168
Medroxypro-gesterone	Aminoglutethi-mide	↓ efficacy of medroxyprogesterone	Due to ↑ hepatic metabolism of medroxyprogesterone via P450 enzymes	Clinical significance may be minimal as both drugs are rarely given concomitantly in clinical practice nowadays.	14
	CYP 3A4 inhibitors[b]	May ↑ levels of medroxyprogesterone	Due to inhibiting hepatic metabolism of medroxyprogesterone via CYP 3A4	Clinical relevance is unknown; monitor for clinical toxicities.	169, 170
	CYP 3A4 inducers[c]	May ↓ levels of medroxyprogesterone	Due to inducing hepatic metabolism of medroxyprogesterone via CYP 3A4	Theoretical concern; clinical relevance is unknown because medroxyprogesterone itself is an inducer; monitor closely for clinical efficacy of medroxyprogesterone.	169-171
	Prednisolone (or other CYP 3A4 substrates[d])	Unbound prednisolone clearance increased by 25% after 2 months of intramuscular medroxyprogesterone therapy; no effect with oral medroxyprogesterone	Induction of hepatic metabolism of prednisolone via CYP 3A4 by IV medroxyprogesterone, but not seen in oral form of medroxyprogesterone.	Clinically significant interaction is unclear; monitor for clinical efficacy.	170

Drug	Interacting agent	Effect	Mechanism	Management	Ref
Melphalan	Cimetidine	Cimetidine ↓ oral bioavailability of melphalan by 30% → ↓ efficacy of melphalan.	Due to change of gastric pH	Avoid concurrent administration of both drugs; or monitor for clinical response and may adjust melphalan dose as needed.	172
	Digoxin	↓ digoxin serum level → ↓ efficacy	High-dose melphalan ↓ absorption of digoxin tablet by 45%.	Substitute liquid form for digoxin tablet; monitor for HR and for CHF symptoms, and check digoxin levels as clinically indicated.	173, 174
Mercaptopurine	Allopurinol	↑ [6-mercaptopurine] → ↑ its toxicity	Inhibits metabolism of oral 6-mercaptopurine by xanthine oxidase → accumulation of toxic metabolites	Dose of oral 6-mercaptopurine should be ↓ to 25%–33% of the usual dose when given concomitantly with allopurinol in clinical practice.	175–177
	Doxorubicin	↑ risk of profound myelosuppression of doxorubicin	Possibly due to liver dysfunction → impair drug metabolism of doxorubicin	Monitor closely for myelosuppression and risk of infection due to profound neutropenia.	178
	Oral methotrexate (20 mg/m²) or high-dose methotrexate	31% ↑ in AUC and 26% ↑ in peak [6-mercaptopurine] → ↑ risk of myelotoxicities	Methotrexate ↑ oral bioavailability of 6-mercaptopurine.	Dose of oral 6-mercaptopurine should be reduced when used with oral methotrexate >20 mg/m² or high-dose methotrexate given IV.	
	Warfarin See Table 4-5				
Methotrexate		See Table 4-7			179–204
Methylprednisolone	CYP 3A4 inhibitors[b]	May ↑ adrenal-suppressive effects	May ↑ levels of methylprednisolone due to inhibiting hepatic metabolism via CYP 3A4	Plasma cortisol level monitoring may be required; monitor for clinical responses and toxicities.	205, 206
	CYP 3A4 inducers[c]	May ↓ adrenal-suppressive or antitumor effects	May ↓ levels of methylprednisolone → due to inducing hepatic metabolism via CYP 3A4	May avoid concomitant use of enzyme-inducing anticonvulsants if methylprednisolone is used as anticancer agent (e.g. in lymphoma setting).	207
	CYP 3A4 substrates[d]	High-dose methylprednisolone may ↓ AUC of CYP 3A4 substrates → may ↓ efficacy of the substrates in one study but no change in another one.	Due to induction of CYP 3A4 by high-dose methylprednisolone	Conflicting results were reported in the literature; clinically significant drug interaction is unclear.	208, 209

Continued

DRUG INTERACTIONS

Table 4-2 Drug Interactions between Anticancer Agents and Other Drugs[4-256]—cont'd

Anticancer Agent	Concurrent Use with	Effect	Possible Mechanisms of Action if Any	Management Options	Ref.
Mitomycin C	Tamoxifen	↑ incidence of anemia and thrombocytopenia and the risk of hemolytic-uremic syndrome	Mitomycin causes subclinical endothelial damage in addition to the thrombotic effect on platelets caused by tamoxifen → hemolytic uremic syndrome.	Monitor clinical signs/symptoms of bleeding and watch closely for renal function.	210
	Vinblastine (other vinca alkaloid such as vinorelbine also reported)	Abrupt pulmonary toxicity in 3%–6% of patients. This toxicity is associated with ≥2 courses of combination therapy.	Unknown; possible additive effect	Monitor closely for pulmonary toxicities (shortness of breath and bronchospasm) when these drugs are used together.	211–214
Mitoxantrone	High-dose cyclosporine level 3000–5000 ng/mL	42% ↓ in clearance of mitoxantrone and ↑ its terminal $T_{1/2}$ by 58% → no toxicity was observed, however.	Due to inhibition by PSC-833 of the multidrug transporter P-glycoprotein in normal tissues	Monitor AUC of mitoxantrone, and dose reduction of mitoxantrone by 40% in pediatric patients is still recommended to achieve similar drug exposure.	215
Mitoxantrone	Valspodar (PSC-833)	↑ elimination $T_{1/2}$ and AUC → severe mucositis and hyperbilirubinemia.	Due to inhibition of the multidrug transporter P-glycoprotein by PSC-833 in normal tissues	Requirement of dose reduction by 20%–66% has been reported for mitoxantrone when given with valspodar.	
Nelarabine	Pentostatin	Pentostatin ↓ conversion of nelarabine to its active moiety → ↓ nelarabine efficacy, and/or after nelarabine adverse event profile.	Pentostatin has been shown to be a strong inhibitor of ADA in vitro. Concurrent administration of nelarabine and pentostatin may result in reduced ADA-dependent conversion of nelarabine to its active moiety.	Concurrent administration of nelarabine with pentostatin is not recommended.	215
Nilutamide	Phenytoin	May ↑ phenytoin level → ↑ risk of toxicity.	Nilutamide may inhibit the activity of hepatic cytochrome P450 isoenzymes.	Monitor phenytoin toxicities (nystagmus, ataxia, lethargy, vertigo, and decreased mental capacity), and check phenytoin levels as clinically indicated.	216, 217
	Warfarin	See Table 4-7			216

Ondansetron	Rifampin (may apply to other CYP 3A4 inducers)	Rifampin ↓ bioavailability of oral ondansetron from 60%–40%; rifampin ↓ AUC of oral ondansetron by 65%; rifampin ↑ clearance of IV ondansetron by 83% and ↓ T$_{1/2}$ of IV ondansetron by 46% and ↓ AUC by 48%.	Induction of the CYP 3A4–mediated metabolism of ondansetron by rifampin	Concomitant use of rifampin or other potent inducers of CYP 3A4 with ondansetron may result in a reduced antiemetic effect, particularly after oral administration of ondansetron. Increasing ondansetron dosage may be required to prevent severe nausea and vomiting especially in patients receiving highly emetogenic chemotherapy; may also consider use of other 5-hydroxytryptamine$_3$ antagonist (dolasetron) with less clinically significant drug interactions with rifampin.	218
Paclitaxel	Carboplatin	Decreased thrombocytopenia was observed in patients receiving a combination of carboplatin and paclitaxel compared with those who received carboplatin alone.	Unknown; no changes in pharmacokinetics of either drugs	Drug selection depends on different cancer settings and different toxicity profile (e.g., carboplatin used alone in ovarian cancer has been shown to achieve similar overall survival compared with the combination of carboplatin and paclitaxel but with a lower nonhematologic toxicity profile).	42–45
	Cisplatin (when paclitaxel infused over 24 hrs was given after cisplatin)	Caused more profound neutropenia	Administration of cisplatin before paclitaxel ↓ paclitaxel clearance by 25%.	Administer paclitaxel first, followed by cisplatin.	65
	Cyclophospha- mide (when paclitaxel in- fused over 24– 72 hrs was ad- ministered before cyclo- phosphamide)	↑ severity of neutropenia, thrombocytopenia, and mucositis	Unknown; as no pharmacokinetic parameters were altered for either drugs with sequential administration of both	Administer cyclophosphamide first, followed by paclitaxel.	77, 78

Continued

DRUG INTERACTIONS

Table 4-2 Drug Interactions between Anticancer Agents and Other Drugs[4-256]—cont'd

Anticancer Agent	Concurrent Use with	Effect	Possible Mechanisms of Action if Any	Management Options	Ref.
Paclitaxel—cont'd	CYP 3A4 inducers[c]	May ↑ metabolism of paclitaxel → ↓ paclitaxel efficacy	Induction of hepatic metabolism of paclitaxel via CYP 3A4	Monitor for clinical efficacy; one study suggested that 50% ↑ dose of paclitaxel may be needed to account for the effects of enzyme induction.	219, 220
	Doxorubicin	↑ risk of neutropenia, stomatitis, and cardiomyopathy	Sequential infusion over 24 hrs followed by 48 hrs continuous infusion doxorubicin → ↓ doxorubicin clearance → possibly due to competition for biliary excretion of both agents.	Doxorubicin should be given before paclitaxel; cumulative doxorubicin doses should also be limited to 360 mg/m² when used concurrently with paclitaxel.	99–101
	Epirubicin	Sequential administration of paclitaxel followed by epirubicin ↑ AUC and ↓ clearance of epirubicin by 37% and 25%, respectively, when compared with alternate sequence → more prolonged neutropenia	Possibly due to (1) altered distribution of epirubicin in plasma and (2) inhibition of P-glycoprotein transporter in normal tissues by Cremophor, the vehicle of paclitaxel formulation → ↓ elimination of epirubicin.	Epirubicin should always be given before paclitaxel in clinical practice.	109
	Trastuzumab	↑ risk of cardiotoxicity compared with trastuzumab used alone.	Possible additive effects	Monitor closely for cardiotoxicity when concurrent use of these drugs is necessary.	80
	Valspodar	↑ [paclitaxel] and its AUC → ↑ hematologic toxicity	Due to inhibition by PSC-833 of the multidrug transporter P-glycoprotein in normal tissues	Dose reductions of paclitaxel by up to 50%–60% if combined with valspodar	221
	Vinblastine	↓ cytotoxic effects, and less toxicities were observed in combination use.	Antagonistic interaction between the drugs	Combination use of vinblastine and paclitaxel is not recommended.	222
	Warfarin	See Table 4-7			223
Pentostatin	High-dose cyclophosphamide in bone marrow transplant settings	Fatal cardiac toxicity has been reported.	Possibly due to interference with adenosine metabolism to cyclophosphamide	Avoid use of this combination outside clinical trials.	79
	Fludarabine	Severe or fatal pulmonary toxicity has been reported.	Unknown; possible additive toxicity	Avoid use of this combination outside clinical trials.	122, 123

Drug	Interacting agent	Effect	Mechanism	Management/Comment	Reference
Nelarabine		Pentostatin ↓ conversion of nelarabine to its active moiety → ↓ nelarabine efficacy, and/or after nelarabine adverse event profile.	Pentostatin has been shown to be a strong inhibitor of ADA in vitro. Concurrent administration of nelarabine and pentostatin may result in reduced ADA-dependent conversion of nelarabine to its active moiety.	Concurrent administration of nelarabine with pentostatin is not recommended.	215
Porfimer	Photosensitizing agents (phenothiazines, sulfonylureas, thiazide diuretics, sulfa products)	May ↑ severity of photosensitivity reactions and tissue damages	Additive effects	Avoid exposure of skin and eyes to direct sunlight for 30 days after porfimer therapy.	224
Prednisolone	CYP 3A4 inhibitors[b]	May ↑ adrenal-suppressive effects	May ↑ levels of prednisolone due to inhibiting hepatic metabolism via CYP 3A4	Plasma cortisol level monitoring may be required; monitor for clinical responses and toxicities.	225
Prednisolone	CYP 3A4 inducers[c]	May ↓ immunosuppressive effects.	↑ elimination of prednisolone→ due to inducing hepatic metabolism via CYP 3A4	Monitor for clinical response, may need to ↑ dose of prednisone to achieve immunosuppressive effect, especially when used in transplant setting.	226–229
Procarbazine	CYP 3A4 inducers[c] (e.g., non–enzyme-inducing anticonvulsants)	↑ risk of procarbazine hypersensitivity reactions in patients with brain tumors	Possibly due to a reactive intermediate generated by CYP 3A isoform induction; strong correlation between therapeutic anticonvulsant level and the hypersensitivity reactions	Consider using non–enzyme-inducing anticonvulsants in patients who receive procarbazine.	230, 231
	High-dose methotrexate	Methotrexate infusion given within 48 hrs of administration of procarbazine ↑ risk of renal impairment.	Procarbazine has a transient effect on the kidneys. If high-dose methotrexate is given before recovery from this change → delays renal excretion of methotrexate and prolongs exposure of the kidneys to methotrexate.	Do not start methotrexate infusion ≤72 hrs after the last dose of procarbazine. Provide aggressive hydration, alkalinize urine to pH >7.0, and monitor renal function closely (BUN, Scr, and fluid status) before, during, and after methotrexate infusion until methotrexate level <0.05 µmol/dL.	195

Continued

DRUG INTERACTIONS

Table 4-2 Drug Interactions between Anticancer Agents and Other Drugs[4-256]—cont'd

Anticancer Agent	Concurrent Use with	Effect	Possible Mechanisms of Action if Any	Management Options	Ref.
Procarbazine—cont'd	MAOIs	↑ risk of hypertensive crisis or seizures	Additive effects	Interactions may be of clinical insignificance because procarbazine is a mild MAOI; monitor blood pressure closely and CNS side effects, especially in patients with a history of uncontrolled hypertension.	230, 232
	Selective serotonin reuptake inhibitors	May ↑ risk of serotonin syndrome[k] and CNS toxicity	Additive effects	Interactions may be of clinical insignificance because procarbazine is a mild MAOI; monitor blood pressure closely and CNS side effects, especially in patients with history of uncontrolled hypertension.	230, 233
	Sympathomimetics[l]	May ↑ risk of hypertension	Additive effects	Interactions may be of clinical insignificance because procarbazine is a mild MAOI; monitor blood pressure closely and CNS side effects, especially in patients with a history of uncontrolled hypertension.	230
	Tyramine-containing food[m]	May ↑ risk of flushing/rash reaction, headache, intracranial bleeding, and hypertensive crisis	High concentration of tyramine achieved in circulation will displace norepinephrine and other catecholamines from presynaptic storage granules → MAOIs like procarbazine may inhibit metabolic degradation of these catecholamines → may trigger profound pressor response.	Interactions may be of clinical insignificance because procarbazine is a mild MAOI; if possible, minimize tyramine-containing food during treatment with procarbazine and watch for the side effects, especially in patients with a history of uncontrolled hypertension.	230
Rituximab	Cisplatin	↑ risk of severe renal failure	Unknown; possibly due to effects of tumor lysis syndrome	Monitor for renal function closely; before, during, and after administration hydrate with at least 2 L of fluid, replenish potassium and magnesium if deficient before administration of both agents.	66
Sorafenib	Doxorubicin	↑ AUC of doxorubicin by 21% → may ↑ risk of toxicity	Unknown	The clinical significance of this interaction is not known; caution is advised when these two agents are coadministered; monitor for signs of doxorubicin toxicity.	234

	Irinotecan	Sorafenib ↑ AUC of irinotecan and its active metabolite SN-38 by 26%–42% and 57%–120%, respectively.	Sorafenib inhibits the UGT1A1 pathway-mediated metabolism of irinotecan and its metabolite SN-38.	Although the clinical significance of this interaction is not known, caution is advised if irinotecan and sorafenib are coadministered; monitor for signs of irinotecan toxicity.	105
	Itraconazole (may apply to other potent CYP 3A4 inhibitors[b])	May ↑ AUC of sorafenib	Inhibit hepatic metabolism of sorafenib via CYP 3A4	Avoid concurrent use of potent CYP 3A4 inhibitors. In the study, the author suggested that since sorafenib is known to have a good tolerability profile, a dosage reduction is not recommended.	234
	Rifampin (may apply to other potent CYP 3A4 inducers[c])	May ↓ AUC of sorafenib	Induce hepatic metabolism of sorafenib via CYP 3A4	Avoid concurrent use of potent CYP 3A4 inducers. If concurrent use cannot be avoided, doses of sorafenib may be considered to be increased in the absence of a severe adverse drug reaction.	234
Sunitinib	Ketoconazole (may apply to other potent CYP 3A4 inhibitors[b])	↑ AUC of sunitinib by 51% → may ↑ risk of toxicity	Inhibit hepatic metabolism of sunitinib via CYP 3A4	Avoid concurrent use of potent CYP 3A4 inhibitors. If concurrent use cannot be avoided, a dose reduction for sunitinib is recommended; consider reducing the dose to a minimum of 37.5 mg daily.	235
	Rifampin (may apply to other potent CYP 3A4 inducers[c])	↓ AUC of sunitinib by 46%	Induce hepatic metabolism of sunitinib via CYP 3A4	Avoid concurrent use of potent CYP 3A4 inducers. If concurrent use cannot be avoided, the sunitinib dose may be increased in 12.5-mg increments, depending on individual safety and tolerability, to a maximum daily dose of 87.5 mg daily.	235
Streptozocin	Doxorubicin	↑ $T_{1/2}$ of doxorubicin and ↓ doxorubicin clearance → ↑ risk of leukopenia and thrombocytopenia	Possibly due to inhibition of hepatic metabolism of doxorubicin	↓ dose of doxorubicin if streptozocin and doxorubicin are used concomitantly.	102
	Phenytoin	Insulin release ↓ → ↓ efficacy of streptozocin	Unknown; phenytoin protects the β cells from cytotoxicity of streptozocin.	Avoid this combination or use other non–enzyme-inducing anticonvulsants for seizure control if clinically applicable.	236

Continued

DRUG INTERACTIONS

Table 4-2 Drug Interactions between Anticancer Agents and Other Drugs[4-256]—cont'd

Anticancer Agent	Concurrent Use with	Effect	Possible Mechanisms of Action if Any	Management Options	Ref.
Tamoxifen	Aminoglutethimide	↓ [tamoxifen] → may ↓ antitumor efficacy of tamoxifen	↑ metabolism via P450 enzymes	Clinical significance may be minimal as both drugs are rarely given concomitantly in clinical practice nowadays.	15
	Letrozole	↓ 38% of [letrozole] → may ↓ efficacy of letrozole	Possibly due to an induction of letrozole-metabolizing enzymes by tamoxifen	Avoid use of this combination outside clinical trials	164
	Mitomycin C	↑ incidence of anemia, thrombocytopenia, and the risk of hemolytic uremic syndrome	Mitomycin causes subclinical endothelial damage in addition to the thrombotic effect on platelets caused by tamoxifen → hemolytic uremic syndrome	Monitor closely for clinical signs/symptoms of bleeding, renal function.	210
	Rifampin (may apply to other CYP 3A4 inducers[c])	↓ [tamoxifen] by rifampin	Possibly due to an induction of metabolism via CYP 3A enzymes	Avoid use of this combination if possible; adjust the dose of tamoxifen and monitor for clinical efficacy of tamoxifen.	237
Teniposide	Warfarin	See Table 4-7			238–240
	Asparaginase	↑ in unbound teniposide → ↑ bone marrow toxicity	Asparaginase ↓ production of albumin → ↓ protein binding of teniposide.	Monitor for drug toxicity, and dosage of teniposide may need to be adjusted.	
	Phenytoin or phenobarbital (may apply to other potent CYP 3A4 inducers[c])	↑ teniposide clearance by 2–3 times → ↓ efficacy of teniposide	Due to an induction of metabolism via CYP 3A enzymes	Monitor for efficacy; may need to ↑ dose of teniposide if anticonvulsants are coadministered.	241
Thalidomide	Darbepoetin alfa	Thalidomide ↑ the thromboembolic risk of darbepoetin alfa patients with myelodysplastic syndrome.	Additive thrombogenic effect	Careful clinical observation is warranted, and thrombosis prophylaxis should be considered.	81
	Dexamethasone	↑ risk of DVT → 15% in patients with multiple myeloma compared with those receiving thalidomide monotherapy.	Unknown; possibly additive thrombogenic activity of thalidomide	Closely monitor for signs and symptoms of DVT and PEs. In patients with a history of VTE, anticoagulation should be considered as secondary prophylaxis.	89

	Interacting agent	Effect	Mechanism	Recommendation	Reference
	Doxorubicin	↑ risk of DVT >6-fold in patients with multiple myeloma compared with those receiving chemotherapy without doxorubicin	Unknown; possibly additive thrombogenic activity of doxorubicin	Avoid use of this combination outside clinical trials.	89, 103, 104
	Fluorouracil	↑ risk of venous thromboembolism	Unknown; possibly due to increased vascular endothelial damage by fluorouracil → initiate thalidomide-mediated thrombosis	Avoid use of this combination as no improved tumor response was observed between fluorouracil, gemcitabine, and thalidomide.	131
Thioguanine	Busulfan	↑ risk of hepatic nodular regenerative hyperplasia of the liver, esophageal varices, and portal hypertension	Unknown	Monitor LFTs; signs/symptoms of liver toxicities (portal hypertension, esophageal varices, ascites, splenomegaly, and gastrointestinal bleeding). *Note:* Clinical significance may be minimal as a combination of both drugs is rarely used in CML.	38
Thiotepa	Aprepitant	Formation clearance of thiotepa by aprepitant was reduced by 33%, and exposures to active metabolite of tepa was ↓ by 20%; 50% inhibitory concentration of aprepitant for inhibition of thiotepa was within therapeutic range.	Inhibit hepatic metabolism of high-dose thiotepa (120 mg/m^2/day for 4 days) via CYP 3A4 and/or 2B6	Interaction between aprepitant and high-dose thiotepa is clinically negligible.	19
Topotecan	Cisplatin	When topotecan dose was given at >0.75mg/m^2 on days 1–5 plus cisplatin dose at >50 mg/m^2, the sequence of cisplatin given on day 1 before topotecan caused more severe bone marrow suppression than the alternate sequence in which cisplatin was given on day 5.	↓ topotecan clearance and subclinical renal toxicity induced by cisplatin.	Administer cisplatin on day 5 after topotecan if 1st dose of topotecan >0.75 mg/m^2 plus cisplatin >50 mg/m^2 is given, with the aid of granulocyte CSFs.	70
	Docetaxel	Administration of topotecan on days 1–4 and docetaxel on day 4 compared with same regimen except docetaxel given on day 1 ↑ incidence of neutropenia.	Due to 50% ↓ in docetaxel clearance; possible inhibition of hepatic metabolism of docetaxel by topotecan via CYP 3A4	Give docetaxel on day 1 and topotecan on days 1–4.	93

Continued

DRUG INTERACTIONS

Table 4-2 Drug Interactions between Anticancer Agents and Other Drugs[1-256]—cont'd

Anticancer Agent	Concurrent Use with	Effect	Possible Mechanisms of Action if Any	Management Options	Ref.
Topotecan—cont'd	Phenytoin	↑ topotecan lactone and clearance of its metabolite by 1.5 times → may ↓ efficacy of topotecan.	Possibly due to induction of hepatic metabolism of topotecan via CYP 3A4 by phenytoin	Consider use of non–enzyme-inducing anticonvulsants if possible; otherwise, consider ↑ dose of topotecan.	242
Toremifene	CYP 3A4 inhibitors[b]	May ↑ levels of toremifene	Due to ↓ hepatic metabolism of toremifene via inhibition of CYP 3A4	Clinical relevance is unknown; monitor for clinical toxicities.	243
	Rifampin (may apply to other CYP 3A4 inducers[c])	Rifampin ↓ AUC of toremifene by 87%, ↓ C_{max} by 55% and $T_{1/2}$ by 44% → may ↓ antiestrogen effects	Due to ↑ hepatic metabolism of toremifene via induction of CYP 3A4	Avoid enzyme-inducing anticonvulsants if possible; monitor closely for clinical efficacy of toremifene and ↑ the dose as indicated if concomitant use of rifampin is unavoidable.	237, 243
Trastuzumab	Cyclophosphamide	May ↑ cardiac toxicities	Unknown; possible additive effects	Monitor for cardiac toxicities closely.	80
	Doxorubicin (apply to other anthracyclines)	↑ 4 times risk of cardiac toxicities when compared with trastuzumab used alone	Unknown; possible additive effects	Avoid concurrent use outside clinical trials.	80
	Paclitaxel	↑ risk of cardiotoxicity compared with trastuzumab used alone.	Unknown; possible additive effects	Monitor for cardiac toxicities closely.	80
Trimetrexate	Azole antifungals (may apply to other CYP 3A4 inhibitors[b])	May ↑ levels of trimetrexate → ↑ risk of toxicity	Due to ↓ hepatic metabolism of trimetrexate via inhibition of CYP 3A4	Monitor for clinical efficacy and toxicities, and adjust the dose of trimetrexate as needed.	244
Vinblastine	CYP 3A4 inducers[c]	May ↓ levels of vinblastine → ↓ efficacy of vinblastine	Due to ↑ hepatic metabolism of vinblastine via induction of CYP 3A4	Monitor for clinical efficacy; may need to ↑ dose of vinblastine as clinically indicated.	245
	Erythromycin (may apply to other potent CYP 3A4 inhibitors[b])	↑ risk of bone marrow toxicity, neurotoxicity, and ileus	Erythromycin may ↓ hepatic metabolism via inhibition of CYP 3A4 and/or drug efflux of vinblastine via P glycoprotein.	Avoid the use of this combination; may consider use of other macrolides (such as azithromycin instead of erythromycin).	246
	Mitomycin C	Abrupt pulmonary toxicity in 3%–6% of patients. This toxicity is associated with ≥2 courses of combination therapy.	Unknown; possible additive effect	Monitor closely for pulmonary toxicities (shortness of breath, bronchospasm) when these drugs are used together.	211-214
	Paclitaxel	↓ cytotoxic effects and less toxicities were observed in combination use.	Antagonistic interaction between the drugs	Combination use of vinblastine and paclitaxel is not recommended.	222

	Interacting agent	Effect	Mechanism	Management	References
Vincristine	Asparaginase	Administering asparaginase concurrently with or before vincristine ↑ risk of neurotoxicity of vincristine.	Possibly due to ↓ vincristine metabolism from the effects of asparaginase on hepatic function.	Administer vincristine before asparaginase.	28
	CSFs (filgrastim or sargramostim)	A high incidence of severe atypical neuropathy (excruciating foot pain associated with marked motor weakness) was observed in one study.	A synergistic effect between administration of CSFs and vincristine to cause neuropathy; most strongly associated with cumulative dose of vincristine (size of individual doses, number of doses given in cycle 1 in the study).	Modification of the study protocol including two doses (given on days 1 and 8) instead of three doses of vincristine given on days 1, 8, and 15 in cycle 1 has been done in the study. Consider limiting maximum individual dose of vincristine to 2 mg; monitor closely for signs/symptoms of neurotoxicity (tingling, numbness, sharp, burning pain, foot drop, and ↓ muscle strength).	247
	High-dose cyclosporine (7.5–10 mg/kg/day IV)	May ↑ levels of vincristine → may ↑ risk of peripheral neuropathy and musculoskeletal pain	Inhibit hepatic metabolism of vincristine via CYP 3A4 and/or due to blockade of P-glycoprotein pump → inhibits vincristine efflux in tumor cells	Monitor for neurotoxicity (muscle pain, numbness, tingling in fingers and toes, jaw pain, abdominal pain, constipation, and ileus) of vincristine.	248, 249
	CYP 3A4 inducers[c]	↓ AUC of vincristine by 43%, its elimination $T_{1/2}$ by 35% and its clearance by 63% in patients with brain tumors → may possibly ↓ antitumor effect observed in brain tumor patients.	Induce hepatic metabolism of vincristine via CYP 3A4	Monitor clinical efficacy of vincristine in patients with brain tumors; may ↑ the dose of vincristine as clinically indicated.	250
	Itraconazole (may apply to other potent CYP 3A4 inhibitors)[b]	May ↑ levels of vincristine → may ↑ risk of peripheral neuropathy	Inhibit hepatic metabolism of vincristine via CYP 3A4 and/or due to blockade of P-glycoprotein pump → inhibits vincristine efflux in tumor cells	Monitor for neurotoxicity (pain, numbness, tingling in fingers and toes, jaw pain, abdominal pain, constipation, and ileus) of vincristine.	251–253
	Nifedipine	↓ metabolism of vincristine → ↑ $T_{1/2}$ and AUC of vincristine → ↑ risk of vincristine neurotoxicity	Due to blockade of P-glycoprotein pump → inhibits vincristine efflux in tumor cells	Monitor for neurotoxicity (tingling, numbness of extremities, foot drop, jaw pain, facial pain, constipation, ileus) of vincristine.	254
Vinorelbine	CYP 3A4 inhibitors[b]	May ↑ levels of vinorelbine → may ↑ risk of neurotoxicity and bone marrow toxicity	Inhibit hepatic metabolism of vinorelbine via CYP 3A4	Monitor for clinical efficacy and toxicities of vinorelbine, and adjust the dose as needed.	245, 255

Continued

DRUG INTERACTIONS

Table 4-2 Drug Interactions between Anticancer Agents and Other Drugs[4-256]—cont'd

Anticancer Agent	Concurrent Use with	Effect	Possible Mechanisms of Action if Any	Management Options	Ref.
Vinorelbine—cont'd	CYP 3A4 inducers[c]	May ↓ levels of vinorelbine → may ↓ antitumor effect	Induce hepatic metabolism of vinorelbine via CYP 3A4	Avoid use of offending drug if possible or change to non-enzyme-inducing anticonvulsants; Monitor for clinical efficacy of vinorelbine, and adjust the dose as needed.	245
	Cisplatin	↑ incidence of grade III and IV granulocytopenia	Possible additive effects	Monitor closely for ↑ incidence of neutropenia and may consider primary prophylaxis of granulocyte CSFs.	71
	Docetaxel	Sequential administration of docetaxel after vinorelbine → ↑ vinorelbine plasma level → ↑ severity of neutropenia compared with alternate sequence.	Plasma level of vinorelbine ↑ due to its lower drug clearance. No difference in changes of C_{max}, clearance, or AUC of docetaxel between two different sequence schedules	Administer docetaxel first, followed by vinorelbine.	94
Vorinostat	Valproic acid	Severe thrombocytopenia and gastrointestinal bleeding	Possible additive effects of both drugs that act as histone deacetylase inhibitor	Monitor platelet count every 2 wks for the first 2 mos of therapy.	256

↓, decrease; ↑, increase; *IL*, interleukin; *AUC*, area under the curve; *CYP*, cytochrome P450; *LFT*, liver function test; $T_{1/2}$, half-time; [ ], serum concentration of the drug; *INR*, international normalized ratio; *GFR*, glomerular filtration rate; *CrCl*, creatinine clearance; *CML*, chronic myelogenous leukemia; *CHF*, congestive heart failure; *PPI*, proton pump inhibitors; *CSF*, colony-stimulating factor; *CBC*, complete blood count; *HR*, heart rate; *DVT*, deep vein thrombosis; *PE*, pulmonary embolism; *VTE*, venous thromboembolism; *IV*, intravenous; *UGT*, uridine diphosphate-glucuronosyltransferase; *ADA*, adenosine deaminase; *BUN*, blood urea nitrogen; *Scr*, serum creatinine; *MAOI*, monoamine oxidase inhibitor; *CNS*, central nervous system.
[a]Protease inhibitors, e.g., amprenavir, indinavir, nelfinavir, ritonavir, and saquinavir.
[b]CYP 3A4 inhibitors, e.g., aprepitant, azole antifungals (fluconazole, itraconazole, ketoconazole, and voriconazole), cimetidine, clarithromycin, imatinib mesylate, diltiazem, erythromycin, grapefruit juice, nifedipine, protease inhibitors (atazanavir, ritonavir, delavirdine, efavirenz, and tipranavir), and verapamil.

^cCYP 3A4 inducers, e.g., rifampin, phenytoin, carbamazepine, phenobarbital, dexamethasone, St. John's wort, nevirapine, efavirenz, ritonavir, and tipranavir.

^dCYP 3A4 substrates: astemizole, cisapride, cyclophosphamide, erlotinib, etoposide, gefitinib, 3-hydroxy-3-methylglutaryl-coenzyme reductase inhibitors, irinotecan, ifosfamide, pimozide, teniposide, terfenadine, and vinca alkaloids.

^eCYP 2C9 substrates, e.g., celecoxib, diclofenac, dronabinol, fosphenytoin, losartan, omeprazole, phenytoin, piroxicam, sertraline, tolbutamide, topiramate, and S-warfarin.

^fCYP 2C19 inhibitors: amprenavir; chloramphenicol, cimetidine, felbamate, fluoxetine, fluvoxamine, indomethacin, ketoconazole, lansoprazole, modafinil, omeprazole, oxcarbazepine, probenecid, ticlopidine, and topiramate.

^gCYP 2C19 inducers: carbamazepine, norethindrone, prednisone, and rifampin.

^hCYP 2B6 inhibitors: efavirenz , ritonavir, and nelfinavir.

ⁱCYP 2B6 inducers, e.g., phenytoin, phenobarbital, primidone, and nevirapine.

^jCYP 2D6 substrates, e.g., β-blockers, clozapine, codeine, cyclobenzaprine, dextromethorphan, donepezil, flecainide, fluoxetine, haloperidol, hydrocodone, maprotiline, meperidine, methadone, methamphetamine, mexiletine, morphine, oxycodone, paroxetine, perphenazine, propafenone, risperidone, thioridazine, tramadol, trazodone, tricyclic antidepressants, and venlafaxine.

^kA serotonin syndrome, a hyperserotonergic state characterized by symptoms such as restlessness, myoclonus, changes in mental status, hyperreflexia, diaphoresis, shivering, and tremor and may even cause death.

^lSympathomimetics, e.g., amphetamine and dextroamphetamine, cocaine, diethylpropion, ephedrine, metaraminol, methylphenidate, phenylephrine, phenylpropanolamine, and pseudoephedrine.

^mFoods rich in tyramine include cheddar and aged cheeses, pickled herring, Chianti wine, beer (alcoholic and nonalcoholic), yeast extract, chicken/beef (nonfresh) liver, avocado, and bananas.

formed from hepatic carboxylesterase, accounts for both its cytotoxic activity and gastrointestinal side effects.[295] The metabolism of SN-38 is catalyzed via induction of CYP 3A4 to a much less active metabolite, aminopentane carboxylic acid.[158] This clinically relevant drug interaction has also been observed in other similar pharmacokinetic studies conducted by Mathijssen et al.[159] and Kuhn.[160] These authors recommended that the dose of irinotecan be increased by 50% in patients who are concurrently receiving enzyme-inducing anticonvulsants to achieve adequate levels of irinotecan and SN-38. Beside irinotecan, the AUC and clearance of vincristine and paclitaxel were also significantly decreased by enzyme-inducing anticonvulsants via the mechanism of hepatic induction.[219,220,250] Because there is no evidence to support the efficacy of prophylactic use of anticonvulsants in patients with newly diagnosed brain tumors in addition to a high incidence of side effects and of drug interactions among anticonvulsants, the Quality Standards Subcommittee of the American Academy of Neurology recommended that anticonvulsant medications should only be used for patients who have experienced a first episode of seizure by the time the brain tumor is diagnosed.[296] Other drugs that have been shown to potentially decrease the efficacy of irinotecan by decreasing the AUC of SN-38 via the CYP 3A4 induction mechanism include dexamethasone administered chronically and a popular herbal product, St. John's wort.[87,161] Similarly, the irinotecan dose should be reduced to 25% in the presence of potent CYP 3A4 inhibitors such as ketoconazole.[156] Although most anticancer agents are substrates for the cytochrome P450 system, some anticancer drugs such as imatinib mesylate (Gleevec) are very potent inhibitors of CYP 3A4, CYP 2C9, and CYP 2D6.[144,150] Other non-anticancer medications known to be substrates for these enzymes include statins (CYP 3A4), warfarin (CYP 2C9), and β-blockers (CYP2D6).[144–152] Rhabdomyolysis, supratherapeutic prothrombin time and possible bleeding, and heart block, respectively, are concerns when the above agents are prescribed for patients who are receiving imatinib mesylate.[144–152] Other isoenzymes that are involved in the metabolism of chemotherapy agents are listed in Table 4-3.

In oncology, drug interactions involving decreased excretion of a drug in a cancer patient can be problematic and may be associated with increased morbidity and even mortality.[30-32,53,61] Among anticancer agents, approximately one third of them exhibit renal clearance of 30% or greater as the active or toxic compound.[297] One of the most relevant examples is methotrexate, of which greater than 80% is excreted unchanged in the kidney.[298] It is well documented that even a minor decrease in renal function can have a profound effect on methotrexate renal clearance and lead to significant toxicity.[299] Several cytotoxic drugs are known nephrotoxins.[61,297,300,327] Cisplatin, a platinum analog used for treatment of various types of cancer, is the most commonly used anticancer agent associated with renal proximal and distal tubular damage.[300] Yee et al.[30] reported that when the cumulative dose of cisplatin is greater than 300 mg/m^2, the total plasma clearance of bleomycin is decreased by 50%. Fatal pulmonary toxicity has been associated with delayed bleomycin elimination as a result of cisplatin-induced renal failure.[31,32] Thus, renal function should be closely monitored in patients receiving concurrent bleomycin and cisplatin. Furthermore, the dose of bleomycin should be reduced when creatinine clearance is less than 60 ml/min.[297]

Similarly, drugs that worsen hepatic metabolism or biliary excretion can increase drug exposure of some cytotoxic drugs. Monitoring liver function and toxicities in patients receiving both hepatotoxic drugs and cytotoxic agents that exhibit biliary elimination is vital for safe administration.[97,98,127] Biliary excretion is a major route of elimination of the anthracyclines, vinca alkaloids, and taxanes.[301–303] Holmes et al.[99] reported higher incidences of neutropenia, stomatitis, and/or cardiomyopathy in breast cancer patients who received sequential administration of paclitaxel infused over 24 hours followed by a 48-hour continuous infusion of doxorubicin compared with the opposite sequence. This phenomenon was explained by the fact that paclitaxel may compete with doxorubicin for biliary excretion, which resulted in 30% decreased clearance of doxorubicin.[99] This sequence-dependent effect on toxicity associated with use of the combination of paclitaxel and anthracyclines in breast cancer patients has been subsequently validated by other investigators. Gianni et al.[100] showed that when a 3-hour infusion of paclitaxel was given before a doxorubicin bolus, the peak level of doxorubicin and its active metabolite, doxorubicinol, along with the AUC were significantly increased. Venturini et al.[109] also documented the fact that sequential administration of paclitaxel given as a 3-hour infusion followed by epirubicin given as an intravenous bolus resulted in an increased AUC and a decreased clearance of epirubicin by 37% and 25%, respectively, compared with the alternate sequence. Based on these data, it is recommended that when these drugs are used together, anthracyclines should be given before paclitaxel to avoid increased toxicities of anthracyclines.

In summary, because the kidneys and liver function as major organs for body clearance of many cytotoxic drugs, renal and hepatic function tests should be performed periodically, and results should be carefully monitored. Because the question of dosing guidelines comes up frequently in oncology, dosing recommendations are provided in Table 4-4.[297,304-322]

Pharmacodynamic Interactions

Pharmacodynamic interactions may occur when two or more drugs acting at a common receptor-binding site affect the pharmacologic action of the object drug, without influencing the pharmacokinetics of each interacting agent. The effects of pharmacodynamic interactions can be additive, synergistic, or antagonistic. It is well known that leucovorin enhances the activity of fluorouracil in the treatment of colorectal cancer by stabilizing the tertiary complex of fluorouracil and thymidylate synthase.[126] In contrast, giving a corticosteroid with the biologic agent interleukin-2 is an example of an antagonistic interaction.[4] It is postulated that corticosteroids inhibit production of interleukin-1, which further blocks the release of interleukin-2 and tumor necrosis factor. In melanoma or renal cancer, in which interleukin-2 plays a major pharmacologic role, the use of corticosteroids is contraindicated. Because dexamethasone is commonly used as an adjunct with serotonin receptor antagonists for prevention and treatment of chemotherapy-induced nausea and vomiting, other antiemetic alternatives should be considered. In terms of additive toxicities that have been observed in the oncology setting, clinical studies have reported that the concurrent administration of trastuzumab and doxorubicin increases the risk of cardiac toxicities fourfold compared with trastuzumab used alone in patients with metastatic breast cancer.[80] Of interest, pharmacodynamic interactions between two drugs may not always produce an adverse drug toxicity profile. Kearns et al.[44] observed that when carboplatin and paclitaxel are used in combination, the incidence of thrombocytopenia is actually less than that when carboplatin is used alone. These investigators concluded that paclitaxel modulates the degree of carboplatin-induced thrombocytopenia, resulting in a platelet-sparing effect.

Pharmaceutic Interaction

Another type of drug-drug interaction, called a *pharmaceutic interaction,* is an incompatibility when drugs are combined in solution or admixed during infusion. One drug may alter the physical or chemical compatibility of another drug. A physical incompatibility may occur when the admixtures of the drugs cause a change in appearance of solution including precipitation, turbidity, and color.[257] A chemical

Table 4-3 Properties of Anticancer Agents That Undergo Metabolism Via Cytochrome P450 Enzymes[257-291]

				CYP P450 SUBSTRATES								
	UGT1A	1A1	1A2	2A6	3A4	3A5–7	2B6	2C8	2C9	2C19	2D6	2E1
All-*trans*-retinoic acid[260]					✓							
Altretamine[261]					✓							
Anastrozole[262,263]					✓							
Aprepitant[20,264,265]			✓ (minor)		✓ (as moderate inducer and inhibitor and as a substrate)			✓	✓ (as inducer)			
Bexarotene[266]					✓							
Bicalutamide[267]					✓							
Bortezomib[33,34]*					✓ > 2C19			✓		✓ (as both inhibitor and substrate)		
Cyclophosphamide[72–75,268,269]		✓			✓ (as both inhibitor and substrate)					✓	✓	
Dacarbazine[270]†			✓ > 2E1									
Dasatinib[82]					✓ (as both inhibitor and substrate)							✓
Dexamethasone[271–273]					✓ (as both inducer and substrate)							
Docetaxel[274]					✓ (as both inhibitor and substrate)							
Dolasetron[275,276]					✓						✓	
Erlotinib[110]			✓ (minor)		✓ (major)							
Etoposide[277,278]					✓							✓ (minor)

Drug						
Exemestane[263]				✓ (as both inhibitor and substrate)		
Flutamide[137,279]			✓ (major)	✓ (minor)	✓ (as a weak inhibitor)	
Gefitinib[138,280]			✓ (as a weak inhibitor)	✓	✓ (as a weak inhibitor)	✓ (as a weak inhibitor)
Granisetron[275,276,281]		✓ (major)		✓		
Ifosfamide[282]				✓ (as both inhibitor and substrate)		
Imatinib mesylate[144-152]		✓ (minor)		✓ (as both inhibitor and substrate)	✓ (as both minor substrate and moderate inhibitor)	✓ (as both minor substrate and moderate inhibitor)
					✓ (minor)	✓
Irinotecan[105,283]	✓ (as substrate)			✓ (as both inhibitor and substrate)		
Ketoconazole[161]				✓	✓ (minor)	
Letrozole[263]			✓ (as both inhibitor and substrate)	✓ (as both inhibitor and substrate)		
Lomustine[284]	✓ (metabolized by cytochrome P450 system but isozymes unknown)					
Medroxyprogesterone[14,169-171]	✓			✓ (as an inhibitor)		

Continued

Table 4-3 Properties of Anticancer Agents That Undergo Metabolism Via Cytochrome P450 Enzymes[257-291]—cont'd

					CYP P450 SUBSTRATES							
	UGT1A	1A1	1A2	2A6	3A4	3A5-7	2B6	2C8	2C9	2C19	2D6	2E1
Methylprednisolone[205-209]					✓ (as both inducer and substrate)							
Nilutamide[216,217]	(metabolized by cytochrome P450 system but isozymes unknown; also as an inhibitor of hepatic cytochrome P450 activity)											
Ondansetron[218,265]		✓	✓		✓						✓ (as an inhibitor)	
Paclitaxel[286-288]					✓			✓ > 3A4				
Palonosetron[275]					✓						✓	
Prednisone[225-229]					✓							
Procarbazine[289]	✓ (metabolized by cytochrome P450 system but isozymes unknown)				✓							
Progesterone[170,171]					✓ (as both inducer and substrate)							
Sorafenib[105,234]	✓ (as inhibitor)				✓		✓ (as inhibitor)	✓ (as inhibitor)				
Sunitinib[235]					✓							
Tamoxifen[290]			✓ (minor)		✓							
Teniposide[251,278]					✓ (major)				✓	✓		
Testosterone[201]					✓							✓

	> 2C19		(as both inhibitor and substrate)
Thiotepa[19,292]			✓
Topotecan[93,242]	✓		
Toremifene[237,243,294]	✓ (as both inhibitor and substrate)	✓	
Vinblastine[245,294]	✓		
Vincristine[245,350,253]	✓		
Vinorelbine[245,255]	✓		

*The major isozymes responsible for the metabolism of bortezomib are CYP 3A4 followed by CYP 2C19.
†Dacarbazine (DTIC) hepatic metabolism: CYP 1A2 is the predominant isozyme; CYP 2E1 contributes to hepatic DTIC metabolism at higher substrate concentrations; and CYP 1A1 catalyzes extrahepatic metabolism of DTIC.

DRUG INTERACTIONS

Table 4-4 Dosing Guidelines for Selected Anticancer Agents in Patients with Renal or Hepatic Dysfunctions[297,304–322]

Agent	Metabolized via	Eliminated via	Dosage Adjustment for Liver Dysfunction	Dosage Adjustment for Renal Dysfunction
Bleomycin	H, GI tract	R (62%)*	ND	CrCl >60 mL/min → 100% full dose CrCl 30–60 mL/min → 50% of full dose CrCl <30 mL/min → do not administer
Capecitabine	H (extensive)	R (95%)*	ND	CrCl >50 mL/min → 100% full dose CrCl 30–50 mL/min → 75% of full dose CrCl <30 mL/min → do not administer
Carboplatin	ND	R (66%)*	ND	CrCl >50 mL/min → 100% of full dose CrCl 10–50 mL/min → 50% of full dose CrCl <10 mL/min → 25% of full dose Alternative method → dosing by Calvert formula
Cisplatin	ND	R (30%)*	ND	CrCl 46–60 mL/min → 50% of full dose CrCl 31–45 mL/min → 25% of full dose. CrCl ≤ 30 mL/min: do not use cisplatin, use an alternative drug
Cyclophosphamide	H (extensive)	R (16%)*	T. bili <1.5 mg/dL or AST <60 international units/L → 100% of full dose T. bili 1.5–3.0 mg/dL or AST 60–180 international units/L → 100% of full dose T. bili >3.1–5.0 mg/dL or AST >180 international units/L → 75% of full dose T. bili >5.0 mg/dL → omit the dose	CrCl < 30 mL/min → 70%–80% of full dose CrCl < 10 mL/min → 50% of full dose
Cytarabine	H, GI tract	R (80%)*	ND Comment: Patients with liver dysfunction receiving cytarabine should be carefully monitored. Doses should be adjusted based on clinical judgment.	CrCl >60 mL/min → 100% of full dose CrCl 40–60 mL/min: If dose >2 g/m²/dose → ↓ to 1 g/m²/dose. If dose = 0.75–1 g/m²/dose → ↓ to 0.5 g/m²/dose CrCl <40 mL/min: If dose >0.75 g/m²/dose → give ≤200 mg/m²/day
Dacarbazine	H (extensive), B (extensive)	R (40%)*	ND Comment: Patients with liver dysfunction receiving dacarbazine should be carefully monitored and the dose adjusted the dose based on clinical judgment.	CrCl >60 mL/min → 100% of full dose CrCl 30–60 mL/min → 75% of full dose CrCl 10–30 mL/min → 50% of full dose CrCl <10 mL/min → omit

Drug				
Daunorubicin	H	R (<18%)* B (40%)	T. bili <1.2 mg/dL or AST <60 international units/L → 100% of full dose T. bili 1.2–3.0 mg/dL or AST 60–180 international units/L → 75% of full dose T. bili >3.1–5.0 mg/dL or AST >180 IU/L → 50% of full dose. T. bili >5.0 mg/dL → omit the dose	Scr >3 mg/dL → 50% of full dose
Decitabine	H	Liver metabolism, granulocytes	If ALT or T. bili ≤2× ULN, do not restart decitabine until ALT and T. bili return to baseline.	Scr >2.0 mg/dl, do not restart until Scr returns to normal.
Docetaxel	H	R (<5%)* B (75–80%)	AST/ALT 1.5× ULN → 100% of full dose AST/ALT 1.6–6.0× ULN → 75% of full dose AST/ALT > 6.0× ULN → physician judgment	ND
Doxorubicin	H (extensive)	R (9%)* B (40%)	T. bili <1.2 mg/dL or AST <60 international units/L → 100% of full dose, AST or ALT 2–3× ULN → 75 % of full dose, T. bili 1.2–3.0 mg/dL or AST or ALT >3 × ULN → 50% of full dose T. bili >3.1–5.0 mg/dL → 25% of full dose T. bili >5.0 mg/dL → omit the dose	CrCl ≤10 mL/min → 100% of full dose; CrCl <10 mL/min → 75% of full dose
Epirubicin	H (extensive)	R (9%)* B (extensive)	T. bili <1.2 mg/dL → 100% of full dose T. bili 1.2–3.0 mg/dL and/or AST 2–4× of ULN → 50% of full dose T. bili >3.0 mg/dL and/or AST >4× of ULN → 25% of full dose	Scr >5 mg/dL → lower doses should be considered.
Etoposide	H	R (30%–50%)* B (<2%)	Albumin <3.5 g/dL dose reduction (depending on severity of hypoalbuminemia) may be considered. Dosage reduction in patients with hyperbilirubinemia still controversial → no prospectively validated studies have been done to support the dose reduction. Comment: Patients with liver dysfunction receiving etoposide should be carefully monitored, and dose may be adjusted based on clinical effects and tolerance of the patient.	CrCl >50 mL/min → 100% of full dose CrCl 10–50 mL/min → 75% of full dose CrCl <10 mL/min → 50% of full dose Or Scr >1.4 mg/dL → 70% of full dose

Continued

DRUG INTERACTIONS

Table 4-4 Dosing Guidelines for Selected Anticancer Agents in Patients with Renal or Hepatic Dysfunctions[297,304-322]—cont'd

Agent	Metabolized via	Eliminated via	Dosage Adjustment for Liver Dysfunction	Dosage Adjustment for Renal Dysfunction
Floxuridine (FUDR)	H (95%)		T. bili and/or alkaline phosphatase 1.2× ULN → 80% of full dose T. bili and/or alkaline phosphatase 1.5× ULN and/or AST/ALT 3× baseline → 50% of full dose	ND
Fludarabine	Intracellular	R (44%)*	ND	CrCl >70 mL/min → 100% of full dose CrCl 30–70 mL/min → 80% of full dose CrCl <10–30 mL/min → 60% of full dose CrCl <10 mL/min → omit
Fluorouracil	H	R (<8%)	T. bili ≤5 mg/dL → give full dose; T. bili >5 mg/dL → omit the dose	ND
Gemcitabine	In plasma	R (–5%)*	T. bili >5 mg/dL → start at 800 mg/m²	ND
Hydroxyurea	H (extensive)	R (35%)*	T. bili 1.5–5.0 mg/dL or AST 60–180 international units/L → 50% of full dose; T. bili >5.0 mg/dL or AST >180 international units/L → omit the dose	CrCl >60 mL/min → 100% of full dose CrCl 10–60 mL/min → 75% of full dose CrCl <10 mL/min → 50% of full dose
Idarubicin	H (extensive)	R (<6%)*	T. bili 2.5–5.0 mg/dL ≥ 50% of full dose T. bili >5.0 mg/dL ≥ omit the dose	Scr ≥2.5 mg/dL → dose reduction is recommended
Ifosfamide	H (extensive)	R (40%)*	ND	CrCl >60 mL/min → 100% of full dose CrCl 30–60 mL/min → 75% of full dose CrCl 10–30 mL/min → 50% of full dose CrCl <10 mL/min → omit
Irinotecan	H (extensive)	R (11%–25%)	Study evaluating the effect of irinotecan given at 350 mg/m² every 3 weeks in patients with hyperbilirubinemia indicates that patients with a bilirubin of >1.5–3× ULN should receive 200 mg/m² or 40% dose reduction or when T. bili 1.5–3.0 mg/dL → 75% of full dose	ND

Drug				
Lenalidomide	ND	R (67%)*	ND	Because patients with renal impairment were excluded in clinical trials, there are no specific dosage recommendations, but the risk of adverse reactions may be increased in patients with renal impairment due to lenalidomide being primarily excreted by the kidney. It is recommended that the dose of lenalidomide be carefully chosen in patients with renal impairment.
Liposomal doxorubicin	H (extensive)	R (5%)*	T. bili 1.2–3.0 mg/dL or AST 60–180 international units/L → 50% of full dose T. bili >3.0 mg/dL or AST >180 international units/L → 25% of full dose	ND
Melphalan	Plasma (extensive)	R (12%)* F (20–50%)	NA	CrCl >50 mL/min → 100% of full dose CrCl 10–50 mL/min → 75% of full dose CrCl <10 mL/min → 50% of full dose
Methotrexate	Intracellular, H	R (77%)* B (10%)	T. bili <1.5 mg/dL or AST <60 international units/L → 100% of full dose T. bili 1.5–3.0 mg/dL or AST 60–180 international units/L → 100% of full dose T. bili 3.1–5.0 mg/dL or AST >180 IU/L → 75% of full dose T. bili >5.0 mg/dL → omit the dose	CrCl >60 mL/min → 100% of full dose CrCl 30–60 mL/min → 50% of full dose CrCl <30 mL/min → omit OR The dose is reduced by the percent reduction of the CrCl below 100 ml/min; e.g., CrCl 70 ml/min mandates a 25% reduction of methotrexate dose.
Mitomycin C	H	R (5%)*	T. bili 1.5–3.0 mg/dL → 50 of full dose T. bili >3.0 mg/dL or hepatic enzymes >3× ULN → 25% of full dose	CrCl <10 mL/min → 75% of full dose
Mitoxantrone	H	R (8%) B (18%)	T. bili <1.5 mg/dL or AST <60 international units/L → 100% of full dose T. bili 1.5–3.0 mg/dL → 50% of full dose T. bili >3.0 mg/dL → 25% of full dose	ND
Oxaliplatin	Plasma (rapid and extensive)	R (50%)	ND	CrCl > 20 mL/min → 100% of full dose

Continued

DRUG INTERACTIONS

Table 4-4 Dosing Guidelines for Selected Anticancer Agents in Patients with Renal or Hepatic Dysfunctions[297,304-322]—cont'd

Agent	Metabolized via	Eliminated via	Dosage Adjustment for Liver Dysfunction	Dosage Adjustment for Renal Dysfunction
Paclitaxel	H (extensive)	R (7%)* B (extensive)	T. bili <1.5 mg/dL and AST/ALT > 2× ULN → 75% of full dose T. bili 1.6–2.9 mg/dL → 40% of full dose	ND
Pentostatin	ND	R (65%)*	T. bili >3.0 mg/dL → 25% of full dose NA	CrCl >60 mL/min → 100% of full dose CrCl 41–60 mL/min → 75% of full dose CrCl 21–40 mL/min → 50% of full dose CrCl <30 mL/min → consider to use alternative drugs if possible Scr > 2.0 mg/dL → dose reduction should be considered.
Procarbazine	H, R	R (<5%)* B (84%)	T. bili >5.0 mg/dL and/or AST/ALT >3× ULN → omit the dose AST/ALT > 1.6–6.0× ULN → 75% of full dose; AST/ALT > 6.0× ULN → physician judgment	
Topotecan	H (extensive)	R (39% in adults and 65% in children)*	No dosage adjustment	CrCl >600mL mL/min → 100% of full dose CrCl 30–60 mL/min → 75% of full dose CrCl 10–30 mL/min → 50% of full dose CrCl <10 mL/min → omit
Vinblastine	H	R (10%)* F (10%)	T. bili <1.5 mg/dL or AST <60 international units/ L → 100% of full dose; T. bili 1.5–3.0 mg/dL or AST 60–180 international units/L →50% of full dose; T. bili >3.1 mg/dL or AST >180 international units/L → omit the dose	ND
Vincristine	H	R (11%)* B (80%)	T. bili <1.5 mg/dL or AST <60 international units/ L → 100% of full dose; T. bili 1.5–3.0 mg/dL or AST 60–180 international units/L →50% of full dose; T. bili >3.1 mg/dL or AST >180 international units/L → omit the dose	ND
Vinorelbine	H (extensive)	R (14%) B (50%)	T. bili <2.0 mg/dL → 100% of full dose; T. bili 2.1–3.0 mg/dL → 50% of full dose T. bili >3.0 mg/dL → 25% of full dose	ND

H, hepatic; *GI*, gastrointestinal; *R*, renal; *ND*, no data; *CrCl*, creatinine clearance; *B*, biliary; *T. bili*, total bilirubin; *AST*, aspartate aminotransferase; *SCR*, serum creatinine; *ULN*, upper the limit of normal; *F*, feces; *NA*, not applicable.

*Percentage of the dose excreted in urine as active or toxic moiety.

incompatibility occurs when the effectiveness of the drug is decreased due to drug inactivation or degradation.[257] For example, the admixture of mesna in cisplatin infusion bags results in inactivation of cisplatin.[323] Refer to Trissel[323] for more information on the subject of parenteral drug-drug admixture interactions.

Other Specific Drug Interactions in Oncology

Methotrexate. Because methotrexate is widely used in oncology, is dependent on folate metabolism for its cytotoxic effects, and is primarily metabolized and cleared by liver and kidneys, respectively, the potential for drug-drug interactions is high. Salicylates, penicillins, sulfonamides, and probenecid all compete for the tubular excretion of methotrexate, leading to increased methotrexate levels and subsequent toxicities. These drugs also displace methotrexate from protein-binding sites on albumin, although this effect is relatively minor. These drugs should not be given concurrently with methotrexate for fear of enhancing toxicity. There have been a few cases in which methotrexate has affected the pharmacodynamics or pharmacokinetics of other drugs.[175–177] For example, the oral bioavailability of 6-mercaptopurine is enhanced by oral methotrexate with a dose greater than 20 mg/m^2 or with concurrent high-dose methotrexate infusion.[175–177] Oral antibiotics and cholestyramine may also potentially decrease the oral absorption of methotrexate, which may in turn decrease its efficacy.[185,188–191] It is recommended that administration of methotrexate and either one of these drugs should be separated by 2–4 hours. Close therapeutic drug monitoring is advised when the cyclosporine is given concurrently with methotrexate.[186] Table 4-5 presents clinical drug interactions associated with methotrexate and other drugs.[26,175–204] For drug interactions resulting in delayed clearance of methotrexate, it is critical that methotrexate levels are monitored and that leucovorin (folinic acid) is prescribed in adequate dosage (Table 4–6) to prevent excessive toxicity to the bone marrow, mucosa, or liver.[324–335]

Warfarin. Thromboembolism is one of the most frequent complications and the second most frequent cause of death in the cancer patient population.[336,337] Warfarin has been shown to be effective in the prevention and treatment of venous thromboembolism in cancer patients.[338–341] After oral absorption, more than 90% of warfarin is rapidly absorbed in the gastrointestinal tract.[342] Warfarin also has high-affinity binding to plasma protein. Warfarin is metabolized primarily by the liver via the cytochrome P450 isoenzymes including CYP 2C9, 2C19, 2C8, 2C18, 1A2, and 3A4.[342] Considering all the pharmacokinetic characteristics of warfarin, use of drugs that affect the degree of absorption, hepatic metabolism via the above isoenzymes, or protein binding of warfarin could potentially lead to changes in its anticoagulant effects.[343] For example, it is well documented that tamoxifen can potentiate the effect of warfarin by inhibiting its metabolism via CYP 3A4.[238–240] On the other hand, Yates et al.[347] did not detect a clinically significant interaction between anastrozole at a dose of 1 mg (a known CYP 1A2, 2C9, and 3A4 inhibitor) and warfarin in a single-dose pharmacokinetic study. GI toxicities (stomatitis and diarrhea) caused by certain chemotherapy drugs may also impair absorption of warfarin, which may result in a subtherapeutic effect. Highly protein-bound drugs such as bicalutamide and flutamide have also been reported to increase the prothrombin time of warfarin by displacing it from protein-binding sites.[29,137] In addition, factors such as thrombocytopenia resulting from the effect of chemotherapy or the disease itself (e.g., acute promyelocytic leukemia) can put cancer patients at higher risk for bleeding.[344] On the other hand, cancer patients who are in a hypercoagulable state or have advanced disease and those who receive hormonal treatment or chemotherapy are also at higher risk for development of

Table 4-5 Clinical Drug Interactions between Methotrexate and Other Drugs

Offending drug(s)	Clinical Interactions/Mechanisms/Subsequent effects	Recommendations if Avoidance of Concurrent Use of the Interacting Drug Is Not Possible	Ref.
Anticonvulsants (enzyme-inducing, such as carbamazepine, phenytoin, phenobarbital)	↓ cytotoxic effect of methotrexate → decrease cytotoxic effects of chemotherapy → may decrease clinical outcomes of the cancer treatment	Avoid use of enzyme-inducing anticonvulsants in patients undergoing chemotherapy if possible.	179
Aspirin/nonsteroidal anti-inflammatory drugs	Aspirin or nonsteroidal anti-inflammatory drugs may ↓ plasma protein binding and renal tubular secretion of high dose methotrexate → ↑ risk of methotrexate toxicity	Do not administer aspirin or nonsteroidal anti-inflammatory drugs within 10 days of high-dose methotrexate therapy.	180–184
Asparaginase	Administration of asparaginase before or concurrently with methotrexate → may ↓ methotrexate efficacy.	Administer asparaginase shortly after methotrexate or 9–10 days before methotrexate.	26
Cholestyramine	Cholestyramine may enhance the nonrenal elimination of oral methotrexate by interrupting the enterohepatic circulation of methotrexate → ↓ methotrexate efficacy.	Separate oral doses of methotrexate from cholestyramine at least 2–4 hrs apart.	185
Cyclosporine	Cyclosporine may interfere with methotrexate renal elimination or vice versa → ↑ risk of toxicities of both drugs.	Monitor methotrexate and cyclosporine levels if clinically applicable. Monitor for both methotrexate and cyclosporine toxicities.	186
5-Fluorouracil	↓ cytotoxic effect of methotrexate when fluorouracil given prior to methotrexate possibly due to interference of conversion of reduced folates to dihydrofolate.	Give methotrexate before fluorouracil.	128
Hepatotoxic agents (azathioprine, retinoids, sulfasalazine)	Possible increased risk of hepatotoxicity	Monitor liver function test results and monitor closely for signs and symptoms of liver failure (flu-like symptoms, abdominal pain, dark urine, pruritus, jaundice, ascites, weight gain, icterus).	187
6-Mercaptopurine	Concomitant administration of oral 6-mercaptopurine at 75 mg/m² and oral methotrexate at 20 mg/m² →31% ↑ in AUC and 26% ↑ in peak [6-mercaptopurine]. Mechanism: Methotrexate is an inhibitor of xanthine oxidase, the enzyme responsible for catabolism of 6-mercaptopurine to its inactive metabolite 6-thiouric acid.	Dose of oral 6-mercaptopurine may need to be increased when used with oral methotrexate >20 mg/m² or in patients on high-dose intravenous methotrexate.	175–177
Oral aminoglycosides (neomycin, paromomycin)	Concomitant administration of oral aminoglycosides ↓ oral absorption of methotrexate by 30%–50%	Separate oral doses of methotrexate from cholestyramine at least 2–4 hours apart.	188
Penicillins	Concomitant use with penicillins → may interfere with the renal tubular secretion of methotrexate → ↓ clearance of methotrexate → ↑ risk of methotrexate toxicity.	Avoid concurrent use with penicillins or monitor for methotrexate levels and clinical toxicities (bone marrow suppression, mucositis, nausea/vomiting).	188–191

Probenecid	Concomitant use of methotrexate and probenecid → ↓ methotrexate clearance by interfering with tubular secretion in the proximal tubule and ↓ plasma protein binding → ↑ [methotrexate] → ↑ risk of methotrexate toxicity.	Avoid use with probenecid. Monitor for methotrexate level and clinical toxicities.	192–194
Procarbazine	Methotrexate infusion given within 48 hrs of administration of procarbazine ↑ risk of renal impairment. Procarbazine has a transient effect on the kidneys. If high-dose methotrexate is given before recovery from this change → delays renal excretion of methotrexate and prolongs exposure of the kidneys to methotrexate.	Do not start methotrexate infusion <72 hrs after the last dose of procarbazine. Administer aggressive hydration, alkalinize urine to pH >7.0, monitor closely for renal function (BUN, Scr, fluid status) before, during, and after methotrexate infusion until methotrexate <0.05 mmol/L.	195
Proton pump inhibitors (PPIs)	Active tubular secretion of methotrexate requires the activity of the proton pump because methotrexate is excreted with hydrogen ions → PPIs can inhibit renal elimination of the hydrogen ion and block the active tubular secretion of methotrexate → ↑ the elimination half-life of methotrexate → which may result in potentially toxic concentrations of methotrexate → ↑ risk of MTX toxicities (myalgias, bone pain, mucositis).	Avoid use of PPIs while patient is receiving high-dose methotrexate.	196–198
Sulfamethoxazole/ trimethoprim	Coadministration of methotrexate with sulfamethoxazole may ↑ free [methotrexate] by displacement of methotrexate from plasma protein binding sites or ↓ renal tubular elimination → ↑ methotrexate toxicity. Trimethoprim inhibits DHFR → additive effects with methotrexate → ↑ methotrexate toxicity.	Avoid coadministration of both drugs or monitor toxicity closely.	199–203
Valproic acid	One case report that high-dose methotrexate (5 g/m² infused over 24 hrs) ↓ serum valproic acid concentration to 25% of the premethotrexate value → poor seizure control. Competitive binding, protein displacement, and decreased absorption were thought to be responsible for decreased valproic acid levels.	Monitor valproic acid administration very closely for clinical signs of seizures.	204

↑, increase; ↓, decrease; [ ], serum concentration of the drug; *AUC*, area under the curve; *BUN*, blood urea nitrogen; *Scr*, serum creatinine; *DHFR*, dihydrofolate reductase.

DRUG INTERACTIONS

Table 4-6 General Guidelines for Modification of Leucovorin Dosage after High-Dose Methotrexate[324-335]

Time After the Start of Infusion	Serum Creatinine	Methotrexate Level	Action
At 24 hrs		If methotrexate is infused as a short infusion (over 0.5–6 hrs), and level is >5 μmol/L,	1) ↑ leucovorin to 100 mg/m² IV every 6 hrs and 2) ↑ fluid to 4–6 L/day. (Leucovorin dosages may be reduced, as indicated, as serum methotrexate level decreases.)
At 48 hrs		If methotrexate is given as continuous infusion for ≥24 hrs and level is >1 mmol/L at 24 hrs postinfusion (i.e., 48 hrs after start of infusion),	adjust leucovorin rescue per recommendation below.†
At 48 hrs		If <1 μmol/L,	continue the same dose as initially started.
		If 1–5 μmol/L,	1) adjust leucovorin to 50 mg IV/PO every 6 hrs, and 2) ↑ fluid to 4–6 L/day.
		If 5–10 μmol/L,	1) adjust leucovorin to 100 mg/m² IV every 6 hrs (leucovorin dosages may be reduced, as indicated, as serum methotrexate level decreases), and 2) ↑ fluid to 4–6 L/day.
		If 10–20 μmol/L,	1) adjust leucovorin to 200 mg/m² IV every 6 hrs (leucovorin dosages may be reduced, as indicated, as serum methotrexate level decreases), and 2) ↑ fluid to 4–6 L/day.
		If >20 μmol/L,	1) adjust leucovorin to 500 mg/m² IV every 6 hrs; consider hemodialysis and hemoperfusion, and 2) ↑ fluid to 4–6 L/day.

At 72 hrs

If serum creatinine is increased by ≥50% from baseline on the next day after methotrexate is infused.

If methotrexate is given as continuous infusion and level is >0.1 μmol/L but <1 μmol/L at 48 hrs, or if methotrexate is given as a short infusion (over 0.5–6 hrs) and level >0.2 μmol/L but <1 μmol/L at 48 hrs,

1) adjust leucovorin to 50 mg IV/PO every 6 hrs until methotrexate level is <0.05 μmol/L (leucovorin dosages may be reduced, as indicated, as serum methotrexate level decreases), and 2) ↑ fluid to 4–6 L/day.

1) adjust leucovorin to 100 mg/m² IV every 6 hrs and continue until methotrexate level is <0.05 μmol/L (leucovorin dosages may be reduced, as indicated, as serum methotrexate level decreases), and 2) ↑ fluid to 4–6 L/day.

*A fluid volume of 2–3 L/day with urinary alkalinization with 50–100 mEq/m² per day should be given before and during methotrexate infusion to ensure urine pH ≥7. Hydration should be continued for 24–48 hrs after the methotrexate infusion is complete.

†ᵇ The following recommendation may apply to both short and continuous infusion of high-dose methotrexate. Doses of leucovorin >50 mg should be given in intravenous form because of the decreased oral bioavailability of leucovorin at doses >50 mg.

Monitor for signs/symptoms of increased methotrexate toxicities: nausea/vomiting, mucositis, low urine pH, low urine output, increased serum creatinine, neurotoxicity, and liver toxicities. Patients who are at high risk of methotrexate toxicity include those with preexisting renal dysfunction, prior cisplatin therapy, "third spacing" (e.g., pleural effusion, or ascites) or gastrointestinal obstruction.

Drugs such as aspirin, penicillins, nonsteroidal antiinflammatory drugs, probenecid, and sulfamethoxazole/trimethoprim should be held during methotrexate infusion and may be resumed when the methotrexate level is .05 mmol/L.

DRUG INTERACTIONS

Table 4-7 **Clinically Significant Drug Interaction between Warfarin and Anticancer Agents**

Antineoplastic or Cancer-Related Agent	↓ Warfarin Effect	↑ Warfarin Effect	POSSIBLE MECHANISMS OF ACTION				
			INHIBIT/INDUCE P450 ISOZYMES			Displace from Protein Binding Sites	Ref.
			2C9	3A4	Nonspecific		
Aminoglutethimide	✓		✓	✓			17, 18
Aprepitant	✓		✓				25
Bicalutamide		✓				✓	19
Capecitabine		✓	✓				39–41
Dasatinib		✓		✓			82
Etoposide		✓				✓	120, 121
Fluorouracil*		✓	✓				132–136
Flutamide		✓				✓	137
Gefitinib		✓	✓	✓			139
Gemcitabine		✓	The case report suggested that reversible hepatotoxicity due to gemcitabine is responsible for the drug interaction.				140
Ifosfamide		✓					143
Imatinib mesylate		✓					144, 150
Mercaptopurine	✓		Unknown mechanism				178
Nilutamide					✓		216
Tamoxifen		✓		✓			238–240

*Parts of the text and tables used in this chapter were originally published in the *Journal of Oncology Pharmacy Practice* 2003;9(2–3):45–85, © 2003 Edward Arnold (Publishers) Ltd..

thrombosis.[345-346] Therefore, it is important to recognize clinically significant drug interactions in those high-risk cancer patients who receive both warfarin and anticancer therapy to prevent a subtherapeutic effect of warfarin or bleeding complications. Table 4-7 lists anticancer agents that have been reported to interact with warfarin and their possible mechanism of actions.

CONCLUSION/RECOMMENDATION

Drug interactions probably occur often in the cancer patient but may go unnoticed. Given the interpatient variability that may alter the pharmacokinetics and the different degrees and types of toxicity profiles of chemotherapy in a cancer patient, it is not surprising that the incidence of oncologic drug-drug interactions has been increasing. Drug-drug interactions may result in favorable or unfavorable clinical outcomes. The mechanisms of such drug-drug interactions can be broadly classified as pharmacokinetic, pharmacodynamic, and pharmaceutic. On the basis of all the interactions reviewed in this chapter, it is estimated that 40% of unfavorable drug interactions are predictable if the clinician recognizes them. To minimize their occurrence, both the clinician and the patient should take responsibility for communicating with each other about the patient's medication history. All oncology clinicians should have a firm understanding of the pharmacology of anticancer agents and other drugs and diseases that may affect positively and negatively the outcomes of drug therapy. The oncology pharmacist may play an important role in the oncology team by identifying any drug-drug interactions in patients at high risk. It is hoped that this chapter will help clinicians familiarize themselves with common drug-drug interactions in oncology and provide guidelines for how to best use the multitude of therapeutic agents currently available in practice. Lastly, patients should be educated about the use of all of their medications and maintain a complete drug history profile on their own.

REFERENCES

1. Nies AS. Principles of Therapeutics. In Hardman JG, Limbird LE, Goodman A, eds. *Goodman & Gilman's The Pharmacological Basis of Therapeutics*, 10 ed. New York, NY: McGraw-Hill Medical; 2001, 45–66.

2. Finley RS. Drug interactions in the oncology patient. *Semin Oncol Nurs* 1992;8:95–101.

3. The FDA Safety Information and Adverse Event Reporting Program. Food and Drug Administration MedWatch Web site. Available at http://www.fda.gov/medwatch/safety.htm. Accessed January 21, 2003.

4. Shiloni E, Matzner Y. Inhibition of interleukin-2-induced tumor necrosis factor release by dexamethasone: does it reduce the antitumor therapeutic efficacy? *Blood* 1991;78:1389–1390.

5. Chabot GC, Flaherty LE, Valdivieso M, Baker LH. Alteration of dacarbazine pharmacokinetics after interleukin-2 administration in melanoma patients. *Cancer Chemother Pharmacol* 1990;27:157–160.

6. Piscitelli SC, Vogel S, Figg WD, et al. Alteration in indinavir clearance during interleukin-2 infusions in patients infected with the human immunodeficiency virus. *Pharmacotherapy* 1998;18:1212–1216.

7. Van Wauwe JP, Coene MC, Goossens J, et al. Ketoconazole inhibits the in vitro and in vivo metabolism of all-*trans*-retinoic acid. *J Pharmacol Exp Ther* 1988;245:718–722.

8. Rigas JR, Francis PA, Muindi JR, et al. Constitutive variability in the pharmacokinetics of the natural retinoid, all-*trans*-retinoic acid, and its modulation by ketoconazole. *J Natl Cancer Inst* 1993;85:1921–1926.

9. Lee JS, Newman RA, Lippman SM, et al. Phase I evaluation of all-*trans* retinoic acid with and without ketoconazole in adults with solid tumors. *J Clin Oncol* 1995;13:1501–1508.

10. Fex G, Larsson K, Andersson A, et al. Low serum concentration of all-*trans* and 13-*cis* retinoic acids in patients treated with phenytoin, carbamazepine and valproate: possible relation to teratogenicity. *Arch Toxicol* 1995;69:572–574.

11. Hande K, Combs G, Swingle R, et al. Effect of cimetidine and ranitidine on the metabolism and toxicity of hexamethylmelamine. *Cancer Treat Rep* 1986;70:1443–1445.

12. Paolini A, D'Incalci M. Effect of phenobarbital pretreatment on the metabolism and antitumor activity of hexamethylmelamine. *Cancer Treat Rep* 1986;70:513–516.

13. Halpern J, Catane R, Baerwald H. A call for caution in the use of aminoglutethimide: negative interactions with dexamethasone and beta blocker treatment. *J Med* 1984;15:59–63.

14. Van Deijk WA, Blijham GH, Mellink WA, et al. Influence of aminoglutethimide on plasma levels of medroxyprogesterone acetate: its correlation with serum cortisol. *Cancer Treat Rep* 1985;69:85–90.

15. Lien EA, Anker G, Lonning PE, et al. Decreased serum concentrations of tamoxifen and its metabolites induced by aminoglutethimide. *Cancer Res* 1990;50:5851–5857.

16. Lonning PE, Kvinnsland S, Bakke OM. Effect of aminoglutethimide on antipyrine, theophylline, and digitoxin disposition in breast cancer. *Clin Pharmacol Ther* 1984;36:796–802.

17. Lonning PE, Kvinnsland S, Jahren G. Aminoglutethimide and warfarin: a new important drug interaction. *Cancer Chemother Pharmacol* 1984;12:10–12.

18. Lonning PE, Ueland PM, Kvinnsland S. The influence of a graded dose schedule of aminoglutethimide on the disposition of the optical enantiomers of warfarin in patients with breast cancer. *Cancer Chemother Pharmacol* 1986;17:177–181.

19. de Jonge ME, Huitema AD, Holtkamp MJ, et al. Aprepitant inhibits cyclophosphamide bioactivation and thiotepa metabolism. *Cancer Chemother Pharmacol* 2005;56:370–378.

20. Product information: Emend (aprepitant) package insert. Whitehouse Station, NJ: Merck & Co., Inc.; 2004.

21. McCrea JB, Majumdar AK, Goldberg MR, et al. Effects of the neurokinin1 receptor antagonist aprepitant on the pharmacokinetics of dexamethasone and methylprednisolone. *Clin Pharmacol Ther* 2003;74:17–24.

22. Majumdar AK, McCrea JB, Panebianco DL, et al. Effects of aprepitant on cytochrome P450 3A4 activity using midazolam as a probe. *Clin Pharmacol Ther* 2003;74:150–156.

23. Shadle CR, Lee Y, Majumdar AK, et al. Evaluation of potential inductive effects of aprepitant on cytochrome P450 3A4 and 2C9 activity. *J Clin Pharmacol* 2004;44:215–223.

24. Nygren P, Hande K, Petty KJ, et al. Lack of effect of aprepitant on the pharmacokinetics of docetaxel in cancer patients. *Cancer Chemother Pharmacol* 2005;55:609–616.

25. Depre M, Van Hecken A, Oeyen M, et al. Effect of aprepitant on the pharmacokinetics and pharmacodynamics of warfarin. *Eur J Clin Pharmacol* 2005;61:341–346.

26. Capizzi RL. Schedule-dependent synergism and antagonism between methotrexate and asparaginase. *Biochem Pharmacol* 1974;23:151–161.

27. Petros WP, Rodman JH, Relling MV, et al. Variability in teniposide plasma protein binding is correlated with serum albumin concentrations. *Pharmacotherapy* 1992;12:273–277.

28. Murphy JA, Ross LM, Gibson BES. Vincristine toxicity in five children with acute lymphoblastic leukaemia [Letter]. *Lancet* 1995;346:443.

29. Product information: Casodex (bicalutamide). Wilmington, DE: Zeneca Pharmaceuticals; 2000).

30. Yee GC, Crom WR, Champion JE, et al. Cisplatin-induced changes in bleomycin elimination. *Cancer Treat Rep* 1983;67:587–589.

DRUG INTERACTIONS

31. Dalgleish AG, Woods RL, Levi JA. Bleomycin pulmonary toxicity: its relationship to renal dysfunction. *Med Pediatr Oncol* 1984;12:313–317.

32. Bennett WM, Pastore L, Houghton DC. Fatal pulmonary toxicity in cisplatin-induced acute renal failure. *Cancer Treat Rep* 1980;64:921–924.

33. Uttamsingh V, Lu C, Miwa GT, Gan LS. Relative contributions of the five major human cytochromes p450, 1a2, 2c9, 2c19, 2d6, and 3a4 to the hepatic metabolism of the proteosome inhibitor bortezomib. *Drug Metab Dispos* 2005;33:1723–1728.

34. Product information: Velcade (bortezomib). Available at: http://www.fda.gov/cder/foi/label/2003/021602lbl.pdf. Accessed October 29, 2006.

35. Hassan M, Ljungman P, Ringden O, et al. The effect of busulfan on the pharmacokinetics of cyclophosphamide and its 4-hydroxy metabolite: time interval influence therapeutic efficacy and therapy-related toxicity. *Bone Marrow Transplant* 2000;25:915–924.

36. Hassan M, Oberg G, Bjorkholm M, et al. Influence of prophylactic anticonvulsant therapy on high-dose busulfan kinetics. *Cancer Chemother Pharmacol* 1993;33:181–186.

37. Buggia I, Zecca M, Alessandrino EP, et al. Itraconazole can increase systemic exposure to busulfan in patients given bone marrow transplantation. *Anticancer Res* 1996;16:2083–2088.

38. Key NS, Kelly PM, Emerson PM, et al. Oesophageal varices associated with busulfan-thioguanine combination therapy for chronic myeloid leukaemia. *Lancet* 1987;2:1050–1052.

39. Product information: Xeloda (capecitabine). Available at: http://www.fda.gov/cder/foi/label/2000/20896lbl.pdf. Accessed October 18, 2006.

40. Janney LM, Waterbury NV. Capecitabine-warfarin interaction. *Ann Pharmacother* 2005;39:1546–1551.

41. Camidge R, Reigner B, Cassidy J, et al. Significant effect of capecitabine on the pharmacokinetics and pharmacodynamics of warfarin in patients with cancer. *J Clin Oncol* 2005;23:4719–4725.

42. Giaccone G, Huizing M, Postmus PE, et al. Dose-finding and sequencing study of paclitaxel and carboplatin in non-small cell lung cancer. *Semin Oncol* 1995;22(Suppl 9):78–82.

43. Bookman MA, McGuire WP III, Kilpatrick D, et al. Carboplatin and paclitaxel in ovarian carcinoma: a phase I study of the Gynecologic Oncology Group. *J Clin Oncol* 1996;14:1895–1902.

44. Kearns CM, Belani CP, Erkmen K, et al. Reduced platelet toxicity with combination carboplatin and paclitaxel: pharmacodynamic modulation of carboplatin associated thrombocytopenia [Abstract]. *Proc Am Soc Clin Oncol* 1995;14:170.

45. The International Collaborative Ovarian Neoplasm (ICON) Group. Paclitaxel plus carboplatin versus standard chemotherapy with either single-agent carboplatin or cyclophosphamide, doxorubicin, and cisplatin in women ovarian cancer: the ICON3 randomized trial. *Lancet* 2002;360:505–515.

46. Dofferhoff AS, Berendsen HH, vd Naalt J, et al. Decreased phenytoin level after carboplatin treatment. *Am J Med* 1990;89:247–248.

47. Selker RG, Moore P, Lodolce D. Bone-marrow depression with cimetidine plus carmustine [Letter]. *N Engl J Med* 1978;299:834.

48. Volkin RL, Shadduck RK, Winklestein A, et al. Potentiation of carmustine-cranial irradiation-induced myelosuppression by cimetidine. *Arch Intern Med* 1982;142:243–245.

49. Dorr RT, Soble MJ. H2-antagonists and carmustine. *J Cancer Res Clin Oncol* 1989;115:41–46.

50. Bjornsson TD, Huang AT, Roth P, et al. Effects of high-dose cancer chemotherapy on the absorption of digoxin in two different formulations. *Clin Pharmacol Ther* 1986;39:25–28.

51. Wolff SN. High-dose carmustine and high-dose etoposide: a treatment regimen resulting in enhanced hepatic toxicity. *Cancer Treat Rep* 1986;70:1464–1465.

52. Levin VA, Stearns J, Byrd A, et al. The effect of phenobarbital pretreatment on the antitumor activity of 1,3-bis(2-chloroethyl)-1-nitrosourea (BCNU), 1-(2-chloroethyl)-3-cyclohexyl-1-nitrosourea (CCNU) and 1-(2-chloroethyl)-3-(2,6-dioxo-3-piperidyl)-1-nitrosourea (PCNU), and on the plasma pharmacokinetics and biotransformation of BCNU. *J Pharmacol Exp Ther* 1979;208:1–6.

53. Komune S, Snow JB. Potentiating effects of cisplatin and ethacrynic acid in ototoxicity. *Arch Otolaryngol* 1981;107:594–597.

54. Kohn S, Fradis M, Podoshin L, et al. Ototoxicity resulting from combined administration of cisplatin and gentamicin. *Laryngoscope* 1997;107:407–408.

55. Riggs LC, Brummett RE, Guitjens SK, Matz GJ. Ototoxicity resulting from combined administration of cisplatin and gentamicin. *Laryngoscope* 1996;106:401–406.

56. Grossman SA, Sheidler VR, Gilbert MR. Decreased phenytoin levels in patients receiving chemotherapy. *Am J Med* 1989;87:505–510.

57. Neef C, de Voogd-van der Straaten I. An interaction between cytostatic and anticonvulsant drugs. *Clin Pharmacol Ther* 1988;43:372–375.

58. Schellens JHM, Ma J, Bruno R. Pharmacokinetics of cisplatin and Taxotere (docetaxel) and WBC DNA-adduct formation of cisplatin in the sequence Taxotere/cisplatin and cisplatin/Taxotere in a phase I/II study in solid tumor patients [Abstract]. *Proc Am Soc Clin Oncol* 1994;13:132.

59. Pronk LC, Schellens JH, Planting AS, et al. Phase I and pharmacologic study of docetaxel and cisplatin in patients with advanced solid tumors. *J Clin Oncol* 1997;15:1071–1079.

60. Hilkens PH, Pronk LC, Verweij J, et al. Peripheral neuropathy induced by combination chemotherapy of docetaxel and cisplatin. *Br J Cancer* 1997;75:417–422.

61. Rossi R, Godde A, Kleinebrand A, et al. Unilateral nephrectomy and cisplatin as risk factors of ifosfamide-induced nephrotoxicity: analysis of 120 patients. *J Clin Oncol* 1994;12:159–165.
62. Pratt CB, Goren MP, Meyer WH, et al. Ifosfamide neurotoxicity is related to previous cisplatin treatment for pediatric solid tumors. *J Clin Oncol* 1990;8:1399–1401.
63. Goren MP, Wright RK, Pratt CB, et al. Potentiation of ifosfamide neurotoxicity, hematotoxicity and tubular nephrotoxicity by prior cis-diamminedichloroplatinum(II) therapy. *Cancer Res* 1987;47: 1457–1460.
64. Beijnen JH, Bais EM, ten Bokkel Huinink WW. Lithium pharmacokinetics during cisplatin-based chemotherapy: a case report. *Cancer Chemother Pharmacol* 1994;33:523–526.
65. Rowinsky EK, Gilbert MR, McGuire WP, et al. Sequences of taxol and cisplatin: a phase and pharmacologic study. *J Clin Oncol* 1991;9:1692–1703.
66. Product information: Rituxan (rituximab). South San Francisco, CA: Genentech, Inc.; 2001.
67. Haas A, Anderson L, Lad T. The influence of aminoglycosides on the nephrotoxicity of *cis*-diamminedichloroplatinum in cancer patients. *J Infect Dis* 1983;147:363.
68. Bergstrom P, Johnsson A, Cavallin-Stahl E, et al. Effects of cisplatin and amphotericin B on DNA adduct formation and toxicity in malignant glioma and normal tissues in rat. *Eur J Cancer* 1997;33:153–159.
69. Christensen ML, Stewart CF, Crom WR. Evaluation of aminoglycoside disposition in patients previously treated with cisplatin. *Ther Drug Monit* 1989;11:631–636.
70. Rowinsky EK, Kaufmann SH, Baker SD, et al. Sequences of topotecan and cisplatin: phase I, pharmacologic, and in vitro studies to examine sequence dependence. *J Clin Oncol* 1996;14:3074–3084.
71. Wozniak AJ, Crowley JJ, Balcerzak SP, et al. Randomized trial comparing cisplatin with cisplatin plus vinorelbine in the treatment of advanced non-small-cell lung cancer: a Southwest Oncology Group study. *J Clin Oncol* 1998;16:2459–2465.
72. Huang Z, Roy P, Waxman DJ. Role of human liver microsomal CYP3A4 and CYP2B6 in catalyzing *N*-dechloroethylation of cyclophosphamide and ifosfamide. *Biochem Pharmacol* 2000;59: 961–972.
73. Yu LJ, Drewes P, Gustafsson K, et al. In vivo modulation of alternative pathways of P-450-catalyzed cyclophosphamide metabolism: impact on pharmacokinetics and antitumor activity. *J Pharmacol Exp Ther* 1999;288:928–937.
74. Oira S, Maezawa S, Irinoda Y, et al. Increased antitumor activity of cyclophosphamide (Endoxan) following pretreatment with inducer of drug-metabolizing enzymes (cytochrome P-450). *Tohoku J Exp Med* 1974;114:55–60.
75. Dorr RT, Soble MJ, Alberts DS. Interaction of cimetidine but not ranitidine with cyclophosphamide in mice. *Cancer Res* 1986;46(4 Pt 1): 1795–1799.
76. Alberts DS, Mason-Liddil N, Plezia PM, et al. Lack of ranitidine effects on cyclophosphamide bone marrow toxicity or metabolism: a placebo-controlled clinical trial. *J Natl Cancer Inst* 1991; 83:1739–1742.
77. Kennedy MJ, Zahurak ML, Donehower RC, et al. Phase I and pharmacologic study of sequences of paclitaxel and cyclophosphamide supported by granulocyte colony-stimulating factor in women with previously treated metastatic breast cancer. *J Clin Oncol* 1996;14:783–791.
78. Tolcher AW, Cowan KH, Noone M, et al. Phase I study of paclitaxel in combination with cyclophosphamide and granulocyte colony-stimulating factor in metastatic breast cancer patients. *J Clin Oncol* 1996; 14:95–102.
79. Gryn J, Gordon R, Bapat A, et al. Pentostatin increases the acute toxicity of high dose cyclophosphamide. *Bone Marrow Transplant* 1993;12:217–220.
80. Slamon D. J., Leyland-Jones B., Shak S. Use of chemotherapy plus a monoclonal antibody against HER2 for metastatic breast cancer that overexpresses HER2. *N Engl J Med* 2001;344:783–792.
81. Steurer M, Sudmeier I, Stauder R, et al. Thromboembolic events in patients with myelodysplastic syndrome receiving thalidomide in combination with darbepoietin-alpha. *Br J Haematol* 2003;121: 101–103.
82. Product information: Sprycel (dasatinib) oral tablets. Princeton, NJ: Bristol-Myers Squibb; 2006.
83. Varis T, Kivisto K, Backman J, et al. The cytochrome P450 3A4 inhibitor itraconazole markedly increases the plasma concentrations of dexamethasone and enhances its adrenal-suppressant effect. *Clin Pharmacol Ther* 2000;68:487–494.
84. McLelland J, Jack W. Phenytoin/dexamethasone interaction: a clinical problem [Letter]. *Lancet* 1978;1:1096–1097.
85. Wong DD, Longenecker RG, Liepman M, et al. Phenytoin-dexamethasone: a possible drug-drug interaction. *JAMA* 1985;254:2062–2063.
86. Privitera MR, Greden JF, Gardner RW, et al. Interference by carbamazepine with the dexamethasone suppression test. *Biol Psychiatry* 1982;17:611–620.
87. Friedman HS, Petros WP, Friedman AH, et al. Irinotecan therapy in adults with recurrent or progressive malignant glioma. *J Clin Oncol* 1999;17:1516–1525.
88. Sanchorawala V, Wright DG, Rosenzweig M, et al. Lenalidomide and dexamethasone in the treatment of AL amyloidosis: results of a phase II trial. *Blood* 2007. in press.

DRUG INTERACTIONS

89. Cavo M, Zamagni E, Tosi P, et al. Superiority of thalidomide and dexamethasone over vincristine-doxorubicin-dexamethasone (VAD) as primary therapy in preparation for autologous transplantation for multiple myeloma. *Blood* 2005;106:35–39.
90. Schuller J, Czejka M, Kletzl H, et al. Doxorubicin (DOX) and Taxotere (TXT): a pharmacokinetic study of the combination in advanced breast cancer [Abstract 790]. *Proc Am Soc Clin Oncol* 1998;17:205a.
91. Royer I, Monsarrat B, Sonnier M, et al. Metabolism of docetaxel by human cytochromes P450: interactions with paclitaxel and other antineoplastic drugs. *Cancer Res* 1996;56:58–65.
92. Engels FK, Ten Tije AJ, Baker SD, et al. Effect of cytochrome P450 3A4 inhibition on the pharmacokinetics of docetaxel. *Clin Pharmacol Ther* 2004;75:448–454.
93. Zamboni WC, Egorin MJ, Van Echo DA, et al. Pharmacokinetic and pharmacodynamic study of the combination of docetaxel and topotecan in patients with solid tumors. *J Clin Oncol* 2000;18:3288–3294.
94. Cattel L, Recalenda V, Airoldi M, et al. Sequence-dependent combination of docetaxel and vinorelbine: pharmacokinetic interactions. *Farmaco* 2001;56:779–784.
95. Rushing DA, Raber SR, Rodvold KA, et al. The effects of cyclosporine on the pharmacokinetics of doxorubicin in patients with small cell lung cancer. *Cancer* 1994;74:834–841.
96. Barbui T, Rambaldi A, Parenzan L, et al. Neurological symptoms and coma associated with doxorubicin administration during chronic cyclosporine therapy. *Lancet* 1992;339:1421.
97. Minow RA, Stern MH, Casey JH, et al. Clinico-pathologic correlation of liver damage in patients treated with 6-mercaptopurine and Adriamycin. *Cancer* 1976;38:1524–1528.
98. Rodriguez V, Bodey GP, McCredie KB, et al. Combination 6-mercaptopurine-adriamycin in refractory adult acute leukemia. *Clin Pharmacol Ther* 1975;18:462–465.
99. Holmes FA, Madden T, Newman RA, et al. Sequence-dependent alteration of doxorubicin pharmacokinetics by paclitaxel in a phase I study of paclitaxel and doxorubicin in patients with metastatic breast cancer. *J Clin Oncol* 1996;14:2713–2721.
100. Gianni L, Vigano L, Locatelli A, et al. Human pharmacokinetic characterization and in vitro study of the interaction between doxorubicin and paclitaxel in patients with breast cancer. *J Clin Oncol* 1997;15:1906–1915.
101. Berg SL, Cowan KH, Balis FM, et al. Pharmacokinetics of taxol and doxorubicin administered alone and in combination by continuous 72-hour infusion. *J Natl Cancer Inst* 1994;86:143–145.
102. Chang P, Riggs CE Jr, Scheerer MT, et al. Combination chemotherapy with Adriamycin and streptozotocin: Clinicopharmacologic correlation of augmented Adriamycin toxicity caused by streptozotocin. *Clin Pharmacol Ther* 1976;20:611–616.
103. Zangari M, Anaissie E, Barlogie B, et al. Increased risk of deep-vein thrombosis in patients with multiple myeloma receiving thalidomide and chemotherapy. *Blood* 2001;98:1614–1615.
104. Zangari M, Siegel E, Barlogie B, et al. Thrombogenic activity of doxorubicin in myeloma patients receiving thalidomide: implications for therapy. *Blood* 2002;100:1168–1171.
105. Mross K, Steinbild S, Baas F, et al. Drug-drug interaction pharmacokinetic study with the Raf kinase inhibitor (RKI) BAY 43-9006 administered in combination with irinotecan (CPT-11) in patients with solid tumors. *Int J Clin Pharmacol Ther* 2003;41:618–619.
106. Sonneveld P, Marie JP, Huisman C, et al. Reversal of multidrug resistance by SDZ PSC833, combined with VAD (vincristine, doxorubicin, dexamethasone) in refractory multiple myeloma: a phase I study. *Leukemia* 1996;10:1741–1750.
107. Advani R, Fisher GA, Lum BL, et al. A phase I trial of doxorubicin, paclitaxel, and valspodar (PSC 833), a modulator of multidrug resistance. *Clin Cancer Res* 2001;7:1221–1229.
108. Murray LS, Jodrell DI, Morrison JG, et al. The effect of cimetidine on the pharmacokinetics of epirubicin in patients with advanced breast cancer: preliminary evidence of a potentially common drug interaction. *Clin Oncol* 1998;10:35–38.
109. Venturini M, Lunardi G, Del Mastro L, et al. Sequence effect of epirubicin and paclitaxel treatment on pharmacokinetics and toxicity. *J Clin Oncol* 2000;18:2116–2125.
110. Product information: Tarceva (erlotinib). Available at: http://www.tarceva.com/tarceva/patient/PI.jsp. Accessed August 18, 2005.
111. Product information: Emcyte (estramustine phosphate sodium). Piscataway, NJ: Kabi Pharmacia; 1999.
112. Lum BL, Kaubisch S, Yahanda AM, et al. Alteration of etoposide pharmacokinetics and pharmacodynamics by cyclosporine in a phase I trial to modulate multidrug resistance. *J Clin Oncol* 1992;10:1635–1642.
113. Bisogno G, Cowie F, Boddy A, et al. High-dose cyclosporin with etoposide-toxicity and pharmacokinetic interaction in children with solid tumors. *Br J Cancer* 1998;7:2304–2309.
114. Yahanda AM, Alder KM, Fisher GA, et al. Phase I trial of etoposide with cyclosporine as a modulator of multidrug resistance. *J Clin Oncol* 1992;10:1624–1634.
115. Lacayo NJ, Lum BL, Becton DL, et al. Pharmacokinetic interactions of cyclosporine with etoposide and mitoxantrone in children with acute myeloid leukemia. *Leukemia* 2002;16:920–927.

116. Rodman JH, Murry DJ, Madden T, Santana VM. Altered etoposide pharmacokinetics and time to engraftment in pediatric patients undergoing autologous bone marrow transplantation. *J Clin Oncol* 1994;12:2390–2397.

117. Keller RP, Altermatt HJ, Donatsch P, et al. Pharmacologic interactions between the resistance-modifying cyclosporine SDZ PSC 833 and etoposide (VP 16–213) enhance in vitro cytostatic activity and toxicity. *Int J Cancer* 1992;51:433–438.

118. Boote DJ, Dennis IF, Twentyman PR, et al. Phase I study of etoposide with SDZ PSC833 as a modulator of multidrug resistance in patients with cancer. *J Clin Oncol* 1996;14:610–618.

119. Kornblau SM, Estey E, Madden T, et al. Phase I study of mitoxantrone plus etoposide with multidrug blockade by SDZ PSC-833 in relapses or refractory acute myelogenous leukemia. *J Clin Oncol* 1997; 15:1796–1802.

120. Le AT, Hasson NK, Lum BL. Enhancement of warfarin response in a patient receiving etoposide and carboplatin chemotherapy. *Ann Pharmacother* 1997;31:1006–1008.

121. Ward K, Bitran JD. Warfarin, etoposide, and vindesine interactions. *Cancer Treat Rep* 1984;68: 817–818.

122. Product information: Fludara (fludarabine). Wayne, NJ: Berlex Laboratories; 1997.

123. Product information: Nipent (pentostatin). Plains, NJ: Morris Plains; 1994.

124. Harvey VJ, Slevin ML, Dilloway MR, et al. The influence of cimetidine on the pharmacokinetics of 5-fluorouracil. *Br J Clin Pharmacol* 1984;18:421–430.

125. Lokich JJ, Pitman SW, Skarin AT. Combined 5-fluorouracil and hydroxyurea therapy for gastrointestinal cancer. *Oncology* 1975;32:34–37.

126. Machover D, Schwarzenberg L, Goldschmidt E, et al. Treatment of advanced colorectal and gastric adenocarcinomas with 5-FU combined with high dose folinic acid: a pilot study. *Cancer Treat Rep* 1982;66:1803–1807.

127. Moertel CG, Fleming TR, MacDonald JS, et al. Hepatic toxicity associated with fluorouracil plus levamisole adjuvant therapy. *J Clin Oncol* 1993;11:2386–2390.

128. Benz C, Tillis T, Tattelman E, et al. Optimal schedule of methotrexate and 5-fluorouracil in human breast cancer. *Cancer Res* 1982;42:2081–2086.

129. Bardakji Z, Jolivet J, Langelier Y, et al. 5-Fluorouracil-metronidazole combination therapy in metastatic colorectal cancer. *Cancer Chemother Pharmacol* 1986;18:140–144.

130. Gilbar PJ, Brodribb TR. Phenytoin and fluorouracil interaction. *Ann Pharmacother* 2001;35: 1367–1370.

131. Desai AA, Vogelzang NJ, Rini BI, et al. A high rate of venous thromboembolism in a multi-institutional phase II trial of weekly intravenous gemcitabine with continuous infusion fluorouracil and daily thalidomide in patients with metastatic renal cell carcinoma. *Cancer* 2002;95:1629–1636.

132. Wajima T, Mukhopadhyay P. Possible interactions between warfarin and 5-fluorouracil [letter]. *Am J Hematol* 1992;40:238.

133. Scarfe MA, Israel MK. Possible drug interaction between warfarin and combination of levamisole and fluorouracil. *Ann Pharmacother* 1994;28:464–467.

134. Brown MC. An adverse interaction between warfarin and 5-fluorouracil: a case report and review of the literature. *Chemotherapy* 1999;45:392–395.

135. Aki Z, Kotiloglu G, Ozyilkan O. A patient with a prolonged prothrombin time due to an adverse interaction between 5-fluorouracil and warfarin [letter]. *Am J Gastroenterol* 2000;95:1093–1094.

136. Chlebowski RT, Gota CH, Chan KK, et al. Clinical and pharmacokinetic effects of combined warfarin and 5-fluorouracil in advanced colon cancer. *Cancer Res* 1982;42:4827–4830.

137. Product information: Eulexin (flutamide). Kenilworth, NJ: Schering Corporation; 2001.

138. Swaisland HC, Ranson M, Smith RP, et al. Pharmacokinetic drug interactions of gefitinib with rifampicin, itraconazole and metoprolol. *Clin Pharmacokinet* 2005;44:1067–1081.

139. Onoda S, Mitsufuji H, Yanase N, et al. Drug interaction between gefitinib and warfarin. *Jpn J Clin Oncol* 2005;35:478–482.

140. Kinikar SA, Kolesar JM. Identification of a gemcitabine-warfarin interaction. *Pharmacotherapy* 1999;19:1331–1333.

141. Longhurst HJ, Pinching AJ. Pancreatitis associated with hydroxyurea in combination with didanosine. *Br Med J* 2001;322:81.

142. Kerbusch T, Jansen RL, Mathot RA, et al. Modulation of the cytochrome P450-mediated metabolism of ifosfamide by ketoconazole and rifampin. *Clin Pharmacol Ther* 2001;70:132–141.

143. Hall G, Lind MJ, Huang M, et al. Intravenous infusions of ifosfamide/mesna and perturbation of warfarin anticoagulant control. *Postgrad Med J* 1990;66:860–861.

144. Peng B, Lloyd P, Schran H. Clinical pharmacokinetics of imatinib. *Clin Pharmacokinet* 2005;44: 879–894.

145. Dutreix C, Peng B, Mehring G, et al. Pharmacokinetic interaction between ketoconazole and imatinib mesylate (Glivec) in healthy subjects. *Cancer Chemother Pharmacol* 2004;54:290–294.

146. Bolton AE, Peng B, Hubert M, et al. Effect of rifampicin on the pharmacokinetics of imatinib mesylate (Gleevec, STI571) in healthy subjects. *Cancer Chemother Pharmacol* 2004;53:102–106.

DRUG INTERACTIONS

147. Frye RF, Fitzgerald SM, Lagattuta TF, et al. Effect of St. John's wort on imatinib mesylate pharmacokinetics. *Clin Pharmacol Ther* 2004;76:323–329.

148. Smith P, Bullock JM, Booker BM, et al. The influence of St. John's wort on the pharmacokinetics and protein binding of imatinib mesylate. *Pharmacotherapy* 2004;24:1508–1514.

149. Smith PF, Bullock JM, Booker BM, et al. Induction of imatinib metabolism by hypericum perforatum. *Blood* 2004;104:1229–1230.

150. Druker BJ, Talpaz M, Resta DJ, et al. Efficacy and safety of a specific inhibitor of the BCR-ABL tyrosine kinase in chronic myeloid leukemia. *N Engl J Med* 2001;344:1031–1037.

151. Peng B, Knight H, Riviere G, et al. Pharmacokinetic interaction between Gleevec (imatinib) and cyclosporin. *Blood* 2002;101:433–34B.

152. O'Brien SG, Meinhardt P, Bond E, et al. Effects of imatinib mesylate (STI571, Glivec) on the pharmacokinetics of simvastatin, a cytochrome p450 3A4 substrate, in patients with chronic myeloid leukaemia. *Br J Cancer* 2003;89:1855–1859.

153. Williams SJ, Baird-Lambert JA, Farrell GC. Inhibition of theophylline metabolism by interferon. *Lancet* 1987;2:939–941.

154. Product information: Retrovir (zidovudine). Research Triangle Park, NC: Glaxo Wellcome Inc.; 1996.

155. Product information: Reyataz (atazanavir). Available at: www.fda.gov/medwatch/SAFETY/2004/ jul_PI/Reyataz_PI.pdf. Accessed August 29, 2005.

156. Kehrer DF, Mathijssen RH, Verweij J, et al. Modulation of irinotecan by ketoconazole. *J Clin Oncol* 2002;20:3122–3129.

157. Wildiers H, Ahmed B, Guetens G, et al. Unexpected interactions between nicotinamide and CPT-11 in a rhabdomyosarcoma tumor model. *Anticancer Res* 2003;23:4055–4059.

158. Murry DJ, Cherrick I, Salama V, et al. Influence of phenytoin on the disposition of irinotecan: a case report. *J Pediatr Hematol Oncol* 2002;24:130–133.

159. Mathijssen RH, Sparreboom A, Dumez H, et al. Altered irinotecan metabolism in a patient receiving phenytoin. *Anticancer Drugs* 2002;13:139–140.

160. Kuhn JG. Influence of anticonvulsants on the metabolism and elimination of irinotecan: a North American Brain Tumor Consortium preliminary report. *Oncology (Huntingt)* 2002;16(8 Suppl 7): 33–40.

161. Mathijssen RH, Verweij J, de Bruijn P, et al. Effects of St. John's wort on irinotecan metabolism. *J Natl Cancer Inst* 2002;94:1247–1249.

162. Gornet JM, Lokiec F, Doclos-Vallee JC, et al. Severe CPT-11-induced diarrhea in presence of FK-506 following liver transplantation for hepatocellular carcinoma. *Anticancer Res* 2001;21:4203–4206.

163. Dresser GK, Spence JD, Bailey DG. Pharmacokinetic-pharmacodynamic consequences and clinical relevance of cytochrome P450 3A4 inhibition. *Clin Pharmacokinet* 2000;38:41–57.

164. Dowsett M, Pfister C, Johnston SR, et al. Impact of tamoxifen on the pharmacokinetics and endocrine effects of the aromatase inhibitor letrozole in postmenopausal women with breast cancer. *Clin Cancer Res* 1999;5:2338–2343.

165. Perez-Gallardo L, Blanco ML, Soria H, Escanero JF. Displacement of rifampicin bound to serum proteins by addition of levamisole. *Biomed Pharmacother* 1992;46:173–174.

166. Product information: Revlimid (lenalidomide) oral capsules. Summit, NJ: Celgene Corporation; 2006.

167. Hess WA, Kornblith PL. Combination of lomustine and cimetidine in the treatment of a patient with malignant glioblastoma: a case report. *Cancer Treat Rep* 1985;69:733.

168. Muller PJ, Tator CH, Bloom ML. Use of phenobarbital and high doses of 1-(2-chloroethyl)-3-cyclohexyl-1-nitrosourea in the treatment of brain tumor-bearing mice. *Cancer Res* 1983;43: 2068–2071.

169. Kobayashi K, Mimura N, Fujii H, et al. Role of human cytochrome P450 3A4 in metabolism of medroxyprogesterone acetate. *Clin Cancer Res* 2000;6:3297–3303.

170. Laine K, Yasar U, Widen J, et al. A screening study on the liability of eight different female sex steroids to inhibit CYP2C9, 2C19 and 3A4 activities in human liver microsomes. *Pharmacol Toxicol* 2003;93:77–81.

171. Tsunoda SM, Harris RZ, Mroczkowski PJ, et al. Preliminary evaluation of progestins as inducers of cytochrome P450 3A4 activity in postmenopausal women. *J Clin Pharmacol* 1998;38:1137–1143.

172. Sviland L, Robinson A, Proctor SJ, et al. Interaction of cimetidine with oral melphalan: a pharmacokinetic study. *Cancer Chemother Pharmacol* 1987;20:173–175.

173. Berns A, Rubenfeld S, Rymzo WT Jr. Hazard of combining allopurinol and thiopurine [letter]. *N Engl J Med* 1972;286:730.

174. Zimm S, Collins JM, O'Neill D, et al. Inhibition of first-pass metabolism in cancer chemotherapy: interaction of 6-mercaptopurine and allopurinol. *Clin Pharmacol Ther* 1983;34:810–817.

175. Balis FM, Holcenberg JS, Zimm S, et al. The effect of methotrexate on the bioavailability of oral 6-mercaptopurine. *Clin Pharmacol Ther* 1987;41:384–387.

176. Innocenti F, Danesi R, Di Paolo A, et al. Clinical and experimental pharmacokinetic interaction between 6-mercaptopurine and methotrexate. *Cancer Chemother Pharmacol* 1996;37:409–414.

177. Schmiegelow K, Bretton-Meyer U. 6-Mercaptopurine dosage and pharmacokinetics influence the degree of bone marrow toxicity following high-dose methotrexate in children with acute lymphoblastic leukemia. *Leukemia* 2001;15:74–79.

178. Spiers AS, Mibashan RS. Letter: Increased warfarin requirement during mercaptopurine therapy: a new drug interaction. *Lancet* 1974;2:221–222.

179. Relling MV, Pui CH, Sandlund JT, et al. Adverse effect of anticonvulsants on efficacy of chemotherapy for acute lymphoblastic leukaemia, *Lancet* 2000;356:285–290.

180. Frenia ML, Long KS. Methotrexate and non-steroidal antiinflammatory drug interactions. *Ann Pharmacother* 1992;26:234–237.

181. Tracy TS, Krohn K, Jones DR, et al. The effects of salicylate, ibuprofen, and naproxen on the disposition of methotrexate in patients with rheumatoid arthritis. *Eur J Clin Pharmacol* 1992;42: 121–125.

182. Maiche AG. Acute renal failure due to concomitant action of methotrexate and indomethacin. *Lancet* 1986;1:1390.

183. Dupuis LL, Koren G, Shore A, et al. Methotrexate-nonsteroidal anti-inflammatory drug interaction in children with arthritis. *J Rheumatol* 1990;17:1469–1473.

184. Furst DE, Herman RA, Koehnke R, et al. Effect of aspirin and sulindac on methotrexate clearance. *J Pharm Sci* 1990;79:782–786.

185. Erttmann R, Landbeck G. Effect of oral cholestyramine on the elimination of high-dose methotrexate. *J Cancer Res Clin Oncol* 1985;110:48–50.

186. Korstanje MJ, van Breda Vriesman CJP, van de Staak WJBM. Cyclosporine and methotrexate: a dangerous combination. *Am Acad Dermatol* 1990;23:320–321.

187. Tung JP, Maibach HI. The practical use of methotrexate in psoriasis. *Drugs* 1990;40:697–712.

188. Cohen MH, Creaven PJ, Fossieck BE, et al. Effect of oral prophylactic broad spectrum nonabsorbable antibiotics on the gastrointestinal absorption of nutrients and methotrexate in small cell bronchogenic carcinoma patients. *Cancer* 1976;38:1556–1559.

189. Liegler DG, Henderson ES, Hahn MA, et al. The effect of organic acids on renal clearance of methotrexate in man. *Clin Pharmacol Ther* 1969;10:849–857.

190. Ronchera CL, Hernandez T, Peris JE, et al. Pharmacokinetic interaction between high-dose methotrexate and amoxycillin. *Ther Drug Monit* 1993;15:375–379.

191. Dean R, Nachman J, Lorenzana AN. Possible methotrexate-mezlocillin interaction. *Am J Pediatr Hematol Oncol* 1992;14:88–92.

192. Aherne GW, Piall E, Mark V, et al. Prolongation and enhancement of serum methotrexate concentration by probenecid. *Br Med J* 1978;1:1097–1099.

193. Howell SB, Olshen RA, Rice JA. Effect of probenecid on cerebrospinal fluid methotrexate kinetics. *Clin Pharmacol Ther* 1979;26:641–646.

194. Basin KS, Escalante A, Beardmore TD. Severe pancytopenia in a patient taking low dose methotrexate and probenecid. *J Rheumatol* 1991;18:609–610.

195. Price P, Thompson H, Bessell EM, et al. Renal impairment following the combined use of high-dose methotrexate and procarbazine. *Cancer Chemother Pharmacol* 1988;21:265–267.

196. Breedveld P, Zelcer N, Pluim D, et al. Mechanism of the pharmacokinetic interaction between methotrexate and benzimidazoles: potential role for breast cancer resistance protein in clinical drug-drug interactions. *Cancer Res* 2004;64:5804–5811.

197. Troger U, Stotzel B, Martens-Lobenhoffer J, et al. Drug points: severe myalgia from an interaction between treatments with pantoprazole and methotrexate. *BMJ* 2002;324:1497.

198. Beorlegui B, Aldaz A, Ortega A, et al. Potential interaction between methotrexate and omeprazole. *Ann Pharmacother* 2000;34:1024–1027.

199. Ferrazzini G, Klein J, Sulh H, et al. Interaction between trimethoprim-sulfamethoxazole and methotrexate in children with leukemia. *J Pediatr* 1990;117:823–826.

200. Thomas MH, Gutterman LA. Methotrexate toxicity in a patient receiving trimethoprim-sulfamethoxazole. *J Rheumatol* 1986;13:440–441.

201. Groenendal H, Rampen FHJ. Methotrexate and trimethoprim-sulphamethoxazole—a potentially hazardous combination. *Clin Exp Dermatol* 1990;15:358–360.

202. Jeurissen ME, Boerbooms AM, van de Putte LB. Pancytopenia and methotrexate with trimethoprim-sulfamethoxazole [letter]. *Ann Intern Med* 1989;111:261.

203. Maricic M, Davis M, Gall EP. Megaloblastic pancytopenia in a patient receiving concurrent methotrexate and trimethoprim-sulfamethoxazole treatment. *Arthritis Rheum* 1986;29:133–135.

204. Schroder H, Ostergaard JR. Interference of high-dose methotrexate in the metabolism of valproate? *Pediatr Hematol Oncol* 1994;11:445–449.

205. Varis T, Kaukonen KM, Kivisto KT, et al. Plasma concentrations and effects of oral methylprednisolone are considerably increased by itraconazole. *Clin Pharmacol Ther* 1998;64:363–368.

206. Varis T, Kivisto K, Neuvonen P. Grapefruit juice can increase the plasma concentrations of oral methylprednisolone. *Eur J Clin Pharmacol* 2000;56:489–493.

207. Stjernholm MR, Katz FH. Effects of diphenylhydantoin, phenobarbital, and diazepam on the metabolism of methylprednisolone and its sodium succinate. *J Clin Endocrinol Metab* 1975;41:887–893.

DRUG INTERACTIONS

208. Konishi H, Sumi M, Shibata N, et al. Influence of intravenous methylprednisolone pulse treatment on the disposition of ciclosporin and hepatic CYP3A activity in rats. *J Pharm Pharmacol* 2004;56: 477–483.
209. Villikka K, Varis T, Backman JT, et al. Effect of methylprednisolone on CYP3A4-mediated drug metabolism in vivo. *Eur J Clin Pharmacol* 2001;57:457–460.
210. Montes A, Powles TJ, O'Brien ME, et al. A toxic interaction between mitomycin C and tamoxifen causing the haemolytic uraemic syndrome. *Eur J Cancer* 1993;29A:1854–1857.
211. Raderer M, Kornek G, Hejna M, et al. Acute pulmonary toxicity associated with high-dose vinorelbine and mitomycin C. *Ann Oncol* 1996;7:973–975.
212. Rivera MP, Kris MG, Gralla RJ, et al. Syndrome of acute dyspnea related to combined mitomycin plus vinca alkaloid chemotherapy. *Am J Clin Oncol* 1995;18:245–250.
213. Rao SX, Ramaswamy G, Levin M, et al. Fatal acute respiratory failure after vinblastine-mitomycin therapy in lung carcinoma. *Arch Intern Med* 1985;145:1905–1907.
214. Hoelzer KL, Harrison BR, Luedke SW, et al. Vinblastine-associated pulmonary toxicity in patients receiving combination therapy with mitomycin and cisplatin. *Drug Intell Clin Pharm* 1986;20:287–289.
215. Product information: Arranon (nelarabine) IV injection. Research Triangle Park, NC: GlaxoSmith-Kline; 2006.
216. Product information: Nilandron (nilutamide). Kansas City, MO: Hoechst Marion Roussel, Inc.; 1996.
217. Babany G, Tinel M, Letteron P, et al. Inhibitory effects of nilutamide, a new androgen receptor antagonist, on mouse and human liver cytochrome P-450. *Biochem Pharmacol* 1989;38:941–947.
218. Villikka K, Kivisto KT, Neuvonen PJ. The effect of rifampin on the pharmacokinetics of oral and intravenous ondansetron. *Clin Pharmacol Ther* 1999;65:377–381.
219. Fetell MR, Grossman SA, Fisher JD, et al. Preirradiation paclitaxel in glioblastoma multiforme: efficacy, pharmacology, and drug interactions. *J Clin Oncol* 1997;15:3121–3128.
220. Chang SM, Kuhn JG, Rizzo J, et al. Phase I study of paclitaxel in patients with recurrent malignant glioma: a North American Brain Tumor Consortium report. *J Clin Oncol* 1998;16:2188–2194.
221. Kang MH, Figg WD, Ando Y, et al. The P-glycoprotein antagonist PSC 833 increases the plasma concentrations of 6—hydroxypaclitaxel, a major metabolite of paclitaxel. *Clin Cancer Res* 2001;7: 1610–1617.
222. Mulatero C, McClaren BR, Mason M, et al. Evidence for a schedule-dependent deleterious interaction between paclitaxel, vinblastine and cisplatin (PVC) in the treatment of advanced transitional cell carcinoma. *Br J Cancer* 2000;83:1612–1616.
223. Thompson ME, Highley MS. Interaction between paclitaxel and warfarin. *Ann Oncol* 2003;14:500.
224. Product information: Photofrin (porfimer). Seattle, WA: QLT Phototherapeutics Inc; 1999.
225. Ulrich B, Frey FJ, Speck RF, et al. Pharmacokinetics/pharmacodynamics of ketoconazole-prednisolone interaction. *J Pharmacol Exp Ther* 1992;260:487–490.
226. McAllister WAC, Thompson PJ, Al-Habel SM, et al. Rifampicin reduces effectiveness and bioavailability of prednisolone. *Br Med J (Clin Res Ed)* 1983;286:923–925.
227. Buffington GA, Dominguez JH, Piering WF, et al. Interaction of rifampin and glucocorticoids: adverse effect on renal allograft function. *JAMA* 1976;236:1958–1960.
228. Brooks SM, Werk EE, Ackerman SJ, et al. Adverse effects of phenobarbital on corticosteroid metabolism in patients with bronchial asthma. *N Engl J Med* 1972;286:1125–1128.
229. Gambertoglio JG, Holford NH, Kapusnik JE, et al. Disposition of total and unbound prednisolone in renal transplant patients receiving anticonvulsants. *Kidney Int* 1984;25:119–123.
230. Product information: Matulane (procarbazine). Nutley, NJ: Roche Laboratories; 1998.
231. Lehmann DF, Hurteau TE, Newman N, et al. Anticonvulsant usage is associated with an increased risk of procarbazine hypersensitivity reactions in patients with brain tumors. *Clin Pharmacol Ther* 1997;62:225–229.
232. Brown CS, Bryant SG. Monoamine oxidase inhibitors: safety and efficacy issues. *Drug Intell Clin Pharm* 1988;22:232–235.
233. Sternbach H. The serotonin syndrome. *Am J Psychiatry* 1991;148:705–713.
234. Product information: Nexavar (sorafenib) oral tablets. West Haven, CT: Bayer Pharmaceuticals Corporation; 2005.
235. Product information: Sutent (sunitinib) oral capsules. New York: Pfizer Laboratories; 2006.
236. Koranyi L, Gero L. Influence of diphenylhydantoin on the effect of streptozotocin [letter]. *Br Med J* 1979;1:127.
237. Kivisto KT, Villikka K, Nyman L, et al. Tamoxifen and toremifene concentrations in plasma are greatly decreased by rifampin. *Clin Pharmacol Ther* 1998;64:648–654.
238. Tenni P, Lalich DL, Byrne MJ. Life threatening interaction between tamoxifen and warfarin. *Br Med J* 1989;298:93–94.
239. Lodwick R, McConkey B, Brown AM. Life threatening interaction between tamoxifen and warfarin. *Br Med J* 1987;295:1141.
240. Richie LD, Grant SM. Tamoxifen-warfarin interactions: the Aberdeen hospitals drug file. *Br Med J* 1989;298:1253.

241. Baker DK, Relling MV, Pui CH, et al. Increased teniposide clearance with concomitant anticonvulsant therapy. *J Clin Oncol* 1992;10:311–315.
242. Zamboni WC, Gajjar AJ, Heideman RL, et al. Phenytoin alters the disposition of topotecan and *N*-desmethyl metabolite in a patient with medulloblastoma. *Clin Cancer Res* 1998;4:783–789.
243. Product information: Fareston (toremifene). Kenilworth, NJ: Schering Corporation; 1999.
244. Heusner JJ, Franklin MR. Inhibition of metabolism of the 'nonclassical' antifolate, trimetrexate (2,4-diamino-5-methyl-6-[(3,4,5-trimethoxyanilino)methyl]quinazoline) by drugs containing an imidazole moiety. *Pharmacology* 1985;30:266–272.
245. Chan JD. Pharmacokinetic drug interactions of vinca alkaloids: summary of case reports. *Pharmacotherapy* 1998;18:1304–1307.
246. Tobe SW, Siu LL, Jamal SA, et al. Vinblastine and erythromycin: an unrecognized serious drug interaction. *Cancer Chemother Pharmacol* 1995;35:188–190.
247. Weintraub M, Adde MA, Venzon DJ, et al. Severe atypical neuropathy associated with administration of hematopoietic colony-stimulating factors and vincristine. *J Clin Oncol* 1996;14:935–940.
248. Weber DM, Dimopoulos MA, Alexanian R. Increased neurotoxicity with VAD-cyclosporin in multiple myeloma. *Lancet* 1993;341:558–559.
249. Bertrand Y, Capdevile R, Balduck N, et al. Cyclosporine A used to reverse drug resistance increases vincristine neurotoxicity. *Am J Hematol* 1992;40:158–159.
250. Villikka K, Kivisto KT, Maenpaa H, et al. Cytochrome P450-inducing antiepileptics increase the clearance of vincristine in patients with brain tumors. *Clin Pharmacol Ther* 1999;66:589–593.
251. Bohme A, Ganser A, Hoelzer D. Aggravation of vincristine-induced neurotoxicity by itraconazole in the treatment of adult ALL. *Ann Hematol* 1995;71:311–312.
252. Gillies J, Hung KA, Fitzsimons E, et al. Severe vincristine toxicity in combination with itraconazole. *Clin Lab Haematol* 1998;20:123–124.
253. Bermudez M, Fuster JL, Llinares E, et al. Itraconazole-related increased vincristine neurotoxicity: case report and review of literature. *J Pediatr Hematol Oncol* 2005;27:389–392.
254. Fedeli L, Colozza M, Boschetti E, et al. Pharmacokinetics of vincristine in cancer patients treated with nifedipine. *Cancer* 1989;64:1805–1811.
255. Bosque E. Possible drug interaction between itraconazole and vinorelbine tartrate leading to death after one dose of chemotherapy. *Ann Intern Med* 2001;134:427.
256. Product information: Zolinza (vorinostat) oral capsules. Whitehouse Station, NJ: Merck & Co., Inc.; 2006.
257. May S. Significant drug-drug interactions with antineoplastics. *Hosp Pharm* 2000;35:1207–1219.
258. Evans WE, Relling MV. Clinical pharmacokinetics-pharmacodynamics of anticancer drugs. *Clin Pharmacokinet* 1989;16:327–336.
259. Canellos GP, Haskell CM, Arseneau J, et al. Hypoalbuminemic and hypocholesterolemic effect of l-asparaginase (NSC-109,229) treatment in man—a preliminary report. *Cancer Chemother Rep* 1969;53:67–69.
260. McSorley LC, Daly AK. Identification of human cytochrome P450 isoforms that contribute to all-trans-retinoic acid 4-hydroxylation. *Biochem Pharmacol* 2000;60:517–526.
261. Damia G, D'Incalci M. Clinical pharmacokinetics of altretamine. *Clin Pharmacokinet* 1995;28:439–448.
262. Grimm SW, Dyroff MC. Inhibition of human drug metabolizing cytochromes P450 by anastrozole, a potent and selective inhibitor of aromatase. *Drug Metab Dispos* 1997;25:598–602.
263. Buzdar AU, Robertson JF, Eiermann W, et al. An overview of the pharmacology and pharmacokinetics of the newer generation aromatase inhibitors anastrozole, letrozole, and exemestane. *Cancer* 2002;95:2006–2016.
264. Shadle CR, Lee Y, Majumdar AK, et al. Evaluation of potential inductive effects of aprepitant on cytochrome P450 3A4 and 2C9 activity. *J Clin Pharmacol* 2004;44:215–223.
265. Sanchez RI, Wang RW, Newton DJ, et al. Cytochrome P450 3A4 is the major enzyme involved in the metabolism of the substance P receptor antagonist aprepitant. *Drug Metab Dispos* 2004;32:1287–1292.
266. Nadin L, Murray M. Participation of CYP2C8 in retinoic acid 4-hydroxylation in human hepatic microsomes. *Biochem Pharmacol* 1999;58:1201–1208.
267. Cockshott ID. Bicalutamide: clinical pharmacokinetics and metabolism. *Clin Pharmacokinet* 2004;43:855–878.
268. Baumhakel M, Kasel D, Rao-Schymanski RA, et al. Screening for inhibitory effects of antineoplastic agents on CYP3A4 in human liver microsomes. *Int J Clin Pharmacol Ther* 2001;39:517–528.
269. Griskevicius L, Yasar U, Sandberg M, et al. Bioactivation of cyclophosphamide: the role of polymorphic CYP2C enzymes. *Eur J Clin Pharmacol* 2003;59:103–109.
270. Reid JM, Kuffel MJ, Miller JK, Rios R, Ames MM. Metabolic activation of dacarbazine by human cytochromes P450: the role of CYP1A1, CYP1A2, and CYP2E1. *Clin Cancer Res* 1999;5:2192–2197.

DRUG INTERACTIONS

271. Tomlinson ES, Lewis DF, Maggs JL, et al. In vitro metabolism of dexamethasone (DEX) in human liver and kidney: the involvement of CYP3A4 and CYP17 (17,20 LYASE) and molecular modelling studies. *Biochem Pharmacol* 1997;54:605–611.

272. Gentile DM, Tomlinson ES, Maggs JL, et al. Dexamethasone metabolism by human liver in vitro: metabolite identification and inhibition of 6-hydroxylation. *J Pharmacol Exp Ther* 1996;277: 105–112.

273. McCune JS, Hawke RL, LeCluyse EL, et al. In vivo and in vitro induction of human cytochrome P4503A4 by dexamethasone. *Clin Pharmacol Ther* 2000;68:356–366.

274. Nallani SC, Genter MB, Desai PB. Increased activity of CYP3A enzyme in primary cultures of rat hepatocytes treated with docetaxel: comparative evaluation with paclitaxel. *Cancer Chemother Pharmacol* 2001;48:115–122.

275. Janicki PK. Cytochrome P450 2D6 metabolism and 5-hydroxytryptamine type 3 receptor antagonists for postoperative nausea and vomiting. *Med Sci Monit* 2005;11:RA322–RA328.

276. Blower PR. 5-HT3-receptor antagonists and the cytochrome P450 system: clinical implications. *Cancer J* 2002;8:405–414.

277. Kawashiro T, Yamashita K, Zhao X.-J, et al. A study on the metabolism of etoposide and possible interactions with antitumor or supporting agents by human liver microsomes. *J Pharmacol Exp Ther* 1998;286:1294–1300.

278. Relling MV, Evans R, Dass C, et al. Human cytochrome P450 metabolism of teniposide and etoposide. *J Pharmacol Exp Ther* 1992;261:491–496.

279. Shet MS, McPhaul M, Fisher CW, et al. Metabolism of the antiandrogenic drug (Flutamide) by human CYP1A2. *Drug Metab Dispos* 1997;25:1298–1303.

280. McKillop D, McCormick AD, Millar A, et al. Cytochrome P450-dependent metabolism of gefitinib. *Xenobiotica* 2005;35:39–50.

281. Nakamura H, Ariyoshi N, Okada K, et al. CYP1A1 is a major enzyme responsible for the metabolism of granisetron in human liver microsomes. *Curr Drug Metab* 2005;6:469–480.

282. Granvil CP, Madan A, Sharkawi M, et al. Role of CYP2B6 and CYP3A4 in the in vitro *N*-dechloroethylation of (*R*)- and (*S*)-ifosfamide in human liver microsomes. *Drug Metab Dispos* 1999;27:533–541.

283. Mathijssen RH, van Alphen RJ, Verweij J, et al. Clinical pharmacokinetics and metabolism of irinotecan (CPT-11). *Clin Cancer Res* 2001;7:2182–2194.

284. Lee FY, Workman P, Roberts JT, Bleehen NM. Clinical pharmacokinetics of oral CCNU (lomustine). *Cancer Chemother Pharmacol* 1985;14:125–131.

285. Dixon CM, Colthup PV, Serabjit-Singh CJ, et al. Multiple forms of cytochrome P450 are involved in the metabolism of ondansetron in humans. *Drug Metab Dispos* 1995;23:1225–1230.

286. Rahman A, Korzekwa KR, Grogan J, et al. Selective biotransformation of taxol to 6-α-hydroxytaxol by human cytochrome P450 2C8. *Cancer Res* 1994;54:5543–5546.

287. Kumar GN, Walle UK, Walle T. Cytochrome P450 3A-mediated human liver microsomal taxol 6-α-hydroxylation. *J Pharmacol Exp Ther* 1994;268:1160–1165.

288. Kostrubsky VE, Lewis LD, Wood SG, et al. Effect of Taxol on cytochrome P450 and acetaminophen toxicity in cultured rat hepatocytes: comparison to dexamethasone. *Toxicol Appl Pharmacol* 1997;142:79–86.

289. Goria-Gatti L, Iannone A, Tomasi A, et al. In vitro and in vivo evidence for the formation of methyl radical from procarbazine: a spin-trapping study. *Carcinogenesis* 1992;13:799–805.

290. Jacolot F, Simon I, Dreano Y, et al. Identification of the cytochrome P450 IIIA family as the enzymes involved in the *N*-demethylation of tamoxifen in human liver microsomes. *Biochem Pharmacol* 1991;41:1911–1919.

291. Choi MH, Skipper PL, Wishnok JS, et al. Characterization of testosterone 11β-hydroxylation catalyzed by human liver microsomal cytochromes P450. *Drug Metab Dispos* 2005;33:714–718.

292. Richter T, Schwab M, Eichelbaum M, et al. Inhibition of human CYP2B6 by N,N ,N `-triethylenethiophosphoramide is irreversible and mechanism-based. *Biochem Pharmacol* 2005;69:517–524.

293. Choi MH, Skipper PL, Wishnok JS, et al. Cytochrome P450 3A enzyme family in the major metabolic pathways of toremifene in human liver microsomes. *Biochem Pharmacol* 1994;47:1883–1895.

294. Zhou-Pan XR, Seree E, Zhou XJ, et al. Involvement of human liver cytochrome P450 3A in vinblastine metabolism: drug interactions. *Cancer Res* 1993;53:5121–5126.

295. Xie R, Mathijssen RH, Sparreboom A, et al. Clinical pharmacokinetics of irinotecan and its metabolites in relation with diarrhea. *Clin Pharmacol Ther* 2002;72:265–275.

296. Glantz MJ, Cole BF, Forsyth PA, Recht LD, Wen PY, Chamberlain MC, Grossman SA, Cairncross JG. Practice parameter: anticonvulsant prophylaxis in patients with newly diagnosed brain tumors. Report of the Quality Standards Subcommittee of the American Academy of Neurology. *Neurology* 2000;54:1886–1893.

297. Kintzel PE, Dorr RT. Anticancer drug renal toxicity and elimination: dosing guidelines for altered renal function. *Cancer Treat Rev* 1995;21:33–64.

298. Breithaupt H, Kuenzlen E. Pharmacokinetics of methotrexate and 7-hydroxymethotrexate following infusions of high dose methotrexate. *Cancer Treat Rep* 1982;66:1733–1741.

299. Bleyer A. The clinical pharmacology of methotrexate: new applications of an old drug. *Cancer* 1978;41:36–51.
300. Daugaard G, Rossing N, Rorth M. Effects of cisplatin on different measures of glomerular function in the human kidney with special emphasis on high dose. *Cancer Chemother Pharmacol* 1988;21: 163–167.
301. Ballet F, Vrignaud P, Robert J, et al. Hepatic extraction, metabolism and biliary excretion of doxorubicin in the isolated perfused rat liver. *Cancer Chemother Pharmacol* 1987;19:240–245.
302. Clarke SJ, Rivory LP. Clinical pharmacokinetics of docetaxel. *Clin Pharmacokinet* 1999;36:99–114.
303. Jackson DV Jr, Castle MC, Bender RA. Biliary excretion of vincristine. *Clin Pharmacol Ther* 1978;24:101–107.
304. Aronoff GR, Berns JS, Brier ME. *Drug Prescribing in Renal Failure. Dosing Guidelines for Adults,* 4th ed. Philadelphia: American College of Physicians; 1999.
305. Patterson WP, Reams GP. Renal and electrolyte abnormalities due to chemotherapy. In Perry MC, ed.: *The Chemotherapy Sourcebook,* 3rd ed. Philadelphia: Lippincott Williams & Wilkins; 2001:494–494.
306. Floyd J, Mirza I, Sachs B, et al. Hepatotoxicity of chemotherapy. *Semin Oncol* 2006;33:50–67.
307. King PD, Perry MC. Hepatotoxicity of chemotherapy. *Oncologist* 2001;6:162–176.
308. Haubitz M, Bohnenstengel F, Brunkhorst R, et al. Cyclophosphamide pharmacokinetics and dose requirements in patients with renal insufficiency. *Kidney Int* 2002;61:1495–1501.
309. Smith GA, Damon LE, Rugo HS, et al. High-dose cytarabine dose modification reduces the incidence of neurotoxicity in patients with renal insufficiency. *J Clin Oncol* 1997;15:833–839.
310. Samur M. Docetaxel and liver dysfunction: is it absolutely contraindicated? *Am J Clin Oncol* 2001;24: 319–321.
311. Baker SD, Ravdin P, Aylesworth C, et al. A phase I and pharmacokinetic (PK) study of docetaxel in cancer patients (PTS) with liver dysfunction due to malignancies [Abstract 739]. *Proc Am Soc Clin Oncol* 1998;17:192a.
312. Joel S, Clark P, Slevin M. Renal function and etoposide pharmacokinetics: is dose modification necessary? *Proc Am Soc Clin Oncol* 1991;10:103.
313. Stewart CF. Use of etoposide in patients with organ dysfunction: pharmacokinetic and pharmacodynamic considerations. *Cancer Chemother Pharmacol* 1994;34:S76–S83.
314. Lichtman SM, Etcubanas E, Budman DR, et al. The pharmacokinetics and pharmacodynamics of fludarabine phosphate in patients with renal impairment: a prospective dose adjustment study. *Cancer Invest* 2002;20:904–913.
315. Falkson G, Hunt M, Borden EC, et al. An extended phase II trial of ifosfamide plus mesna in malignant mesothelioma. *Invest New Drugs* 1992;10:337–343.
316. Raymond E, Boige V, Faivre S, et al. Dosage adjustment and pharmacokinetic profile of irinotecan in cancer patients with hepatic dysfunction. *J Clin Oncol* 2002;20:4303–312.
317. Batchelor T, Carson K, O'Neill A, et al. Treatment of primary CNS lymphoma with methotrexate and deferred radiotherapy: a report of NABTT 96-07. *J Clin Oncol* 2003;21:1044–1049.
318. Lathia C, Fleming GF, Meyer M, et al. Pentostatin pharmacokinetics and dosing recommendations in patients with mild renal impairment. *Cancer Chemother Pharmacol* 2002;50:121–126.
319. Massari C, Brienza S, Rotarski M, et al. Pharmacokinetics of oxaliplatin in patients with normal versus impaired renal function. *Cancer Chemother Pharmacol* 2000;45:157–164.
320. Takimoto CH, Remick SC, Sharma S, et al. Administration of oxaliplatin to patients with renal dysfunction: a preliminary report of the national cancer institute organ dysfunction working group. *Semin Oncol* 2003;30(4 Suppl 15):20–25.
321. Zamboni WC, Heideman RL, Meyer WH, et al. Pharmacokinetics (PK) of topotecan in pediatric patients with normal and altered renal function [Abstract 371]. *Proc Am Soc Clin Oncol* 1996; 15:180.
322. O'Reilly S, Rowinsky E, Slichenmyer W, et al. Phase I and pharmacologic studies of topotecan in patients with impaired hepatic function. *J Natl Cancer Inst* 1996;88:817–824.
323. Trissel LA, ed. *Handbook on Injectable Drugs,* 11 ed. Bethesda, MD: American Society of Health-System Pharmacists; 2001.
324. Crom WR, Evans WE. Methotrexate. In Evans WE, Schentag JJ, Jusko WJ, eds: *Applied Pharmacokinetics: Principles of Therapeutic Drug Monitoring,* 3rd ed. Vancouver, WA; Applied Therapeutics, Inc.; 1992.
325. Ackland SP, Schilsky RL. High-dose methotrexate: a critical reappraisal. *J Clin Oncol* 1987;5: 2017–2031.
326. Treon SP, Chabner BA. Concepts in use of high-dose methotrexate therapy. *Clin Chem* 1996;42: 1322–1329.
327. Goldie JH, Price LA, Harrap KR. Methotrexate toxicity: correlation with duration of administration, plasma levels, dose and excretion pattern. *Eur J Cancer* 1972;8:409–414.
328. Relling MV, Fairclough D, Ayers D, et al. Patient characteristics associated with high-risk methotrexate concentration and toxicity. *J Clin Oncol* 1994;12:1667–1672.

329. Evans WE, Crom WR, Abromowitch M, et al. Clinical pharmacodynamics of high-dose methotrexate in acute lymphocytic leukemia. *N Engl J Med* 1986;314:471–477.
330. Stoller RG, Hande KR, Jacobs SA, et al. Use of plasma pharmacokinetics to predict and prevent methotrexate toxicity. *N Engl J Med* 1977;297:630–634.
331. Rosen G, Caparros B, Huvos AG, et al. Preoperative chemotherapy for osteogenic sarcoma: selection of postoperative adjuvant chemotherapy based on the response of the primary tumor to preoperative chemotherapy. *Cancer* 1982;49:1221–1230.
332. Skarin AT, Zuckerman KS, Pitman SW, et al. High dose methotrexate with folinic acid in the treatment of advanced non-Hodgkin lymphoma including CNS involvement. *Blood* 1977;50:1039–1047.
333. Nixon PF, Bertino JR. Effective absorption and utilization of oral formyltetrahydrofolate in man. *N Engl J Med* 1972;286:175–179.
334. Delepine N, Delepine G, Cornille H, et al. Dose escalation with pharmacokinetics monitoring in methotrexate chemotherapy of osteosarcoma. *Anticancer Res* 1995;15:489–494.
335. Frei E III, Blum RH, Pitman SW, et al. High dose methotrexate with leucovorin rescue: rationale and spectrum of antitumor activity. *Am J Med* 1980;68:370–376.
336. Donati MB. Cancer and thrombosis. *Haemostasis* 1994;24:128–131.
337. Sorensen HT, Mellemkjaer L, Olsen JH, et al. Prognosis of cancers associated with venous thromboembolism. *N Engl J Med* 2000;343:1846–1850.
338. Zacharski LR, Henderson WG, Rickles FR, et al. Effect of warfarin anticoagulation on survival in carcinoma of the lung, colon, head and neck, and prostate. *Cancer* 1984;53:2046–2052.
339. Falanga A, Levine MN, Consonni R, et al. The effect of very-low-dose warfarin on markers of hypercoagulation in metastatic breast cancer: results from a randomized trial. *Thromb Haemost* 1998;79:23–27.
340. Levine M, Hirsh J, Gent M, et al. Double-blind randomized trial of very-low-dose warfarin for prevention of thromboembolism in stage IV breast cancer. *Lancet* 1994;343:886–989.
341. Rajan R, Gafni A, Levine M, et al. Very low-dose warfarin prophylaxis to prevent thromboembolism in women with metastatic breast cancer receiving chemotherapy: an economic evaluation. *J Clin Oncol* 1995;13:42–46.
342. Package insert: Coumadin (warfarin sodium). Wilmington, DE: DuPont Pharma; 1996.
343. Wells PS, Holbrook AM, Crowther NR, et al. Interactions of warfarin with drugs and food. *Ann Intern Med* 1994;121:676–683.
344. Kwaan HC, Wang J, Boggio LN. Abnormalities in hemostasis in acute promyelocytic leukemia. *Hematol Oncol* 2002;20:33–41.
345. Goodnough LT, Saito H, Manni A, et al. Increased incidence of thromboembolism in stage IV breast cancer patients treated with a five-drug chemotherapy regimen: a study of 159 patients. *Cancer* 1984;54:1264–1268.
346. Saphner T, Tormey DC, Gray R. Venous and arterial thrombosis in patients who received adjuvant therapy for breast cancer. *J Clin Oncol* 1991;9:286–294.
347. Yates RA, Wong J, Seiberling M, et al. The effect of anastrozole on the single-dose pharmacokinetics and anticoagulant activity of warfarin in healthy volunteers. *Br J Clin Pharmacol* 2001;51:429–35.

Considerations in Preventing Medication Errors

Robert J. Ignoffo

One of the most devastating events that can happen to a cancer patient and his or her health care provider is the occurrence of a chemotherapy error that results in serious harm or death. Richard Knox, a reporter and colleague of Betsy Lehman and health journalist for *The Boston Globe,* brought this issue to national attention in 1995.[1] Unfortunately, two women with breast cancer who were enrolled on a clinical trial received a fourfold amount of cyclophosphamide over the intended dose; Lehman was one of the women. The order was written "4 g/sq m over 4 days." Although pharmacists and nurses did not misinterpret the dose, they failed to recognize the amount of drug as an overdose. The intended dose was 1 g per square meter daily for 4 days. A clinical research associate who had been abstracting clinical trial data from their charts discovered the error. This error occurred at Dana-Farber Cancer Institute, an institution with a prestigious reputation. In response to the error, an internal and external peer review committee was convened, and this committee agreed that clinical leadership within the institution needed to be strengthened and that specific steps in processing chemotherapy orders needed improvement. The hospital made several public statements that were aired on network TV. Soon thereafter, editorials[2,3] and review articles appeared in the literature recommending strategies that an institution might use to prevent chemotherapy errors.[4,5] This prompted another major cancer center to examine its practices and those of 123 other hospitals to ascertain methods used for processing chemotherapy orders.[6] Most programs had a process in place to prevent chemotherapy errors. The recommendation was that when chemotherapy was used as a modality, the team should include well-trained physicians, nurses, and pharmacists. Since 1995, medication safety has been a pressing concern to those of us practicing oncology, including administrators of cancer centers. The Institute of Medicine Report (IOM) on medication errors in the United States was published in 2000[7] and called for major reform in health system design to prevent medication errors. Lucian Leape, a long time researcher in medication errors, and his colleague Donald Berwick stated in their recent article[8] that "Since the IOM report *To Err Is Human: Building a Safer Health System,* small but consequential changes have gradually spread through hospitals." These improvements are largely due to the concerted activities by hospital associations, professional societies, and accredited bodies, especially The Joint Commission (TJC). Their efforts have motivated thousands of practitioners in hospitals and clinics to become more alert to patient safety issues and implement methodologies for quality improvement. However, Leape and Berwick thought that progress had been too slow and that patient safety goals should be more explicit and ambitious. They strongly recommended that the Agency for Healthcare Research and Quality (AHRQ) bring all stakeholders together to agree on patient safety goals that can be reached by the year 2010. In the oncology arena, the pressure for change may come from accrediting organizations such as the JCAHO and American College of Surgeons (ACOS) as well as from third-party payers that may invoke payment incentives for quality care (note the recent decision by payers in the state of Minnesota to withhold payments from hospitals if a serious preventable adverse drug event occurs).[9] Leaders in the field are calling for health care payers to adopt this approach nationwide.

The U.S. Pharmacopeia (USP) standard USP 797, which is now an enforceable document, gives the U.S. Food and Drug Administration (FDA), state boards of pharmacy, and accrediting organizations such as JCAHO a standard when evaluating the appropriate preparation of high-risk compounded sterile products, such as cytotoxic chemotherapy drugs.[10] Although USP 797 does specifically mention chemotherapy, Darryl Rich of JCAHO has discussed the possibility that products which are premixed for use at a later time could be surveyed to comply with this standard.[11] Compounded sterile products that are prepared and administered immediately do not fall under USP 797. One of the problems with implementing USP 797 is that it does not address safe handling issues for cytotoxic agents. This may be changed by the time of this publication, but as of March 2006, JCAHO was not considering safe handling of these drugs as part of a survey under USP 797.

Although medication error reporting has improved since the rollout of the FDA's MedWatch Web-based program in 1996[12] and the Medication Errors Reporting Program, a cooperative effort of the USP and the Institute for Safe Medication Practices (ISMP),[13] serious errors continue to occur in the oncology setting. From March to December 2000, a prospective cohort study of more than 2700 visits to the ambulatory oncology clinic was done at Dana-Farber Cancer Institute. The results showed that 3% of the 10,110 chemotherapy orders reviewed prospectively contained errors, 82% of which could have produced potential harm with one third of these classified as serious.[14] Fortunately, 45% of the errors were detected before the patient received the treatment, and no patients died. This audit has led to further refinements in the chemotherapy process at that institution.

Perhaps the most ambitious reporting system comes from the state of Minnesota. Minnesota has led the way in adopting a patient safety initiative by approving in 2003 its Adverse Health Events Reporting Law, which is mandated by the Minnesota Alliance for Patient Safety. The Alliance generates a summary report from adverse event submissions from all Minnesota hospitals and publishes its findings annually. As of the writing of this chapter, its February 2006 report[15] included six events classified as serious morbidity and one death that were associated with a medication error. It is uncertain whether any of these events were associated with cancer chemotherapy.

CAUSES OF CHEMOTHERAPY ERRORS
The list below is taken from actual published reports of chemotherapy errors.

1. **Name confusion (substituting an incorrect drug for another).** A patient with ovarian cancer was given a dose of cisplatin rather than carboplatin.[16] The dose of cisplatin was given at the dose intensity for carboplatin, the equivalent of a three- to fourfold overdose. Thus, this patient not only received the wrong drug but also the wrong dose. Another patient received a dose of vincristine that was used instead of vinblastine, leading to a 10 times overdose, severe paralysis, and death.[17] A third case involved the inadvertent substitution of docetaxel for paclitaxel, which resulted in a substantial overdose of docetaxel. The patient died 5 days later, but the error could not be identified as the inciting cause of death because the patient was very debilitated from metastatic disease.[18]

2. **Vial overfills.** Twenty-one reports of dosing errors due to vial overfills have occurred with Taxotere. Taxotere for injection concentrate contains 23.6 and 94.4 mg for the 20- and 80-mg vials. The diluent vials also contain overfills. These overfill amounts should not be used for withdrawing the intended dose because the final strength may be miscalculated. Instead, the package insert directions should be followed.[18]

3. **Administering the drug by the wrong route of administration.** Despite repeated warnings about the danger of administering vincristine intrathecally,[19] several case reports continue to appear in the literature. Unfortunately, inadvertent intrathecal injection has led to 26 deaths and severe neurologic

complication in 37 patients.[19a] While no standard treatment is recommended, one patient was treated with cerebrospinal fluid exchange by ventriculostomy with prevention of neurologic sequelae.[19b] Preliminary research in animals using hypochlorous acid is ongoing to determine if this agent might be useful antidote for accidental intrathecal of vincristine.[19c]

In a woman with acute lymphoblastic leukemia, inadvertent doxorubicin administration intrathecally caused severe, life-threatening, acute encephalopathy with high-pressure hydrocephalus. This patient was managed with ventriculo-peritoneal shunting that led to complete reversal of hydrocephalus and progressive disappearance of the acute encephalopathy.[20]

4. **Confusion with the chemotherapy regimen.** An inadvertent overdose of chemotherapy may occur if the chemotherapy regimen in not written in a clear manner. Despite being care for at a major cancer center, two patients who were in a high-dose chemotherapy stem cell transplant program received a four-times overdose. The total dose (4 grams/m^2) of cyclophosphamide was given daily for 4 days rather than the intended 1 gram/m^2 for 4 days. Both patients died of serious heart damage.[21] These errors were heralded for the next 3 years in many newspapers and led to considerable change in institutional practice. Today, the Dana Farber Cancer Institute, the institution involved in these unfortunate errors, re-tooled there entire system and has been recently distinguished for its remarkable record of safety record since the date the errors occurred in 1994.

5. **Poor packaging or labeling.** The initial packaging for irinotecan was poorly designed (the mg/mL concentration was often mistaken to be the total amount of drug per vial). This has resulted in the drawing up of a 5 times overdose of the drug. Several patients received overdoses as a result of this problem in package design. The manufacturer has since redesigned the packaging to clearly indicate the concentration and amount of drug in the vial.

6. **Look-alike, sound-alike drugs.** Examples include Doxil and doxorubicin, Neupogen and Neulasta and Neumega, docetaxel and paclitaxel, and cisplatin and carboplatin. Preparers can mistakenly select the wrong product from the shelf. Several manufacturers are now using "Tall-Man Lettering" on the labels of these products.

7. **Use of abbreviations.** Abbreviations of chemotherapy names, such as MTX, VCR, VLB, NH2, and CPT-11, can be misinterpreted to be a nonintended drug.

8. **Decimal-point errors.** Doses should be rounded to a full integer (e.g., 160 mg rather than 159.5 mg) so as not to present the potential for a 10-fold overdose. Similarly, the use of a leading decimal without a preceding 0 can also lead to a 10-fold overdose.

9. **Illegible prescriber orders.** In addition to poor handwriting, the faxing of chemotherapy orders can result in decimal point errors and potential overdosing or underdosing.

10. **Erroneous publication of drug dosages or regimens in records of professional meetings, journals, or books.** Unfortunately, errors in dosage frequently appear in publications that are used as references by practitioners. It is recommended that more than one reference be used to verify whether the order is for an appropriate dose. A textbook by this chapter's author included an incorrect dosage formula for carboplatin. Rather than calculating a dose in milligrams, the formula printed on p. 30 of this book calculated the dose as mg per m^2.[22] In a popular Lexi-Comp series (edition 2005–06) a dosage regimen that included days 1 and 15 was published. The regimen as

published by the investigator is "irinotecan 180 mg/m² over 90 minutes should be given on days 1, 15, and 22...."[23] Misprints can also occur in journal articles. One such case involved a vincristine overdose.[24]

11. **Frequent interruptions during compounding of chemotherapy.** Preparation of cytotoxic chemotherapy requires the full attention of the pharmacist, nurse, or technician.

12. **Miscommunication between health care providers.** Verbal orders may be misinterpreted and transmitted incorrectly to the nurse or pharmacist.

13. **Lack of appropriate warnings on chemotherapy products.** Information about products that are to be given by a unique route of administration or using a particular infusion device should be highlighted clearly on the label. For example, vincristine is sometimes prepared in a small volume similar to other drugs intended for administration by the intrathecal route. Vincristine should be clearly labeled "FATAL IF GIVEN INTRATHECALLY, FOR INTRAVENOUS USE ONLY."

STRATEGIES FOR PREVENTING CHEMOTHERAPY ERRORS

At both Memorial Sloan-Kettering Cancer Center and Fox Chase Cancer Center, several rules have been in place as policy since 1996. These rules were published in Pharmacy Practice News Oncology Special Edition[25] (McMahon Publishing Group) and are intended to improve care through a systems approach. Most of these rules have been endorsed (albeit not formally) by the American Society of Health-System Pharmacy's (ASHP) Council of Professional Affairs. Several of these rules have resulted in outcome improvements and thus should be beneficial to institutions.

Some institutions have participated in the multi-institutional collaborative effort of the Institute for Healthcare Improvement under the leadership of Lucian Leape on Reducing Adverse Drug Events and Medical Errors, which began in 1996 and culminated in a national congress in March 1997.[26] Successful institutions were able to use a rapid change methodology to pursue their aims, choose practical interventions, and make early process changes. They did not spend months collecting data before beginning a change. Leape stated, "Changes that were most successful were those that attempted to change processes, not people."

Whether an institution uses a rapid change method or chooses to study their error processes more systematically, the following list of rules may be used to assist the quality improvement plan. Some of these rules are reproduced with the permission of the authors and the publisher (McMahon Publishing Group), whereas others have been modified to incorporate some newer concepts and suggestions from other institutions and organizations.[25]

Rule 1. Mandate the use of preprinted order forms or standardize computerized order sets.[27]

In the absence of a computerized medication order system, the use of preprinted order forms decreased the risk of medication errors at Walter Reed Memorial Hospital, a major Army medical center.[28] At Walter Reed Army Medical Center, the study was carried out to assess the effect of using printed standardized order forms on prescribing error rate and antiemetic costs. Over a 4-month period, improvements were seen in both the antiemetic costs and the antiemetic error rate. Specifically, the error rate decreased from 1.5% to 0.33%. A smaller but similar, audit was performed at the University of California, San Francisco (UCSF) Comprehensive Cancer Center with similar results. In the UCSF system, the use of more than 100 standardized order sets based on published chemotherapy regimens in the literature has been instituted. As at Walter Reed Memorial Hospital, the

UCSF Comprehensive Cancer Center outpatient infusion center pharmacy service is responsible for the development of the standardized forms, which are then approved by an attending oncologist and administrative nurse of the infusion center before use. An approval date is included as a footnote on each order set. Order sets for the inpatient setting are reviewed by the attending hematologist/oncologist, pharmacist, and a nursing team. Order sets are then generated on an individual basis, according to protocol and are not preprinted in advance.

Rule 2. Generate and implement chemotherapy prescribing guidelines.

The following is a list of do's and don'ts for writing chemotherapy orders:

- Use full drug names.
- Avoid abbreviations.
- Express doses in milligrams.
- Prohibit the use of doses prescribed in terms of units (U), micrograms (μg), and daily.
- Avoid trailing zeros after a decimal point.
- Use a leading zero before a decimal point.
- Round all doses over 5 mg to the nearest whole number.
- Require that multiday regimens specify the dose per m^2 per day, dose per day, and number of days of therapy.

Rule 3. Prohibit the use of verbal orders for the initiation of chemotherapy.

The only exception should be to discontinue therapy in the event of an adverse reaction.

Rule 4. Educate new practitioners (nurses, pharmacists, oncology fellows, and residents).

The institution should hold periodic educational sessions to update practitioners on new drugs, procedures, and improvements for patient safety.[19,29] Chemotherapy drug information should be made available or be easily accessible to all practitioners. UCSF provides an embossed information chemotherapy card (ChemoCard) that describes each drug, its usual dose, diluent, and stability and whether or not it is a vesicant to all fellows and oncologists who write chemotherapy orders. Ideally such information should also be available electronically on the institution's intranet.

Rule 5. All fellows or residents in training who write chemotherapy orders must have their orders co-signed by a qualified attending oncologist.

Redundant review of chemotherapy orders is important for the prevention of chemotherapy errors. A policy should be in place to state that the prescription for chemotherapy written by a fellow or resident is valid only with the inclusion of an attending oncologist co-signature and date on the chemotherapy order.

Rule 6. Before preparation and administration of chemotherapy, all appropriate laboratory data should be reviewed.

In addition to the oncologist, the pharmacist or nurse preparing or administering cytotoxic chemotherapy should review the patient's current blood chemistry data including the white blood cell count, hemoglobin, hematocrit, platelet count, and absolute neutrophil count. Depending on the drug, other laboratory data, such as electrolyte levels or liver function test results, may be required, (e.g., for carboplatin, the serum creatinine level is required to calculate a dose using the standard Calvert formula).

SUPPORTIVE CARE

Rule 7. Before preparation of a cytotoxic agent, assess the vial integrity, clarity of the labeling, and other labels with the intent of avoiding confusion and potential error.[30]

Some products may be available from multiple suppliers or manufacturers. An assessment of the product and its safety should be performed.

Rule 8. Self-assessment and error reporting.[31]

As suggested by Kohn et al. in the IOM report *To Err Is Human: Building a Safer Health System,*[7] human error is always possible, so a culture of safety should be promoted. All errors (prescribing, preparation, dispensing, and administration types) should be discussed with a multidisciplinary group in a nonpunitive manner. Serious errors should be report to the FDA MedWatch program. A quality improvement committee may be formed to address the issue of medication errors or chemotherapy error in particular. UCSF provides report cards to our practitioners in an anonymous manner. Practitioners may request more education to improve their skills, depending on the nature of the error. A continuous improvement process may assist institutions in ensuring that safe chemotherapy practices are used throughout the hospital.[29]

Rule 9. Distribute alerts from the ISMP and JCAHO to all practitioners involved in the chemotherapy process.

Administrators of institutions should remain abreast of the errors that are reported by other institutions. The ISMP maintains a log of medications errors on its Web site (www.ismp.org), and both the ISMP and JCAHO report medication error alerts on their respective Web sites on a regular basis. Current information should be publicized and emphasized, especially for new drugs or devices.

Rule 10. Assessment and documentation of competency of all staff should be performed on an annual basis.

This rule may be applicable to the USP 797 requirement for programs in which sterile chemotherapy is prepared several hours in advance of drug administration.

Rule 11. Educate patients about their chemotherapy.

It is important that patients be involved in the patient safety program because they might be able to detect something that is out of the ordinary. Furthermore, they should be informed about the names of their chemotherapy drugs, the planned treatment schedule, the method of chemotherapy administration, and potential side effects of each of the agents along with suggested strategies to treat or minimize their occurrence.

Rule 12. Implement technologic advances that are proven to decrease medication errors, such as computerized prescriber order entry (CPOE) and bar coding for chemotherapy orders.[32]

The use of CPOE programs has the potential for avoidance of errors of omission or dosing irregularities. Protocols or approved institutional chemotherapy regimens can be built into the program to prompt the prescriber to include all appropriate orders for not only the chemotherapy but for premedications, such as antiemetics, medications to prevent allergic reactions, the need for hydration, and medications for acute emesis or other acute drug-induced effects. Patient-specific parameters such as height, actual weight, or adjusted weight with a corresponding calculated body surface area that is generated by the computer is one of the advantages of CPOE system. The program should be able to apply existing policies into the order set such as the rounding up or down of chemotherapy doses. Furthermore, it should be able to keep a running tab of cumulative lifetime doses of particular drugs, such as doxorubicin and bleomycin. All order sets should be easily accessible as a "read-only" file on the institution's intranet. Changes to orders should be requested by the chief pharmacy officer and approved by the oncology practice committee (made up of the chief physician, administrative nurse, and managing pharmacist). However, as advanced as a CPOE system may sound, medication errors can still occur and even increase if a system lacks decision support for drug selection, dosing, and monitoring.[33]

The generic name of the drug must be on the order. Acceptable exceptions are for Doxil and Abraxane. It is useful to also include the trade name to decrease confusion with look-alike, sound-alike drugs (e.g., docetaxel and Taxotere).

Bar coding is another technologic advance that, if developed with appropriate controls, could decrease the potential for medication errors in all areas, including oncology.[34,35] This technology has the benefit of interfacing with systems involved in drug prescribing, drug preparation, and drug administration.

Rule 13. Be cautious of outsourcing preparation and administration services.
The American Society of Clinical Oncology (ASCO) produced a position statement on this topic.[36] ASCO recommended that if an oncologist refers a patient to an outside agency, such as an infusion center or home care agency, for chemotherapy administration the agency should meet the following standards:

1. Administration should be overseen by a physician qualified in oncology.
2. Administration should be performed by professionals qualified in such procedures.
3. Physicians or nurses should be certified in cardiopulmonary resuscitation (CPR).
4. Medications for managing acute allergic reactions or chemotherapy extravasation should be immediately available.
5. The facility should have safeguards and double-checking systems to prevent over- or underdosing of chemotherapy or supportive care drugs.

For drugs prepared by outside sources, the referring oncologist should ensure that the agency uses appropriate preparation techniques and that the drug dispensed is the drug that was ordered, that the dose drawn up is correct, and that double-checking procedures are used by the agency to minimize medication errors.

CONCLUSIONS
Chemotherapy errors have resulted in fatal consequences. It behooves those of us practicing in this area to use all our resources to minimize the risk of chemotherapy errors. Incorporating a patient safety initiative at institutions involved in the treatment of cancer should be a primary focus and endeavor.

REFERENCES
1. Knox RA. Response is slow to deadly mixups: too little done to avert cancer drug errors. *Boston Globe* June 26, 1995:29–33.
2. Cohen MR. Medication error report analysis: cancer chemotherapy needs improved quality assurance —so where are the pharmacists? *Hosp Pharm* 1995;30:258–259.
3. Ignoffo RJ. Preventing chemotherapy errors. *Am J Health-Syst Pharm* 1996;53:733
4. Attilio RM. Caring enough to understand: the road to oncology medication error prevention. *Hosp Pharm* 1996;31:17–26.
5. Cohen MR, Anderson RW, Attilio RM, et al. Preventing medication errors in cancer chemotherapy. *Am J Health-Syst Pharm* 1996;53:737–746.
6. Fischer DS, Alfano S, Knobf MT, et al. Improving the cancer chemotherapy use process. *J Clin Oncol* 1996;14:3148–3155.

SUPPORTIVE CARE

7. Kohn LT, Corrigan JM, Donaldson MS. *To Err Is Human: Building a Safer Health System.* Washington, DC: National Academies Press; 2000.

8. Leape LL, Berwick DM. Five years after *To Err Is Human*: what have we learned? *JAMA* 2005;293: 2384–2390.

9. Kazel R. Minnesota insurer won't pay hospital for "never events." *American Medical News.* November 8, 2004. Available at www.ama-assn.org/amednews/11/08.htm.

10. Kastango ES. Blueprint for implementing *USP* chapter 797 for compounding sterile preparations. *Am J Health Syst Pharm* 2005; 62:1271-1288.

11. Rich D. JCAHO Update on Auditing institution. American Society of Health System Pharmacy. Symposium Presentation. December 5, 2004.

12. FDA MedWatch—Reporting of adverse events/reactions to medications, drug products or medical devices to the Food and Drug Administration voluntary reporting system. www.fda.gov/medwatch/

13. Institute For Safe Medication Practices. Provides information about adverse drug events and their prevention to healthcare practitioners and institutions, regulatory agencies, www.ismp.org/

14. Gandhi TK, Bartel SB, Shulman LN, et at. Medication safety in the ambulatory chemotherapy setting. *Cancer* 2005;104:2477–2483.

15. Minnesota Alliance for Patient Safety (MAPS) - Promoting optimum patient safety through collaborative and supportive efforts among health care organizations in Minnesota. www.mnpatientsafety.org/. Report on Medication Errors 2003.

16. *New York Post*, April 14, 1992. Confusion over chemotherapy drug leads to patient's death.

17. Garloch K. Wrong drug killed boy. *Charlotte Observer.* May 11, 1991; Metro Section:1B.

18. Medication safety errors associated with Taxotere and Taxol. ISMP Medication Safety Alert. February 7, 2001. Accessed December 7, 2006.

19. Inadvertent intrathecal vincristine. Institute for Safe Medication Practices (ISMP) Newsletter, 1996.

19a. Australian Council on Safety and Quality in Healthcare. High-risk medication alert—vincristine. 2005. Available at www.safetyandquality.org.

19b. Michaelagnoli MP, Bailey CC, Wilson I, Livingston J, Kinsey SE: Potential salvage therapy for inadvertent intrathecal administration of vincristine. *Br J Haematol* 1997;99:364-67.

19c. Ozgen U, Soylu H, Onal SC, et al. Potential salvage therapy for accidental intrathecal vincristine administration: A Preliminary Experimental Study. *Chemotherapy* 2000;46:322-326.

20. Arico M, Nespoli L, Porta F, Caselli D, Raiteri E, Burgio GR. Severe acute encephalopathy following inadvertent intrathecal doxorubicin administration. *Med Pediatr Oncol* 1990;18(3):261-3.

21. Ignoffo RJ, Viele CM, Venook A, Damon L. Carboplatin dosing. In *Cancer Chemotherapy Pocket Guide.* Philadelphia, PA: Lippincott Raven; 1997:30.

22. Institute for Safe Medication Practices. Irinotecan (Camptosar) dosing print error in Lexicomp's 2005–06 *Drug Information Handbook*. Available at http://www.ismp.org/Errata/camptosar.asp.

23. Cohen MR. Misprint in journal article leads to vincristine overdose. *Hosp Pharm* 1994;29: 294–302.

24. Muller RJ and Kloth. Pharmacy Practice News Oncology Special Edition 2005;8:224-230.

25. Leape LL, Kabcenell A, Gandhi TK, et al. Reducing adverse drug events: lessons from a breakthrough series collaborative. *Jt Comm J Qual Improv* 2000:26:321–331.

26. Dinning C, Branowicki P, O'Neill JB, et al. Chemotherapy error reduction: a multidisciplinary approach to create templated order sets. *J Pediatr Oncol Nurs* 2005;22:20–30.

27. Sano HS, Waddell JA, Solimando DA Jr, et al. Study of the effect of standardized chemotherapy order forms on prescribing errors and anti-emetic cost. *J Oncol Pharm Pract* 2005;11:21–30.

28. Goldspiel BR, DeChristoforo R, Daniels CE. A continuous-improvement approach for reducing the number of chemotherapy-related medication errors. *Am J Health-Syst Pharm* 2000;57 (Suppl 4): S4–S9.

29. ASHP Council on Professional Affairs. ASHP guidelines on preventing medication errors with antineoplastic agents. *Am J Health-Syst Pharm* 2002;59:1648–1668.

30. Bonnabry P, Cingria L, Ackermann M, et al. Use of a prospective risk analysis method to improve the safety of the cancer chemotherapy process. *Int J Qual Health Care* 2006;18:9–16.

31. Kozakiewicz JM, Benis LJ, Fisher SM, Marseglia JB. Safe chemotherapy administration: using failure mode and effects analysis in computerized prescriber order entry. *Am J Health-Syst Pharm* 2005;62:1813–1816.

32. Nebeker JR, Bennett CL. Reducing adverse drug events in the outpatient chemotherapy setting: attention must be paid. *Cancer* 2005;104:2289–2291.

33. Neuenschwander M, Cohen MR, Vaida AJ, et al. Practical guide to bar coding for patient medication safety. *Am J Health-Syst Pharm* 2003;60:768–779.

34. Wright AA, Katz IT. Bar coding for patient safety. *N Engl J Med* 2005;353:329–331.

35. American Society of Clinical Oncology Statement Regarding the Use of Outside Services to Prepare or Administer Chemotherapy Drugs. *J Clin Oncol* 2003;21:1882–1883.

**Occupational Exposure
to Hazardous Drugs**

Dominic A. Solimando, Jr.

ASSESSING THE RISK

Many antineoplastic agents are known to be either mutagenic or carcinogenic.[1,2] The potential risks of long-term exposure to low levels of such drugs is a concern to health care workers. It has been estimated that workplace exposure to antineoplastic agents *could possibly* result in an annual increase of up to 60 additional cases of cancer per 1 million health care workers in all practice settings.[3,4] However, so far, no studies documenting an actual increase in the incidence of malignant diseases have been published. When one is evaluating such reports, several factors should be considered:

- The difference in dose and intensity between therapeutic use and workplace exposure is extremely large.
- No method for relating short-term, high-intensity exposure in patients with long-term, low level exposure in health care workers has been established.
- Oncology patients are predisposed to cancer and are at much higher risk of developing a second malignancy than are "healthy" workers.
- Oncology patients have impaired immune systems, both from the underlying disease and from therapy.

Additionally, a variety of acute adverse effects of exposure to antineoplastic agents (including sore throat, cough, infections, dizziness, eye irritation, and headaches)[5,6] and increases in fetal abnormality, fetal loss, and fertility impairment[7] have been associated with workplace exposure to antineoplastic agents.

Despite intense investigation of the issue, there is no definitive evidence of a causal relationship between prolonged exposure to low levels of antineoplastic agents in the workplace and development of malignancies, nor have "safe" or "nonhazardous" exposure levels been established. *There is also no conclusive evidence that such exposure is not hazardous.* Given this uncertainty about a potentially serious consequence, most organizations have adopted a "zero tolerance" approach to the problem, seeking to eliminate any possible exposure.[8,9] Although the concern has been primarily with exposure to antineoplastic agents, a number of non-antineoplastic compounds are also included in current definitions of "hazardous agents." The U.S. Environmental Protection Agency's (EPA) list of regulated hazardous chemicals contains twice as many non-antineoplastic agents as antineoplastic drugs (Table 6–1). Accordingly, these principles of safe handling should be applied to *all hazardous agents throughout the entire institution.*

Several problems are associated with attempts to define the actual risk posed by working with antineoplastic agents, including various definitions of hazardous agent, poor quality of data, and conflicting conclusions concerning the efficacy of proposed protective measures. These are discussed in the following sections.

Definitions

The American Society of Health-System Pharmacists (ASHP), the EPA, and the National Institute of Occupational Safety and Health (NIOSH) have formal definitions of hazardous agents (Table 6–2). Unfortunately, these definitions do not agree. Some criteria are extremely vague (e.g., EPA's "appears on one of the following lists," ASHP's "causes serious organ or other toxic manifestation at low doses," and NIOSH's "acutely toxic to an organ system").

The EPA list of hazardous chemicals includes 723 compounds. Of the 24 therapeutic agents listed, only 8 are antineoplastic agents. NIOSH lists 60 drugs on its "incomplete and not all-inclusive" listing of hazardous drugs; 13 are

Table 6–1 Drugs Listed as Hazardous

EPA		NIOSH		
Antineoplastic	**Non-Antineoplastic**	**Antineoplastic**	**Non-Antineoplastic**	**Product Labeling**
Arsenic trioxide	Dichlorodifluoro-methane	Altretamine	Anesthetic agents	Cidofovir
Chlorambucil	Diethylstilbestrol	Aminoglutethimide	Cyclosporin	Finasteride
Cyclophospha-mide	Epinephrine	Azathioprine	Diethylstilbestrol	Ganciclovir
Daunomycin	Hexachlorophene	Asparaginase	Estradiol	Mycophenolate
Melphalan	Lindane	Bleomycin	Ethinyl estradiol	Nicotine gum
Mitomycin	Nitroglycerin	Busulfan	Ganciclovir	
Streptozotocin	Paraldehyde	Carboplatin	Isotretinoin	
Uracil mustard	Phenacetin	Carmustine	Medroxyprogesterone	
	Physostigmine	Chlorambucil	Nafarelin	
	Physostigmine salicylate	Chloramphenicol	Pentamidine	
	Reserpine	Chlorozotocin	Plicamycin	
	Resorcinol	Cisplatin	Ribavirin	
	Saccharin	Cyclophosphamide	Testolactone	
	Selenium sulfide	Cytarabine	Vidarabine	
	Trichloromonofluoro-methane	Dacarbazine	Zidovudine	
	Warfarin	Dactinomycin		
		Daunorubicin		
		Doxorubicin		
		Estramustine		
		Etoposide		
		Floxuridine		
		Fluorouracil		
		Flutamide		
		Hydroxyurea		
		Idarubicin		
		Ifosfamide		
		Interferon-A		
		Leuprolide		
		Levamisole		
		Lomustine		
		Mechlorethamine		
		Megestrol		
		Melphalan		
		Mercaptopurine		
		Methotrexate		
		Mitomycin		
		Mitotane		
		Mitoxantrone		
		Pipobroman		
		Procarbazine		
		Streptozocin		
		Tamoxifen		
		Thioguanine		
		Thiotepa		
		Uracil mustard		
		Vinblastine		
		Vincristine		

Table 6–2 **Criteria for Defining Hazardous Agents**

EPA	NIOSH	ASHP
Meets one of the following criteria:	Designated as Therapeutic Category 10:00 (Antineoplastic Agent) in the American Hospital Formulary Service Drug Information	Genotoxic
Ignitability—create fire under certain conditions or are spontaneously combustible and have a flash point <600° C		
Corrosivity—acids or bases (pH <2 or >12.5) capable of corroding metal containers	Manufacturer suggests use of special techniques in handling, administration, or disposal	Carcinogenic
Reactivity—unstable under "normal" conditions; can cause explosions, toxic fumes, gases, or vapors when mixed with water	Mutagenic	Teratogenic or impairs fertility
	Carcinogenic	Causes serious organ or other toxic manifestation at low doses
Toxicity characteristic—when disposed of on land, contaminated liquid may drain or leach from the waste and pollute ground water		
	Teratogenic or reproductive toxicant	
OR	Acutely toxic to an organ system	
Appears on one of the following lists:	Investigational drugs	
F—wastes from certain common or industrial manufacturing processes from nonspecific sources		
K—wastes from certain specific industries from specific sources.		
P—wastes from pure or commercial grade formulations of certain specific unused chemicals		
U—wastes from pure or commercial grade formulations of certain specific unused chemicals		

From *Safe Handling of Hazardous Drugs.* Lexi-Drugs Online. Lexi-Comp Clinical Reference Library OnLine. Copyright © 1978–2006 Lexi-Comp, Inc. Used by permission.

non-antineoplastic agents. Some manufacturers recommend special precautions for handling certain non-antineoplastic medications (Table 6–1).

Poor Quality of Data

Most studies of occupational exposure in medical personnel have been small, uncontrolled trials or anecdotal reports. In addition, the biologic and analytical procedures used to measure exposure in many of the early studies were lacking in specificity and sensitivity. In a review of 63 studies published between 1979 and 1996, the conclusion was that the methods used were not "sufficiently reliable or reproducible for routine monitoring of exposure in the workplace."[10] A concern is that the studies reviewed included many that are the basis for recommending common protective measures such as biologic safety cabinets, gloves, gowns, and aseptic technique.

Large scale, prospective, controlled trials of occupational exposure to health care personnel and the efficacy of various protective measures have never been conducted. Despite more than a quarter century of work, a nonhazardous exposure threshold has not been established, nor are practical, reliable, "real-time" techniques to monitor exposure available.

Conflicting Conclusions

Although often overlooked and not mentioned in the guidelines, not all studies showed that health care workers were exposed to hazardous agents. Of the studies reviewed by Baker and Connor,[10] only 45% of the biologic studies were positive for exposure. In addition, 48% showed no exposure, and 7% were equivocal. Seventeen percent of the urine analysis studies were also negative for exposure.

ROUTES OF EXPOSURE

Proposed mechanisms by which health care personnel may be exposed to hazardous agents include inhalation, accidental injection, ingestion of contaminated food, mouth contact with contaminated hands, and dermal absorption. The role of the various mechanisms is uncertain.

Air samples have been reported to show low or undetectable levels of hazardous drugs, suggesting that inhalation may not be a primary means of exposure.[11–14] However, other reports suggest that lack of efficacy in sampling methods[15] or volatility of the marker drug(s)[15–18] may have affected the results. Although some antineoplastic agents may be absorbed through the skin, at least one report failed to detect such absorption.[19–21] Oral ingestion is also a possible route of exposure.[22,23]

Recent reports have identified contamination of the outer surface of medication vials and packaging during the manufacturing process. These reports raise the concern that workplace contamination may not be solely the result of compounding or administration procedures within the pharmacy or clinic but may originate, at least partially, outside the institution. Such external contamination may require additional procedures for decontaminating drug containers at the point of entry, rather than in the preparation or administration areas.[24,25]

PROTECTIVE MEASURES

A variety of protective measures, primarily physical barriers, have been recommended to reduce potential exposure of health care personnel to the hazardous medications they handle. The most common measures include:

Separation

Many institutions, particularly ones in which a large number of antineoplastic doses are prepared, have a separate area for preparation of antineoplastic agents. For a variety of reasons, these oncology sections are often located some distance from the main pharmacy area. Although such separation limits exposure to antineoplastic agents to a minimum number of individuals, it may not be completely adequate. As noted previously, not all hazardous agents are antineoplastic medications. Also, unless the oncology section operates 7 days a week, personnel not assigned to the oncology service occasionally may be required to prepare or administer antineoplastic agents.

Biologic Safety Cabinets

A class II biologic safety cabinet with an exhaust outside the facility is currently recommended for preparation of hazardous agents.[8,9] Isolators, glove boxes, and class III biologic safety cabinets have also been suggested for preparation of hazardous agents; however, they are not formally recommended by ASHP or NIOSH.

Protective Clothing

Protective gloves, gowns, and eye protection are universally recommended while one is handling hazardous agents; even though many studies supporting their efficacy may have been flawed.[10]

Gloves. Gloves are available in a variety of materials, but no one type appears to be preferred. ASHP currently recommends changing gloves, or at least the outer glove, every 30 minutes.[8] Some investigators have reported test drugs permeating the glove within 10 minutes, suggesting that more frequent glove changes may be appropriate.[26] ASHP also recommends double-gloving, although no studies demonstrating a reduction in exposure with double-gloving over single-gloving have been published.

Generally, powder-free gloves are recommended to reduce particulate matter; handwashing before gloving and after removal of gloves is also recommended. Although such precautions may help reduce operator exposure, they are not in accordance with the sterile preparation guidelines mandated by the U.S. Pharmacopeia (USP). If nonsterile gloves are worn, the standards of sterile product preparation in USP Chapter 797 mandate washing or decontaminating of the gloves after they have been donned and before sterile product compounding is begun.[27]

Gowns. Use of gowns that have "a closed front, long sleeves, and tight-fitting elastic or knit cuffs" is recommended.[8] Like gloves, protective gowns are available in a variety of materials. Polypropylene or vinyl-coated materials have been shown to be more protective than polyethylene; however, these gowns are also reported to be uncomfortable, and health care personnel are prone to resist using them.[28–31]

Other Protective Clothing. Many institutions dispense with the requirement for wearing face shields or respirators when medications are prepared in a biologic safety cabinet equipped with a glass front. A recent revision of the ASHP guidelines now includes use of face shields and NIOSH-approved respirator masks when one is working with hazardous agents, although the added benefit of such devices has not been well documented.[8] To comply with the USP's "clean room" standards for compounding sterile products, head and foot coverings should also be worn.[27]

Closed System Devices

An additional safety precaution available to minimize workplace contamination is a closed system transfer device. Such systems have been available on packages of injectable antibiotics for some time but are not amenable to use with antineoplastic agents for which precise dosing precludes development of a limited number of package sizes. An external system (PhaSeal) is available and is used in many institutions. PhaSeal is a multicomponent system that incorporates a double membrane enclosing an injection cannula. A number of studies have documented decreased environmental contamination when the PhaSeal system is used.[32–36] Although the PhaSeal system is the prevalent system in the United States, other systems are available. The Genie vial access system (ICU Medical Systems), Tevadaptor system (Teva) and Texium adaptor and SmartSite needle-less valve system (Cardinal) have recently been introduced. At present, little information about these newer systems, and no comparisons among the various systems are available.

ASEPTIC TECHNIQUE

Three reports attributed low or undetectable levels of exposure to hazardous drugs to the experience level or skill with aseptic technique of the individual worker.[37–39] Procedures for generation and maintenance of a partial vacuum ("negative pressure") by removal of air from drug vials and careful avoidance of generating drug aerosols during compounding procedures have been described.[39] Use of these procedures has been suggested as a possible cause of failure to detect workplace exposure in one institution.[38]

MONITORING

The NIOSH and ASHP recommendations for handling hazardous agents include monitoring personnel who handle hazardous agents.[8,9] Implementation of surveillance programs has been difficult for a variety of reasons, including lack of accepted standards for interpreting examination and laboratory results, concerns over privacy, confidentiality and data security, and cost.

Procedures to monitor contamination of the work area are somewhat more successful, although a practical, real-time monitoring system is not available. Results of urine drug level studies, surface wipe tests, or airborne drug levels require sophisticated laboratory support that is not available at many institutions. Such monitoring is most commonly performed as part of a research project, rather than as a routine quality assurance procedure.

Use of ultraviolet light to detect occult drug spills and assess individuals' handling technique has been reported.[39,40] Training and testing kits incorporating this concept are available, but the procedure has several limitations. Only a few hazardous agents will fluoresce when exposed to ultraviolet light. The procedure also lacks specificity: if contamination is detected, neither the particular drug(s) nor the amount spilled can be determined. The surveillance procedure is done after completion of drug compounding, precluding determination of contamination, and institution of corrective measures at the time of the occurrence. Although not practical for continuous monitoring, fluorescence testing can be useful in training and periodic performance evaluation of personnel.

DECONTAMINATION

The possibility of contamination of the medication vials and packaging during the manufacturing process necessitates that appropriate precautions be taken when one is handling drug containers.[24,25] Measures such as protective clothing, segregated receiving or storage areas, and dedicated storage and transportation containers have all been recommended for personnel involved in the receipt, storage, and transport of hazardous agents.[8]

At the time of receipt, all drug containers should be examined carefully. Any container with evidence of damage should be handled with caution. Damaged containers should be quarantined and decontaminated before being placed in stock or returned to the manufacturer.[8,24]

All equipment and, as necessary, drug containers should be decontaminated. Alcohol should not be used as a disinfectant because it will not inactivate hazardous agents. Use of sodium hypochlorite and sodium thiosulfate solutions is recommended for decontamination[8]; but only a limited number of hazardous agents have been demonstrated to be inactivated by these compounds.

CONCLUSION

Health care personnel who routinely handle hazardous agents may be at risk of developing a variety of adverse effects from exposure to these drugs. Achieving an appropriate balance between personnel protection and overreaction to a poorly defined threat remains a challenge. Available guidelines are based on presumptions of risk extrapolated from data obtained from exposure to therapeutic doses of agents in patients. Because of the continued uncertainty, the a zero tolerance philosophy has been adopted for most guidelines. Recommendations for many of the protective measures used are based on short-term studies in very small populations and "prudent practice" rather than on large, controlled trials.

REFERENCES

1. *IARC Monographs on the Evaluation of the Carcinogenic Risk of Chemicals to Humans.* Geneva, Switzerland: World Health Organization; 1981.
2. Benedict WF, Baker MS, Haroun L, et al. Mutagenicity of cancer chemotherapeutic agents in the Salmonella/microsome test. *Cancer Res* 1977;37:2209–2213.
3. Sessink PJM, Kroese ED, van Kranen HJ, et al. Cancer risk assessment for health care workers occupationally exposed to cyclophosphamide. *Int Arch Occup Environ Health* 1995;67:317–323.

4. Ensslin AS, Stoll Y, Pethran A, et al. Biological monitoring of cyclophosphamide and ifosfamide in urine of hospital personnel occupationally exposed to cytostatic drugs. *Occup Environ Med* 1994; 51:229–233.

5. Valanis BG, Hertzberg V, Shortridge L. Antineoplastic drugs: handle with care. *AAOHN J* 1987;35: 487–492.

6. Valanis BG, Vollmer WM, Labuhn KT, et al. Association of antineoplastic drug handling with acute adverse effects in pharmacy personnel. *Am J Hosp Pharm* 1993;50:455–462.

7. Valanis BG, Vollmer WM, Steele P. Occupational exposures to anti-neoplastic agents: self-reported miscarriages and stillbirths among nurses and pharmacists. *J Occup Environ Med* 1999;41:632–638.

8. American Society of Hospital Pharmacists. *ASHP Guidelines on Handling Hazardous Drugs.* Prepublication version. Available at: www.ashp.org, Accessed December 22, 2005.

9. *Preventing Occupational Exposure to Antineoplastic and Other Hazardous Drugs in Health Care Settings.* NIOSH Publication No. 2004-165. Available at: www.cdc.gov/niosh/docs/2004-165. Accessed August 20, 2005.

10. Baker ES, Connor TH. Monitoring occupational exposure to cancer chemotherapy drugs. *Am J Health-Syst Pharm* 1996;53:2713–2723.

11. Sessink PJM, Boer KA, Scheefhals APH, et al. Occupational exposure to antineoplastic agents at several departments in a hospital: environmental contamination and excretion of cyclophosphamide and ifosfamide in urine of exposed workers. *Int Arch Occup Environ Health* 1992;64:105–112.

12. Sessink PJM, Van de Kerkhof MCA, Anzion RB, et al. Environmental contamination and assessment of exposure to antineoplastic agents by determination of cyclophosphamide in urine of exposed pharmacy technicians: is skin absorption an important exposure route? *Arch Environ Health* 1994;49:165–169.

13. Sessink PJM, Wittenhorst BCJ, Anzion RBM, et al. Exposure of pharmacy technicians to antineoplastic agents: reevaluation after additional protective measures. *Arch Environ Health* 1997;52:240–244.

14. Nygren O, Lundgren C. Determination of platinum in workroom air and in blood and urine from nursing staff attending patients receiving cisplatin chemotherapy. *Int Arch Occup Environ Health* 1997;70: 209–214.

15. Larson RR, Khazaeli MB, Dillon HK. A new monitoring method using solid sorbent media for evaluation of airborne cyclophosphamide and other antineoplastic agents. *Appl Occup Environ Hyg* 2003;18: 120–131.

16. Opiolka S, Schmidt KG, Kiffmeyer K, et al. Determination of the vapor pressure of cytotoxic drugs and its effects on occupational safety [abstract]. *J Oncol Pharm Pract* 2000;6:15.

17. Kiffmeyer TK, Kube C, Opiolka S, et al. Vapor pressures, evaporation behavior and airborne concentrations of hazardous drugs: implications for occupational safety. *Pharmt J* 2002;268:331–337.

18. Connor TH, Shults M, Fraser MP. Determination of the vaporization of solutions of mutagenic antineoplastic agents at 23 and 36° C using a desiccator technique. *Mutat Res* 2000;470:85–92.

19. Sessink PJM, Van de Kerkhof MCA, Anzion RB, et al. Environmental contamination and assessment of exposure to antineoplastic agents by determination of cyclophosphamide in urine of exposed pharmacy technicians: is skin absorption an important exposure route? *Arch Environ Health* 1994;49:165–169.

20. Kromhout H, Hoek F, Uitterhoeve R, et al. Postulating a dermal pathway for exposure to antineoplastic drugs among hospital workers: applying a conceptual model to the results of three work-place surveys. *Ann Occup Hyg* 2000;44:551–560.

21. Dorr RT, Alberts DS. Topical absorption and inactivation of cytotoxic anticancer agents in vitro. *Cancer* 1992;70(Suppl.):983–987.

22. Bos RP, Leenaars AO, Theuws JLG, et al. Mutagenicity of urine from nurses handling cytostatic drugs, influence of smoking. *Int Arch Occup Environ Health* 1982;50:359–569.

23. Evelo CTA, Bos RP, Peters JGP, et al. Urinary cyclophosphamide assay as a method for biological monitoring of occupational exposure to cyclophosphamide. *Int Arch Occup Environ Health* 1986;58: 151–155.

24. Connor TH, Sessink PJ, Harrison BR, et al. Surface contamination of chemotherapy drug vials and evaluation of new vial-cleaning techniques: results of three studies. *Am J Health-Syst Pharm* 2005;62: 475–484.

25. Kiffmeyer TK, Ing KG, Schoppe G. External contamination of cytotoxic drug packing: safe handling and cleaning procedures. *J Oncol Pharm Prac* 2000;6:13.

26. Sessink PJM, Cerna M, Rossner P, et al. Urinary cyclophosphamide excretion and chromosomal aberrations in peripheral blood lymphocytes after occupational exposure to antineoplastic agents. *Mutat Res* 1994;309:193–199.

27. Pharmaceutical considerations—sterile preparations (general information Chapter 797). In: *The United States Pharmacopeia,* 27th rev., and *The National Formulary,* 22nd ed. Rockville, MD: The United States Pharmacopeial Convention; 2004:2350–2370.

28. Connor TH. An evaluation of the permeability of disposable poly-propylene-based protective gowns to a battery of cancer chemotherapy drugs. *Appl Occup Environ Hyg* 1993;8:785–789.

29. Harrison BR, Kloos MD. Penetration and splash protection of six disposable gown materials against fifteen antineoplastic drugs. *J Oncol Pharm Pract* 1999;5:61–66.

30. Laidlaw JL, Connor TH, Theiss JC, et al. Permeability of four disposal protective-clothing materials to seven antineoplastic drugs. *Am J Hosp Pharm* 1985;42:2449–2454.

31. Valanis B, Shortridge L. Self protective practices of nurses handling antineoplastic drugs. *Oncol Nurs Forum* 1987;14:23–27.

32. Sessink PJM, Rolf ME, Ryden NS. Evaluation of the PhaSeal hazardous drug containment system. *Hosp Pharm* 1999;34:1311–1317.

33. Vandenbroucke J, Robays H. How to protect environment and employees against cytotoxic agents, the UZ Gent experience. *J Oncol Pharm Pract* 2001;6:146–152.

34. Nygren O, Gustavsson B, Strom L, et al. Exposure to anti-cancer drugs during preparation and administration: investigations of an open and a closed system. *J Environ Monit* 2002;4:739–742.

35. Connor TH, Anderson RW, Sessink PJ, et al. Effectiveness of a closed-system device in containing surface contamination with cyclophosphamide and ifosfamide in an IV admixture area. *Am J Health-Syst Pharm* 2002;59:68–72.

36. Spivey S, Connor TH. Determining sources of workplace contamination with antineoplastic drugs and comparing conventional IV drug preparation with a closed system. *Hosp Pharm* 2003;38:135–139.

37. Wilson JP, Solimando DA. Antineoplastics: a safety hazard? (letter) *Am J Hosp Pharm* 1981;38:624.

38. Staiano N, Gallelli JF, Adamson RH, Thorgeirsson SS. Lack of mutagenic activity in urine from hospital pharmacists admixing antitumour drugs (letter). *Lancet* 1981;1:615–616.

39. Wilson J, Solimando D. Aseptic technique as a safety precaution in the preparation of antineoplastic agents. *Hosp Pharm* 1981;16:575–581.

40. Solimando D, Wilson J. Demonstration of skin fluorescence following exposure to doxorubicin. *Cancer Nurs* 1983;6:313–315.

Table 6–3 **Teratogenic Agents**

PREGNANCY RISK FACTOR X		PREGNANCY RISK FACTOR D	
Antineoplastic	**Non-Antineoplastic**	**Antineoplastic**	**Non-Antineoplastic**
Abarelix	Alprostadil	Alitretinoin	Amitriptyline and chlordiazepoxide
Bexarotene	Amyl Nitrite	Altretamine	Amitriptyline and perphenazine
Bicalutamide	Atorvastatin	Aminoglutethimide	Aspirin and codeine
Goserelin	Bosentan	Anastrozole	Aspirin and dipyridamole
Megestrol	Carboprost tromethamine	Arsenic trioxide	Aspirin and meprobamate
Methotrexate	Cetrorelix	Azacitidine	Atenolol and chlorthalidone
Thalidomide	Chorionic gonadotropin (recombinant)	Bleomycin	Butabarbital
Leuprolide	Clomiphene	Busulfan	Clidinium and chlordiazepoxide
Tositumomab	Danazol	Capecitabine	Demeclocycline
	Dihydroergotamine	Carboplatin	Doxycycline
	Ergonovine	Carmustine	Efavirenz
	Ergotamine	Chlorambucil	Fosphenytoin
	Estazolam	Cisplatin	Hydrocodone and aspirin
	Estradiol	Cladribine	Meprobamate
	Estrogens (conjugated A /synthetic)	Cyclophosphamide	Methimazole
	Estrogens (conjugated/ equine)	Cytarabine	Minocycline
	Estrogens (esterified)	Cytarabine (liposomal)	Nicotine
	Estropipate	Daunorubicin citrate (liposomal)	Orphenadrine, aspirin, and caffeine
	Finasteride	Daunorubicin hydrochloride	Oxycodone and aspirin
	Fluoxymesterone	Docetaxel	Penicillamine
	Flurazepam	Doxorubicin	Perindopril erbumine
	Fluvastatin	Doxorubicin (liposomal)	Phenobarbital
	Follitropins	Epirubicin	Potassium iodide
	Ganirelix	Etoposide	Primidone
	Histrelin	Etoposide phosphate	Propoxyphene
	Isotretinoin	Floxuridine	Propylthiouracil
	Leflunomide	Fludarabine	Secobarbital
	Levonorgestrel	Fluorouracil	Streptomycin
	Lovastatin	Flutamide	Tolbutamide
	Lutropin alfa	Fulvestrant	Valproic acid and derivatives
	Medroxyprogesterone	Gefitinib	Voriconazole
	Menotropins	Gemcitabine	Zoledronic acid
	Methyltestosterone	Gemtuzumab ozogamicin	
	Mifepristone	Hydroxyurea	
	Miglustat	Idarubicin	
	Misoprostol	Ifosfamide	
	Nafarelin	Imatinib	
	Nandrolone	Irinotecan	
	Norethindrone	Letrozole	
	Norgestrel	Lomustine	
	Oxymetholone	Mechlorethamine	
	Oxytocin	Melphalan	
	Podophyllum Resin	Mercaptopurine	
	Pravastatin	Mitomycin	
	Quinine	Mitoxantrone	
	Raloxifene	Oxaliplatin	
	Ribavirin	Paclitaxel	
	Rosuvastatin	Pemetrexed	
	Simvastatin	Pentostatin	
	Stanozolol	Procarbazine	
	Tazarotene	Streptozocin	
	Temazepam	Tamoxifen	

Table 6–3 **Teratogenic Agents—cont'd**

PREGNANCY RISK FACTOR X		PREGNANCY RISK FACTOR D	
Antineoplastic	Non-Antineoplastic	Antineoplastic	Non-Antineoplastic
	Testosterone	Temozolomide	
	Triazolam	Teniposide	
	Triptorelin	Thioguanine	
	Warfarin	Thiotepa	
		Topotecan	
		Toremifene	
		Tretinoin	
		Trimetrexate glucuronate	
		Vinblastine	
		Vincristine	
		Vinorelbine	

From *Safe Handling of Hazardous Drugs.* Lexi-Drugs Online. Lexi-Comp Clinical Reference Library OnLine. Copyright © 1978–2006 Lexi-Comp, Inc. Used by permission.

Table 6–4 **AHFS Category 10:00 Antineoplastic Agents**

Abarelix	Dacarbazine	Hydroxyurea	Paclitaxel
Aldesleukin	Dactinomycin	Ibritumomab	Pegaspargase
Alemtuzumab	Daunorubicin	Idarubicin	Pemetrexed
Anastrozole	Denileukin	Ifosfamide	Pentostatin
Arsenic trioxide	Docetaxel	Imatinib	Procarbazine
Asparaginase	Doxorubicin	Interferon alfa-2a	Rituximab
Azacytidine	Epirubicin	Interferon alfa-2b	Streptozocin
Bevacizumab	Erlotinib	Irinotecan	Tamoxifen
Bexarotene	Estramustine	Letrozole	Temozolomide
Bicalutamide	Etoposide	Leuprolide	Teniposide
Bleomycin	Exemestane	Lomustine	Testolactone
Bortezomib	Floxuridine	Mechlorethamine	Thioguanine
Busulfan	Fludarabine	Megestrol	Thiotepa
Capecitabine	Fluorouracil	Melphalan	Topotecan
Carboplatin	Flutamide	Mercaptopurine	Toremifene
Carmustine	Fulvestrant	Methotrexate	Tositumomab
Cetuximab	Gefitinib	Mitomycin	Tretinoin
Chlorambucil	Gemcitabine	Mitotane	Triptorelin
Cisplatin	Gemtuzumab	Mitoxantrone	Valrubicin
Cladribine	Goserelin	Nilutamide	Vinblastine
Cyclophosphamide	Histrelin	Oxaliplatin	Vincristine
Cytarabine			

BODY SURFACE AREA (BSA) (DUBOIS BODY SURFACE AREA)

$$BSA = 0.007184 \times weight \ (kg)^{0.425} \times height \ (cm)^{0.725}$$

It is easiest to use the MedMath program on a handheld calculator or computer or go online and Google a program for BSA.

BSA in Amputees

The following formula and table may used to estimate BSA in an amputee:

$$BSA \ (m^2) = BSA - (BSA \times \% \ BSA \ part \ amputated \ (from \ table)$$

Body Part	% Surface Area
Hand	3
Lower part of arm	4
Upper part of arm	6
Foot	3
Lower part of Leg	6
Thigh	12

Data from Colangelo PM. Two methods for estimating body surface area in adult amputees. *Am J Hosp Pharm* 1984; 41:2650–2655.

APPENDICES

CREATININE CLEARANCE (CrCl)

Although there are many methods available to calculate creatinine clearance, the most commonly used and inexpensive methods are the Cockroft and Gault formula and the Jelliffe formula. These formulas appear below. Both of these formula have significant variation (mean prediction error of about 20%), but for noncachectic cancer patients with serum creatinines of 0.7 mg/dL or higher, the Cockroft and Gault formula is the most accurate.

Cockroft and Gault (C&G) Formula

Most practitioners use this formula for bedside calculation of CrCl. It is primarily used in the modified Calvert formula below. This formula tends to underestimate values determined by a collected creatinine clearance method and also underestimates glomerular filtration rate (GFR), which is used in the traditional Calvert formula. However, when the Jaffe method is used for assaying serum creatinine, as is the case for many clinical laboratories, the C&G formula more accurately estimates GFR.

$$CrCl \ (mL/min) = [(140 - age) \times weight \ (kg)/(72 \times Cr_s)] \times (0.85 \ if \ female)$$

$$C\&G \ CrCl \ corrected \ for \ BSA \ (mL \times min^{-1} \times 1.73 \ m^{-2}) = CrCl \ by \ C\&G \times (1.73/BSA)$$

Jelliffe Formula

Although this formula is less accurate than the C&G formula, it is often used in Gynecologic Oncology Group Clinical Studies:

$$CrCl \ (mL/min) = [98 - 0.8 \times (age - 20)/Cr_s] \times (0.90 \ if \ female)$$

The non-BSA–adjusted formula above is required in GOG protocols:

$$Jelliffe \ CrCl \ corrected \ for \ BSA \ (mL \times min^{-1} \times 1.73 \ m^{-2}) = CrCl \ Jelliffe \times (1.73/BSA)$$

519

Modification of Diet in Renal Disease (MDRD) Formula

This is a complicated bedside formula that has been shown to be less accurate than the C&G formula in the noncachectic cancer patient. It is recommended for patients who are severely malnourished or who have severe inflammation.

Male: GFR $= 170 \times [S_{Cr}]^{-0.999} \times [age]^{-0.176} \times [1.0] \times [race] \times [S_{urea}]^{-0.170} \times [S_{albu}]^{+0.318}$

Female: GFR $= 170 \times [S_{Cr}]^{-0.999} \times [age]^{-0.176} \times [0.762] \times [race] \times [S_{urea}]^{-0.170} \times [S_{albu}]^{+0.318}$

where S_{Cr}, serum creatinine in mg/dL; S_{urea}, blood urea nitrogen in mg/dL; S_{albu}, serum albumin in mg/dL.

CARBOPLATIN FORMULAS

Traditional Calvert Formula

This formula is used in Europe as laboratories perform GFR tests.

Carboplatin (mg) = Area under curve (AUC) × [GFR + 25]

The usual AUC for gynecologic cancers ranges between 4.5 and 6.0.

Modified Calvert Formula

This formula is used primarily in the United States as practitioners perform bedside calculation of CrCl.

Carboplatin (mg) = Area under curve (AUC) × [CrCl (mL/min) + 25]

The Usual AUC $= 5$–7 for solid tumors and may be as high as 9 for high-dose therapy as in stem cell transplant therapy.

Carboplatin Dosing in Obese Patients

The use of the modified Calvert formula in obese cancer patients receiving carboplatin may result in exceedingly large doses of carboplatin that could result in high AUCs and excessive toxicity. This is due to the weight variable in the C&G formula used for calculating a patient's creatinine clearance. The definition for obesity is a body mass index (BMI) greater than 30 kg/m^2. No one method has been studied adequately in this patient population.

To resolve this situation, one may perform a number of adjustments to the calculation including (1) capping the creatinine clearance at 120–150 mL/min or (2) substituting an adjusted body weight (Adj.BW) for actual body weight (ABW) in the C&G formula by making the following simple calculations:

Adj.BW (in kg) = Ideal body weight (IBW) + 0.4 × (ABW − IBW)

IBW (in kg) = 45 + 2.3 (patient's height in inches − 60 inches) in females

IBW (in kg) = 50 + 2.3 (patient's height in inches − 60 inches) in males

IBW is ideal body weight

HOW TO FIND A REGIMEN FOR VERIFICATION OF CHEMOTHERAPY ORDERS

Because regimens change so frequently in the treatment of malignancies, we have elected not to publish dosage regimens for specific cancers except in the pediatric oncology chapter. The reader is directed to go to the following Web sites to obtain the latest information on chemotherapy regimens, dosing, and other helpful information.

American Cancer Society: *www.cancer.org*
National Cancer Institute: *www.cancer.gov*
Abramson Cancer Center of the University of Pennsylvania: *www.oncolink.com*
American Society of Clinical Oncology: *www.asco.org*
Oncology Nursing Society: *www.ons.org*
Hematology/Oncology Pharmacy Association: *www.hoparx.org*
BC Cancer Agency Care and Research: *www.bccancer.bc.ca* (Click on the Health Professionals Info link.)
The Doctor's Lounge: *www.thedoctorslounge.net/oncology/regimens/index.htm* (Select the disease state to get regimens from various institutions.)
Avon, Somerset and Wiltshire Cancer Services: *www.aswcs.nhs.uk/pharmacy/ChemoHandbook/STCP/index.htm*

APPENDICES

Patients who may need help with insurance coverage for drugs used in the treatment of their cancer may apply to the particular pharmaceutical company for assistance. On the Web site for the company, look for a link or contact information to patient assistance programs.

A useful Web site that has a link for patient assistance programs is *www.phrma. org.* This site can help patients and prescribers determine whether patients are eligible for assistance in filling prescriptions. In the table is a list of pharmaceutical companies and Web sites for many of commonly used anticancer drugs.

The Partnership for Prescription Assistance (PPA) is a national initiative to make it easier for consumers to access patient assistance programs. Qualifying patients who lack prescription coverage now have a single point of contact to access information about the public and private programs that may be right for them.

The PPA consists of a coalition of the pharmaceutical companies, physicians, and patient advocates in the United States and represents the largest ever private-sector program to help bring medicines to Americans who lack prescription drug coverage and are having difficulty affording their prescription medicines. More than 475 public and private patient assistance programs are available through the PPA, including more than 150 programs offered by pharmaceutical companies.

Although eligibility requirements may vary, the patient assistance programs generally offer free medication to patients with incomes up to 200% of the Federal Poverty Guidelines. To find out whether they may qualify for one or more programs, patients can visit a user-friendly Web site (*www.pparx.org*) or call toll-free 1-888-4PPA-NOW (1-888-477-2669) to speak with a trained specialist who can provide application assistance in English, Spanish, and approximately 150 other languages.

APPENDICES

(Table for Appendix 3)

Company	Contact Information	Other Information
Amgen	*www.amgen.com.* Go to the "Patients" link, then in the drop-down menu, click on "Patient assistance." SAFETY NET Program: Write to Post Office Box 13158, LaJolla, CA 92039-3185, or call 1-800-272-9376 or fax 1-888-508-8090, Reimbursement Connection®. Go to the particular drug of interest and click. Extensive information is available including application forms.	Product covered: Aranesp Epogen Kepivance Neulasta Neupogen
Astra Zeneca	*www.astra-zeneca-us.com.* Patient Assistance Link. Patient Assistance Program call 1-800-424-3727, Monday through Friday, 9:30 am to 6:30pm EST. Together Rx Access™ Program is a free drug card program that offers savings from 25% to 40% and sometimes more on prescriptions for more than 275 brand-name drugs for qualified, low-income Americans who are not eligible for Medicare and have no prescription drug insurance. A member of PPA	Drug products: Arimidex Casodex Faslodex Iressa Nolvadex Zoladex
Bristol-Myers Squibb	*www.bms.com.* Company oncology and virology products are available to eligible patients without charge through the Bristol-Myers Squibb/ AmeriCares Oncology Virology Access Program. Call 1-800-332-2056 for information about the Patient Assistance Foundation; call 1-800-272-4878 for the Oncology/Virology Access Program.	Drug products: Erbitux Taxol

Continued

(Table for Appendix 3)—cont'd

Company	Contact Information	Other Information
Celgene	*www.celgene.com.* Patient Support Link on Web site Patent Support Solutions (PSS) program. The PSS^{SM} program is provided by Celgene to simplify reimbursement support. The PSS program allows a health care provider to inquire about and arrange for reimbursement and insurance assistance on a patient's behalf if he or she has been prescribed or is being treated with select Celgene products. Call 1-888-423-5436 and press 3 at the main menu.	Drug products: Revlimid Thalomid Alkeran
Chiron	*www.chiron.com.* The Proleukin and Tobi patient assistance programs are consistent with Chiron's belief that no patient should be denied treatment because of financial status. These programs cover the Food and Drug Administration–approved labels for U.S. citizens only. The programs are designed to assist patients who do not have health care insurance or have exhausted their insurance coverage and other resources. To receive assistance, a patient's physician must request application materials from Chiron's Reimbursement Service. PROLEUKIN® Patient Assistance Program: 1-866-385-4729 TOBI® Patient Assistance Program: 1-866-598-8624	Drug product: Proleukin
Genentech	*www.gene.com.* Click on "Products," then on "Patient Access Programs" The Genentech® Access to Care Foundation. For eligible patients who are treated in the United States, Genentech will provide product to those who cannot afford to pay. All of Genentech's products are covered by the Genentech Access to Care Foundation, except for Pulmozyme (dornase alfa, recombinant), which is covered by the Genentech Endowment for Cystic Fibrosis. *Reimbursement.* Genentech provides a service called Single Point of Contact (SPOC) for reimbursement support. SPOC provides one-stop access to a broad array of reimbursement information, support and services.	SPOC covers: Avastin Tarceva Rituxan Herceptin
Lilly	*www.lilly.com.* Lilly Cares™ is a patient assistance program provided by Lilly through the Lilly Cares Foundation. As part of the company's efforts to provide access to products for legal U.S. residents regardless of their ability to pay, it created a program to offer free medication, through physicians, to patients who are otherwise unable to obtain its products. Lilly Cares assists patients who are uninsured and whose income is less than 200% of the federal poverty level. In 2004, the Lilly Cares program responded to 275,000 requests, valued at $167 million, for Lilly products. Most Lilly products are available through the program. Eligibility is based on the patient's inability to pay and lack of third-party drug payment assistance, including insurance, Medicaid and government, community, or private programs; patients cannot be eligible for Medicare. Applications are available to anyone and must be completed and signed by the patient and the physician. Patients can download a blank application from the Lilly Cares Web site or applications can be faxed by calling 1-800-545-6962.	Drug products: Alimta
Merck	*www.merck.com.* Patients may be eligible for discounted Merck medicines regardless of age and income. Patients may be eligible for free Merck medicines through the Merck Patient Assistance Program. If enrolled in Medicare, patients are eligible to enroll in the new Medicare Prescription Drug Coverage Program.	Oncology products: Cancidas Emend Fosamax Fosamax Plus D
MGI Pharma	*www.mgipharma.com.* No link to a patient assistance program detected.	
Millenium	*www.millennium.com.* Go to the "Clinicians" link and click on "Velcade" and then on "Reimbursement." Reimbursement Assistance Program: Call 1-866-VELCADE. Millennium Pharmaceuticals, Inc. provides customer resources to health care providers, patients, and caregivers through its VELCADE information line, in the following categories: • Medical information • Clinical trial information • The VELCADE Reimbursement Assistance Program information, which is available to health care providers, patients, and caregivers to assist with reimbursement issues, including the following:	Drug product: Velcade

Company	Contact Information	Other Information
	Insurance verification Coding and billing Claims appeal support Alternative funding searches Patient Assistance Program The program is easily accessed by calling 1-866-VELCADE, option 2. Reimbursement specialists are available from 9 AM to 8 PM, Eastern Standard Time.	
Novartis	*www.us.novartisoncology.com/info/index.jsp*. Go to the Novartis Oncology site and click on "Coping with Cancer" and then "Payment for Treatment." *Reimbursement*. Here is information on Novartis Oncology Reimbursement Support Services, as well as general information on insurance and paying for cancer treatment. Novartis Oncology is committed to supporting the care of eligible patients. Novartis has a number of reimbursement support services available to assist the patients by: • Verifying insurance for cancer coverage • Locating participating pharmacies and/or distributors • Providing billing and coding assistance • Identifying alternative sources of coverage • Evaluating eligibility for Novartis patient assistance programs • Reimbursement information for Novartis Oncology Products may be found on our individual product sites.	Products covered: Femar Glevec Sandostatin Zometa
Onyx	*www.onyx-pharm.com*. No information	Drug product: Nexavar
Ortho Biotech	*www.orthobiotech.com*. Member of Together Rx Access™ Program; also supports the PPA program.	
Pfizer	*www.pfizer.com*. Click link on "How we Help," then click "Access to Medicines," and then link to "US Programs" or "International Programs," which will bring one to I. Pfizer Patient Assistance Programs • Pfizer Helpful Answers™ is a family of programs to help Americans without prescription coverage save on many Pfizer medicines, no matter what their age or income. People with limited incomes may even qualify to get their Pfizer medicines for free. • Connection to Care provides Pfizer medicines for free to qualified patients through their doctor's office. • Sharing the Care provides Pfizer medicines for free to eligible patients through participating community health centers. • The Pfizer Hospital Partnership Program provides Pfizer medicines for free to eligible patients through participating disproportionate-share hospitals. • Pfizer Pfriends provides savings on Pfizer medicines at the pharmacy to qualified patients without prescription coverage, regardless of age or income. • Other product-specific patient assistance programs provide medicines for low-income, uninsured patients including those suffering from particularly complex diseases that require case management and complex drug regimens. II. Industry Programs • The PPA is an industry program that offers a single point of access to more than 475 patient assistance programs, including over 180 programs offered by pharmaceutical companies, such as Pfizer Helpful Answers. • Together Rx Access™ is a prescription savings program sponsored by 10 pharmaceutical companies, including Pfizer. It provides savings on a wide range of prescription products at the pharmacy counter to eligible patients without prescription coverage. III. Government Programs • Medicare Prescription Drug Coverage was set up to help people with Medicare pay for their prescription drugs. Medicare has contracts with private insurance companies who offer prescription drug plans. Each company has set up its own plan. People with Medicare can choose whether or not they want to join a plan. • There are many patient assistance programs offered, depending on what state a patient lives in.	

EXPOSURE TO HAZARDOUS DRUG

Continued

(Table for Appendix 3)—cont'd

Company	Contact Information	Other Information
Sanofi-Aventis	*www.oncology.sanofi-aventis.us/home.do; www.taxotere.com.* No patient assistance programs are listed on the Sanofi or Aventis oncology Web site. However, on the Taxotere Web site, the oncology resources link has Web links to: General Oncology Resources Breast Cancer Resources Lung Cancer Resources Prostate Cancer Resources Treatment Guidelines Journals	

Index

Entries can be identified as follows: drugs in all bold indicate generic names and Cap/lowercase indicate trade names. Page numbers followed by "b," "f," and "t," indicate boxes, figures, and tables, respectively.

IV Compatibilities

Drug	Cimetidine (Tagamet)	Famotidine (Pepcid)	Granisetron (Kytril)	Ondansetron (Zofran)	Palonosetron (Aloxi)	Dexamethasone (Decadron)	Diphenhydramine (Benadryl)
Cimetidine							
Famotidine	Y-site						
Granisetron	Y-site	Y-site					
Ondansetron	Y-site	Y-site	N/A				
Palonosetron	Y-site	Y-site	N/A	N/A			
Dexamethasone	Yes	Yes	Yes	Yes	Yes		
Diphenhydramine	Yes	Yes	Y-site	Y-site	Y-site	No	

Yes: compatible in either dextrose 5% in water (D5W), normal saline (NS), dextrose 5% in ½ normal saline (D51/2NS) as IV admixture and Y-site; Y-site: Y-site and physically compatible for at least 2-4 hours in NS, drug was diluted in NS or D5W; No: The two drugs are incompatible, precipitants have been observed when mixed. N/A: not applicable.
Data from *King Guide to Parenteral Admixtures*. Thomson Micromedex Healthcare Series, Powered by Trissel's™2 Clinical Pharmaceutics Database. Fall 2006.